THE PRINCIPLES & PRACTICE

OF

HOMŒOPATHY

BY

RICHARD HUGHES.

L.R.C.P., Ed., M.R.C.S., Eng., M.D. (*Hon.*), N.Y., Phila., St. Louis, U.S.A.

AUTHOR OF

"A manual of Pharmacodynamics," "A Manual of Therapeutics,"
"The Knowledge of the Physician," "Hahnemann as a
Medical Philosopher," "The Cyclopædia of
Drug Pathogenesy," &c., &c.

B. Jain Publishers (P) Ltd.

USE — EUROPE — INDIA

THE PRINCIPLES & PRACTICE OF HOMOEOPATHY

13th Impression: 2020

NOTE FROM THE PUBLISHER
Any information given in this book is not intended to be taken as a replacement for medical advice. Any person requiring medical attention should consult a qualified practitioner or a therapeutist.

No part of this book may be reproduced, stored in a retrieval system or transmitted, in any form or by any means, mechanical, photocopying, recording or otherwise, without any prior written permission of the publisher.

© with the publisher

Published by Kuldeep Jain for
B. JAIN PUBLISHERS (P) LTD.
D-157, Sector-63, NOIDA-201307, U.P. (INDIA)
Tel.: +91-120-4933333 • Email: info@bjain.com
Website: www.bjain.com
Registered office: 1921/10, Chuna Mandi, Pahargani, New Delhi-110 055 (India)

Printed in India

ISBN: 978-81-319-0248-6

PREFACE TO THE THIRD EDITION.

The second edition of this book had been sold out rapidly and the book remained out of print for a considerable time. Now the call for a third edition has come. This gives us much gratification.

The third edition is virtually unchanged from the second edition and the arrangement that is made in it is the same as that of the second edition. Though great care has been taken to avoid printer's errors, a number of them have unfortunately crept it. We sincerely regret for this and ensure their correction in the next edition.

The paper and press difficulties, the high cost of labour and materials, and the other pressing circumstances, arising out of the peculiar time we are passing through, have made delay in the publication of the book. The same reasons have compelled us to make unwillingly a slight increase in its price.

It is hoped that in spite of this, this third edition will receive the same reception from the profession and lovers of Homœopathic Science as the previous editions have done.

PREFACE TO THE FOURTH EDITION

The great popularity of this immortal work of Dr. Hughes has once again incited us to bring out its Fourth Edition, the earlier one having been exhausted sooner than ever.

Along with a display of better types, this Fourth Edition has been thoroughly revised for certain improvements in its get up, such as :— (1) Better display of types ; (2) Improvements in general arrangement ; (3) Corrections of printer's errors as crept in previous editions ; (4) Better binding and (5) The volume has been brought out in two parts for easier handling, as has been suggested by a number of its learned readers.

An indispensable guide for students and practitioners alike as it is, we doubt not that this Fourth Edition will also be received with a fervour equal to its predecessors by the profession and lovers of Homœopathy here and abroad, and in fact, wherever Homœopathy is adored.

FOREWORD.

We have the pleasure to announce the publication of this immortal work of Dr. Hughes, which according to the celebrated Dr. Dudgeon is "Unrivalled in Homœopathic Literature and which must long serve as the text-book for Homœopathic Students and Practitioners," and "a complete survey of all diseases and their rational Homœopathic Treatment."

The special characteristic of this book is that Dr. Hughes, himself a great physician, has thoroughly availed himself of the experiences of his predecessors and colleagues all over the world, enriched by his own, and has never been wanting in recommending the findings of others, whenever necessary. In short, the votaries of Homœopathy will find in this book of reference, the methods of treatment of all the great Homœopaths of the 18th and 19th centuries, with a man of Dr. Hughes' skill and experience to guide them.

We have made no change from the original, save for the improvement of the printing. For convenience of reading, we have printed this book all through in bigger types than in the original, the names of medicines in italics, and the more important ones in antiques. All important passages or words are in small cap, and the names of diseases which were in antiques in the original are in antique cap, in this book.

Our heartfelt gratitude is due to Messrs. Leath & Ross, London, for giving us the privilege of being its publishers in India.

PREFACE.

The present work is much more than a revised edition of the "Therapeutics," the last edition of which was published in 1878. The plan on which it is constructed is the same, but every subject treated of has been, when not entirely re-written, brought up to the latest date of general medical and special Homœopathic knowledge.

Dr. Hughes's experience and skill as a physician, and his thorough acquaintance with all medical literature, has enabled him to produce a work of cyclopædic character unrivalled in Homœopathic literature and which must long serve as the text-book for Homœopathic students and practitioners.

Cut off suddenly in the very flower of his age and at the height of his intellectual ability, he had not completed more than one-half of the task of correcting the proof-sheets of this colossal work. But fortunately the whole of the manuscript was in the printer's hands, so that the work is complete just as it would have appeared had its author lived to see it through the press. His family having confided to me the labour of love to complete the task its author was destined to leave unfinished, I have scrupulously avoided making any alterations or additions to the author's text. My task has been confined to proof-correcting and index-making, so that the reader may be assured that he has the work exactly as it would have been under the author's own superintendence.

In the present work Dr. Hughes makes frequent reference to his other great work on "Pharmacodynamics," which is in the hands of most Homœopathic practitioners, and which all who desire to gain a knowledge of Homœopathic medicines will do well to study. That other magnificent work of Dr. Hughes's, "The Cyclopædia of Drug Pathogenesy," is frequently utilized in the present volume for the purpose of demonstrating the perfect Homœopathicity of the remedies recommended.

The inestimable value of works on the theory and practice of Homœopathy contributed by Dr. Hughes during his all too short career, their scientific character and their strenuous advocacy of pure and unadulterated Homœopathy mark him as by far the greatest, ablest and most faithful exponent of the great Therapeutic truth revealed by Hahnemann, and the most zealous, enthusiastic, indefatigable and clear-headed disciple of the illustrious Founder of the great Medical Reformation. That some who are not distinguished for their strict adhesion to the teachings of Hahnemann should insinuate doubts as to the value of Dr. Hughes's colossal and disinterested work and the sincerity of his zeal for Homœopathy reminds us of Juvenal's sneer at Gracchi for complaining of sedition.

It would ill become me to write either eulogy or criticism of the work which it has by a strange fatality fallen to my lot to prepare for publication; but I cannot forbear calling attention to a singular and original feature in this book, to wit the masterly account of the origin and development of Hahnemann's method, which occupies the first fourteen lectures. This will be found to constitute a perfect introduction to the Therapeutics of the remaining lectures, and is of great value to all enquirers into Homœopathy.

The rest of the work is devoted to the Homœopathic treatment of all the diseases in the nosology. The author, while giving his own experience, which was very extensive, in the treatment of most diseases, gives full consideration to the practice and opinion of others, not even omitting to describe those of other than Homœopathic practitioners, when these seemed to him to be of any practical value and of Homœopathic character. As the experience of no single physician could extend to all diseases, Dr. Hughes has been careful to give that of others, who have had the opportunity of observing and treating diseases which had been denied to himself. Thus the book will be found to be a complete survey of all that is known up to the date of its publication about diseases and their rational Homœopathic treatment.

I may be permitted here to correct an erroneous impression entertained by Dr. Hughes (v. p. 17, note) with regard to a Greek quotation made by Hahnemann in his "Medicine of Experience." The translation which was adopted by me in the "Lesser Writings," erroneously ascribed the words to Gregory the Great, whereas Hahnemann in the original correctly attributes them to Gregory Nazianzen. Of course, I am to blame for passing this undoubted press error when I included the translation in my collection, so no blame can be attached to Hahnemann for the substitution by the translator of "Greg Mag." for Hahnemann's "Greg. Naz." Possibly few will care whether a Greek saying came from Pope Gregory the Great, who, though he is credited with the conversion of Britain to Christianity, probably only wrote in Latin, or from the Nazianzen Gregory, who, though a saint like the other, was never a pope, but only a bishop, and probably knew no language but Greek; but I am unwilling that any slur should be put on Hahnemann's reputation for classical knowledge, which has hitherto never been truthfully impugned.

R. E. DUDGEON

Some of the more familiar Homœopathic periodicals quoted in this work are indicated by abbreviations. Thus:—

"*Annals*," stands for *Annals of the British Homœopathic Society*.
"*B.J.H.*"   „   *British Journal of Homœopathy*.
"*H.W.*"   „   *Homœopathic World*.
"*J.B.H.S.*"   „   *Journal of the British Homœopathic Society*.
"*M.H.R.*"   „   *Monthly Homœopathic Review*.
"*N.A.J.H.*" „   *North American Journal of Homœopathy*.

CONTENTS.

PART ONE

Lecture.		Page.
I.	HOMŒOPATHY : ITS NATURE AND ORIGIN	1
	NOTES TO LECTURE 1.	9
II.	THE "ORGANON"	12
III.	THE "ORGANON" (Concluded)	23
IV.	THE KNOWLEDGE OF DISEASE	38
V.	THE KNOWLEDGE OF MEDICINES	53
VI.	"SIMILIA SIMILIBUS"	69
VII.	THE SELECTION OF THE SIMILAR REMEDY	82
VIII.	THE SELECTION OF THE SIMILAR REMEDY (Concluded)	94
IX.	THE ADMINISTRATION OF THE SIMILAR REMEDY	107
X.	THE ADMINISTRATION OF THE SIMILAR REMEDY (Concluded)	122
XI.	HOMŒOPATHIC PRACTICE	136
XII.	THE PHILOSOPHY OF HOMŒOPATHY	148
	APPENDIX TO LECTURE XII.	163
XIII.	THE HISTORY OF HOMŒOPATHY	164
XIV.	THE PHILOSOPHY OF HOMŒOPATHY	179
XV.	GENERAL DISEASES.—*The Acute Infectious Disorders*	193
XVI.	GENERAL DISEASES.—*The Acute Infectious Disorders (Concluded).* – *The Exanthemata. Variola.*	205
XVII.	GENERAL DISEASES.—*The Exanthemata* (Concluded).—Vaccinia. Varicella. Morbilli. Rubella. Scarlatina. Dengue. Miliaria.	220
XVIII.	GENERAL DISEASES.—*The Continued Fevers.*— Typhus. Typhoid or Enteric Fever.	231
XIX.	GENERAL DISEASES.—*The Continued Fevers.* (*Concluded*)—Febricula. Simple Continued Fever. Relapsing Fever. Yellow Fever. Cerebro-spinal Fever. Mediterranean Fever. Plague. *The Malarial Fevers* or *Agues*. Remittent Fever. Bilious Remittent.	242

CONTENTS

Lecture		Pages
XX.	GENERAL DISEASES.—Cholera. Diphtheria. Influenza.	262
XXI.	GENERAL DISEASES.—*The Blood Infections.*—Erysipelas. Phagedæna, Malignant Pustule. Glanders. Pyæmia. Septicæmia. Actinomycosis. *The Arthritic Affections.*—Gout. Rheumatism. Rheumatic Gout. Gonorrhœal Rheumatism.	280
XXII.	GENERAL DISEASES.—*Diathetic Vices*—Scrofula. Cancer. *Blood Disorders.*—Scurvy. Purpura. Plethora. Anæmia. Chlorosis. Pernicious Anæmia. Leucocythæmia.	301
XXIII.	GENERAL DISEASES.—*The Venereal Maladies.*—Syphilis. Gonnorrhœa. Soft Chancre. Sycosis.	319
XXIV	DISEASES OF THE NERVOUS SYSTEM.—*Maladies Affecting The Brain.*—Cerebral Congestion. Meningitis. Cerebritis. Cerebral Softening. Cerebral Tumours. Apoplexy.	334
XXV.	DISEASES OF THE NERVOUS SYSTEM.—*Maladies Affecting The Brain* (Concluded). *Mental Disorders.*—Mania. Malancholia. Dementia. General Paresis. Hypochondriasis. Delirium Tremens. *Of Various Origin.*—Headache. Vertigo. Derangements of Sleep. Concussion of the Brain. Spinal Irritation. ..	346
XXVI.	DISEASES OF THE NERVOUS SYSTEM.—*Maladies Affecting The Spinal Cord.*—Spinal Congestion. Spinal Irritation. Spinal Meningitis. Myelitis. Spinal Paralysis. Labio-glosso-laryngeal Paralysis. Multiple Spinal Sclerosis. Lateral Spinal Sclerosis. Locomotor Ataxy. Progressive Muscular Atrophy. Spinal Softening. Hydrophobia. Tetanus.	366
XXVII.	DISEASES OF THE NERVOUS SYSTEM.—*The Neuroses.*—Epilepsy. Chorea. Tremor. Hysteria. Catalepsy. Neurasthenia.	380
XXVIII.	DISEASES OF THE NERVOUS SYSTEM.—*Local Nervous Affections.*—Neuritis. Neuralgia. Megrim. Local Spasms. Facial Palsy.	392

End of Part One

PART TWO

Lecture		Pages
XXIX.	DISEASES OF THE EYE—*Of the Ocular Appendages.*—Blepharitis. Hordeolum. Blepharospasm. Ptosis. Chalazion. Dacryo-cystitis. Fistula Lachrymalis. Lachrymation. *Of the Conjunctiva.*—Conjunctivitis Simplex. Purulent Conjunctivitis. Gonorrhœal Ophthalmia. Strumous Ophthalmia. Phlyctenular Conjunctivitis. Conjunctivitis Membranosa. Conjunctivitis. Trachomatosa. Pterygium.	410
XXX.	DISEASES OF THE EYE.—*Of the Sclera.*—Scleritis. *Of the Cornea.*—Keratitis. Corneal Opacities. *Of the Iris.*—Iritis. *Of the Choroid.*—Choroidal Congestion. Choroiditis. Glaucoma. *Of the Retina.*—Retinal Hyperæmia. Retinal Hæmorrhage. Retinitis. Detachment of the Retina. Retinal Hyperæsthesia.	423
XXXI.	DISEASES OF THE EYE (Concluded.).—*Of the Vision.*—Amblyopia. Hemiopia. Nyctalopia. *Of the Lens.*—Cataract. *Of the Ocular Muscles.*—Asthenopia. Oculo-motor Paresis. Myopia. Strabismus. Nystagmus. *Of the Refraction.*—Astigmatism. *Of the Orbit.*—Orbital Cellulitis. Orbital Periostitis.	436
XXXII.	DISEASES OF THE EAR.—*Of the Auricle.*—Erysipelas Aurium. Eczema Aurium. *Of the External Meatus.*—Otitis Externa. Otorrhœa. Polypus Aurium. Exostoses. *Of the Tympanic Cavity.*—Affections of the Membrana Tympani. Throat-deafness. Otalgia. Tympanitis. Deafness. *Of the Audition.*—Tinnitus Aurium. Meniere's Disease.	444
XXXIII.	DISEASES OF THE DIGESTIVE ORGANS.—*Of the Mouth.*—Stomatitis. Fœtor Oris. Glossitis. Ulcers of the Tongue. Syphilis of the Tongue. Cancer of the Tongue. Toothache. Gumboil. Mumps. Salivation. Ranula. Angina Ludovici. *Of the Throat.*—Angina Faucium. Quinsy. Enlarged Tonsils. Chronic Pharyngitis. *Of the Œsophagus.* Œsophagitis. Spasmodic Stricture of Œsophagus.	460

CONTENTS

Lecture		Pages
XXXIV.	DISEASES OF THE DIGESTIVE ORGANS.—*Of the Stomach.*—General Disorders. Gastritis. Ulcer of the Stomach. Cancer of the Stomach. Gastralgia. Acute Indigestion. Chronic Dyspepsia. Pain after Food. Acidity. Heartburn. Water-brash. Flatulence. Vomiting. Hæmatemesis.	472
XXXV.	DISEASES OF THE DIGESTIVE ORGANS.— *Of the intestines.*—Enteritis. Muco-Enteritis. Duodenitis. Typhlitis. Peri-typhlitis. Proctitis. Ulceration of the Bowels. Intestinal Cancer. Hæmorrhage from the Bowels. Colic. Diarrhœa. Dysentery.	489
XXXVI.	DISEASES OF THE DIGESTIVE ORGANS.— *Of the Intestines* (Concluded).—Constipation. Intestinal Obstruction. Hernia. Chronic Constipation. Hæmorrhoids. Fissure of the Anus. Prolapsus Ani. Fistula-in-Ano. Worms. Proctalgia. Paresis Ani.	499
XXXVII.	DISEASES OF THE DIGESTIVE ORGANS. *Of the Peritoneum.*—Peritonitis. Ascites. *Of the Pancreas.*—Pancreatitis. *Of the Liver.*—Hepatic Congestion. Hepatitis. Acute Atrophy of the Liver. Cirrhosis of the Liver. Fatty Liver. Waxy Liver. Pigmentary Degeneration. Cancer of the Liver. Jaundice. Gall-stones, Functional Derangements of the Liver.	512
XXXVIII.	DISEASES OF THE RESPIRATORY ORGANS. —*Of the Nose.*—Rhinitis. Coryza. Ozœna. Hay Fever. Epistaxis. Polypus Narium. Sneezing.	524
XXXIX.	DISEASES OF THE RESPIRATORY ORGANS. *Of the Larynx* :—Laryngitis. Œdema Glottidis. Aphonia. *Of the Bronchial Tubes.*—Bronchitis. Capillary Bronchitis. Toxœmic Bronchitis. Chronic Bronchitis. Bronchiectasis. Emphysema Pulmonum. Asthma.	538

Lecture		Page
XL.	DISEASES OF THE RESPIRATORY ORGANS. *Of the Lungs.*—Pneumonia. Abscess of the Lungs. Gangrene of the Lungs. Pulmonary Congestion. Œdema Pulmonum. Hæmoptysis.	552
XLI.	DISEASES OF THE RESPIRATORY ORGANS. —*Of the Lungs* (Concluded).— Phthisis Pulmonalis. Pulmonary Syphilis. Pulmonary Cancer. *Of the Pleura.*—Pleurisy. Hydrothorax. *Of the Diaphragm.*—Diaphragmatitis. Acute Rheumatism of the Diaphragm. *Of the Thoracic Walls.*—Pleurodynia.	563
	APPENDIX TO LECTURE XLI .. .	579
XLII.	DISEASES OF THE CIRCULATORY SYSTEM.— *Of the Heart.*—Functional Derangements. Palpitation. Hypertrophia Cordis. Dilatatio Cordis. Adipositas Cordis. Pericarditis. Endocarditis. Valvular Disease of the Heart. Cardiac Dropsy. Angina Pectoris.	580
	APPENDIX TO LECTURE XLII.	597
XLIII.	DISEASES OF THE CIRCULATORY SYSTEM. *Of the Arteries.*—Arteritis. Aneurism. Arterial Degeneration. *Of the Veins.*— Phlebitis. Varicosis. *Of the Lymphatics.*—Lymphangitis. Lymphadenoma. *Of the Blood Glands :* *Spleen.* — Leucæmia. *Of the Suprarenal Capsules.*—Addison's Disease. *Of the Thyroid* —Bronchocele. Myxœdema. Exophthalmic Goitre.	604
XLIV.	DISEASES OF THE URINARY ORGANS.— *Of the Kidneys.*—Bright's Disease. Nephritis Albuminosa. Granular Degeneration of the Kidneys. Amyloid Degeneration of the Kidneys. Fatty Degeneration of the Kidneys. Albuminuria.	617
XLV	DISEASES OF THE URINARY ORGANS— *Of the Kidneys* (Continued).—Diabetes Mellitus. Diabetes Insipidus. Chyluria. Azoturia. Gravel.	628

CONTENTS

Lecture		Page
XLVI.	DISEASES OF THE GENITO-URINARY ORGANS.—*Of the Kidneys* (Concluded).—Renal Congestion. Suppression of Urine. Hæmaturia. Hæmoglobinuria. Suppurative Nephritis. Pyelitis. *Of the Bladder.*—Cystitis. Irritable Bladder. Strangury. Paralysis of the Bladder. Stone in the Bladder. Cancer of the Bladder. Tubercle of the Urinary Tract. *Of the Urethra.*—Stricture of the Urethra *Of the Male Sexual Organs.*—Diseases of the Testicles.—Orchitis. Sarcocele. Irritable Testicle. Neuralgia Testis. Satyriasis. Impotency. Sterility. Spermatorrhœa. Hydrocele. *Of the Spermatic Cords.*—Varicocele. Retraction of the Testicles. *Of the Seminal Vesicles.*—Seminal Vesiculitis. *Of the Prostate Gland.*—Chronic Enlargement of the Prostate Gland. Prostatitis. *Of the Penis and Scrotum.*—Chancroid. Balanitis. Epithelioma. Inflammation of the Scrotum.	639
XLVII.	DISEASES OF THE FEMALE SEXUAL SYSTEM.—*Of the Ovaries.*—Ovaritis. Ovarian Neuralgia. Ovarian Dropsy. *Of the Fallopian Tubes.*—Salpingitis. *Of the Menstruation.*—Menorrhagia. Amenorrhœa. Vicarious Menstruation. Dysmenorrhœa.	655
XLVIII.	DISEASES OF THE FEMALE SEXUAL SYSTEM.—*Of the Uterus.*—Chronic Metritis. Hysteralgia. Endo-Metritis. Cervico-Metritis. Leucorrhœa. Displacements of the Uterus. Uterine Fibroids. Uterine Polypi. Uterine Cancer.	670
XLIX.	DISEASES OF THE FEMALE SEXUAL SYSTEM.—*Of the Uterus* (Concluded). Metrorrhagia. Hydrometra and Physometra. Perimetritis. Pelvic Hæmatocele. Pelvic Cellulitis. Pelvic Abscess. *Of the Vagina and Vulva.*—Vaginitis. Vaginismus. Prolapsus Vaginæ. Vulvitis. Acute Labial Abscess. Cancer Pudendi. Nymphomania.	

CONTENTS

Lecture.		Page
XLIX. (Contd.)	Vascular Tumour of the Urethra. Sterility. *Of the Mammæ.*—Inflammation of the Mammæ. Mammary Scirrhus. *Of the Coccyx.*—Coccygodynia.	683
L.	DISEASES OF THE FEMALE SEXUAL SYSTEM.—*Disorders of Pregnancy.*—Miscarriage. Disorders of Parturition. Post-partum Hæmorrhage. Puerperal Convulsions. *Disorders of the Puerperal State.* Puerperal Fever. Puerperal Insanity. Disorders of Lactation. Mastitis. Phlegmasia Alba Dolens.	692
LI.	DISEASES OF THE SKIN.—*Of the order Exanthemata.*—Erythema. Urticaria. *Of the order Papulæ.*—Lichen. Prurigo. *Of the order Vesiculæ.*—Eczema. Herpes. Pemphigus. *Of the order Pustulæ.*—Impetigo Ecthyma. *Of the order Squammæ.*—Pityriasis. Psoriasis. Icthyosis.	709
LII.	DISEASES OF THE SKIN (Concluded).—*Of the Papillæ.*—Verruca. *Of the Sebaceous Glands.*—Seborrhœa. Molluscum. Acne. *Of the Sweat Glands.*—Hyperidrosis. Bromidrosis. *Of the Hair Pollicles.*—Mentagra. Alopecia. *General Diseases.*—Lupus. Rodent Ulcer. Leprosy. *Local Affections.*—Furuncle. Carbuncle. Ulcers. *Of the Nails.*—Mal-nutrition. Onychia. Paronychia. *Parasitic Infections.*—Tinea. Scabies. Elephantiasis. Actino-Mycosis. Pruritus.	722
LIII.	DISEASES OF THE LOCOMOTIVE ORGANS —*Of the Muscles.*—Myositis. Myalgia. Lumbago. Stiff-neck. Omodynia. *Of the Bones.*—Periostitis. Nodes. Ostitis. Caries. Necrosis. Exostosis. Mollitis Ossium. Acromegaly. Enchondroma. *Of the Joints.*—Synovitis. White Swelling. Arthralgia. Bursitis. Ganglion.	737
	CASUALTIES.—Wounds. Contusions. Strains. Burns and Scalds. Chilblain. Stings. Fractures. Sun-stroke. Shock. Emotional Disturbances.	745

Lecture		Page
LIV.	DISEASES OF CHILDREN.—*General Diseases.*— Infantile Remittent Fever. Rickets. Infantile Syphilis. *Of the Nervous System.*—Tubercular Meningitis. Hydrocephaloid. Hydrocephalus. Convulsions. Infantile Paralysis.	751
	APPENDIX TO LECTURE LIV.	760
LV.	DISEASES OF CHILDREN (Concluded).—*Of the Eyes.*—Opthalmia. Neonatorum. *Of the Digestive Organs.*—Stomatitis. Thrush. Cancrum Oris. Stammering. Morbid Dentition. Diarrhœa. Cholera Infantum Colic. Constipation. Prolapsus Ani. Tubercular Peritonitis. *Of the Respiratory Organs.*—Laryngismus Stridulus Pertusis. Croup. Broncho-Pneumonia. *Of the Circulatory Organs.*—Lymph-Adenitis. Tabes Mesenterica. *Of the Urinary Organs.*—Enuresis Nocturna. *Of the Genital Organs.*—Leucorrhœa Noma Pudendi. *Cutaneous Diseases.*— Intertrigo. Crusta Lactea. Purrigo Capitis. Strophulus. Ringworm. *Miscellaneous Affections.*— Cephal Hæmatoma. Nævus. Hernia. Mastitis Neonatorum. Icterus Neonatorum. Scleroderma Neonatorum. Trismus Neonatorum.	763
	APPENDIX—The Menopause or Critical Age. ..	786
	INDEX.	787

LECTURE I.

HOMŒOPATHY: ITS NATURE AND ORIGIN

I am to endeavour, in the ensuing course of Lectures, to tell you what Homœopathy can do in the various recognised forms of diseases, and with what instruments it effects the doing. But before I come to such exposition, it is necessary that you and I should arrive at a mutual understanding as to what Homœopathy is, and as to some at least of the questions that arise out of its theoretic conceptions and practical applications.

Briefly, then, let me define what is contained in the word we are using. Homœopathy, I would say, is a therapeutic method, formulated the rule SIMILIA SIMILIBUS CURENTER—let likes be treated by likes. The two elements of the comparison herein implied are the effects of drugs on the healthy body and the clinical features of diseases; in either case all being taken into account, which is appreciable by the patient or cognizable by the physician, but hypothesis being excluded. Medicines selected upon this plan are administered single (*i.e.*, without admixture), and in doses too small to excite aggravation or collateral disturbance.

I believe that nine-tenths at least of the adherents of Homœopathy would accept this as a true account of all that is essential to it. If it be so, it is obvious that the thing with which we shall have to do is a METHOD—not a doctrine or a system. It belongs to the art of medicine rather than to its science. Of course, the rules of art need not be, should not be, merely empirical: they should be in harmony with philosophy and science, and framed with correct conception and from sound induction. I shall try to shew you that Hahnemann's method fulfils these requirements; that his way of regarding disease and drug action is eminently philosophical, that his direction to treat likes with likes results logically from a true induction from the facts of the matter and his reduction of dose follows as a necessary corollary thereto. But it remains a method still, and nothing more. It takes a particular aspect of disease and of drug-action—not denying that there are others—as the opposing surfaces: and of the possible modes of applying the one to the other which we shall see to be three in number, it selects that which is expressed by SIMILIA SIMILIBUS. Observe also that this expression—in its completeness as constituting the Homœopathic formula—is (in our definition) worded as a rule of art rather than a law of science. It does not say, SIMILIA SIMILIBUS CURENTER—likes are cured by likes, which (to say nothing of its dubious Latinity) would be inadequate, if meaning merely that such cure may be, unwarrantable if implying that all cure is, so wrought. It says, SIMILIA SAMILIBUS CURENTER—let likes be treated by likes,* which is good Latin and tenable direction.

I am well aware that the affirmative form of the phrase has long been current among Homœopathists; † and that, so rendered, it has been taken as equivalent to a law of Nature, or even of morals. ‡ It is however, quite unwarranted by history, and must no longer be suffered to mislead. I know also how tempting it is to give to a method a philosophic body, to connect what is in itself purely practical with theoretic conceptions—in the present case of life, disease, and of the MODUS OPERANDI of drugs. This has been attempted by many adherents of Homœopathy, from its founder onwards; and with theories of dynamism and such like, they have built up a system as ambitious as those which reigned in the seventeenth and eighteenth centuries. It is natural that the enquiring mind of man, "looking before and after," should seek so to round his conceptions. But these thinkers have too often become so enamoured of their speculations that they have required—or seemed to require—that the profession should accept all, if they are to take any, should adopt the philosophy as well as the creed. In so doing, they have seriously prejudiced the cause they have sought to advance. The notions of Physiology and Pathology current eighty years ago, and with which therefore the earlier Homœopathists were imbued, are now greatly changed, and are not acceptable to the present generation. That Homœopathy has been linked with these, has needlessly multiplied its vulnerable points; and it is at these that the attack of its hostile critics is generally made— their success at such outworks favouring in themselves and others the belief that they have made the citadel untenable.§ Our wisdom would rather have been to have kept on the ground chosen with such general acclamation by Dr. Geddes Scott, in his Prize Essay of 1848, which you will find in the Sixth Volume of the BRITISH JOURNAL OF HOMŒOPATHY. He there shewed the great value of Homœopathy to be that it was a theory of CURE rather than of DISEASE, and led direct to practise without the intervention of any further theory; in

---

* In the discussion as to the true reading of the Homœopathic formula, it has sometimes been overlooked that the subjunctive mood is used here, not in its potential (likes MAY BE treated by likes) but in its imperative force. It is like the well-known CEDANT ARMA TOGŒ where the same grammatical form is employed.

† See Note 1 to this Lecture (p. 9).

‡ See Note 2 (p. 11).

§ See for instance the "Examen du systeme de S. Hahnemann : le spiritualisme et le mader alisme en Medicine" Par Dr. Stapparts, Brussels, 1881; the article on Homœopathy by Dr Glover in the Last Edition of the ENCYCLOPŒDIA BRITANNICA; and that of Professor Palmer in the NORTH AMERICAN REVIEW of March, 1882.

short, that it was a therapeia, complete in itself, and independent of allied sciences of Physiology and Pathology, so far as these consist of doctrines and conceptions, and are more than CATALOGUES RAISONNES of facts.

It appears, therefore, from what has been said, that Homœopathy is essentially a practical method. It is, as its originator called it, an organon—an instrument for effecting in the best manner a certain end, viz.: The cure of disease. It answers to machines like the steam-engine and the spinning-jenny; and like these must have had an inventor. That inventor was SAMUEL HAHNEMANN.

That the idea of fitting likes to likes in the treatment of disease had occurred to men's minds prior to Hahnemann may be freely acknowledged. It may be found here and there in medical literature from Hippocrates downwards. But when examination is made into the nature of these similarities, they will be found in most instances something very different from those which Homœopathy uses as its fulcra. That vomiting should be checked by an *emetic*, in an emetic dose (VOMITUS VOMITU), was treatment by similars in the eyes of the father of Medicine; and his successors wandered still further from the mark. Their notions on the subject have been fully exhibited by Dr. Dudgeon, in his "Lectures on Homœopathy," and by Dr. Burnett, in his "Ecce Medicus!" Signatures—the resemblance in form or colour of parts of plants to parts of the body; analogies yet more imaginary between the constituents of the macrocosm of the world and the microcosm of the organism; the use of preparations of the organs of animals for disorders of the same organs in man—a practice at present undergoing a curious revival; the application of certain theoretical qualities of bodies—dryness, coldness, and so forth—to corresponding rath r than opposite characters of disease—these were the similars of t' mediæval physicians. A few later writers—Stahl the Dane, Stoerck, de Haen—noticed the occasional or possible curative operation of measures * which caused disorder similar to that of the patient; but there they left the matter. Hahnemann's distinction is that he grasped this similarity as the only real and fruitful one; and, seeing reason for suspecting it to be a general and not an exceptional basis of cure, tested and worked out his thought until he formulated it as a standing rule for the best medical practice.

This Hahnemann, of whom I am now speaking, was a German physician whose long life extended from 1755 to 1843. The story of it I need not tell you here, you can read it, if you know it not already,

* I say "measures," and not drugs, for Stahl's instances of cure by similars are all of external applications, like heat to burns, save one—the use of *Sulphuric acid* for Acidity of stomach ; and this, as the *acid* is not shewn to be capable of causing VITAL Acidity, such as that which it cures, is no better Homœopathy than that of the mediævalists.

in the pages of the two books I have mentioned, or yet more fully in the Memoir by our able Russian colleague, Dr. Brasol, which was contributed to the International Homœopathic Congress of 1896, and may be found in its Transactions. I will only say that the man who lived this life was no common character—Jean Paul Richter's phrase for him, "a double-headed prodigy of genius and erudition," being amply borne out by his doings. Perhaps the best way to get an unprejudiced idea of the manner of man he was, is to read, in Dr. Dudgeon's collection of his "Lesser Writings," his earlier works on medical and allied topics. Of these I cannot now dwell, my present business is with the genesis in his mind of the thought which led him to Homœopathy. It arose when, in 1790, he was rendering Cullen's "Materia Medica" into German. He felt dissatisfied with the Scotch professor's explanation of the febrifuge properties of *Cinchona*, and his consideration of the subject led him to the results which—as was his wont in translating—he expressed in a footnote.* "It will not" he writes, "be such an easy matter to discover the still lacking principle according to which its action may be explained. Nevertheless, let us reflect on the following. Substances such as very strong *Coffee, Pepper, Arnica, Ignatia* and *Arsenic,* that are capable of exciting a kind of fever, will extinguish types of Ague. For the sake of experiment, I took for several days four QUENTSCHEN of good *Cinchona* twice a day. My feet, the tips of my fingers, etc. first became cold, and I felt tired and sleepy; then my heart began to beat, my pulse became hard and quick. I got an insufferable feeling of uneasiness, a trembling (but without rigor), a weariness in all my limbs, then a beating in my head, redness of the cheeks, thirst; in short, all the old symptoms with which I was familiar in Ague appeared one after the other. Also, those particularly characteristic symptoms which I was wont to observe in Agues—obtuseness of the senses, a kind of stiffness in all the limbs, but especially that dull disagreeable feeling which seems to have its seat in the periosteum of all the bones of the body—these all put in an appearance. This paroxysm lasted each time for two or three hours, and came again afresh whenever I repeated the dose, not otherwise. I left off, and became well."

I have said in another place, when speaking of this experiment, that Hahnemann "proved *Cinchona* to discover on what principle it acted" in Intermittents. † It would be better perhaps, to say— "whether it, like the other febrifuges, excited a kind of fever." But I must maintain that this is the true account of it, and not that which is put forward by the representatives of a certain school amongst us, who rather read into his doings their own later ideas. Thus Dr. Adolf Lippe writes:—"Hahnemann was sitting at Leipzig, with his midnight lamp before him, translating Cullen's 'Materia

---

* See Vol. II., p. 108.

† Manual of Pharmacodynamics, p. 395. The references to this work are made to the Fourth and later Editions, the pagination of which is uniform.

Medica,' which was then a standard work. He came to *Cinchona officinalis*, and found Cullen say that this bark possessed specific febrifugal actions, because it was both the most aromatic and bitter substance known. Hahnemann laid down his quill and exclaimed, 'Preposterous!' There are more substances, more barks, possessing more, both bitter and aromatic properties, and *Cinchona* is not a specific for Ague. He argued, while it does cure some cases, it does not cure other cases. There must be a way to find out under what conditions the *bark* cured and did not cure. It was at that moment that this good and benevolent man had an 'Inspiration.' He concluded to take the drug himself, and whether light could not be brought into the prevailing darkness. Bright and early in the morning, Hahnemann went to the 'Apotheke zum Goldenen Loewen' on the marketplace of Leipzig, and there and then selected some fresh *Cinchona* bark, and obtained some vials and Alcohol. He prepared a tincture, took it, and behold, the symptoms he observed on himself shewed a marked similarity to cases of Ague cured by him by the same drug, and it was then that a new light broke upon him! That light was this:—A drug will cure such ailments as its sick-making power will produce similarity to."

To do him full justice, I have given Dr. Lippe's IPSISSIMA VERBA; and, as he expressly writes to correct the account I have presented of the matter, I must hold him to them. Contrast now his narrative with Hahnemann's own; and it will be seen at a glance that the two are incompatible. The school Dr. Lippe represented are careless about similarity between disease itself and drug-action, so long as the "conditions" of the two correspond. To favour their view, therefore, Hahnemann must have proved *Cinchona* bark to ascertain under what conditions it cured Ague; whereas he himself tells us that he did so to find out whether, like other febrifuges, it was febrigenic at all, and that his result was to find it productive of all the symptoms, general and characteristic, of the Intermittent paroxysm.

This is a digression, to clear Hahnemann's proceeding from misrepresentation on the part of his own followers. It is still more important to vindicate it from the objection made by opponents, that it is a wholly insufficient—nay, a false basis of a curative method. This challenge is supported by the allegation, first, that *bark* has no real power of causing in the healthy such a fever as that imagined by Hahnemann: and, secondly, that it cures Ague by an action, not on the body of the patient, but on the minute organisms of which MALARIA consists, so that its therapeutic power is independent of any it may exert on the healthy frame. In reply to these statements, I would ask you to suspend your judgment till we come to the treatment of the Malarious Fevers, when it will be fully discussed. In the meantime, however, I may be permitted to refer you to the article on *Cinchona* in my "Manual of Pharmacodynamics," where you will find numerous instances of the febrigenic power of the drug and its alkaloid, ending with a description of the *Cinchona*-fever by Bretonneau, warranted by Trousseau and Pidoux, which quite corresponds to that of Hahnemann; you will also see it demonstrated that Ague may be cured by *Quinine* in doses far too small to affect the vitality of microzymes. But even were no such evidence forthcoming, no amount of doubt cast upon Hahnemann's *Cinchona*-experiment and his inference therefrom would impeach SIMILIA SIMILIBUS CURENTER: for this was suggested by it, not built upon it. It might have been found that Newton's apple (to which it has been happily compared), fell to the ground for other reasons than because of gravitation, but that would not alter the fact, subsequently ascertained by him, that matter as such attracts matter in proportion to its mass. Following up the hint afforded him by his apple, Hahnemann (like Newton with moon's motions) tested his hypothesis by application to all other congruous instances—by seeing how far it would explain the recorded successes of the past and lead to fresh ones in the future. It is on a body of evidence of this kind that his method ultimately rests, and not on the single experiment which originally led him to it; and deductive verification is as good evidence of truth as the graduated induction urged by Bacon. Buckle has well-argued this in one of his essays; and has shown that, INTER ALIA, it was the way in which Kepler arrived at his great discoveries.

Hahnemann's further procedure may best be related in his own words. "I now commenced to make a collection of the morbid phenomena which different observers had from time to time noticed as produced by medicines introduced into the stomachs of healthy individuals, and which they had casually recorded in their works. But as the number of these was not great, I set myself diiigently to work to test several medicinal substance of the healthy body, and see! the carefully observed symptom they produced corresponded wonderfully with the symptoms of the morbid states they would easily and permanently cure." * The first fruit of this task was the "Fragmenta de Viribus Medicamentorum Positivis," published in 1805, and containing pathogeneses more or less complete of twenty-seven medicines. This was, as its name implies, in Latin; but in 1811, Hahnemann began to issue in successive volumes his German "Reine Arzneimittellehre," containing (in its First Edition) fifty-eight drugs, proved on a much larger scale.† He continued to add to his old and take part in new provings for some time yet, and altogether furnished materials for the knowledge of at least ninety medicines, besides giving an impetus to the work of experimenting on the healthy body which has never lost its force, and has been and is most fruitful in results.

* Lesser Writings (tr. Dudgeon), p. 586.

† The six volumes of the First Edition appeared at intervals from 1811 to 1821; those of the Second Edition from 1822 to 1827; and a Third Edition of the first two volumes saw the light in 1830 and 1833.

The provision for working the new method supplied in the "Fragmenta de Viribus" was followed up by an exposition of its theory and rules for its practical working. These first took the form of an essay in HUFELAND'S JOURNAL for 1806, entitled "The Medicine of Experience," and finally, in 1810, of a separate treatise, the "Organon of Rational Medicine." Of the latter work I hope to give some account in my next lecture. Suffice it now to say that in it Hahnemann leaves no point untouched which conduces to the working of the machine he has invented. Besides a full discussion of the theory of his method, and demonstration of its philosophical and scientific soundness, he gives minute rules for the examination of patients, for the proving of drugs, and for the selection of remedies upon the Homœopathic principle. He enquires what should be done when only imperfect similarity can be obtained, when more than one medicine seems indicated, and when the symptoms are too few to guide to a satisfactory choice. He considers the treatment in the new method of local diseases (so-called), of mental disorders, and of the great class of intermittent affections.

There are yet two features of the method of Hahnemann which have not come before us—the single remedy and the reduced dose. The first is obviously a necessary corollary of the rule: as the drug is proved, so it must be administered, if it is a true SIMILE. Hahnemann saw this at once, and in the trials which substantiated the soundness of his therapeutic rule used none but single remedies. "Dare I confess," he wrote in 1797,* "that for years I have never prescribed anything but a single medicine at once, and have never repeated the dose until the action of the former one had ceased—a venesection alone, a purgative alone, and always a simple, never a compound remedy, and never a second until I had got a clear notion of the operation of the first? Dare I confess, that in this manner I have been very successful, and given satisfaction to my patients, and seen things which otherwise I never would have seen?" The necessity for reduction of dose was not so self-apparent. In 1796 we find Hahnemann thus expressing himself †:—"The cautious physician, who will go gradually to work, gives this remedy (the Homœopathic one) only in such a dose as will scarcely perceptibly develop the artificial disease to be looked for (for it acts by virtue of its power to produce such an artificial disease), and gradually increases the dose, so that he may be sure that the intended internal changes in the organism are produced with sufficient force, although with phenomena vastly inferior in intensity to the symptoms of the natural disease: thus a mild and certain cure will be effected." In the "Medicine of Experience" and the "Organon," however, the logical consequences of the new method in the direction of posology are perceived

* Lesser Writings, p. 373.
† Ibid., p. 312.

and started. The dose of a Homœopathically-selected remedy he there argues, must obviously be smaller than one intended to act in an opposite direction to the disease. It should be so far reduced that its primary aggravation (which he supposed a necessary occurrence) should be barely perceptible and very short. This last direction involves a theory as to the action of similar remedies, which may well admit of question; but that comparatively small dosage is essential to them is a fact beyond dispute. It characterizes not only the practice of the avowed disciples of Hahnemann, but also that modified Homœopathy which (after the distinguished Professor at University College) may be called Ringerism. Drop doses of *Ipecacuanha wine* were unheard of till it began to be given to check vomiting instead of to excite it; and while the twelfth of a grain of *Corrosive sublimate* was deemed sufficiently fractional for all previous purposes, the reduction went to hundredths when the drug was administered in Dysentery.

Small dosage, then, speaking comparatively, is an essential element of the Homœopathic method. But that such dosage should be what is known as infinitesimal—that it should habitually deal with fractions from millionth upwards—to this Homœopathy does not compel either logically or practically. There are and always have been multitudes of its warmest adherents and most eminent practitioners who never employ these attenuations. I shall hereafter, indeed, have to exhibit the activity of infinitesimal quantities as a discovery of Hahnemann's to discuss the evidence for it and the theories which have been put forward to account for it. But, whatever be its value, it stands on its own merits, its connection with Homœopathy as method is historical, and not vital.

The sum of what has now been said is thus: Homœopathy is a therapeutic method, an instrument for the selection of the most suitable remedy for each case of disease. Hahnemann is to it that which Watt was to the steam-engine and Arkwright to intellectual sphere— that which Bacon was to induction by graduated generalisation. He is the author of the method : To him belongs the merit of all it has accomplished, and with his name it must ever be indissolubly connected. But in adopting this method of Hahnemann as our chief guide in Therapeutics, we do not necessarily become followers of his, in other departments of thought : We are Homœopathists, not Hahnemannians. He was more than a therapeutist, and so are we; but in those wider regions he is but one master among many, and we may— as I confess I do—prefer the guidance of Fletcher in Physiology and of Tessier in Pathology to his. Nor must his METHODUS MEDENDI itself be conceived of as insusceptible of improvement. The steam-engine of today is not altogether that of Watt. Homœopathy, like the candlestick of the Hebrew tabernacle, has been shaped by hammering not by casting: or rather, it is a vital thing, growing as the years go on, and legitimately influenced by its environments. It is in our hands somewhat different from what it was when it dropped from Hahnemann's; but it is Hahnemann's still. All study, exposition, practice of it must start from him: and the results it achieves must be accounted a monument reared to his honour.

It is with such a mind that I invite you to follow me in my attempt to expound the Principles of Homœopathy.

NOTES TO LECTURE I.
Note 1, Page 2.

It is not easy to say how the alteration of "curentur" into "curantur" came to be made. Hahnemann used the former in the "Organon," from its First Edition in 1810 onwards; and again in a letter written in 1835 to the French Minister of Public Instruction,"* —these being the only two places in which the formula is employed by him. The change occurred in his life-time, for Mr. Everest, his English pupil, stated that he was much annoyed by the substitution of "curantur"—which is not surprising, since this is (as I have said) obvious Latin, as well as a misrepresentation of his intention. He may be said to have condoned it, however; for among the articles we found on his body when we exhumed it in 1899, to give it more fitting sepulchre, was a gold medal presented to him by the French Homœopathic Society, which bore the formula in its later form. That was certainly the current phase when Homœopathy began to flourish in this Island, and was accordingly adopted as its motto by the BRITISH JOURNAL OF HOMŒOPATHY on its appearance in 1843. In 1862, Dr. Ryan—who was a fine classical scholar—took exception † to the phrase, and urged a reversion to Hahnemann's original wording. The then editors of the BRITISH JOURNAL opposed the change,‡ but their argument throughout proceeds on the assumption that "curantur" is generally understood to mean "are treated," whereas there can be no doubt that nine hundred and ninety-nine persons in every thousand would render it "are cured." I was myself convinced by Dr. Ryan's reasoning; and in my "Manual of Therapeutics" published in 1869, expressed my preference for "curantur," which I have ever since adopted.§

* MONTHLY HOM. REVIEW, FEB., 1802.

† BRIT. JOURN. OF HOMŒO., xxxviii., 64.

‡ BRIT. JOURN. OF HOMŒO., xx., 314.

§ The "curantur" on pp. 2 and 45 of the Fourth Edition of my "Pharmacodynamics" was a would-be improvement of the printer, made after the return of the last proof. It has been corrected in subsequent editions—of like origin, is doubtless the "curantur" which Dr. C. Wasselhœft has been made to put into Hahnemann's mouth in his translation of "Organon."

Of late, the "curentur" having been espoused and defended by the weighty authority of Dr. Dudgeon, more attention has been directed to it. The displeasure which has been evinced by the more ardent Hahnemannians at the proposed return to its use may have arisen from the mistranslation I have already adverted to. Thus Dr. Reinke, of Jamaica, in the UNITED STATES MEDICAL INVFSTIGATOR for March 24th, 1883, asks "Why do some of our doctors say CURENTUR? Are they not sure?" His question would have been spared had he understood that the subjunctive is used in its imperative force.* The true reading has now however, been irrevocably affirmed—written with an iron pen, and graven in the rock for ever. The Committees which have erected in Hahnemann's honour the tombstone of Pere Lachaise and the cenotaph which adorns the city of Washington have both been convinced that SIMILIA SIMILBUS CURENTUR was what the Master wrote, and have inscribed it accordingly upon those memorials of his fame.

Note 2, Page 2

In writing thus, I was referring to an Article in the NORTH AMERICAN JOURNAL OF HOMŒOPATHY for August, 1878, by my venerable friend Dr. P. P. Wells, of Brooklyn. He has long ago gone to his rest, and his pronouncement on the subject is probably forgotten; but as it may express the thoughts of many others I briefly notice it here. Dr. Wells stigmatized the reduction of Homœopathy to a mere rule of practice as a "crime for which our language fails to give a designation sufficiently condemnatory." In maintaining it to be a law, however, he confuses the sense in which science uses this term and that which belongs to it in the sphere of ethics and politics. He says—"It is an important element in the nature of law, that it is wholly mandatory. It commands, it neither solicits nor permits." Now this is true enough of a moral or a criminal law, but it is entirely incorrect when applied to a so-called law of Nature. The latter is simply an expression of a certain general fact which we perceive in the order of the universe; and it takes the form, not of a mandate, but of an affirmation. "Thou shalt not kill"—here is the law of conscience and of citizenship: The law of Nature is such as that all matter attracts all other matter in direct proportion to its mass and

§ Dr. Peck, of Providence, in a paper presented to the American Institute of Homœopathy at its meeting of 1900, has well-appreciated the significance of this fact, and shewn that pure Homœopathy is the gainer by its recognition.

in inverse proportion to the square of its distance. The real question is whether Homœopathy is such a law as that of gravitation. It is an inference from certain observed facts : Shall we state the inference by an affirmation, universal, exclusive, unchanging, that "likes are cured by likes," or by a practical conclusion, admitting of qualification and exception—"let likes be treated by likes?" Dr. Wells, and those who think with him, declare for the former alternative. I must follow Hahnemann himself in thinking the latter the utmost for which we have warrant. It requires a vast number of observations and experiments ere we can formulate a law of Nature, while a rule of art can be deduced from a very few particulars—its application being a speedy test of its validity. I cannot think we are justified in affirming that all morbid states are curable by their similars or better cured thus than by any other means : I can only feel borne out by the facts when I affirm that my practical wisdom lies in following the rule "let likes be treated by likes" as fully as I am able.

LECTURE II.

THE "ORGANON"

During my tenure of a chair in the London School of Homœopathy, I occupied the Summer Session of 1881 by reading with my class the "Organon" of Hahnemann, expounding and commenting as I went. I collated, for this purpose, the five editions through which the work had passed. Being called upon, in the October of that year, to deliver the then annual Hahnemannian Lecture, I utilised the studies of the Summer, and discoursed on Hahnemann as a Medical Philosopher, with especial reference to the Organon. The lecture was published, but is probably long ago out of print; and its subject is of so much importance to our present enquiry that I think I cannot do better than reproduce its substance here.

1. The Organon was first issued in 1810. A Second Edition appeared in 1819; a Third in 1824: a Fourth in 1829; and a Fifth and last in 1833. Each of these is described as "augmented" (2nd), "improved" (3rd), or both "augmented and improved" (4th and 5th); and in truth all save the Third, shew considerable changes as compared with their immediate predecessors. It is quite impossible to form an adequate estimate, either of the work or of its author, without some knowledge of the changes it has undergone in its successive stages. Without this, neither foe can criticise it nor disciple learn from it aright. For instance, the hypothesis of the origin of much Chronic Diseases in Psora, which hostile critics are never weary of ridiculing as one of the fundamental principles of Homœopathy, first appeared in the Fourth Edition, *i.e.*, in 1829. Theory of the dynamization of medicines—*i.e.*, of the actual increase of power obtained by attenuation, when accompanied by trituration or succussion—is hardly propounded until the Fifth Edition. Again, there is the doctrine of a "vital force," as the source of all the phenomena of life, as the sphere in which disease begins and medicines act. This has been regarded by many of Hahnemann's followers as an essential part of his Philosophy. "Voici donc" exclaims M. Leon Simon (the

first of the three who have made this name distinguished) "la pensee fondamentale de Hahnemann, la pierre angulaire du system!" But the earliest mention of this conception occurs in the Fourth Edition; and the full statement of it with which we are familiar in the Fifth (§ 9-16) appears there for the first time.

You may ask how you are to get a knowledge of this development of our text-book. To some extent, I shall give it to you in the present Lecture; but you may all obtain for yourselves, and in full detail, by gaining possession of the translation of the "Organon" by Dr. Dudgeon, issued by the Hahnemann Publishing Society in 1893. In this volume, besides a revision of his version of 1849, our learned colleague has supplied an Appendix containing a full exhibition of the changes the work has undergone between 1810 and 1833; so that we have its growth before us at a glance. This is not the least of the many boons Dr. Dudgeon has bestowed upon Homœopathic literature.

II. The "Organon" is Hahnemann's exposition and vindication of his therapeutic method. It had been preceded by a number of essays in HUFELAND'S JOURNAL—the leading medical organ of the time, in Germany. Of these the most noteworthy were—"On a New Principle for ascertaining the Curative Powers of Drugs" (1792); "Are the obstacles to certainty and simplicity in Practical Medicine insurmountable?" (1797); and "The Medicine of Experience" (1806). The time seemed now to have come when there should be published separately a full account of the new departure he was advocating; and hence the "Organon" of 1810.

Why did he give his treatise this name? He must, there can be little doubt, have had Aristotle in memory, whose various treatises on Logic were summed up under the common title "Organon." Logic —the art of reasoning—is the INSTRUMENT of research and discovery: Hahnemann designed his method as one which should be a medical logic, an instrument which the physician should use for the discovery of the best remedies for diseases. But the example immediately before his mind, and through whom he was probably led to Aristotle, must have been Bacon. The second treatise of the "Instauratio Magna" of the English Chancellor is entitled "Novum Organum": it was the setting forth of a new mode of reasoning, which in scientific research should supersede that of Aristotle, and lead to developments of knowledge hitherto unattained. That Hahnemann should aspire to do such work for medicine as was done for science in general by Bacon has been scouted by his enemies, and even deprecated by his friends, as presumption. And yet no comparison could better illustrate the real position of the man both in its strength and in its weakness. If he erred as to special points of Pathology, and even of practice, we must remember that Bacon was a doubtful acceptor of the Copernican Astronomy and ridiculed Harvey's doctrine of the circulation, while he saw no difficulty in the transmutation of metals

But, on the other side, how truly Baconian is the whole spirit and aim of the "Organon"! Like his great exemplar, Hahnemann sought to recall men from the spinning of thought-cobwebs to the patient investigation of facts. Like him, he set up the practical—which in this case is the healing of disease—as the proper aim of medical Philosophy; not seeking "in knowledge a terrace, for a wandering and variable mind to walk up and down with a fair prospect," but rather accounting it "a rich store-house, for the glory of the Creator, and THE RELIEF OF MAN'S ESTATE." Like him, his chief strength was devoted to the exposition and perfecting of his proposed method of further progress towards this end, leaving to the future the carrying it into effect. Another Descartes may arise in medicine whose perception of special fields of knowledge may be keener, and who may leave his mark more clearly traced on certain branches of our art. But Hahnemann, when once his method shall have won the acceptance we claim for it will ever be reckoned as the Bacon of Thearpeutics—the fruitful thinker who taught us what was our great aim as physicians and how we should best attain to it.

Hahnemann first called his work "Organon of the Rational Medical Science!"* (HEILKUNDE); but from the Seuond Edition onwards the title was changed to "Organon of the Healing Art" (HEILKUNST)—the "rational" being here, and in all other places of its occurrence, either dropped or replaced by "true" or "genuine" (WAHRE). Why this alteration? The elimination of the term "rational" has been supposed to "imply that his followers were required to accept his doctrines as though they were the revelations of a new Gospel, to be received as such, and not to be subjected to rational criticism." † I cannot think so. To me the clue of it seems to be afforded (and the Preface to the Second Edition bears out my view) by the coincident change from "Heilkunde" to "Heilkunst." The name "science," the epithet "rational," were in continual use for the hypothetical system of the day. The promulgation of his views had arrayed the advocates of all these in bitter opposition against him. Hahnemann was accordingly anxious to make it clear that, in entering the lists of conflict, he came armed with quite other weapons. He was seeking, not the consistency of a theory, but the success of a practical art: to him it mattered little whether a thing commanded itself or not to the speculative reason, his one concern was that it should be true.

III. On the title-page of his First Edition, Hahnemann placed

* In my Hahnemannian Lecture, I rendered "Kunde" by "doctrine". A consideration of the discussion on the subject carried on in the HOMŒOPATHIC WORLD of 1881 suggests that I shall be more closely adhering to the German, while not weakening my argument, if I now translate it "science."

† BRIT. JOURN. OF HOMŒO., XXXVI., 63.

a motto from the poet Gellert, which has been rendered into English thus:

> "The truth we mortals need
> Us blest to make and keep
> The All-wise slightly covered o'er
> But did not bury deep."

This was replaced in subsequent Editions by the words "Aude sapere"; but it continued to denote the profound conviction and motive inspiration of Hahnemann's mind. It was the same thought as that which he expressed in the "Medicine of Experience":—"As the wise and beneficent Creator has permitted those innumerable states of the human body differing from health, which we term diseases. He must at the same time have revealed to us a distinct mode whereby we may obtain a knowledge of diseases that shall suffice to enable us to employ the remedies capable of subduing them; He must have shewn to us an equally distinct mode whereby we may discover in medicines those properties that render them suitable for the cure of diseases—if He did not mean to leave his children helpless, or to require of them what was beyond their power. This art, so indispensable to suffering humanity, cannot therefore remain concealed in the unfathomable depths of obscure speculation, or be diffused through the boundless void of conjecture; it must be accessible, READILY ACCESSIBLE to us within the sphere of our external and internal perceptive faculties." Hahnemann believed in the illimitable possibilities of medicine, because he believed in God.

I lay more stress on this faith of Hahnemann's, from the contrast presented to it by the language of the only fair and calm examination (to my knowledge) which the "Organon," has received in this country. I refer to the Address in Medicine delivered before the British Medical Association in the same year already referred to (1881) by the late Dr. Bristwoe. The able and candid physician asks—"What grounds of reason and experience have we to justify the belief that for every disease an antidote or cure will sooner or later be discovered?" and going further still, declares it to be in his judgment "utopian to expect that diseases generally shall become curable by therapeutical or any other treatment." That this melancholy Pyrrhonism is of extensive prevalence appeared also that year at the International Congress in London, where—according to the LANCET *—"therapy" was conspicuous by its absence. It was not so at the Homœopathic Convention which preceded it; and this just stamps the difference between the two attitudes of mind. I cannot prove—at any rate here—that the faith of the founder of Homœopathy was sound, and the scepticism of its critics otherwise; but it is

---

* Aug. 27, 1881.

evident which is the more fruitful. As a lover of my kind, and not a mere man of science, I can say MALO CUM HAHNEMANNO ERRARE QUAM CUM—well, it would be personal, as well as difficult, to Latinise the rest, but my hearers will supply it.

IV. Hahnemann, whose heart was indeed bubbling up with his good matter, and whose tongue was certainly the pen of a ready writer, wrote a separate Preface for each edition of his work. I cannot give any account of them here, but they are all well worth reading. The Second especially deserves notice as a full statement in brief, of the author's view of the existing state of medicine; nowhere does Bacon speak more clearly through him than in his emphatic statements here regarding the relation of reason to experience in the study of the subject. I pass on to the Introduction which in every edition forms a considerable proportion of the whole volume. It has altered very much, however, between its earliest and latest appearance. In the first three editions, it consists of a series of unintentional Homœopathic cures (so considered) taken from medical literature, with a few preparatory and concluding remarks. But in the Second and Third, Hahnemann had introduced into the body of the work a long section of destructive criticism on existing theories and modes of treatment; and this, when he issued the Fourth, seemed to him to find a more appropriate place in the Introduction. Thither, accordingly, it was transferred, forming—under the title "Survey of the Allopathy* of the hitherto-prevailing School of Medicine"—a first part; while the "Instances of Involuntary Homœopathic Cures" took place as a second. In the Fifth Edition, these last disappeared altogether, being merely referred to in a note; and the Introduction became a continuous essay, its subject being the medicine of the author's contemporaries and predecessors.

I think that no one who is acquainted with the state of medical thought and practice in Hahnemann's day will question the general justice of the strictures he here makes upon it. The critic to whom I have referred admits, "the chaotic state of therapeutical theory and practice at that time prevalent"; but he hardly appreciates Hahnemann's merits in proscribing and stigmatizing it as he did. Chaos itself, to the habitual dwellers in it, seems to be cosmos:" it can only be apprehended for what it is by those who have the cosmos in their souls Thus it was with Hahnemann's. He saw all around him two things which he cites, Gregory Nazianzen as pronouncing ἄιgλgs—λόγοs

* So written in the Fourth Edition of the original, but in the Fifth more correctly given as "Allœopathy," which I think the translators should have reproduced. "Αλλοιον παθος. not ολλο, is Hahnemann's antithesis to ομοιον πα'θος; and as the latter forms Homœopathy, the former should be Allœopathy.

ἀπραειOs and ἀλογος πραγις.* On the one side were the men of note—
the Stahls and Hoffmanns and Browns and Cullens building up their
ingenious and ambitious systems on hypothetical data; on the other
were the mass of practitioners, quite unable to utilise these imagin-
ings, and treating disease according to empirical maxims or the directions of the prescription-book. The physician's art was the butt of
every satirist, the dread of all who fell ill, the despair of the minds that
formed a nobler ideal of it. Hahnemann himself, as you may read in
his life, for a time gave himself up to such despair, till his experiment
with *Cinchona*-bark proved the clue of Ariadne which suggested the
true law of the phenomena and led the way to better things.

If we were going through the Introduction in detail, there would
be many points on which criticism and correction would be necessary;
but the general soundness of its attitude must be sufficient for us to-day.
It bears to the body of the work the same relation as Bacon's "De
Augmentis" to his "Novum Organum" and the treatise on "Ancient
Medicine" to the "Aphorisms" of Hipprocrates. Before leaving it, I
must say a few words about the instances of cure, which, though dropped by himself were inserted from the Fourth Edition in Dr. Dudgeon's
first version of the Fifth, and are therefore familiar to us all.† His critic
has singled out the first and last of these, and has no difficulty in dis-
posing of them as without bearing on the point to be proved. But a
more thorough examination would shew that "A DOUBUS DISCERE
OMNES" was hardly a safe mode of proceeding. Of the forty-five references made (I speak from consultation of the original sources) six
are indeed quite worthless, and fifteen more dubious; but the remaining twenty-four will stand the most searching scrutiny. The cures were
reported by the best observers of their time; the remedies employed
were undoubtedly Homœopathic to the disorders present, and have
no other mode of action to which their benefits could by any plausibility be ascribed. We could multiply and perhaps improve upon
them now; but such as they are, they do speak the language as utterers
of which Hahnemann cited them.

V. We come now to the 'Organon' proper. It consists of a series
of aphorisms—in its latest form 294 in number, to which are appended
numerous and often lengthy notes. This is a form of composition

---

* Lesser Writings, p. 501. Hahnemann ascribes the phrase to "Greg. Mag."
but surely Gregory the Great did not write in Greek.

† In the translation of 1849, Dr. Dudgeon, not having the original of the
Fourth Edition at hand, transferred these instances from an older version
(Devrient's). Several errors crept in accordingly, but these have of course
been corrected in the revision of 1893, where the cases in question will be
found in the Appendix.

eminently suggestive and stimulating. It is endeared to many of us by Coleridge's "Aids to Reflection"; but Hahnemann must have taken it from the 'Novum Organum,' perhaps also with a recollection of the father of Medicine which derives its name therefrom.

While each aphorism is complete in itself, and might be made the text of a medical discourse, the work they collectively constitute has a definite outline and structure, which remains unchanged through the successive editions, and is as evident in the first as in the last. This outline is given in the third aphorism, which—with the exception of "rational" for "true" (practitioner) in the first—is identical in all editions:

"If the physician clearly perceives what is to be cured in diseases, that is to say, in every individual case of disease (KNOWLEDGE OF DISEASE, INDICATION); if he clearly perceives what is curative in medicines, that is to say, in each individual medicine (KNOWLEDGE OF MEDICINAL POWERS); and if he knows how to adapt, according to clearly-defined principles, what is curative in medicines to what he has discovered to be undoubtedly morbid in the patient, so that recovery must ensue—to adapt it as well in respect to the suitableness of the medicine most appropriate according to its mode of action to the case before him (CHOICE OF THE REMEDY, THE MEDICINE INDICATED), as also in respect to the exact mode of preparation and quantity of it required (proper DOSE), and the proper period for repeating the dose; if, finally, he knows the obstacles to recovery and is aware how to remove them, so that the restoration may be permanent: Then he understands how to treat judiciously and rationally, and he is a true practitioner of the healing art."

The three desiderata, then, are—

1st. The knowledge of the morbid state—which supplies the indication:

2nd. The knowledge of medicinal powers—which gives the instrument:

3rd. The knowledge how to choose and administer the remedy—which is the thing indicated.

The First Part of the Organon (down to § 70) treats of these points doctrinally, by way of argument*; the Second practically, in

* § 5-18 discuss knowledge of disease, 9-21 knowledge of medicines, 22-27 knowledge of application of one to the other; and 28-69 are an explanation and defence of the mode of application by similarity.

the form of precept. The summing up of the doctrinal portion is contained in § 70, in these words:—

"From what has been already adduced we cannot fail to draw the following inferences:

"That everything, of a really morbid character, and which ought to be cured, that the physician can discover in diseases consists solely of the sufferings of the patient and the sensible alterations in his health—in a word, solely of the totality of the symptoms, by means of which the disease demands the medicine requisite for its relief.

"That this derangement of the state of health, which we term disease, can only be converted into health by another revolution effected in the system by means of medicines, whose curative powers, consequently, can only consist in altering a man's state of health— that is, in a peculiar excitation of morbid symptoms, and can be learned with most distinctness and purity by proving them on the healthy body.

"That, according to all experience, a natural disease can never be cured by medicines whose power is to produce in the healthy individual an alien morbid state (dissimilar morbid symptoms) DIFFERING from that of the disease to be cured (never that is, by an Allœopathic mode of treatment); and that even in Nature, no cure ever takes place in which an inherent disease is removed, annihilated and cured by the addition of another disease dissimilar to it, be the new one ever so strong.

"That, moreover, all experience proves that by means of medicines which have a tendency to produce in the healthy individual an arttificial morbid symptom ANTAGONISTIC to the single symptom of disease sought to be cured, the cure of a long-standing affection will never be effected, but merely a very transient alleviation, always followed by its aggravation; and that, in a word, this antipathic and merely palliative treatment in long-standing diseases of a serious character is absolutely inefficacious.

"That, however, the third and only other possible mode of treatment (the HOMŒOPATHIC), in which there is employed for the totality of the symptoms of a natural disease a medicine capable of producing the most similar symptoms possible in the healthy individual, given in suitable dose, is the only efficacious remedial method, whereby diseases, which are purely dynamic, deranging irritations of the vital force are overpowered, and being thus easily, perfectly, and permanently extinguished, must therefore cease to exist and for this mode of procedure we have the example of unfettered

Nature herself, when to an old disease there is added a new one similar to the first, whereby the old one is rapidly and for ever annihilated and cured."

Then in § 71, Hahnemann propounds the practical questions which in the remainder of the Treatise he seeks to answer, thus:

1st. How is the physician to ascertain what is necessary to be known in order to cure the disease?

2nd. How is he to gain a knowledge of the instruments adapted for the cure of the natural disease—the pathogenetic powers of medicines?

3rd. What is the most suitable method of employing these artificial morbific agents (medicines) for the cure of natural diseases?

In reply to the first question, he gives rules for the examination of the patient; to the second, for the proving of medicines upon the healthy: to the third, for the determination of similarity, the choice and repetition of the dose, the preparation of drugs, the diet and regimen to be observed, and so forth.

This is, in the author's own words (crabbed and gnarled, yet weighty with thought), the ground-plan of the 'Organon'. Of course, each position needs justification on its own merits; and this we shall enquire, as we proceed, how far we can award. But I would first call your attention to the simplicity of Hahnemann's conception, to its entire freedom from hypothesis and completeness within itself. All other medical systems had been based upon certain doctrines of life and disease: Hahnemann's method was utterly independent of them. His whole argument might be conducted, as indeed it is in the first three editions of his work, without any discussion of Physiological and Pathological questions. I would again impress this fact upon such of his disciples as represent Homœopathy to be a complete scheme of medical Philosophy; who would make the dynamic orgin of all maladies a plank of the platform on which we must stand, and call the Psora-hypothesis "the Homœopathic doctrine of Chronic Disease." This is an entire mistake. There are certain views in Physiology and Pathology which seem more harmonious than others with Homœopathic practice; Hahnemann thus came to hold them, and most of us tend in the same direction. But they might all be disproved and abandoned, and Homœopathy would still remain the same: we should still examine patients and prove drugs and administer remedies on the same principle and with the same success.

But I would commend this consideration also to Hahnemann's

critics. He has had critics from the first,* though nothing is wide of
the mark than to speak of "the contempt which experienced physicians
felt and freely expressed for him and his whimsical doctrines." Not
thus did Hufeland and Brera and Trousseau and Forbes write of the
new method and its author. But the first-named of these made a
remark which is full of significance: He said that if Homœopathy succeeded in becoming the general medical practice, it would prove "the
grave of science." Now this I make bold to claim as an unintentional
complement; for it describes our system as being true medicine, which
is not science, but art. This is a truth very much forgotten now-a-days.
Hahnemann, in the opening paragraph of the 'Organon,' proclaims
that the physician's high and sole mission is to restore the sick to
health—to cure, as it is termed. It is with this direct aim that he is
to study disease and drug-action, and the relation between the two.
He is not, primarily, a cultivator of science: He is a craftsman, the
practiser of an art and skill, rather than knowledge in his qualification.
HIS ART, INDEED, LIKE ALL OTHERS, HAS ITS ASSOCIATED SCIENCES.
PHYSIOLOLGY AND PATHOLOGY ARE TO IT WHAT CHEMISTRY IS TO
AGRICULTURE AND ASTRONOMY TO NAVIGATION. SO FAR AS THEY
BRING REAL KNOWLEDGE, THE MORE VERSED THE PHYSICIAN IS
IN THEM THE BETTER FOR HIMSELF AND FOR THOSE IN WHOSE
AID HE WORKS. But he was before they had being, and his art
should have a life of its own, independent of the nourishment they
bring. They must, being progressive, consist largely of uncertainties
—working hypotheses and imperfect generalisations, destined ere long
to be superseded by more authentic conceptions. Medicine should
not vary with their fluctuations, or hold its maxims at the mercy of
their support. While grateful for any aid they bring, it should go on
its own separate way and fulfil its distinctive mission.

One great value of the method of Hahnemann is that it dwells in
this sphere of art. It is "the grave of science"; for science as such,
has no existence here—it dies, and is buried. But its corpse enriches
the ground which covers it, and thereon grass springs up and fruits
ripen for practical use. On the other hand, the great weakness of the
general medicine of today is that, so far as it is more than blind
empiricism, it is an applied science rather than an art. It shifts from
heroism to expectancy, and from spoilation to stimulation, with the
prevailing conceptions of the day as to life and disease. Maladies are
studied with the eye of the naturalist rather than of the artist; and
the student is turned out thoroughly equipped for their diagnosis, but
helpless in their treatment. Hence the Nihilism of so much of modern
teaching; hence, at the Congress I have referred to, the miserable half-

---

*An answer to one of them, Hecker, was written nominally by Hahne-
mann's son, Friedrich, actually by himself. It has lately been Englished by
Dr. Dudgeon (Philadelphia; Boericke and Tafel, 1896). In it Hecker survives as does Celsus' attack on Christianity in the pages of Origen's defence
of it.

penny-worth of therapeutic bread to the gallons of scientific sack. It would have been well for its three thousand members if they had gone home to meditate the words of the man they ignored—"the physician's high and sole mission is to restore the sick to health"; if they would recognise Medicine as the art of healing, and cultivate it accordingly.

I must adjourn the further consideration of the 'Organon' for our next meeting.

LECTURE III.

THE "ORGANON" (concluded)

In my last Lecture I sketched the ground-plan of Hahnemann's "Organon." Let us now consider the three positions he takes up—his attitude (1) towards disease, (2) towards drug-action, and (3) towards the selection and administration of remedies.

1. In the RESUME of his conclusions which I have quoted (§70), Hahnemann speaks of the sum total of the symptoms of a patient as the only curative indication which the physician can discover. In this he hardly does himself justice; for in § 5 he has pointed to the knowledge of the CAUSES of the malady as important, and § 7 and its note has assumed as obvious that any exciting or maintaining cause which is discoverable and accessible shall be removed. He has further reminded us, in § 3 and 4 that both to prevent disease, and to make his curative treatment unobstructed and permanent, the physician must also be a hygienist. It would hardly be necessary to mention such points, but that Dr. Bristowe has said that "for him, preventive medicine which deals specially with the causes of disease, and has been successful only in proportion to its knowledge of them, would have been a mockery and a snare."

With these qualifications, however, Hahnemann's doctrine is that the totality of the symptoms—the sum of the sufferings the patient feels and the phenomena he exhibits—constitutes, FOR ALL PRACTICAL PURPOSES, the disease. He does not say that they alone are the disease. On the contrary, he constantly speaks of them as the "outwardly reflected picture," the "sensible and manifest representation," of what the essential alteration is. His point is that at this last you cannot get, and, to cure your patient, need not get. If you can find means for removing the sum total of his symptoms, he will be well, though you may know as little as he wherein, essentially, he was ill (§ 6-18).

Now what objection can be taken to this thesis? No one can seriously maintain that symptoms and morbid changes are not correlative; that there is any way of inferring the latter except from the former, or any way of removing the former, as a whole, except by righting the latter—their proximate cause. The critic we have now in view is too acute to say much of this kind. His main charge against Hahnemann's view of disease is that it ignores Pathology and more especially morbid Anatomy, so that the "laborious investigations conducted in our dead-houses, which we fondly imagine to add to our knowledge of diseases," would be "looked upon by him with contempt." But in so speaking he forgets Hahnemann's aim. He is laying down what are the curative indications in disease, what the physician can and should know of it in order to remove it. Do the investigations of the dead-house help us here? The changes they discover are the results—generally the ultimate results—of morbid action; but in this stage of the process such action is no longer amenable to remedies. If it is to be cured, it must be taken at an earlier period, before there has occurred that "serious disorganization of important viscera" which Hahnemann speaks of as an "insuperable obstacle to recovery."* And how shall it then be recognised, except by its symptoms? No microscope can see the beginning of CIRRHOSIS of the Liver or of SCLEROSIS in the Brain and Cord; but the patient may feel them, and may even exhibit them. Some slight hepatic uneasiness, some dart of pain or altered temper or gait, may and often do supervene long before the pathognomonic physical signs of such maladies appear. It is impossible to say how much suitable remedies applied at this time may not do—may not have done—to arrest the morbid process then and there. The Hahnemannic Pathology is a living one, because it seeks to be a helpful one. It was wisely pointed out by Clotar Muller that the contemplation of disease, mainly in the light of its final organic results had a discouraging effect; whereas, if we would just apply our method fully to each "TOUT ENSEMBLE" of disorder as it came before us, our possibilities were boundless. †

But Hahnemann has been accused of ignoring Pathology in another way, viz., by "objecting to all attempts on the part of systematic writers and practical physicians to distinguish and classify diseases." He is supposed to have been—and the utterances of some of his own disciples lend colour to the charge—a mere individualiser, regarding the maladies which affect mankind as "with a few exceptions, simply groups of symptoms, mosaics of which the component pieces admitted of endless re-arrangement." But this, again, is a great mistake, as I endeavoured to prove in a paper on "Generalisation and Individualisation" which I submitted to our International Congress of 1881, and which you may see in its Transactions. I there shewed, by numerous quotations, that Hahnemann recognised as freely as any

* Lesser Writings, p. 261.

† Carroll Dunham's Essay on the "Relation of Pathology to Therapeutics" (HOMŒOPATHY, THE SCIENCE OF THERAPEUTICS, p. 99) makes the same point.

other physician the existence of definite types of disease, of fixed character because resulting from unvarying cause, to which distinctive appellations might be given and specific remedies (or group of remedies) allotted. He varied from time to time, as Pathology itself varied, in the list of those to which he would assign such place; but at the lowest estimate they cannot fairly be described as "a few exceptions." They embrace the whole field of "specific" disease—acute and chronic. Take the instance of Intermittent Fever, which has been cited. Hahnemann is supposed to have declared these fevers innumerable, and each instance of them that came before him, an independent disease. But read the Section of the 'Organon' expressly devoted to the subject (§235-244). You will see there, that it is only sporadic Intermittents occurring in non-Malarious districts that he thus describes. The true endemic Marsh-ague he recognises as a disorder of fixed type, always curable by *bark* if the patient is not otherwise unhealthy: while the epidemic Intermittents, though distinct among themselves, have each a specific character so as to be amenable to one common remedy. It is in these (and the sporadic cases) only that he reprobates the blind *Cinchona*-giving practised in his day.

Here also, then, Hahnemann must be vindicated from the charge of ignoring any real Pathology, however little he valued the speculations of his own time which laid claim to that title. It is in the First Part of the Second Division of the 'Organon' that his views on the subject are expressed; and, allowing for the fact that they are nearly a century old, and therefore possibly to some degree antiquated, there is nothing in them unworthy of a learned and sagacious physician. I reserve his theory about "Psora" intercalated in the Fourth and Fifth Editions, which must subsequently receive a few words on its own account.

Hahnemann concludes this portion of his subject with some suggestions as to the examination of patients (§ 83-104), of which all that need be said is they are, as becomes their object, thorough. The Homœopathic physician does not listen and enquire merely to find out to what class of maladies his patients are to be relegated. For this end but few symptoms are necessary, and the rest can be left. He has to get at their totality, that he may cover them with a medicine capable of producing them on the healthy subject; and in pursuit of this aim he must not account any detail superfluous. It has been objected that we should come off badly upon such a method with Mrs. Nickleby for a patient. But happily all patients are not Mrs. Nicklebys; and when we do meet them, common-sense must deal with them accordingly. Of course, proportion must be observed; and anything we KNOW to be merely incidental must be omitted. Our colours must be mixed, like Opie's, "with brains, sir." But if we only THINK a detail unimportant, our wisdom will be to give the patient the benefit of the doubt, and insert it in our picture.

2. Such is Hahnemann's attitude towards disease; and I think it comes out from examination proof against every objection, and fitted at all points for its object. Still more incontrovertibly can this be said of the position he takes up with reference to drug-action (§ 19-22). His one insistence is that this can only be ascertained, by experiment on the healthy human body. Few now-a-days question the value of this proceeding; but Hahnemann has hardly yet been awarded the merit which belongs to him, as its pioneer. Haller had indeed preceded him in affirming its necessity, and Alexander and a few others had essayed tentatively—very tentatively—to carry it out; but Hahnemann developed Haller's thought into a doctrine, and multiplied a hundred-fold Alexander's attempts at proving. When the profession comes to know him at his worth, he will be recognised by all as the father of Experimental Pharmacology.

The great value of choosing the human subject for our provings is, that thereby their subjective symptoms—the sufferings as well as the phenomena they cause—can be ascertained. There is of course the inevitable shadow here—the counter-peril that a number of sensations of no moment shall be reported by the experimenters and cumber our our pathogeneses. This is inevitable; but Hahnemann at least saw the inconvenience, and did his best to avoid it. Let his rules for proving in the 'Organon' (§ 105-145) be read, and the information we have elsewhere as to his manner of proceeding be considered, and it will be seen that he did all that his lights suggested to make experimentation of this kind pure and trustworthy.

3. We pass now to the third division of the "vocation of the true physician," as conceived by Hahnemann. How is he to use his knowledge of drug-action in the treatment of disease? How is he to wield the potencies the former gives him for the favourable modification of the latter?

To the answer to these questions are devoted forty-eight aphorisms (§ 22-69) of the first and a hundred-and-forty-seven (§ 146-292) of the second division of the 'Organon.' Hahnemann argues that there are only three conceivable relations between the Physiological effects of a drug and the symptoms of disease, and therefore only three possible ways of applying the one to the other. The two may be altogether diverse and heterogeneous, as the action of a purgative and a congestive headache; and if you use the former to relieve the latter, you are employing a foreign remedy—you are practising Allœopathy (ἀλλοῖον πάθος). Or the may be directly opposite, as the influence of a *Bromide* and the sleeplessness of mental excitement: then to give *Bromide of Potassium* to induce slumber is to act upon the enantiopathic or anti-pathic principle (εναvίλον, αvIl, πaoos). Or thirdly, they may be similar, as *Strychnine*-poisoning to TETANUS or that of *Corrosive sublimate* to DYSENTERY. If such drugs are used for their corresponding disorders, you are evidently Homœpathizing (όμ3ivπάθos). Now of these, Allœopathic medication must be condemned, both on the ground of its uncertainty, and on that of the positive injury it does by disordering healthy parts and by flooding the system with the large doses of drugs necessary to produce the desired effects. Antipathic treatment is certainly and rapidly palliative; but the inevitable reaction which follows, leads to a return of the evil, often in greater force. It can rarely moreover, deal with more than a single symptom at a time; and even then its capabilities are limited by the very few really opposite states which exist between natural disease and drug-action. Antipathy may do tolerably well for immediate needs and temporary troubles; but it is not competent to deal with complex, persistent or recurrent maladies. For these we are shut up to the Homœopathic method, if we are to make any rational use of drugs in disease at all. This operates "without injury to another part and without weakening the patient." It is of inexhaustible fertility, for the analogies between natural and medicinal disorders are endless. It is complete, for the one order of things may cover the other in its totality. It is gentle, for no large and perturbing dosage is required for its carrying out. It is, lastly, permanent; for the law of action and re-action, which makes the secondary effects of antipathic palliatives injurious, here operates beneficially. The primary influence of the drug being in the same direction as the morbid process, the secondary and more lasting recoil will—after (it may be) a slight aggravation—directly oppose and extinguish it. It is thus that Hahnemann explains the benefit wrought by Homœopathic remedies—thus, and also by the theory (§ 28-52) of the substitution of the medicinal for the actual disease, of which he cites parallels in nature.

Here again we pause to ask what objections have been taken to Hahnemann's position. His doctrine of the three relations between drug-action and disease seems too simple for certain minds. One (Anstie) calls it Metaphysical; another (Ross) Geometrical; a third exclaims "how curious, how ingenious, how interesting!" and seems to think that in so designating it he excludes the possibility of its conformity to Nature. But why should it not have these features and yet be true? What other alternative is possible? What fourth term of comparison can be found between (be it remembered) the effects of drugs on the healthy and the symptoms of disease? If you use the one for the other, you must do so Allœopathically, antipathically, or Homœopathically. Medical men seem very fond now-a-days for disclaiming any system in their practice, and announcing themselves as altogether lawless and empirical. But they can no more help practising upon one or other of these principles than M. Jourdain could help speaking prose unless he launched into verse. If they would only analyse their own thoughts, they would see that as soon as they learn the Physiological action of a drug, they consider what morbid states it can indirectly modify or directly oppose. These are two of the members of Hahnemann's triad; and the difference between us and them is that our first thought seeks out what disorders the drug phenomena most resemble. We would not neglect the other two directions in which the medicine might be utilised, if we had reason to think it advantageous to follow them; and our complaint is that the profession at large do neglect and ignore the third, to the great loss of their patients.

Why should they do so? Some have answered that the method is really practicable, that real parallels between disease and drug-action are rare. To speak thus, however, implies a very deficient knowledge of Pharmacodynamics. Others have expressed a more general and natural objection when they have argued that medicines which are truly similar must aggravate rather than benefit, if they act at all. It would seem so; and it is not surprising that in the older works on Materia Medica morbid states analogous to the action of drugs are set down as contra-indicating their employment. But this difficulty SOLVITUR AMBULANDO. Let any one take an obvious instance of such a contra-indicating condition—a sick stomach for *Ipecacuanha*, a congested brain for *Opium*, a dry febrile tongue for *Belladonna*. If he gives a quantity capable of exciting such states in the healthy, he may undoubtedly aggravate. But let him reduce his dose somewhat below this point, and he will get nothing but benefit. This has been tested again and again and no one has reported adversely to it: on the contrary, uses of medicines derived from the method are now becoming as popular in general practice as they have long been in ours. Why should this benefit result? We have heard Hahnemann's explanation, that such remedies work by substitution and by exciting reaction. It is one in which it is not difficult to pick holes, and he himself says, in propounding it, that he does not attach much importance to it (§ 28). Any discredit, however, resulting from its disproval must attach equally, as regards substitution, to Bretonneau and Trousseau; as regards reaction, to more than one ingenious thinker of our own country, as Fletchers, Ross, Rabagliati. * More recently, the hypothesis has been advanced, that medicines have, even in health, an opposite action in large and small quantities, so that the reduction of dose necessary to avoid aggravation gives you a remedy acting in a direction

---

* See MONTHLY HOM. REVIEW, xxiii, 600-2.

contrary to that of the disorder, while its choice by similarity secures practicability and complete embracement. I myself feel great difficulty in acceding to this theory as a general account of Homœopathic cure; but there is no justification for representing its adoption as an abandonment of the Homœopathic position. It is an attempt at explanation, that is all: the fact that likes are cured by likes is the all-important thing, account for it how we may. So Hahnemann said, and so all we Homœopathists believe.

The side of Hahnemann's position on which he is most vulnerable is his exclusiveness; in which he maintains his method to be applicable to all non-surgical diseases, and to render all other ways of employing medicines superfluous and hurtful. This led him, as has been fairly urged, to regard intestinal worms as product of the organism, and to ignore the acarus as the exciting cause of Scabies; it has resulted among his followers in a deinal of palliatives to their patients by which much suffering might have been spared. In the first matter, however, he erred in common with most of his contemporaries; and in the second he is not responsible for the excesses of disciples who are often more Wilkesite than himself. The rational Homœopathist recognises, indeed, the inferior value and limited scope of antipathic palliation. He knows that it is only properly applicable to temporary troubles; but in these he makes full use of it. He does not allow his patients to endure the agonies of Angina pectoris, when he knows that *Amyl nitrite* will relieve them: he does not refuse them *Chloroform* during the passage of a calculus any more than during that of a fœtus. Hahnemann's exclusiveness is not to be justified: but it may fairly claim excuse as the enthusiasm of a discoverer, full of the sense of the power of his new method, and naturally led to apply it everywhere and to esteem it without rival.

The treatment of his subject in the second part of the 'Organon' is purely practical. It gives instructions for the selection of remedies upon the Homœopathic principle, and for their judicious employment when selected. It enquires what should be done when only imperfect similarity can be obtained, when more than one medicine seems indicated, and when the symptoms are too few to guide to a satisfactory choice. It considers the treatment on the new method of local diseases (so called), of mental disorders, and for the great class of Intermittet affections. It gives directions for diet and regimen; for the preparation of medicines; for the repetition of doses, and for their size.

It is on the last of these points only that I can touch here: for the rest I must refer to the work itself. Hahnemann's treatment of the subject of dose had not had justice done to it, in consequence of our knowing only the Fifth Edition of the 'Organon.' In the year 1829, after the publication of the Fourth Edition, he unfortunately determined to secure uniformity in Homœopathic usage by having one dilution for all medicines, and this the decillionth—the 30th of the centesimal scale. Our present 'Organon' represents this view; but the first four editions make no such determination, and are entirely moderate and reasonable in the principle of posology they lay down. The dose of a Homœopathically selected remedy, they say, must obviously be smaller than one intended to act antipathically or Allœopathically. If too large, it will excite needless aggravation and collateral suffering. It should be so reduced, that its primary aggravation (which Hahnemann supposed a necessary result) should be hardly perceptible, and very short-lasting. How far this must be, varies with the medicine used; and for suggestions on this point he refers to his MATERIA MEDICA PURA, where the dosage recommended ranges from the mother-tincture upwards, the 30th being a dilution of exceptional height. He alleges experience alone as having led him to attenuate as far as he has; but argues the reasonableness of so doing from the increased sensitiveness of the diseased body, pointing out that dilution does not diminish the power of a substance in proportion to the reduction of its bulk. Excluding the specific doses mentioned in the other work referred to, which are simply matters of fact and experience, there is nothing in this part of the 'Organon'—in its essential structure—to which fair exception could be taken.

I wish I could have stopped here; that there had been in the volume I am now expounding nothing more difficult to defend than what has gone before. In its first three editions—i.e., up to 1824—there is not. Almost everything in Hahnemann's work during the first quarter of this century is of enduring worth; it is positive, experimental, sound. But from this time onwards we see a change. The active and public life he had led at Leipzig, with the free breath of the world blowing through his thoughts, had been exchanged, since his exile to Coethen in 1821, for solitude, isolation, narrowness. The reign of hypothesis began in his mind—hypothesis Physiological, Pathological, Pharmacological. The theories he was led to form in all these branches of thought found their way into the later editions of the 'Organon', and so demand some consideration from us here. But let it be remembered throughout that they are not of the essence of its argument; that its structure and substance were complete before they appeared, and—in the judgment of many of us—are rather injured by their interpolation. Without them, all is inductive reasoning or avowedly tentative explanation; they, dogmatically asserted but all unproven, introduce a new and questionable element, they constitute what Drs. Jousset and Gailliard have well called the "romance of Homœopathy."

The first of these hypotheses is that of a VITAL FORCE, as being the source of all the phenomena of life, and the sphere in which disease begins and medicines act. Hahnemmn would probably at all times have called himself a vitalist, in distinction alike from the animism of Stahl (which made the immortal soul the principle of life), and from the views of those who would bring all vital phenomena under the laws of Physics and Chemistry. He early, moreover, employed the term "dynamic" to denote the sphere in which true disease took its origin and those effects of drugs which require vitality for their production. Disease has its "materies morbi" and organic changes; but all these may be—Hahnemann would have it always were—secondary products and effects, the primary derangement being invisible and intangible, manifest only in altered sensations and functions. Drugs, again, produce—many of them—chemical and mechanical effects; but these might occur in the dead as in the living body. The exclusively vital reactions they set up in the crucible of the organism belong to another sphere: they correspond with the beginnings of disease, like them are revealed by altered sensations and functions, like them are to be characterized as "dynamic."

Had he gone no further all would have been well. It is easy to read into his language the present protoplasmic doctrine of life; while the frequent commencement of disease in molecular rather than molar changes,* and the dynamic—as distinct from the mechanical and the chemical—action of drugs, are recognised by all. But in his later years Hahnemann advanced from this thoroughly tenable position into one far less easy to maintain. He adopted the view that vitality was a "force," analogous to the physical agencies so called, without which the material organism would lack sensation and functional activity, which animates and energises it during life and leaves it at death. It is this "vital force" (LEBENSKRAFT) which is primarily deranged in illness, and on which morbific potencies—both natural and medicinal—act through the sensory nerves. Its behaviour under medicinal influence is ingeniously imagined and elaborately described (§ 127); and in the Fifth Edition of the 'Organon' it is frequently mentioned as the actor or sufferer where previously the author had been content to speak of the organism (as in § 148).

Now Hahnemann can hardly be thought the worse of for entertaining this view, since, in some form or other, it was almost universally prevalent in his day. If the advice of the present Pope has been taken, it is still the teaching of all Roman Catholic colleges; for it is simply

---

* Hahnemann himself would have allowed this "frequent" to be more correct than "invariable"; for he considered Cholera due to the invasion of a cloud of minute organisms, and on this ground advised *Camphor* to be used so freely for it (see Lesser Writings, p. 851, 854). He is thus granting, IN PRINCIPLE, the germ-theory of infectious disease, and the propriety of parasiticide treatment in them.

the Thomist doctrine—itself derived from Aristotle—under another name. But the tendency of recent science is to regard the organism as no monarchy, wherein some "archæus" lives and rules, but as a republic in which every part is equally alive and independently active, the unity of the whole being secured only by the common circulation and the universal telegraphic system of nerves. It is unfortunate, therefore, that Hahnemann should have committed himself and his work to another conception. Either or neither may be wholly true; but one would have been glad if the 'Organon' had kept itself clear of such questions, and had occupied only the solid ground of observation and experiment.

And now of the PSORA-THEORY. This is far too large a subject for justice to be done it here. It has been fully handled elsewhere;* and any one who would desire to deal fairly with Hahnemann on the point has abundant material for so doing. I can only say a few words as to what it purports to be and what it really is.

It is sometimes averred by Hahnemann's critics that he made all Chronic Disease—or at least seven-eighths of it—orginate in from the category of true chronic maladies those which arise from unhealthy surroundings, noxious habits, and depressing influences (§. 77) for these, he says, disappear spontaneously when the LŒDENTIA are removed. Neither will he allow the name to the medicinal affections which the heroic treatment of his day made so common (§. 74-6), and which he regards as incurable by art. True Chronic Disease consists of such profound disorders as Asthma, Phthisis, Diabetes, Hypochondriasis, and the like—disorders insusceptible of cure by Hygiene, and tending to permanent stay and even increase. A certain proportion of the affections so characterized were traceable to venereal infection—Syphilitic or "Sycotic" (*i.e.*, *Gonorrhœal*); and it seemed to him that the remaining seven-eighths (it is here that these figures come in) must have some analogous "miasmatic" origin. In the

* See Dudgeon's LECTURES ON HOMŒOPATHY, IX and X and my own PHARMACO-DYNAMICS, pp. 87, 90 and 839. A thoughtful paper on the subject was presented to our International Congress of 1896 by Dr. Goldsborough; and, with the discussions following, may be read in its Transactions. Dr. Goldsborough differs from me as to the range of cutaneous disease covered by the name "Psora" in Hahnemann's writings, and indeed so extends it as to include itching eruptions of all kinds. He makes him explicitly contained for a doctrine of "herpetism" which I have viewed as only implicitly contained in his thought. He is thus unable to agree with me that Hahnemann "based the logical superstructure of his Psora-theory upon the distinct entity Scabies." I have carefully weighed what my able colleague has written, but am unable to modify the judgment expressed in the text, and in the references given in this note.

medical literature of his day he found numerous observations (he cites ninety-seven of them) of the supervention of such diseases upon the suppressing of cutaneous eruptions among which Scabies—then very prevalent—held a prominent place. In this last he had found the "Miasm" he wanted. It resembled Syphilis in its communication by contact, its stage of incubation, and its local development, while it was far more general. He thereupon propounded it as—together with the other contagious skin affections, the Tineæ, etc., which he regarded as varieties of it—the source of the non-specific Chronic Diseases, understood as defined.

Now it is easy for us, knowing what we know (or suppose we know) about Itch, to make merry over this theory of Hahnemann's. But to condemn or ridicule him for it, is a gross anachronism. We forget that the modern doctrine of Scabies dates only from Hebra's writings on the subject in 1844. Before that time men like Rayer and Biett could deny the existence of the acarus; and it was quite reasonable to regard it as only the product of the disease. Hahnemann, who was one of the most learned physicians of his time, knew all about it, and had, in 1792, written up on it.* He nevertheless, in 1816, described Scabies as a specific, miasmatic disorder, forming itself in the organism after contagion (as Syphilis does), and announcing by the Itch-vesicle its complete development within. It was thus regarded that he propounded it as the origin of so much Chronic Diseases. We, understanding it better, must refuse it such a place. But when we look beneath the surface of his doctrine, we find it far from being bound up with his view of Scabies. It rests upon the broader ground of morbid diathesis, and especially upon that form of it associated with cutaneous disorder which has led the French Pathologists to speak of a DIATHESE HERPETIQUE OR DARTREUSE. Translate Hahnemann's "Psoric," now into these terms, now into "scrofulous," and you have the substance of his thought, which is absolutely true and of the utmost importance. It was for therapeutic purposes that he arrived at it, and these it has subserved in no common degree, giving us a wealth of new remedies, of long and deep action, which are our most valued means in chronic disorders. Compare, for instance, our use of *Sulphur* with that which generally obtains—with that even which obtained in our own school before the Psora-doctrine was enunciated, and you will see what we have gained by it.

Here again, then, we cannot allow Hahnemann to be deprecated on account of his hypothesis, strange as it may seem to us. But we must regret that he incorporated it in his 'Organon.' Neither it nor its practical consequences form any part of his method, as such; and Pathological theory is out of place in the exposition of a mode of pro-

* See B. J, H., xxi, 670.

ceeding which is wholly independent thereof. In reading the 'Organon', let us determine to ignore it, or to translate its language in the way I have suggested: We shall then do greater justice to the main argument of the Treatise.

And now a few words upon the theory of DYNAMIZATION, which is a subject quite distinct from that of infinitesimal dosage. We have seen that Hahnemann was led to adopt and defend the latter on grounds whose legitimacy all must admit, whatever they may think of their validity. For the first quarter of a century of his practice in this way (he began it in 1799) he thus regarded and justified it. He maintained, as I have said, that by the mulptiplication of points of contact obtained, dilution does not weaken in proportion to the reduction of bulk; but, in so speaking, he admitted that it did weaken. He even attempted to fix the ratio of the two processes, estimating that each quadratic diminution of quantity involved loss of strength by only one-half; and this calculation remains unaltered in all editions of the Organon (note to § 284). In the Third Edition, however (i.e., in 1824), there appears for the first time the note we now read as appended to § 287. He here speaks of the unfolding of the spirit of a medicine as effected by the pharmaceutic processes of trituration and succussion, and in proportion to the duration of the one and the repetition of the other. By regulating these, accordingly, we can secure either moderation of excessive crude power on development of finer or more penetrating medicinal energy. In publications of 1825 and 1827, he carries yet further this new thought. At first he had ascribed the increase of power to the more intimate mixture effected by his processes; but now he declares it to be something over and above this—a change, a liberation of the dynamic, a development of the spiritual powers of the drugs, analogous to the production of heat by friction. Treated in this way, he affirms, "medicines do not become by their greater and greater attenuation weaker in power, but always more potent and penetrating"; there is "an actual exaltation of the medicinal power, a real spiritualisation of the dynamic property, a true, astonishing, unveiling and vivifying of the medicinal spirit."

These views were so little in accordance with those expressed in the 'Organon', that we find scant further trace of them in the Edition of 1829. In the note before-mentioned "refined" (VERFEINERT) becomes "potentised," as we have it now; and in the directions for proving medicines a note is added to § 129, saying that recent observation pointed to greater attenuation and potentisation rather than larger quantity as best giving the strength required for the purpose. This is all. In 1833, however, the pharmaceutical portion of the treatise has two new aphorisms (269, 270) embodying them. Its posological section remains unchanged, save in § 276. Here Hahnemann had said, in former editions, "a medicine, even though it may be Homœopathically suited to the cure of disease, does harm in every dose that is too large, the more harm the larger the dose, and by the magnitude of the dose it does more harm the greater its Homœo pathicity." In the Fifth Edition he adds, "and the higher the potency selected," which obviously changes the meaning of what has gone before, and makes dose a mere question of number of drops or globules. I mention all this to shew how entirely the doctrine of dynamization was an after-thought, and how little the 'Organon' proper (with which we are immediately concerned) has to do with it.

But what shall we say of the theory itself, in its bearing on Hahnemann's worth as a thinker? This must depend very much upon the stand-point from which we regard it. Was it a gratuitous hypothesis, at best a mere logical consequence of the other views of the originator? Or, was it an attempt to account for facts—these being in themselves genuine? Hostile critics assume the former position, and judge accordingly. We, however, cannot do this. Whatever our own preferences in the matter of dosage, it is impossible to read the history of Homœopathy, still more to be acquainted with its periodical literature, without recognising that highly attenuaed medicines have an activity SUI GENERIS. They show this in provings on the healthy as well as in the treatment of the sick; and not here and there only, but in such multitudinous instances as to make coincidence and imagination utterly inadequate as accounts of the phenomena. The Hahnemannic processes certainly do develope virtues in drugs which in their crude state are altogether latent. Brimstone, oyster-shell, flint, charcoal, table-salt—these substances in mass have a very limited range of medicinal usefulness; but what cannot Homœopathy do, what has it not done, with *Sulphur, Calcarea, Silicea, Carbo vegetabilis* and *Natrum muriaticum*, in the dilutions from the 6th to 30th? In this form they are in our hands as well-tried agents as any on which ordinary medicine depends. Their potency is a fact to us; how are we to account for it? Hahnemann's dynamization, in the light of later science, must be held untenable; but to this day we have nothing to put in its place. And even if we had, we should not the less honour the philosopher who perceived the necessity of the explanation, who brought to light the hitherto unknown phenomena, and set us to work at giving a scientific account of them.*

---

* Dr. Gatchell, in a very interesting essay, brought before the Paris congress of 1900 the views now entertained about the effects of solution, as substantiating Hahnemann's dynamization. In a complete solution of a complex body, he writes, there are no molecules, but only "ions" into which the molecules have dissociated. These ions are electrically active while molecules are passive, and so a fresh force may be said to have been imparted to the original substance. These views may be helpful to our conceptions, so far as com-

I have now completed my exposition of Hahnemann's Medical Philosophy as contained in his 'Organon.' But we are accustomed now-a-days to demand more of Philosophy than that it shall be sound in method: It must also show its power in bearing fruit. Hahnemannians need not fear the challenge. There is a fine passage in Macaulay's Essay on Bacon, in which he recounts the numerous gains to mankind which the science of the last two hundred years has contributed. If the writer of the 'Novum Organum' could have looked forward, he says, he might well have rejoiced at the rich harvest which was to spring up from the seed he had sown. In like manner has even the immediate future responded to the impulse given by our Organist. Could he have foreseen the medicine of to-day, how much there would have been to gladden his heart. He lived in a time when heroic antiphlogisticism was in full force; when physicians "slew," as in Addison's day, "some in chariots and some on foot"; when every sufferer from acute diseases was drained of his life-blood, poisoned with *Mercurials,* lowered with *Antimonials,* and raked by PURGATIVES. He denounced all this as irrational, needless, injurious; and it has fallen—never, we trust, to resume its sway. The change thus wrought even in the practice of the old school would be a matter for thankfulness on his part; but how his spirit would have bounded when he looked upon the band of his own followers! The few disciples made during his life-time have swelled into a company of over twelve thousand practitioners, who daily, among the millions of their CLIENTELE, in their hundreds of hospitals and dispensaries and charitable homes, carry out his beneficient reform, making the treatment of disease the simple administration of a few (mostly) tasteless and inodorous doses, and yet therewith so reducing its mortality that their patients' lives can be assured at lower rates. He would see the *Aconite* and *Belladonna,* the *Bryonia* and *Rhus,* the *Nux vomica* and *Pulsatilla,* the *Calcarea, Silicea, Sulphur,* which he created as medicines, playing their glorious part on an extensive scale, robbing acute diseases of their terrors and chronic maladies of their hopelessness. He would see his method ever developing new remedies and winning new victories—evoking *Lachesis, Apis, Kali bichromicum, Gelsemium,* and earning laurels in Yellow Fever as green as those which crowned it in the visitations of CHOLERA. He would see his principles gaining access one by one to the minds of physicians at large —the proving of medicines, the single remedy, the fractional dose already accepted, and selection by similarity half-adopted under other explanations and names. He might well feel, like Bacon, about the "Philosophia Secunda" which should end his Instauratio Magna.

pound salts and solvent processes are concerned, but they hardly aid us for other substances and modes of preparation; and as a solution of one part in the thousand is considered a "perfect" one, we do not even for the salts get far on in Hahnemann's scale.—Dr. Gatchell's paper may be read in English in the MEDICAL ERA for April, 1901.

He had given its "Prodromisive Anticipationes": "The destinies of the human race must complete it—in such a manner, perhaps, as men looking only at the present would not readily conceive." The destinies of the human race, in respect of disease and its cure, are completing it; and will be yet more profoundly modified for the better as that completion goes on.

LECTURE IV.

THE KNOWLEDGE OF DISEASE

Hitherto, in dealing with three elements of the method of Hahnemann—the aspect it takes of disease, the mode in which it ascertains drug-action, and the principles on which it fits the one to the other—I have confined myself to exposition and vindication of Hahnemann's own deliverances on the subject, and these mainly as contained in his 'Organon'. There is still, however, a criticism to be made on his positions from the standpoint of the medicine of to-day; and to this, I must now address myself.

In the opening words of the definition of Homœopathy which formed the starting-point of my First Lecture, I said Homœopathy is "a therapeutic method." It is, I might have added, so described by its author. We find the name, the formula and the full statement of it in the First Edition of the 'Organon.' "Hitherto," he writes in the Introduction, "the diseases of human being have been treated not rationally, not on fixed principles, but according to various curative intentions, among others by the palliative rule CONTRARIA CONTRARIIS CURENTER. Directly opposite to this lies the truth, the real road to cure, to which I give the guide in this work: To cure mildly, rapidly, and permanently, choose in every case of disease a medicine which can of itself produce an affection similar ($\H{o}\mu\varsigma\iota o\nu$ πa os) to that it is wished to cure (SIMILIA SIMILIBUS CURENTUR)." Homœopathy is a therapeutic method; and it belongs, avowedly at least, exclusively to that part of the therapeutic sphere in which drugs are our instruments. "To cure" . . . "choose in every case of disease a medicine." It gives no instruction as to the other resources of the physician's art—diet, regimen, temperature, climate, the use of water and electricity and so forth. Some analogies among these and even among psychical affections, to the operation of similars have been pointed out by various writers from Hahnemann downwards; but, whatever be their value,* that at any rate find no place here. For our present purpose, Homœo-

---

* Hahnemann's suggestions of the kind have been criticised by Dr. Dudgeon in his Lectures (p. 71-4), and by Dr. Sharp in his "Essays on Medicine" (1874), Essay VI. On the other side see Dr. Percy Wilde in the M. H. R., for 1896, pp. 116, 149.

pathy is a method of drug-therapeutics; and while it has the advantages, must also share the limitations, of its materials. These limitations are of several kinds, but are mainly imposed by the superior claims of other remedial measures. SIMILIA SIMILIBUS may be the best mode of choosing medicines, but medicines are not always the chief or the most appropriate means of treating the sick. Such a thought was hardly so familiar to the age of Hahnemann as it is in our own. The ordinary medical attendant was then in fact as in name an apothecary— one who served out drugs from a store; his only variation upon this theme occurring when he bled or blistered. Of the natural history of disease nothing was known, and the idea of trusting to it was before Skoda and Dietl unheard-of. Hygiene played as little part in the doctor's prescription as it did in the patients' lives; and the TOLLE CAUSAM on which we now lay so much stress was then directed only to those hypothetical morbid states—obstructions, spasms, altered humours, and so forth—which were assumed as the foundations of disease. With the advance of knowledge on these subjects a corresponding encroachment has been made on the sphere of drug-therapeutics; and Homœopathy occupies a less prominent part in the practice of Homœopathists, not because they trust to it less as a guide to drug selection, but because they have less need of drug-action itself

In a lecture "On the Place of Drugs in Therapeutics," delivered at the London Homœopathic Hospital in 1895, which is readily accessible,* 1 traced the progressive adoption of this position from Hahnemann himself through Caroll Dunham, Dudgeon and Dake. In assuming it on my own part, I reminded my hearers of the potency of diet in Scurvy and of regimen in Lithæmia; and of the benefit of the exposure to Nature's influences as seen in Pfarrer Kneipp's system (to which might now be added the fresh air treatment of Phthisis). I showed the wide range of the maxim TOLLE CAUSAM ("that royal road," as Hahnemann calls it), applying it to the abuse of the tea, coffee, tobacco and Alcohol which—to say nothing of coca, kola and absinthe—play so large a part in present-day life; and also to the place occupied by the reflex action in the etiology of disease. I recognised the aid brought to the healing art by Surgery, by Hydrotheraphy, by Electricity, by gymnastics and massage (I might have added, by heat and cold). I need not further enlarge on this subject. I only mention it here to show that I am not unmindful of the wide field of therapeutic work which lies outside the special plot of ground we cultivate; and of our right and duty, as physicians and not merely Homœopathists, to labour in it.

* See M. H. K. xl. 14.

Proceed, therefore, with my comments on our original definition, Homœopathy is a therapeutic method, formulated in the rule SIMILIA SIMILIBUS CURENTER—let likes be treated by likes. The two elements of the comparison here implied are the effects of drugs on the healthy body and the clinical features of disease; in either case "all being taken into account which is appreciable by the patient or cognizable by the physician but hypothesis being excluded." We shall have more yet to say upon SIMILIA SIMILIRUS; but must first dwell further on what I have called the elements of comparison, and will begin with the aspect of disease which is selected for it.

I suppose that all lecturers on the Practice of Physic commence the account of particular diseases by describing their clinical features. "Every now and then," as my former teacher at King's College—Dr. George Budd—used to say, "we meet with" cases presenting such and such groups of phenomena and sensations. He would then give the name by which the malady thus constituted is styled, and would proceed to relate how it came about, and wherein essentially consisted, so far as these points were known. But observe the difference involved in this "so far." The etiology and Pathology of the disease were more or less uncertain, and our conception of them was liable to vary as new facts came into view. But its clinical features remained. They were those which perchance Sydenham, or even Hippocrates, had described as graphically as any modern physician: they, amid all shiftings of conceptions about them, were permanent and sure.

Hahnemann, as we have seen, took these features as the disease-basis of method. Simplicity and certainty were his aims in practical medicine. He could not conceive that the obstacles to them were insurmountable, and we have heard him* expressing—out of his profound Theism—his faith that as the Creator has permitted disease in its numerous forms* He must also have to reveal to us a distinct mode whereby it may be known and combated. This "distinct mode" was, he considered, the clinical. He was indeed far from refusing the aid of etiology to such extent as it was available. The 'Organon' has shewn him pointing out that it is obviously part of the physician's duty to ascertain the presence or incidence of any exciting causes of disease, that he may remove them now and ensure their avoidance in future. It is also desirable, according to his teaching, to discover the past causes—both predisposing and exciting—of the patient's morbid condition, as certain medicines are found specially suitable when disease has originated in certain ways—*Arnica* when from in-

---

* See p. 15.

juries *Rhus* and *Dulcamara* when from cold damp and so on. Pathology, however, Hahnemann absolutely rejected for therapeutic purposes. It was in his day far more a matter of guess-work than it is now, and was too much of a quicksand for a sure foundation to be laid in it. But he went further, and maintained that a knowledge of the essential nature of disease was both unattainable and useless. His views on this subject are best expressed in § 5 and 6 of the Fourth Edition of the 'Organon' (they were omitted, I know not why, in the Fifth):—"It may be conceded that every disease is dependent on an alteration in the interior of the organism. But the alteration is only guessed at by the understanding in a dim and illusory manner from what the morbid symptoms reveal concerning it (and there are no other data for it in non-surgical diseases); and the exact nature of this inner-invisible alteration cannot be ascertained in any reliable manner. The invisible morbid alteration in the interior and the alteration in the health perceptible to our senses together constitute to the eye of creative Omnipotence what we term disease : But the totality of the symptoms is the only side of the disease turned towards the practitioner—this alone is, that is perceptible to him, that is the main thing he can know respecting the disease, and that he needs to know to help him to cure it." The side of disease which Pathology explores was thus to Hahnemann its NOUMENON in the strict sense of the word—recognised metaphysically as existent, but taken no practical account of for all purposes, but those of thought represented by the phenomena. "The totality of the symptoms" is to the therapeutist, the disease.

Is this position tenable? Most persons would at once answer in the negative; they would do so, I think without regard to the end set before us, in thus limiting our apprehension of disease. If we were dealing with it as an object of science, a branch of natural history, it is certain that symptomatology would be an insufficient basis for our knowledge. No one has better shown this than Liebermeister, in his Introduction to the section on 'Infectious Diseases' in Zeimssen's "Cyclopædia."[22] The basing unities of disease on symptoms gave us such Pathological entities as Hydrops, Icterus, Apoplexy, and the like; and "from this symptomatic stand-point Quotidian Fever was a different malady from the Tertian or the Quartan form, while on the other hand Ascites and Tympanites were only different forms of the same disease." He goes on to argue that the most scientific—because the most real—rule of classification must refer to CAUSES, must be etiological. The Quotidian and Quartan types of fever are one, because they both originate from Malaria; they are to be differentiated from pyæmic febrile attacks, though these may have a similar rhythm and similar symptoms, but are to have grouped with the other Malarial affections which differ greatly in symptoms, such as Malarial Neuralgia, Malarial Diarrhœa, Malarial Cachexia. "The lightest form of Varioloid is regarded as essentially identical with the most severe form of Variola; on the other hand, Vaccinia and Varicella are separated from it. The simplest Diarrhœa arising from the poison of Asiatic Cholera is to be ascribed to this disease : On the other hand, a very severe and deadly Cholera Morbus is to be marked as another malady."

Nor is it for classification only that such scientific knowledge of morbid states can be turned to account. It avails for prognosis. That we are able to distinguish true Typhus from other forms of Continued Fever, and that we know its natural history enables us to affirm, that if the patient survives the nadir of his prostration between the fourteenth and seventeenth day, and then displays an upward tendency, he will pretty certainly recover. It avails for the general management of the patient. To recognise Relapsing Fever as present leads to a care being taken after the first apparent recovery which would otherwise be needless, but which here materially influences the course of the second paroxysm: It also suggests the use of antiseptics, during the interval for the possible prevention of the recurrence, as carried out so successfully by Dr. Dyce Brown in Aberdeen.* It avails, again, for estimating the influence of treatment. Of old, every Chancre which disappeared without secondaries supervening went to the credit of the *Mercury* given, or to the demonstration of its needlessness if it had been omitted. We now know that the Soft Chancre—which occurs by far the more frequently of the two—has no such significance, and is naturally without SEQUELÆ.

Now if medicine were an applied science only, it would be with such knowledge and its utilisation entirely that we should be concerned. But it is (as we have seen) the merit of Homœopathy that in it medicine assumes its true place in being an art—the art of healing. It should have, as I have said, a life of its own, independent of the nourishment its associated sciences bring. The method of Hahnemann gives it this, by taking the clinical aspect of disease as its working basis. Pathological knowledge has little to do with drug-selection so determined. It has taught us—for instance—to recognise Enteric Fever as specifically distinct from Typhus, and for many purposes this differentiation is highly important. But the indications for its Homœopathic remedies were just as plain when it was classed merely as "Typhus Abdominalis,"

*See B. J. H. xxxi, 355,

and were as well given of old by Wolf and Trinks, as they are new by Jousset and Panelli.

Again, if our aim be the ascertainment of the particular organ affected in a given case, symptomatology is certainly insufficient. Not, indeed, because it is to be distinguished from physical diagnosis, and has to do with "rational" signs merely. The phenomena requiring a 'scope or speculum' for their perception, the sounds elicited only by percussion and auscultation, are as truly symptoms, as is a dilated pupil or a wheezing respiration. Not thus, but because to ascertain the seat of disease we have to bring in the aid of morbid Anatomy. This is the science of LESIONS, while clinical medicine takes account of MALADIES—which, in the words of Tessier, are "constituted by an assemblage of symptoms and lesions undergoing a definite evolution." The one speaks of Hepatisation of the Lung, the other of Pneumonia ; the one of Herpes, the other of Shingles. Now the lesion—save where, as in the last instance, it is on the surface—is a thing inferred only, not perceived or experienced ; and hence is not strictly included within the range of the knowledge of disease required by the Homœopathic method which—again to quote Tessier—is one of "positive indications." To many minds, accustomed to make physical diagnosis their chief aim as physicians, this is a very unacceptable feature of our practice. But let us look at the matter dispassionately. What do you gain by inferring, from certain signs, that a given group of symptoms means the presence of inflammation of the air-cells proper, as distinguished from the bronchial mucous membrane or the pleura ? Something, it may be, for prognosis: You know better what the patient has to expect and both he and you feel more security from being able to follow the morbid process as it were with your mind's eye through all its stages. In other cases, as where the digestive organs are at fault, a knowledge of the precise seat of the malady aids you in general management : You can order such food only to be taken as will give the affected portion rest—farinaceous where the stomach, animal where the duodenum, is involved. In neither instance, however, have you gained anything as regards drug-treatment, especially if you are going to conduct this on the principle of SIMILIA SIMILIBUS. Your medicine must indeed act on the same parts as those affected by the disease, and in the same manner. But, if it produce a like group of symptoms, the inference is that it does so. As Hahnemann wrote in the 'Organon' (§ 148)—"A medicine which has the power and tendency to produce symptoms the most similar possible to the disease to be cured, affects those very parts and points in the organism now suffering from the natural disease." It is from the phenomena that in diagnosis, you infer the noumena : Quite as surely, in treatment, if drug and disease have the same phenomena, it may be concluded that their noumena are also identical. You are indeed in this way more certain of your aim ; for your diagnosis may be wrong, as the autopsy not uncommonly proves, but your comparison of symptoms—if intelligent and painstaking cannot err of the mark. And further, it must be remembered that our object, is to select not a SIMILE only, but the SIMILIMUM—the medicine whose action on the healthy correspond to the particular case in its individuality, in the finer features and more minute ramifications of the malady here presented. Identity of lesion is insufficient for this : "We want" as Dr. Drysdale has said, "a Pathological simile far more exact and qualitatively like than that afforded by mere coarse morbid Anatomy, which is common to all cases alike." We get this by fitting together the variety of phenomena manifested in disease and in drug-action by "covering" the one with the other. We may not be able to explain why certain symptoms are present in certain cases ; but we must believe that each has its proximate cause, and that the combination of such causes constitutes the individual malady from which the patient is suffering, and to which our drug must be fitted.

For drug-therapeutics on the Homœopathic principle, therefore, symptomatology may justly supersede diagnosis, as being in many cases surer and in all more thorough. It gives us a further advantage (which I have already touched upon), in that it often enables us to attack maladies in their forming stage, before they have developed such lesions as physical signs can manifest. The totality of symptoms is intended to be a curative indication ; and if disease is to be cured it should be taken as early as possible, before such results have occurred as become the subjects of morbid Anatomy POST MORTEM, or even of Pathology during life. In such early stages maladies are often recognisable by rational signs alone, and mainly by symptoms of a subjective nature. This point has been forcibly made by Carroll Dunham, in his Essay entitled, "The Relation of Pathology to Therapeutics"; and I would take the opportunity of commending the writings of this "beloved physician" (by no name less tender can those who knew him speak of him) to your most earnest attention. His lucid style is but an index to the clearness of his thought ; and in him Hahnemann finds an expositor who knows how to reconcile him to science and expound him in reason without sacrificing an iota of his essential principles. In the Essay I have mentioned he shews, that as Physiology takes cognisance, not of life, but of the results of life, so that with which Pathology is concerned is the result of the abnormal and perverted life which we call disease. The products of disease Pathology sees, hears, or infers : It knows nothing of disease itself. Hence, to base Therapeutics upon Pathology alone is to make the former merely palliative —a pumping out a leaking ship instead of stopping the leak. It may be said that we do not know where the leak—the primary disturbance —is, and that if we knew we could not reach it to stop it. But by the proving of medicines we obtain agents which their powers to cause similar inundations, and therefore presumably, similar breaches, which —upon the principle SIMILIA SIMILIBUS—it is the hypothesis that they can repair. If then, the comparison between the results of disease and of drug-influence be thoroughly and accurately made, the parallelism of action must reach also to that which originates either. "And here," Dr. Dunham writes, "I cannot refrain from tendering homage to the wonderful prevision of genius by which, in an age when Pathology, as we understand it, was unknown. Sammuel Hahnemann anticipated all that we have said, and all that the most advanced thinkers of our day have taught, respecting the scope and influence of Pathology in relation to Therapeutics. The symptoms of the urinary organs in connection with the discharge of morbid urine would at one time have been regarded as the proper subject of treatment. But Pathology has now taught us to trace these symptoms back to the kidneys and beyond the kidneys to the blood, and beyond the blood to the nutrition and the destruction of all the organised tissues. As Dr. Carpenter remarks, —'When, for example, the urine presents a particular sediment, our enquiries are directed not so much to the sediment itself, as to the constitutional state which causes an undue amount of the substance in question to be carried off by the urinary excretion, or which prevents it from being (as usual) dissolved in the fluid.' To confine the attention, therefore, in prescribing for a given cause, to the immediate organ the perversion of whose functions is most obviously pointed out by the prominent symptoms, is to disregard the clearest indications of Pathology. We must analyse these prominent symptoms, and must include their remotest elements in our indications. Nay, these remotest elements—the constitutional disturbances of which Carpenter speaks —are even more—important indications for treatment than the more obvious and objective symptoms. But how can we analyse these more obvious symptoms, and ascertain those 'constitutional disturbances' in which they have their origin ? In no other way than by a study of the functions of the entire organism—in what way and to what extent they are performed in an abnormal manner. And this brings us at once to that rule on which Hahnemann so strongly insisted, that the entire organism of the patient should be examined in every possible way, and that the 'totality of symptoms' should be made the basis of the prescription ; nay, that the constitutional, general symptoms are often more conclusive as to the proper treatment than the more obvious local symptoms. The grand old master reached at a single bound the same conclusions to which the labours of a half century of able Pathologists have at last, with infinite research, brought the medical profession."

All this time we have been dealing with general principles : but let us look at special forms of disease, and see whether or not the

Hahnemannian mode of regarding them is sufficient for their treatment.

1. The FEVERS constitute a group which plays a large part in daily practice. They are maladies in which morbid increase of temperature exists prior or out of proportion to any local inflammation which may be present. The theory of this state is still a moot one. According to some Pathologists it depends upon excessive heat-production; according to others upon deficient heat-radiation; while yet another class (with whom I venture to think the truth resides) believe that both factors operate at one time or another in the process.* But whatever be the genesis of fever, it remains a positive fact, a clinical entity, with which we have to deal. Upon the Homœopathic principle, we have to treat it with drugs capable of producing fever. How they do so, we may not know; but our ignorance of the process matters little if we are sure about the result. "An infinitesimal quantity of *Atropia*—a mere atom," writes Dr. John Harely "as soon as it enters the blood, originates an action which is closely allied to, if it be not identical with, that which induces the circulatory and nervous phenomena accompanying Enteric or Typhus Fever." This is sufficient; and as soon as we learn it to be a fact from Hahnemann's proving of *Belladonna* (made, I may add, before Dr. Harely was born), yet minuter quantities of *Atropia* (in the form of the juice of its mother plant) became in our hands trusted remedies for these very fevers. Again, the classification of fevers of which we have already spoken, so necessary for science and so valuable for general purposes, has but the smallest influence upon drug-selection. The old divisions of Synocha, Synochus, and Typhus (the last with its "nervous" and "putridus"), worthless as they are from a scientific point of view, are much more useful for our practice than those of Typhus, Typhoid, Relapsing, and Ephemeral. They denote the KIND of fever with which we have to do, its quality and mode of life; and to us it is all important that our drugs, next to being really febrigenic, should correspond in their action to the kind of fever present. They can hardly set up a whole Typhoid, in its complete evolution; but the febrile state they develope is certainly either a Synocha, a Synochus, a Typhus nervosus versatilis or stupidus, or a Typhus putridus; and if we find these states existing, in the essential fevers, the exanthemata, or elsewhere, in them we shall have our remedial means.

---

*See my "Knowledge of the Physician," Lecture V.

2. After FEVERS, the most important group of disease consists of the INFLAMMATIONS. To the Pathology of this morbid process many pages are devoted at the commencement of every treatise on Medicine or Surgery. Whether, after all that has been written, we know much about it in its essence, may well be doubted; but even if we do, of what avail is our knowledge for treatment—at any rate for medicinal treatment? The old phenomenal signs, DOLOR, CALOR, RUBOR, TURGOR, still for all practical purposes constitute INFLAMMATION, when externally manifested and when it is internal, and so invisible, the facts which lead us to infer its presence and seat are no less of the symptomatic order, as I have already argued. To treat Inflammation Homœopathically, it is only necessary to find a drug capable of setting it up, at the same spot, and in the same manner, as evidenced by the symptoms.

3. The NEUROSES, of which I would in the third place speak, are still—as Libermeister says symptomatic groups. Their unity is one neither of cause nor of lesion; it is clinical only. It is of much interest to know what is the seat and process of the Epileptic paroxysm; but our choice of Anti-epileptic remedies must be determined mainly by the power they have of inducing similar paroxysm in the healthy subject, explain it or not as we can. In like manner is it with Cholera and Tetanus and Hysteria; no conceivable knowledge we can gain as to their intimate nature would make us better able to fit Homœopathic remedies to them than we should be, if we possessed their symptomatic analogues in drugs.

It thus appears that of the three elements which exist in all knowledge—phenomena, laws, and causes, it is the first which for positive therapeutic action, chiefly concerns us in disease. Not that the other two are worthless to us, even for this end. Our laws here are classification—the recognition in morbid states of genera, species and varieties analogous to those of animated nature. These enable us to form groups of remedies associated with them, instead of having to wander through the whole Materia Medica for each prescription: They also give a continuity to medicinal treatment, without which the USUS IN MORBIS were of no avail. Hahnemann led the way here, by constantly insisting on the existence of fixed and definite types of disease, to which standing remedies should be applied; and by giving us group of "Antipsorics." I fear, however, that he must be considered as having rejected all enquiry into causes—I mean, proximate causes, the noumena of the phenomena—in this sphere. In so doing we need not follow him. His ground for taking symptoms as the element of parallelism between disease and drug-action was that they only were surely known in his day this was true, and his selection of them was most prudent. But to maintain that they alone were knowable was unwarrantably to bar the progress of science. His stricter followers have acted on the DICTUM, and have looked askance on the positive Pathology of the present day, with its physical diagnosis and post-mortem confirmations. They have always been a decade or more behindhand in their recognition of such distinction as those between Typhus and Typhoid, between Chancre and Chancroid, and in their use of such means as auscultation and thermometry. Now this is altogether wrong. An inference from symptoms, if sure, is as good a basis for treatment as symptoms themselves. This sureness is assumed in the prognosis given and the general management instituted : Why should it not be also for purposes of drug-selection ? By proceeding upon it we secure another route to the SIMILE we desiderate. We use symptoms to reach it, because they are its most certain expression; but if it can be otherwise attained, the alternative access may often be useful. Morbid lesions sometimes occur almost, if not quite, without symptoms, as for instance Caries of the Vertebræ and Senile Pneumonia. To attempt to "cover" these from the results of the proving of drugs would be futile. But Toxicology and experiments on animals here come to our aid and give us in *Phosphorus* a substance capable of inflaming alike the cancellous structure of bone and the pulmonary air-cells ; so that with it we can combat these diseases, however latent and expressionless they may be. There is indeed something fascinating about similarities of this kind ; and our late colleague Dr. Sharp proposed (following in the footsteps of Paracelsus and Rademacher) to make seat of action instead of symptoms the basis of our methed, which accordingly he would call "Organopathy." That remedies so led to may prove effectual is undoubted ; We have a good example of them in the *Ceanothus Americanus* which, though never proved on the healthy, and only known to "act upon" the spleen, has been found strikingly effective in pains, enlargements, and other disorders of this organ. But we should never, if possible, rest content with identity of seat between disease and drug : We should aim also at making their kind of action the same, and this can only be done by securing similarity in their symptoms. In this way we elevate the SIMILE to a SIMILIMUM, and proportionately enhance its energy in cure.

We thus come back to the phenomena as our mainstay in practice ; for therapeutic purposes, the totality of symptoms, constitutes the disease. As a result of this view, the examination of patients by the Homœopathic prescriber is far more minute than that ordinary practised. He can hardly, indeed, inspect and explore for himself more thoroughly than does the well-trained practitioner of to-day ; but he listens to and questions the sick person with greater patience and more painstaking completeness. He pays more regard to subjective symptoms. I have already more than once indicated the large part played by sensations in Homœopathic proving and prescribing of medicines: I am glad now to support our appreciation of these from an Address delivered by the late Dr. Russel Reynolds in 1874.

"Is it not coming to this," he protested, "that but little attention is often paid to the accounts which patients give of themselves, their ideas, emotions, feelings and physical sensations? These are things which we cannot weigh in our most guarded balances—measure by our finest scales—split up by our crucibles—or describe in any terms save those which are peculiar to themselves and which we cannot decompose. These symptoms are often disregarded and set aside : And the patient, whose story of disease is made of them, is thought fanciful, hypochondriacal, hysterical, nervous, or unreal : because, forsooth, we have physically examined thorax, abdomen, limbs and excretions, and have found in them nothing wrong; because we have looked at the retinæ, examined the limbs electrically, traced on paper the beatings of the pulse, weighed the patient and not found him wanting. Still he is miserable, in spite of placebo and assurance that there is nothing organically wrong ! There may be in him a consciousness of a deep unrest ; or of a failing power which he feels, but which we cannot see ; or of a something worse than pain, a sense of impending evil that he is conscious of in brain or heart; a want of the feeling of intellectual grasp, which he may call failure of memory, but which memory—when we test it—seems free from fault ; a want of the sense of capacity, for physical exertion, which seems, when we see him walk or run, to be a mere delusive notion, for he can do either well or easily to our eyes and those of others ; and so he is called nervous, and told to do this or that, and disregard those warnings which come to him from the very centre of his life. And let me ask whether or no it has not again and again happened in the course of such a history as that which I have only faintly sketched, that some terrible catastrophe has occurred : Do we not see minds gradually breaking down while we say there is no organic change in the brain ? Hearts suddenly ceasing to do their work, when after careful auscultation we have said there was nothing to fear ? Suicide or sudden death sometimes disturbs the calm surface of our scientific prognosis of no evil : We may be startled, and may then see all that we ought to have before, But when the ripples that such unforseen events have occasioned on that smooth surface have subsided, we go on as we have already done, and still pay but little attention to what the patient feels, and delight ourselves in the precision of our knowledge with regard to physical conditions of which he may know nothing and may care still less. No one can appreciate more highly than I do the value of precise observation, but I do not believe that minute, delicate, and precise observation is limited to a class of facts which can be counted, measured or weighed. No one can see more distinctly than I do, the wrong conclusions at which a physician may arrive at by accepting as true the interpretations which fanciful patients may offer of their symptoms; but I am sure that if we pay no heed to these mistaken notions of a suffering man, we loose our clue to the comprehension of the real nature of his malady. Morbid sensations and wrong notions are integral parts of the disease we have to study as a whole, and we are bound to interpret their value for ourselves; but we can ill afford to set them aside, when we are as yet but in the dawn of scientific Pathology, and are endeavouring to clear away the obstacles that hide the truths we hope hereafter to see more clearly about the mystery of disordered life. The value of such symptoms may be slight in some kinds of diseases, when compared with that of those phenomena which may be directly observed; but we are bound to remember that there are many affections in which they furnish the earliest indication, and there are not a few of which they are throughout the only signs."

In the light of this, which is but one among the many advantages of Hahnemann's mode of observing disease, I think we may make claim for it as being, not only the one safe thing for his own time, but also a mode of procedure most important in itself, and never to be left behind. It needs especially to be emphasised at the present day. It is with us as before the Reformation, when the Bible was used by the Church as a rule of faith only—a source whence were to be inferred the doctrines and practices obligatory on her children. What Luther and his followers did was—as Dr. Robertson Smith has well shown—to recover the Book itself in the totality of its thoughts and words, as a means of grace to each individual soul. The fruitful results thus achieved in the spiritual sphere will be paralleled in the medical as the clinical study of disease is allowed its due preponderance, and is made the direct road to Therapeutics. Of this reformation Hahnemann was the preacher in his day: And his voice must ever be echoed by his disciples when they see the profession straying into the alluring, but less practical, paths of Pathological speculation.

In support of thus acting, they could cite the words of another acknowledged leader in English medicine, also now deceased—Sir Andrew Clark. In his Presidential Address at the Clinical Society of London in 1883, this distinguished physican said:—*

"Another great work of our Society has been and continues to be, the unfolding of the exact relations which morbid Anatomy and incidentally, Experimental Pathology should hold to clinical medicine. These two chief servants of our art, excited and carried away by their marvellous successes, and assuming a joint sovereignty over our art, look down with condescending superiority upon clinical medicine, ridicule her claims to supremacy, scoff at her empirical distinctions, reproach her with being unscientific, and strive to torture her into a slavish subjection to their theories. But the true relation is not this : It is, indeed, the converse of it. For the structural change is not disease, it is not co-extensive with disease; and even in those cases where the alliance appears the closest, the Statical or Anatomical alteration is but one of other effects of Physiological forces, which, acting under unphysiological conditions, constitute by this new departure the essential and true disease. For disease in its primary condition and intimate nature is in the strict language dynamic; it precedes, underlies, evolves, determines, embraces, transcends, and rules the Anatomical state. It may consist of mere changes in the relations of parts, of re-arrangements of atomic groupings, of recurring cycles of vicious chemical substitutions and exchanges, of new conditions in the evolution and distribution of nerveforce; and any or all of them may be invisible to the eye, inseparable from life, and undiscernible in death. Undoubtedly the appearance of a structural alteration in the course of disease introduces a new order of events, sets in action new combinations of forces, and creates disturbances which must be reckoned with, even as mechanical accidents of the Pathological processes. But always behind the Statical lies the Dynamic condition; underneath the structural forms are the active changes which give them birth, and stretching far beyond the limits of Pathological Anatomy, and pervaded by the actions and interactions of multitudinous forces, there is a region teeming with manifold forms of disease unconnected with structural change and demanding the investigation which it would abundantly reward. It is in this mysterious and fertile region of dynamic pathogenesis that we come face to face with the primitive manifestations of disease, and learn how much knowledge from all sources is needed to understand it aright ; it is here that we see how, without the help from Physics, Chemistry, and Biology, collecting, converging, and meeting in a common light, no single problem in disease can be completely solved; it is here that we are made to comprehend how the nature of a Pathological product cannot be determined by its structural character, but by the life-history of the processes of which it is only a partial expression; it is here that we observe how, in therapeutic

*LANCET, Feb. 3, 1883.

experiments, the laws of the race are conditioned and even traversed by the laws of the individual; and it is here that we discover how clinical medicine is to become a science, and how she is already, beyond all question, at once the mother and the mistress of all the medical arts."

* It is pleasant to find Dr. Clifford Allbutt following in this direction his eminent predecessor. "Mere observation of disease," he said in his inaugural lecture at the Middlesex Hospital School in 1900, "and morbid Anatomy have taken us almost as far these means can do. ... We must track our morbid processes in their earliest dynamic irritation, so as to arrest them at these stages." (BRIT. MED. JOURN., Oct. 6, 1900).

LECTURE V.

THE KNOWLEDGE OF MEDICINES

At our last meeting we spoke of the knowledge of disease required for the practice of Homœopathy. We saw that the phenomena we call "clinical"—the symptoms of maladies, subjective and objective, rational and physical, in their connection, conditions, and order of evolution—form for this purpose the main object of our study. They do more than enable Nosology to classify their sum and Pathology to diagnose their seat; they directly avail, under the guidance of the method of Hahnemann, for the choice of their remedies. Nosology aids in this, by grouping drugs around definite morbid species, and Pathology by utilising their local affinities; but both need completing by symptomatology to determine finally the one medicine which shall be the SIMILIMUM of the disorder we have to treat. We heard some of the ripest medical thinkers of our time bearing witness indirectly to the validity of this mode of procedure, recognising the dynamic origin of disease, the importance of subjective symptoms as indicating its beginnings, and the necessity of taking all symptoms into account if we are to arrive at a true conception of a case. The inference is that to the clinical study of disease the Homœopathic student and practitioner should devote his chief attention. He should learn, indeed, all that Pathology, which is the science of disease, can tell him about it in various forms; but should use the light of such knowledge, not so much to gaze upon in scientific interest, as to illumine his perception of the actual features of that with which he has to do.

Our subject today is the KNOWLEDGE OF MEDICINE, which are the tools of the healing art, as disease is the material on which it works. What are medicines? I do not know that any better definition of them can be given than that which was put forth by Hahnemann in 1805, in the Preface to his "Fragmenta de Viribus Medicamentorum positivis":—Quæ corpus mere nutriunt, ALIMENTA, quæ vero sanum hominis statum (vel parva quantitate ingesta) in ægrotum—ideoque et ægrotum in sanum—mutare valent, MEDICAMENTA appellantur." My own difference with him would be that I should place the corollary foremost, and define a medicine as a substance which has the power of changing sickness into health, and therefore —on the principle, 'nil prodest quod non lœdit idem'—of altering health to sickness.

Now on what ground is any substance to be reckoned a medicine? And how is it to be ascertained what are the morbid conditions and processes it can favourably modify? There are but two ways by which to arrive at such conclusions, the empirical and the rational.

1. Many, perhaps most, of the ordinary remedial uses of drugs, have been stumbled upon by chance. It has generally been the "common man" (as Hahnemann calls him), sometimes even the still lower brute, that has discovered them; and the professional healer has taken the hint and adopted the practice. After this manner has been gained *Bark* as a remedy for Ague, burnt Sponge for Goitre, *Arnica* for the effects of falls and strains, *Graphites* for Tetters, *Sulphur* for the Itch. Not less empirically, though among the practitioners of medicine, has arisen the use of *Mercury* and *Iodide of Potassium* in Syphilis, of *Bismuth* in Gastralgia, of *Arsenic* in Psoriasis. Theories of the MODUS OPERANDI of such remedies have often been subsequently framed; but it is certain that their original adoption grew out of no such theories; but was an accidental discovery.

Now it would be the height of unwisdom to neglect information from this source. A remedy is a remedy, however, comes at, and whether conforming or not to any laws of action we may suppose to prevail. Experience is the test even of medicines rationally ascertained to be such : It is but beginning the process a little lower down when experience itself discovers them. But on the other hand it is obvious that the empirical method is a very uncertain one, and affords no guarantee of further additions to our remedial wealth. Indeed, it is no method at all, but mere guess-work and chance picking-up. It is only hopelessness as to rational therapeutics which has led such writers as Wilks and Druitt in the past to make empiricism a matter for satisfaction and a standard of advance, and it is with regret that we see it rampant in the highest ranks of the medicine of today. Sir William Gowers has for sometime been regarded as one of the leading authorities upon Nervous Diseases, and as a Neurological specialist is in great request for consultative purposes. In an Address published in the LANCET of 1895 (November 23rd) he has shewn us what is in this case the "scientific medicine" on the possession of which that periodical so often felicitates the profession. "It has not been my privilege," he says, "to add much to our therapeutical resources," but the few agents I have recommended have been based on pure empiricism." He gives as examples his employment of *Borax* in Epilepsy and of *Aluminium* for the pains of Locomotor Ataxy. Of the former his words are—"It was one of many things I tried, simply as a peasant might try in succession a number of herbs"; of the latter, "I had no better reason for trying it than the fact that Arsenic is a metal, and so is Aluminium."* If this is the only mode of progress that "regular" medicine at its best can adopt, we may be content to remain "irregular."

2. There are certain pseudo-rational modes of discovering remedies which have brought undeserved slight on those truly bearing the name. Such is the doctrine of "signatures," and much of the iatro-mechanical and iatro-chemical theory of former and later times. When a real medicine has been gained by these means—as *Chelidonium* in disorders of the liver and *Euphrasia* in those of the eye, as *Iron* in Anæmia and *Muriatic acid* in Low Fevers—it has been by coincidence, not from induction: The result is practically empirical. The truly rational method is that which infers the place and the power of a drug in disease from its behaviour in health. Every such substance, on being introduced into the animal organism, causes certain disturbances, certain changes. Each has its proper series of effects; each selects certain organs and tissues, or certain tracts and regions of the body, and there sets up phenomena of a definite kind. This is the only source of information about them which is certainly and infinitely fruitful. If from observing the Pathogenetic effects of a substance we can conclude (subject to the teachings of experience) as to its therapeutic virtues, we have but to experiment with fresh poisons to gain as many additional remedies.

In two of his Essays—the "Suggestions" of 1796, and the "Examination of the Sources of the common Materia Medica" of 1817—Hahnemann has fully considered the empirical and pseudo-rational ways of arriving at the knowledge of medicines, and has proved them wanting. In the latter he discusses the ascription of general therapeutic virtues, as when drugs are styled resolvent, tonic, and so forth; the inference from sensible properties, as those of the bitters and aromatics, or from chemical qualities; and the USUS IN MORBIS, shewing conclusions from this source to be vitiated by polypharmacy and lack of individualisation. In the former Treatise he also enquired how far Botanical affinity

* It is rather curious that the very unusual Aluminium should have been the first metal thought of by Sir W. Gowers as a succedaneum to Arsenic. Is it possible that the fact had reached him (it is mentioned in my "Therapeutics") that Bœnninghausen many years ago published two cases of Tabes dorsalis in which a cure had been effected by *Aluminium metallicum* in the 200th dilution?—See AMER. HOM. REVIEW, I. 107.

could guide to medicinal virtues. His conclusion is that none of these sources is trustworthy, and that the only sure one is the effect produced by drugs on the healthy organism.

It is needless at the present day to vindicate the wisdom of Hahnemann's rejection of the fanciful modes of apprehending drug-action mentioned above. We still, indeed, hear of "tonics" (though not of "resolvents"); but that three such incongruous substances as *Iron, Quinine* and *Arsenic* should stand at the head of the list of these shews how little of scientific worth there is in the conception. The USUS IN MORBIS of course maintains its ground, but it is confessed to be only available as a guide when freed from the elements which in Hahnemann's day made it useless. A steadily growing usage, together with ever-multiplying admissions, shews that the proving of drugs on the healthy will ere long be recognised as being all that Hahnemann claimed for it. But in the meantime there is on the part of many such a tendency to look askance at it, and with all so much grudging of Hahnemann's merits as its initiator, that its exposition—if not justification—here becomes a necessity and a duty. We have also, on the other side, to present some critical estimate of the manner in which the work has been done by himself and his disciples, and of the materials we have gained thereform for our practice.

The organisms on which the effects of drugs can be ascertained are those of the lower animals and of man.

1. There was a time when the CORPUS VILE of brutes was thought the only ground on which FIET EXPFRIMENTUM; and even now it plays by far the largest part in the pharmacological research of the profession at large. If this were sound practice, Hahnemann would be somewhat discredited; for he, recognising that it was available, deliberately rejected it. But have his arguments against its adequacy ever been answered ? The first is that the effects of drugs are different on them and on us, and different as between themselves. "A pig can swallow a large quantity of *Nux vomica* without injury, and yet men have been killed with fifteen grains. A dog bore an ounce of the fresh leaves, flowers and seeds of monkshood: what man would not have died of such a dose ? Horses eat it, when dried, without injury. Yew leaves, though so fatal to man, fatten some of our domestic animals. . . . The stomach of a wolf poisoned by monkshood was found inflamed, but not that of a large and a small cat, poisoned by the same substance."*
Thus Hahnemann, and similar facts have come to light in later times, among which I may mention the impunity with

---

* Lesser Writings, p. 299.

which the rabbit may be fed for days upon *Belladonna* leaves. The argument from them has been urged afresh in the Forty-first Volume of the BRITISH JOURNAL OF HOMŒOPATHY, and shewn to be borne out by the contradictory results of later pharmacological research on animals. The second is yet more destructive: It is that we cannot obtain subjective symptoms from dumb creatures, and we have learnt how important these are in the knowledge—for curative purposes—of disease and therefore also of drugs. We may see this by the instance of *Aconite*. In experiments on animals, loss of sensibility of the surface is always noted ; hence the drug is supposed to be an anæsthetic, and suited for employment in Neuralgia and other simple pains, for which must be given in Physiological doses, or—where the affected parts can be reached—applied locally. But consult human poisonings, or—still better—provings, and another tale is told. While the surface may be insensible to external impressions, it is not so to the patients' own consciousness. It is a Dysæsthesia, an Anæsthesia dolorosa, from which he is suffering, which —as in the case of Schroff's provers—may devolope into actual Neuralgic pain, to which therefor *Aconite* is truly Homœopathic, and which it will cure by internal administration and in non-perturbing dosage.

These objections are surely fatal to any exclusive to even predominant reliance on experiments upon animals for ascertaining the properties of drugs. But on the other hand they have a place, which Hahnemann himself was ready to acknowledge (thirty years before Magendie began their systematic institution) and which the provings of his school, when thorough, have always given them. Besides the induction of the more violent effects of the drugs, we can learn upon these subjects the results of their long-continued employment in doses sufficient to change without killing. In this way, Wegner has ascertained the power of *Phosphorus* to induce a plastic irritation of periosteum, and of the interstitial tissue of the stomach and liver ; and Eugene Curie has shown *Bryonia* capable of exciting pseudo-membranous deposit and *Drosera* that of Tubercle. Again experiments on animals lend themselves to analysis and interpretation. Sir Lauder Brunton has well-shown how in this way the rapid circulation of *Atropia* has been proved to be due to paresis of the terminal extremities of the vagi in the heart; and the opposite effect of *Digitalis* has been demonstrated to result from stimulation of the same inhibitory fibres at at their origin. It is not always that here LE JEU VAUTLA CHANDELLE—that we have taken much by our knowledge : but assuming it to be worth having, it is certainly from experiments on animals that we must obtain it.

II. Such experiments, then, being of subsidiary value only, turn to the action of drugs on the human body as the main source of our knowledge of them. Thus knowledge must be gained here, as elsewhere, by observation and by experiment.

I. Observation, in the present instance, has for its field poisoning of healthy and over-dosing of sick persons; and each of these subdivisions requires separate discussion.

a. Poisoning is obviously limited to the comparatively small class of drugs sufficiently virulent to produce such effects. Here, however, it is of great value. It supplies the more violent disturbances and the POST-MORTEM changes induced by medicinal substances better (because more surely) than experiments on animals can do: It aids us greatly in arriving at the lessons they can produce and in obtaining similarity of seat between drug-action and disease. Records of poisoning and works on Toxicology have therefore been always largely employed, from Hahnemann downwards, in the construction of our pathogeneses; and nothing can be said against this source of knowledge save that it is, as it were, illegitimate. Poisonings are the product of crime or of carelessness, and in the progress of society should become more and more rare: So that we may not lean too confidently upon them as materials of future information.

b. Overdosing may also be said to be a remediable error: but as long as traditional medicine is practised, it will be liable to occur again and again, as it has occurred in the past. The object, both of Antipathic and of Allœopathic medication being to induce the Physiological actions of drugs, these are continually being observed; while even in "alterative" treatment the ponderable doses deemed necessary, and the occasionally quick susceptibilities of patients, occasion the development of collateral effects. The older Treatises on Materia Medica draw largely on such observations, partly for knowledge as to pathogenetic action, and partly for warning as to excessive doscage. They formed, as we have seen, Hahnemann's earliest source of symptoms; and continued to occupy a prominent place in all his collections. Ere long, indeed, they assumed a position there, which our present knowledge must declare unwarrantable. Their obvious weakness in the uncertainty which belongs to them, owing to their exhibitor being already the subject of disease. Of course, if this be of a definite and limited character, and consisting with fair general health; and if all symptoms conceivably resulting from it, or occupying the same seat, are excluded, and likewise all phenomena previously observed in or by the patient during his illness—then pathogenetic effects of drugs may be observed almost as well as upon healthy subjects. Some of our best records of the effects of

Atropia, as those of Grandi, Michea and Lussana, have been in this manner obtained; and without it we should know next to nothing of the Physiological action of the *Bromide* and *Iodide* of Potassium and so *Salicylic acid*. But Hahnemann, though he perceived the necessity for such precautions, soon came practically to ignore them. An exaggerated notion of the potency of drugs led him to set down well-nigh all the phenomena and sensations noted in patients from day to day by their physicians as effects of the drugs they were taking; and this in the presence of other sufficient causes and often in the face of the most glaring improbability. I have shown how he has treated the cases of Greding, Storck, Carrere, and Collin in this way*; and these are but specimens of his pervading practice. At first, it was only from the writings of physicians of the old school that symptoms so obtained were taken; for the Homœopathic dosage was conceived as reducing the power of drugs to do harm. When, however (about 1824), the theory of dynamisation began to influence his mind, and attenuations became potencies, there seemed no reason why these should not produce pathogenetic effects, and they became credited with the changes observed in patients taking them as previously had been Stork's *Conium* and Greding's *Veratrum*. The pathogeneses of the 'Chronic Diseases,' and the new symptoms of the Third Edition of the 'Materia Medica Pura,' are—so far as they are Hahnemann's—exclusively due to this source, and are untrustworthy in proportion.

This verdict must be passed still more decisively on another mode in which Hahnemann, in later years, utilised the sick in the construction of his pathogeneses. I refer to aggravations, real or supposed, of their symptoms. In 1813, he expressed the opinion that such aggravation "most probably indicates that the medicine given can itself also excite similar symptoms," but he would not have such symptoms set down as pathogenetic. In the 'Chronic Diseases,' however, there is good reason to believe that he departed from his salutary caution; and many of the apparently wonderful effects of drugs which experience has proved of the 'Materia Medica Pura,' are—so far as they are Hahnemanner obtained.

2. We come now to experiment, which here, as in other departments of research, should be our principle resource. Very little use, however, had been made of it before the time of Hahnemann. Haller's insight had perceived its need; and he had written—"It is upon the healthy body first that the medicine, free from any foreign admixture, is to be tested: 1st taste and odour to be ascertained, and

* See my "Pharmacodynamics," p. 28-30.

then, small doses being swallowed, their effects to be fully noted, how the pulse behaves, how the temperature, how the breathing, how the excretions." * But his words have fallen on barren ground; for there is no trace of any connection between them and the few provings which were extant at the end of the last century. Stork (1750-1760) had swallowed a few doses of *Aconite, Conium,* and *Colchicum*—merely, however, to ascertain whether and how far they could be administered with impunity. Alexander (1768) had tested on his own person *Castor, Suffron, Nitre* and *Camphor;* but here again as much to try whether these substances had any activity at all (which in the case of the first two he was led to answer in the negative) as to ascertain their "doses and effects" if really operative. Grimm (1767), Crumpe (1793) and Bard (1765) had made some experiments with *Opium,* Coste and Willemet some with *Asarum,* and Wasserberg one with *Belladonna.* These were the only forerunners of Hahnemann; and how few and (mostly) feeble were their efforts! He, on the other hand, once persuaded of the necessity for therapeutics of drug-provings on the healthy human body proceeded to institute them on the most extensive scale. I have already mentioned the publications in which his results appeared; and two of these—the "Fragmenta de Viribus" and the "Reine Arzneimittellehre"—are mainly made up of provings. The pathogeneses of the "Chronischen Krankheiten" consist, as I have said largely of observations on the sick; but the contributions thereto of others besides himself are in most instances the product of experiments made in health. Of the subjects, manner and mode of presentation of these provings I have now to say a few words.

a. For the provings whose results are given in the 'Fragmenta' (1805), and in the First Volume of the First Edition of the 'Reine Arzneimittellehre' (1811), Hahnemann had as subjects only himself and some members of his family—"some others" as he describes them "whom I knew to be perfectly healthy and free from all perceptible disease." By the time, however, that the Second Volume of the latter work was published (1816), he had gathered round him a band of disciples, and enlisted them in the task. The names of thirty-seven appear in the subsequent issues; and for the Pathogeneses of the 'Chronic Diseases' he can acknowledge the co-operation of twenty-six more. These men conducted their trials of drugs mostly under Hahnemann's eyes, and on their own persons; in some instances, however, as internal evidence shews, they experimented on others, and

---

* Pharm Helv., Preface.

THE KNOWLEDGE OF MEDICINES   61

those who lived at a distance communicated their results by letter. In all cases the Master, being responsible for his disciples' work, supplied the fullest instruction and the most watchful superintendence, so that the results are as genuine as he could make them.

b. As regards doses and mode of administration, it is to be regretted that more definite information has not been vouchsafed to us. We may infer, however, from hints which are dropped, that the symptoms of the 'Fragmenta'· were the result of single full doses of the several drugs; and that the provings of the 'Reine Arzneimittellehre' —at least up to 1826—were conducted with the first trituratoins (*i, e,* 1 to 100) of insoluble substances and the mother tinctures of vegetable drugs, repeated small doses being taken until some effect was produced. Towards the end of the first quarter of the century, Hahnemann had began to entertain his later views about dynamisation; so that we find the three medicines added to the Second Edition of the Sixth Volume (1827), *viz.*: *Ambra, Carbo animalis* and *vegetabilts,* proved in the third trituration, and the symptoms of *Natrum muriaticum* supplied by three persons to the Fourth Volume of the First Edition of the 'Chronic Diseases' (1830) were obtained from the thirtieth dilution. As in the Fifth Edition of the 'Organon' (1833) Hahnemann recommends that provings be ordinarily made with this potency, as yielding the best results, we may fairly suppose that it was used in all the fresh experiments whose results are contributed to the Second Edition of the 'Chronic Diseases,' which appeared between 1835 and 1839.

It is only this last mode of proceeding which needs—if it bears—defence. The question is part of the general one of the infinitesimals of Homœopathy, which I shall have to discuss when I come to the administration of the similar remedy.* I shall there adduce good evidence to show that attenuation of a potent drug like *Arsenic*, even to degrees representing fractions ranging from the hundred millionth to the quintillionth, does not destroy its pathogenetic activity; while in the case of common Salt, almost inert in its crude state, but VIRES ACQUIRENS EUNDO, such activity positively increases at least up to a certain point, so that the provings made with it at Vienna, more abundant results were obtained from the higher, than from the lower dilutions. Others among the Austrian provings exhibit the same thing, positively if not comparatively, and later experiments furnish numerous corroborations. I may mention, EXEMPTI GRATIA, Dr. Conrad Wesselhœft's results from *Iris versicolor*, as reported to the American Institute in 1868. The tincture, in repeated doses of ten to fifty drops, produced little but local effects,

* Lecture X.

whereas the 5_x dilution developed a genuine (though not severe) Sciatica, which was renewed a month later by the 3_x and intensified by the 1_x, under which last Rheumatic and Neuralgic pains occurred in other parts also. These, he expressly says, were not developed by the tincture. Dr. Wesselhœft has so little of the fanciful about him that this experience of his is of special value. I am quite aware that such results are exceptional; that you may give attenuations to twenty students, and one or two only shall report effects from them. I recognise also that special care must here be taken to avoid illusion, and to eliminate the working of expectant attention. But when all this is said, it remains that potencies will produce medicinal effects which crude drugs cannot excite, and which we of all men, heirs of this great discovery of Hahnemann's must not neglect.

The symptoms thus obtained, moreover, are of a class especially suitable to Homœopathic practice. They are of the "contingent" kind (to use Dr. Drysdale's nomenclature)—dependent upon special susceptibility, rather than "absolute"—producible on all subjects if only sufficient doses are given; and they present, as a rule, those resemblances to the minuter features of idiopathic disease which enable us to select SIMILLIMA instead of SIMILIA only. I shall not be suspected of undervaluing the importance of Pathological lesions and pathognomonic symptoms when I urge the claims, in their own place, of these finer shades of the morbid picture. Let us indeed get images of sicknesses in our drug pathogenesy, but let us also get images of sick persons, in all the variety they display; and this we can sometimes best do by experimenting with infinitesimal quantities. I do not mean such "airy nothings" as the hundredth, thousandth and millionth dilutions employed (or supposed to be employed) by the extreme left of our school. I do not mean "fluxion potencies" of any one's manufacture. I am speaking of the graduated attenuations of Hahnemann's scale, carried up to any reasonable height the experimenter may choose, the same lattitude being given here which we allow in clinical reports.

c. The mode of presentation adopted by Hahnemann in his provings is less defensible. Instead of giving us in detail the records of the experiments, he has distributed the symptoms obtained in a schema, mainly Anatomical, proceeding from head to extremities, and ending with generalities and physical phenomena.* The names of the observers, and frequently the time of occurrence after a dose, are affixed to each; but beyond this no information is given as to connection and sequence in which they occurred. The result is a mass of DISJECTA MEMBRA which impresses on the mind of its

* In his later pathogeneses these last were placed first.

would-be student a sense of utter confusion and discouragement. As has been said (in allusion to the order of the schema), he begins with Vertigo, and ends with Rage.

This unfortunate procedure has been fatal to any acceptance of Hahnemann's provings on the part of the profession at large; and it has been almost universally lamented among his own followers. I may quote Dr. Dudgeon's caustic description of the schema. "It is," he says, "as unnatural and artificial an arrangement of the features of many allied morbid portraits as though an artist should paint a family group, arranging all the eyes of all the members of the family in one part of the picture, all the noses in another, the ears all together, the noses all together, and so on. From such a picture, correct though each feature might be, it would be a difficult matter for us to build up each separate portrait, and it is equally difficult for us to ascertain the various morbid portraits from the TABLEAUX, Hahnemann has presented us with in his Materia Medica." * The fact is that he never intended his disciples to discover such portraits A PRIORI, but only A POSTERIORI, from the treatment of disease. His ideal of Homœopathic practice was that the symptoms of the patient should be ascertained and recorded, in the order of the schema, and then compared with the Materia Medica to see what medicine has produced all, or the greatest number, or the most characteristic of them. For such a proceeding the schema-form would seem to suffice. But the Master forgot that his disciples had not the clue to the maze which he possessed in the knowledge of the original-provings, and did not recognise that without it they were liable to go astray and find out false resemblances without end. To use the Materia Medica aright even upon this plan it is necessary to know the significance of the several symptoms as fully as may be, and to be acquainted with the general sphere and character of the medicine. A mere mechanical symptom-covering is as likely to miss as to hit the mark.

This is one of the points in which we have improved upon Hahnemann, even in the structure of his own machine. SIMILIA SIMILIBUS is our aim, as it was his; but we desire to trace our similarities where possible A PRIORI in the Physiological action of drugs. The schema is very useful, as a CATALOGUE RAISONNE in which we may find individual symptoms, and to cover cases as anomalous and incoherent as itself. But it should supplement the details of provings, not be substituted for them. To give the latter, in the narratives of the experimenters, has been the rule in Homœopathic literature ever since the Austrian Society (1842)

* Lectures, p. 234.

showed this more excellent way; and exceptions are to be found only in the limited circle which calls itself Hahnemannian, and copies with Chinese accuracy the defects as well as the merits of its eponym. The vicious procedure will call down its own punishment; for in the Materia Medica of the future their uninteresting and uninstructive contributions, if admitted at all, will receive the comparative discrediting of smaller type.

The members of his party have wrought another great evil in the field of Materia Medica. Hahnemann, in his later years, made too large use of patients (as we have seen) for eliciting symptoms. Not only were fresh sensations and phenomena occurring in the course of their treatment set down to the medicines they were taking, but aggravations of their existing troubles were ascribed to these, and registered as pathogenetic effects accordingly. But here the Master has been quite outdone by the disciples. When in a prover some existing deviation from health disappeared under the influence of a drug, Hahnemann recorded it, adding "Heilwirkung" (curative action). Only in the case of *Iodine* has he done this with definite maladies (as Goitre and Enlarged glands) treated with the medicine. But the Hahnemannians have seized upon the proceeding, and carried it to lengths from which he would have shrunk aghast. They have freely admitted "clinical symptoms" into our pathogenetic lists, cutting up the cases which have recovered under the action of a remedy into their component parts, and showing these in the appropriate divisions of the schema. They at first denote such symptoms by a sign (° or *), but soon grew careless about affixing it and at last (as in Lippe's "Text-book" and Hering's "Condensed Materia Medica" and "Guiding Symptoms"), avowedly omitted it altogether.

I have spoken of "the Materia Medica of the future." The antithesis in the past which I contemplate is not Hahnemann's work —which, for good and for evil, must stand as it is—but the collections of pathogenesy which serve for daily study and reference. Provings, as made, are published ordinarily in Journals; it is obvious that the practitioner cannot thus have them to his hand. Accordingly, certain amongst us have from time to time set themselves to make a digest of this material, and to present it in a compact and accessible shape. The names of Jahr and of Noack and Trinks are well-known in this connection, and they supplied the wants of the second generation of Homœopathists. For us, the third, a similar but far more extensive work was done (1874-9) by Dr. T. F. Allen, of New York, and our Materia Medica of yesterday was contained in his ten well-filled volumes. But alas! they presented the same bewildering and repelling appearance as those of Hahnemann.

their symptomatology was given almost throughout in schema. This was pardonable, and perhaps unavoidable, in the older works, where the great preponderance of material existed only in this form. But Dr. Allen had to his hand a wealth of detailed provings, the translation and collation of which would have been an incalculable boon to the profession : And I must keenly regret that he should have cut up these, and also the records of poisoning he has employed, into the fragments of the Hahnemannic arrangement. His last Volume suggests that the same regret has been growing on his own mind; for the fresh material given in its Appendix has suffered no such distortion.

For this reason, and for many others, bearing on questions of trustworthiness and accuracy, it became our persuasion in this country that the work must be done over again, and the British Homœopathic Society determined to undertake it. It made overtures to the American Institute of Homœopathy, which also had the subject on its mind; and the result was the appointment of editors and consultative committees from the two countries, and an agreement as to the principles on which the new Materia Medica was to be constructed. This was in 1884 ; and, the work being at once taken in hand, by the end of 1891 the "Cyclopædia of Drug Pathogenesy" was completed. Leaving Hahnemann's work in this department to stand on its own merits, it collated all available material accruing since his time or from outside his sphere in such a form as to make it alike genuine and intelligible. Genuine, because all versions and copies have been (where possible) traced back to their ultimate originals, and verified, corrected, or reproduced therefrom ; because all "clinical" (*i.e.*, merely cured) symptoms and supposed medicinal aggravations have been excluded, and phenomena observed in patients taking drugs accepted only on amply sufficient evidence ; because provings themselves have been critically scrutinised, and not admitted (at any rate to full-sized type) unless their source and method seemed free from objection. And intelligible, because all observation and experiments have (again where possible) been related in detail or sufficient summary, so as to preserve the order of evolution of the drug's effect; and, where this could not be, the symptoms of each prover given separately, so that some approximation might be made to the same type. We thus have a series of individual pictures of the morbid conditions induced by our medicines ; and have only to fit these to idiopathic disease on the principle SIMILIA SIMILIBUS, to have the Homœopathic method at our full disposal.

When I say this, I am thinking of disease as clinically studied ; for here again the phenomena, in their totality, are those which claim our most earnest attention. The aspect of disease chiefly utilised for Homœopathic Therapeutics must have its complement in the acquaintance we make with medicines: to obey the Law of Similars we must have wholes to compare with wholes. In the ordinary practice men aim at knowing what drugs can do, that in disease they may induce such effects with them when they deem it desirable. In old days, accordingly, they cared only to learn whether a given one could purge, or puke, or sweat, that they might class it as cathartic, emetic, or sudorific; and now they correspondingly limit their investigation to the question whether it is an excitant or depressant of certain nerve-tracts. For such purpose dumb creatures suffice; and hecatombs of these unfortunates are now annually sacrificed in enquiries as to drug-action. The differences of result, and therefore of opinion, are endless; and the gain is proportionately small: as our General Medical Council, by banishing "Pharmacology" from the place they had given it among subjects for students' examinations, seems to have come to think. We on the other hand, have wanted the whole picture of the effects of drugs for comparison with the phenomena of disease, and have gone to work accordingly. As it is human disease to which we need SIMLIA, and as this is largely made up of subjective symptoms, it is on the human subject that we experiment; and we faithfully record the whole series of morbid changes which occur after the ingestion of a drug. We test the effect of single full doses to get analogues of acute disease; and of long-continued small ones, that chronic maladies may find their anti-types. Thus our pathogenetic knowledge, when truly obtained and registered, is like a picture-gallery, in which the discerning eye may perceive the lineaments of all morbid conditions known of likely to occur. Our provings minister to medicine as an art: They are synthetic and sensuous, full of colour and detail. Those of the other camp are analytic, appealing to the reason; and are available only so far as morbid processes are scientifically understood. The record of the one recalls the graphic picture of Hippocraces, Sydenham and Watson, to whose ever-fresh lineaments the mind returns with pleasure, wearied with the merely intellectual refinements of modern Nosography. The work of the Physiological laboratory goes hand in hand with that of the deadhouse. Hahnemann's Pharmacology and Pathology alike move in the region of life.

But you will remember that, when speaking of the knowledge of diseases, we saw that their clinical aspect is not the only one in which we should regard the ills which flesh is heir to. From Pathology—the science of disease—its phenomena are always illuminated, and sometime even rendered transparent so that through them we can see the noumena. Pharmacology should

THE KNOWLEDGE OF MEDICINES   67

seek a standpoint no less advanced. Provings correspond with our studies at the bedside or in the consulting room; but as to interpret these we go to the dead-house, so to provings we must add—where possible—poisonings and experiments on animals, that the lesions wrought by drugs may be positively ascertained. Records of this kind should find place in the actual Materia Medica of Homœopathy. This, in the "Cyclopædia," has been done; but yet our work is not over. We must use these facts also as materials for inductive generalisation; we must seek to connect, classify and interpret them, to ascertain their laws, to trace them to their causes. In proportion as we do so, we make our Pharmacology a worthy mate for the Pathology which is growing into maturity beside it. In neither do we content ourselves with generalisations alone; the clinical history of diseases and the detailed provings of drugs must ever form the basis—and the visible basis—of any super-structure which may be reared. But while (to employ another figure) these are the text of our Materia Medica, we should read it with the help of a commentary which may illuminate it by the best available lights. There are some who think they are best following Hahnemann by shutting their eyes and ears to all that has been learned since his time; by recognising nothing in disease but the patient's sensations and obvious appearances, and nothing in drug-action but a scattered heap of symptoms of like kind. We should not go to the other extreme, and ignore any aid which may thus be gained in practice. But we should regard the human body, whether idiopathically or medicinally disordered, as one of whose order we are not wholly ignorant—as a sphere in which we are to some degree at home, and where we may speak and act as no mere strangers. In studying the Materia Medica we are to be more than symptom-rememberers, in applying it more than symptom-coverers; we are CLERI and not LAICI here, and we fall short of our vantage ground if we work mechanically only.

Whether such commentary should form part of the "Materia Medica Homœopathica" is a moot question. The editors of the "Cyclopædia of Drug Pathogenesy" have thought it should not. They have had the records of provings, poisonings, and experiments on animals given apart by themselves just as elicited from Nature without touch of human hand in the way of either explanation or transposition of features. But as on the side the last is required in the form of a schematic index, for the needs of the practitioner, so on the other student should have an introduction and companion to the text, supplying him with illuminative and exegetical commentary. In monographs on medicines, like those of the Hahnemann Publishing Society, all will go together; but for the Materia Medica at large separate treatises seem necessary. I have done what I could in this way in my

"Pharmacodynamics"; Dr. Hempel, in his "Lectures," had preceded me, and Dr. Burt, in his "Physiological Materia Medica," has followed me. Under the guidance of one or other of us, and in the new form in which our pathogenetic records are now presented, we hope that the student may find these, though perhaps "a mighty maze," yet "not without a plan."

LECTURE VI.

SIMILIA SIMILIBUS

We have studied together the two elements contained in the maxim SIMILIA SIMILIBUS CURENTUR—the phenomena and sensations of disease and of drug-action respectively. It now becomes our task to see how we are to put the SIMILIA together so as to CURARE by their means. Before we can do so, however, we must enquire if the whole series of drug-effects on the healthy are available for the treatment of the sick after this manner; and we shall soon find that some of them are by their nature excluded from the category. Thus :—

1. Drugs, being material substances, must, if introduced in sufficient quantity into the body, act MECHANICALLY, by their bulk and weight, and so forth. Such properties of theirs have found little use in medicine—the swallowing of crude *Mercury* to overcome Intestinal Obstruction, of *Olive oil* to detach Biliary Calculi, being the only familiar instances. Whatever its value—and the latter practice seems effective and is certainly harmless—it has nothing to do with our present subject; SIMILIA SIMILIBUS has no application here.

2. Drugs, when taken from the mineral kingdom, have CHEMICAL properties; and they exert these within the organism as they do outside it, with such modification as the higher laws of life there reigning impose upon their action. An *Alkali* will neutralise an *Acid* in the stomach as in a test-tube, and so may give immediate relief to heart-burn. A solvent of *Uric acid*—such as the *Boro-citrate of Magnesia* seems, and *Piperazin* is reputed, to be—will act thus upon it in the kidney almost as well as in the apparatus of the laboratory. These are examples of the chemical action of medicines. They might be multiplied largely, and would bring us at last into more debatable regions, as the treatment of Rheumatic fever by *Potash salts* because of a presumed excess of *Lactic acid* in the blood. Stopping short of these, in the cases I have instanced it is obvious that Homœopathicity plays no part, and yet that they are rational enough in themselves. We have better remedies for the tendency to Gastric Acidity and to Renal Calculus; but when these products are formed, and are causing distress by their presence, if we can remove the symptoms by chemically-acting drugs we are bound to use them.

3. We are thus shut up, for the sphere of Homœopathic action, to the third and last kind of drug-energy, which may be called DYNAMIC from its analogy with the forces of Nature generally VITAL from its manifestation only in the presence of life. It is the reaction which drug-stimuli excite in living matter. But even here we must recognise a limitation. Vital action which is exclusively topical does not necessarily, or even ordinarily, conform to the Law of Similars. It may do so. The local application of *Nitrate of Silver* in inflammations of skin and mucous membrane, which Trousseau cited as the cardinal example of "the great therapeutic principle of substitution which at present rules supreme in medical practice",—this is obviously an illustration of SIMILIA SIMILIBUS, as the same writer admits. "It was soon perceived," he writes, "that the primary effects of such agents were analogous to that produced by inflammation; and it was easy to understand that inflammation artificially induced in tissues already inflamed led to a cure of the original inflammatory attack." If Anstie* and James Ross,† with Fletcher‡ before them, are right, a similar explanation is to be given of the effects of counter-irritation. Blisters are not revulsives, but substitutive agents, acting through continuous and contiguous parenchyma, or through the nerves along the paths of reflex action. But if we follow up our topical agents, we shall find the relation of similarity to fail us. The action of *Arnica* in easing the pain and promoting the resolution of contusions is a dynamic one; but no such condition can be induced by applying *Arnica* to a healthy part. *Calendula* is a vulnerary by no chemical or mechanical properties it possesses; it cannot act otherwise than vitally; yet it has no power of causing wounds on the unbroken skin. And conversely, it does not follow that because the fumes of *Osmium* set up Eczema on the parts exposed to them, that metal taken internally will act upon idiopathic Eczema as *e.g., Arsenic* will. The latter inflames the skin, however introduced into the system; it is therefore constitutionally Homœopathic to Dermatitis, while the other is (so far as we know at present) only locally so.

Dynamic action, to be available according to the Law of Similars, must thus not to be topical only. It must further be exerted on the living matter of the patient's self, and not on that of guests to which he is against his will playing the part of host. It is not by Homœopathic action that *Sulphur* ointment cures the Itch, for its influence is exerted on the Acarus scabiei rather than on the skin

---

* PRACTITIONER, iv., 156.

† "On Counter Irritation" (Churchill).

‡ "Elements of General Pathology" (1842), p. 484. See also Dr. Drysdale's Exposition of Fletcher's Doctrine, in B. J. H., xxvii, 494.

that parasite irritates. The same statement may be made as to the living creatures which infest the intestines. *Santonine* kills the round worm, *Filix mas* the Tænia, by dynamic toxic power directly exerted; the practice is as rational as that which we follow in Scabies, but there is nothing in it which lends itself to the rule SIMILIA SIMILIBUS. And so of more complex morbid states, whose causation is traceable to agents of this kind. The pernicious Anæmia of the East, known as "Beri-beri," is now believed to depend on the presence of the Ankylostoma duodenale at the seat its name imports. If we were to treat it symptomatically with *Arsenic*, or to attack its cause with *Thymol*, we should in either case be acting on living matter, but in the former only should be giving a Homœopathic remedy. You will think at once of the applicability of such reasoning to Malarial fevers, as now understood; but I must reserve that question till I me to their treatment.

Once again, there are drugs, like *Mercury* and *Iodine*, which have peculiar solvent, loosening effect upon organic substance, melting it down and favouring its ready deportation by the absorbents. The action is a vital one, and we utilise it when we give such drugs in small doses for similar conditions of relaxation and wasting. But we may also employ it directly. New growths and adventitious products are susceptible to this influence as well as the ordinary tissues; they may, indeed, feel it and give way to it before the latter are appreciably affected. It is in this way, I opine, that the lymph of plastic Iritis disappears under Mercurialisation, the Gumma of Syphilis from the administration of *Iodide of Potassium*. Whether the good done here outweighs the evil I do not now attempt to decide. I only give the instance to illustrate what I mean by vital actions of drugs which are outside the possible range of the method of Hahnemann.

It is, nevertheless, within this sphere that the method finds its place; it is dynamically acting drugs influencing living matter which is neither parasitic nor adventitious, and doing this constitutionally and not merely topically, which can become Homœopathic remedies. From their list we reach these, ordinarily, by the rule "let likes be treated by likes." The similarity here required is, as we have seen, to be found in the pathogenetic effects of drugs as compared with the phenomena of disease. To establish it, therefore, a collection of such of these effects as had been hitherto observed, and a systematic eliciting and recording of fresh ones, was necessary. This task was initiated by Hahnemann, and has been continued by his followers, in the manner I have already described. From the four large volumes of his "Materia Medica Pura" and "Chronic Diseases," and the similar number complementary thereto of the "Cyclopædia of Drug Pathogenesy, a full acquaintance with the disease-producing energies of drugs can be obtained by the English reader; and now it only needs the discovery among them of similar conditions to make them also disease-curing.

We have got, then, our dynamic constitutionally-acting drugs; we have the record of their effects of this kind in health; and now we wish to apply our knowledge. There are, Hahnemann has pointed out, three modes, and three only, in which such application can be made.

1st. Having ascertained that a given substance has the power (say) of exciting any bodily function, you give it in disease of other parts when you think such excitation desirable. Thus, you administer diuretics in Hydrothorax, and purgatives in Apoplexy. It is not that kidney or bowels are inert and require raising to their normal activity, but it is that you think an exaggeration of their ordinary function likely to benefit the water-logged pleura, or the congested brain. There is here no relationship between the Physiological effects of the drug and the phenomena of disease. They are foreign ἀλλοιος, the one to the other; we may fairly call the practice so exemplified Allœo- or Allo-pathic. *

2nd. The same discovery having been made, you apply your knowledge in dealing with opposite conditions of such functions themselves. You give your diuretic in Ischuria, and your purgative in constipation; you administer paralysing agents for Spasm and anæsthetics for pain. Here you are acting directly on the part affected, and the symptoms of drug and disease admit of true comparison. The relation between them is expressed by the ancient formula "CONTRARIA CONTRARIIS" εναντία εναντίοις: The practice is Enantio- or Antipathic.

3rd. But there is yet a third alternative. Still acting upon the part affected, you may give your drug in morbid states thereof similar instead of opposite to its Physiological effects. You may administer your diuretic in Polyuria, your cathartic in Diarrhœa: you may treat Mania with *Stramonium* and Tetanus with *Strychnia*. If you do so, you are, as Sir Thomas Watson recognised in regard of the latter piece of practice (which yet he suggests), acting "according to the Hahnemannic doctrine—

---

* I have mentioned (p. 16) that Hahnemann, at least in the Fifth Edition of the Organon, always employs the more correct form, Allœopathic"; but his followers having dropped into the more convenient "Allopathic," Dr. Dudgeon has adopted this term in his translation. It is, of course, only partially correct to use it, as ordinarily, to describe traditional medicine as a whole, this being multiform in character.

SIMILIA SIMILIBUS CURANTUR—a doctrine much older, however than Hahnemann."* SIMILIA SIMILIBUS is the Greek ὁμοία ὁμοίοις : your procedure is Homœopathic.

It is of the third mode of procedure that Homœopathy avails itself. Before I show you how it does so, let me say a few words in comparative commendation of its action. You must pardon me if in so doing I go again over the ground already trodden while we considered the Organon together.

Hahnemann's objections to Allœopathic medication are two. There is, first, its uncertainty : You MAY do something by your evacuant and derivative measures, but it is quite as likely that you will not ; your procedure is indirect, roundabout, and one guessing at the problem rather than solving it. Secondly, it is actually injurious : it disorders healthy parts, and floods the system with large and poisonous doses of drugs—these being necessary to produce the desired effects. It disobeys that sage counsel which Dr. Paris used to give to his students : "If you cannot heal your patient, gentlemen, at least do not hurt him." It is a doing evil that good may come, which, if not so absolutely banned in medicine as in morals, should at least be ventured on but rarely and for very good cause.

The Antipathic use of drugs has more in its favour, in that it is certainly and rapidly palliative, while it is as direct as the Homœopathic. No one would hesitate to employ it in cases of acute poisoning, to antidote—for example—*Morphia* by *Atropia*; and no one refuses *Chloroform* to the parturient woman because it is on this principle that it allays her labor-pangs. Why then should there be any prejudice against it in other brief and sudden sufferings ? Why should not the deadly spasm of Angina be relaxed by *Nitrite of Amyl*, and the keen agony of the passage of calculi receive what solace it may from a kindly *Opiate* or even anæsthetic ? I must hold that the man who denies his patients such relief is sacrificing them to his prejudices, is preferring system to humanity, and is unworthy of the name of physicians. I thus entirely go with Dr. Kidd † in holding CONTRARIA CONTRARIIS to be equally with SIMILIA SIMILIBUS, a law of therapeutics. It is the law of palliation ; and such palliation is often, in temporary disorders, all that need be done, ‡ while in incurable disease it is sometimes all that can be done.

But the very fact that it is palliation to which it guides, and not cure, limits its range of usefulness. It is helpful only for immediate

* Lectures, 4th Ed., i., 591.

† "The Laws of Therapeutics," 2nd Ed., 1881.

‡ See Hahnemann's introduction to *Opium*, MAT. MED. PURA, tr. by Dudgeon, H.

needs and passing troubles : it is not competent to deal with complex, persistent, or recurrent maladies. It is here rarely practicable, from the few really opposite states which exist between natural disease and drug-action : It is inadequate, from being seldom able to deal with more than a single symptom at a time ; and the inevitable reaction which follows from its being put in operation leads to a return of the evil, often in greater force. These are Hahnemann's arguments against Antipathy (or, as he more correctly called it Enantiopathy) and they seem to me quite unanswerable.

By cognate reasons it is easy to show the (at least theoretical) superiority of the third, or Homœopathic method. Like the Antipathic, it acts directly on the affected parts, leaving healthy regions unharmed ; but this last end it is more certain to secure, from the non-perturbing dosage which answers its purpose. It is thus gentle in its manner, opening the closed door of the diseased body, not by smashing the lock with a crowbar, but by finding the proper key. Again, it is of inexhaustible fertility. The fevers, the inflammations, the neuroses, which constitute the greater number of typical diseases, are all more or less plainly figured in drug-pathogenesy : And quite as readily can those unclassifiable morbid states which so often meet us in practice be covered therefrom, though their interpretation remain unknown. Homœopathic treatment, moreover, is complete ; it does not, like its rival, employ bits of Physiological action, but opposes wholes to wholes, tracking—by its investigation of the totality of symptoms—the malady in its entire evolution, and so reaching it in root as well as in branches. It is lastly, permanent ; for the law of action and re-action which makes the secondary effects of Antipathic palliatives injurious here oparates beneficially. The primary influence of the drug being in the same direction as the morbid process, any recoil there may be will directly oppose and extinguish it. Hahnemann, as we shall see when we come to the Philosophy of Homœopathy, supposed that such secondary action always took place, and explained by means of it the MODUS OPERANDI of similar remedies. We may not be able to agree with him on this point ; but at least it is clear that any benefit wrought by a Homœopathically-acting medicine is in its nature lasting, and liable to no injurious reaction.

These are arguments which, in substance, I have already cited from the 'Organon,' I would fix your attention to-day on three further points—the safety of the method ; the superiority IN KIND of the remedies it educes ; and the success which it has uniformly displayed when fairly contrasted with traditional medication.

1. The Antipathic and the Homœopathic modes of applying

the pathogenetic effects of drugs to the treatment of disease have this advantage in common over the Allœopathic, that they act directly on the affected parts, and avoid disturbing those that are healthy. But then, of the two, the Homœopathic use commends itself to us by its greater gentleness. The Antipathic drug has to oppose the morbid process that is going on. It must do this by force, by inducing its own equally morbid condition in the suffering organ, without pledge that this shall subside when that is neutralised. It must therefore be given in full doses; and it is not easy so to proportion these that some side-action shall not be exerted elsewhere as they circulate in the blood. In Allœopathic and Antipathic medication alike you have to induce the Physiological action of drugs—that is, you employ them as poisons: In the Homœopathic we convert them into medicines. "Their whole Physiological action" as our lamented Drysdale used to say, "is absorbed into their therapeutic." Their influence is mild; it solicits and persuades rather than compels; the patient is conscious of nothing save the amelioration of his distress. Acting thus, they need no large quantities; and here comes in one characteristic feature of Homœopathy—the smallness of its dosage. I am not now alluding to infinitesimals: they form a subject by themselves to be hereafter discussed. They are fully capable of defence; but their use forms no essential of Homœopathy: The small dose does. In employing this term, I am thinking of such an obvious inference as led *Ipecacuanha wine* to be given by single drops only when administered to check vomiting instead of to excite it; and to such experience as Dr. Ringer relates with *Amyl nitrite*. In treating with this substance flushes like that it causes, "the author," he writes, "began with minim dose, but was obliged to reduce this quantity, and he ultimately found that, for the most part, these patients can bear one third of a minim without any disagreeable symptoms, but that a tenth, nay, even a thirtieth of a minim will in some patients counteract the flushing." Dr. Murell has had similar results from *Drosera* in Spasmodic Cough and Sir L. Brunton from *Opium* in Constipation; and it has been the almost uniform experience of those who have used Homœopathically-acting remedies, so that to the gentleness of their working is added the smallness of their necessary dosage.

The result is comfort and peace to the patient is manifest; and this is no slight advantage, especially with children. Had such non-perturbative treatment been available in the days of Montaigne, he would not have written as he did of doctors and physic. "I have," he says, "a contemptuous indifference to medicine at ordinary times; but when I am taken ill, instead of coming to terms with it I begin more thoroughly to hate and fear it, and reply to those who press me to take physic that they must wait, at any rate, until I am restored to my usual health and strength, that I may be better able to stand the potency and danger of their compounds." I would emphasize these last words, and would claim for Homœopathy the high merit that it obeys, that cardinal maxim of medicine, PRIMO NON NOCERE, which ordinary treatment does not. Against the benefits which our profession has undoubtedly rendered to the world must be set, I fear, a long array of ills produced by drugging. The "Cyclopædia of Drug Pathogenesy," of which I have spoken, finds copious material for its "Poisonings" section in the records of over-dosing with medicines. Nor is this a thing of the past. Physicians no longer, perhaps, lead their patients into *Opium*-taking; and a Coleridge with his poetic power blighted, his philosophising emitted only in fragments, and—worst of all—his moral life wrecked, may not be extant now, though we have heard of a *Morphia*-Mania which is hardly less distressing. But those who knew Rossetti best have hinted plainly that what made him the melancholy and unfruitful recluse of the last ten years of his life was the abuse of *Chloral*; and a lesser, though true, poet—Sydney Dobell—has told us himself how all motive power was paralysed in him by the *Bromide of Potassium* forced upon him by his medical advisers. "He had hoped" writes his biographer, "to abandon the habitual use of a sedative medicine which he took always under protest, with a sense that it poisoned life and fettered the use of his brain, but which, during the last eight years had been prescribed for him by every physician consulted. The result of medical experiment and observation now led to its being prescribed in larger quantities. This was a severe disappointment, as during the few days of its discontinuance he believed that his mind worked more freely and easily."* The picture here presented, of a noble "life poisoned" and a creative "brain fettered" by the constant administration of a fashionable sedative, tells its own sad story, and points its burning moral. Of how many private tragedies may not these public ones be indices! Medicinal Mercurialism—so disastrous in the past—is rarely seen now, though a recent observation of Mr. Hutchinson's† warns against its possibility; and Iodism, in its constitutional form, does not seem to affect other people as Coindet and Rilliet observed it in the sensitive Genevese. But Aresenicism has been in full process during the last generation : It is from the medical use of this substance that we have learned its Homœopathicity to Shingles, to Pemphigus, and to Cancer. ‡ *Iodine*, moreover, in the form of its compound with *Potassium*, so lavishly employed during the last sixty years, has done almost as much harm as good. To the

* Life and Letters of Sydney Dobell (1878), Vol. ii. See his own words quoted in M. H. R., xxiii., 321.

† Cycl. of Drug Path., iv., 644.

‡ Ibid., i., 448; ii., 726.

older observations of its noxious effects left us by Wallace, Ricord and Langston Parker, we have later ones to add collected by Lewin and Morrow.* They exhibit its injurious effects upon the skin, the tongue, and the nervous system; and it is shrewdly suspected that the kidneys do not escape damage while eliminating the mass of chemicals in this shape introduced into the circulation. Men speak lightly of the Deafness and tinnitus characteristic of *Quinine;* but the aurists are beginning to cry out against the wrong thus done to the delicate structures of the ear, and I have more than once seen Labyrinthine Vertigo resulting from the abuse of the drug. The Coaltar products which have come into such large use of late as heat-reducers and pain-killers have already an extensive pathogenesis, and much of the severity and even mortality of the recent Influenza has been traced to the *Antipyrin* so freely employed to subdue its fever. Antisepsis, too, with all its virtues, has opened a new source of medicinal poisoning, and its *Carbolic acid* and *Corrosive sublimate,* used to bring local death to bacteria, have proved by absorption indefinitely harmful to the patients they would protect against them. Drugging has increased of late, is increasing, and must be diminished. Better expectancy than this! Skoda, Dietl and Hughes-Bennett in Pneumonia, Gull and Sutton in acute Rheumatism, many practitioners in Typhoid and other self-limiting diseases, have left their patients almost, if not altogether, to Nature, with results far from satisfactory. It is often charged against Homœopathic medication that it is a pretentious doing-nothing. If it were so, it might be worse. Doctor and patient are sustained by the idea that treatment is being adopted, and the one may lay the flattering unction to his soul that at least the other has not been harmed by him.

2. But Homœopathy has further claims than such negative ones as these. Its remedies are inoffensive; they are non-perturbative; they are liable to do no injury from too liberal or long-continued use; but they are also positive agents, of a kind which forms, the highest DESIDERATA of medicine. Sprengel, the greatest historian of our art, writes:—"Hahnemann, by a true induction, demonstrated that most of those potent medicines known under the name of specifics are useful just because they set up an artificial excitement which often produces phenomena very like those of the malady." It is so; and, conversely, the medicines given in Homœopathic practice—given because they set up in health an artificial excitement producing phenomena very like those of the malady—display that potent kind of action known as "specific." Homœopathy is specific medication, and SIMILIA

Ibid., ii. 713-6; iv. 627.

SIMILIBUS is an instrument for the discovery of specific—not for types of disease merely, but for each individual case. Hahnemann claimed this place for his method, (which till 1808 he called) simply "specific;" and even after he had begun, in that year to use the term "Homœopathic," he often conjoined the other with it. Hufeland, the head of German medicine in Hahnemann's day, allowed the claim. He said that the knowledge of medicines which produce in a healthy state symptoms similar to those of disease may be very well profited of, in order to discover specifics; and in another place, that "the aim of Homœopathy is to find specifics for individual forms of disease, by doing which it may render great service to medicine."*

I am quite aware that at the present day to claim the possession of specific positively prejudices our cause in the minds of the profession. Medicine, they have decided, is to be an applied science, and is not to run before the knowledge by which it works, while specifics belong to the sphere of pure art. The result is fairly expressed in the following passage from a recent Editorial in the LANCET.†

"Bacteriologists may be fairly asked to furnish us with definite knowledge as to whether a characteristic micro-organism uniformly present in Pneumonia, and if so, whether its lifehistory affords any clue to the phenomena of the disease. While this question remains in abeyance, the treatment of Pneumonia —always one of the most disputable and difficult in the whole range of medicine—becomes more difficult than ever. If the disease be truly parasitic, and if the destruction of the parasite be the true object of therapeutics, then it is evident that the Antiphlogistic treatment of former days and the stimulant treatment of the present day are alike mistaken and futile. . . . . At another point the uncertainty overhanging the Pathology of Pneumonia is very embarrassing. Is the Pyrexia the reaction of the organism to the action of a morbid substance—whether bacillary or not—in the blood? Is it simply the effect of such a poison, or is the effort of the organism to rid itself of the poison? In other words, as Dr. Hale White puts it, is the Pyrexia one of the defensive mechanisms of the body?" We cannot answer these questions with any confidence or certainty in the present state of our knowledge, and yet until they are answered our treatment must remain halting and tentative."

* For this subject of "Specifics," see Dudgeon's Lectures, Lecture iii., and Russell's "History and Heroes of the Art of Medicine," pp. 194, 267.

† July 27, 1895.

If those who think thus would look into the literature of Homœopathy, they would find a treatment of Pneumonia there recognised for many decades past, which is neither Antiphlogistic nor stimulating, which is uninfluenced by theories of the bacterial origin of the inflammation or the "defensive" part played by the fever; but which apportions individual specifics to the different forms and stages of the disease, with results in diminishing its mortality and lessening its duration which no other treatment, positive or negative, can show.*

Happily (perhaps) for their patients, the readers of the LANCET do not really wait till these theories have settled their conflicts, but are quite ready to try any remedy which professes to be good for this or that, whether they understand its action or not. If they did not, indeed, they would soon be deserted by their patients, who wish to be cured, and care little for the mode in which this end is attained. Men like Bacon and Boyle have made themselves their spokesmen, and they have urged upon the profession from without the search for remedies of this kind. Sydenham, from within full of the fresh sense of the blessings of specifics gained from the introduction of *Bark* in the treatment of Agues, believed in their existence and advocated their cultivation. But the leading physicians generally, from Hippocrates onwards, in their desire to be rational instead of empirical, have aimed at treating patients according to systems which they have excogitated, and have left specifics to quacks—who have thriven accordingly. Hahnemann once more bent attention in the true direction; while, by discovering the law of specific action, he rescued it from empiricism and haphazard, and made it as rational as it is beneficial. I say, beneficial; for would it not be an immense boon for suffering humanity if all diseases could be treated as Ague is treated with *Quinine*? It is because Homœopathy is working towards this end—and indeed towards something still more perfect, for to give *Quinine* in every intermittent without discrimination is but rough practice—it is for this reason among others that its method is not only positively but comparatively desirable.

3. There could only be one challenge to this inference—the appeal to facts. If, in spite of its pleasantness and harmlessness, and of the theoretic promise of the remedies it employs, Homœopathy had failed to hold its own in actual practice, we should have to keep silence about it, and at the best wait for a brighter day. But it has been very far otherwise. The early battles over it in this country were fought (at least on our side) largely on the ground of statistics. I

---

* See Dr. Pope's articles on the treatment of this disease in the MONTHLY HOM. REVIEW of 1892.

do not propose to renew the combat in detail; but this gage I must throw down, prepared to maintain it A OUTRANCE, that never has the method of Hahnemann had fair opportunity of pitting itself against its rival that it has not come off victorious in the contest. It was so when Tessier had half the beds in the Hospital St. Marguerite at Paris; it was so when Fleischmann handled his Cholera patients at Vienna with such comparative success as to win from the Government the long-withheld toleration of the practice; it was so when similar results obtained in this disease in the London Homœopathic Hospital (then in Golden Square) had the honour of being stifled by the official reporters, lest they should reflect upon the less favourable statistics of other institutions. It has been so since, when the Michigan and Illinois State Prisons were served by the two systems in successive terms of years; when the mortality of the one Orphan Asylum of New York which has Homœopathic treatment was set against that of the six others during the same time; when the Homœopathic portion of the Cook County Hospital at Chicago recently compared notes with the other wards of the charity. To come nearer home, when the National Temperance Hospital was able to show better results than the metropolitan hospitals generally, it was obliged to except the London Homœopathic. It could only account for so surprising a fact by the supposition (which was, of course, entirely unfounded, and was promptly contradicted) that we did not admit acute cases! Is there any failure to set against these triumphs? There is none; and yet, on the assumption of the nullity of Homœopathy, every such trial ought to have ended in discomfiture—that is, if the ordinary treatment were itself of any value. If the same assumption be persisted in, in face of the facts, then the higher mortality which the figures show for ordinary treatment means simply that it is to this extent positively murderous. I do not myself draw this conclusion; but then I do not believe that the rival method is merely expectancy.

The conclusion arrived at is that Homœopathic remedies are, from their nature, from their negative advantages, and from the comparative results obtained with them, the best that can be employed, and such as should always be resorted to when practicable. I could enlarge more fully, did time allow, on the argument from their nature. I could show that they are constitutional SUBSTITUTIVES, acting by elective affinities instead of topical application, and so of much more penetrating influence and grasp of disease as a whole. * I could exhibit them as

* Dr. George Wood, in his "Pharmacology and Therapeutics," maintains that this is the MODUS OPERANDI of *Quinine* in Intermittent Fever—the standing type as I have shown and have yet to show of a Homœopathic specific.

ALTERATIVES, having all the merits of the drugs so called—silently and peacefully, without evacuation or other intermediate action, extinguishing the morbid process at the seat of mischief; the only trace of their working being that where there was a storm there is calm, where there was pain there is ease, where there was weakness there is strength. But I must pause. I have said enough, I think, to vindicate Hahnemann's choice of the Homœopathic, as distinguished from the Antipathic and Allœopathic methods of utilising drug-action in therapeutics. We have yet to study the mode of selecting the similar remedy : And this will occupy us at our next meeting.

LECTURE VII.

THE SELECTION OF THE SIMILAR REMEDY

That likes should—wherever practicable—be treated by likes, and that the elements of the comparison should ordinarily be the clinical features of disease and the symptoms produced by drugs in the healthy—these points have now been established. Can we—as it would seem we could—proceed at once to select our remedies ?

It might have appeared to Hahnemann at first that the problem was thus simple. But in the Fourth Edition of the 'Organon' (1829) he introduced a paragraph which recognised the necessity for wider considerations. It is that numbered § 5 in the Fifth Edition, which is the one we have in our hands as translated by Dr. Dudgeon. Let me read it to you :—

"Useful to the physician in assisting him to cure, are the particulars of the most probable exciting cause of an acute disease, as also the most significant points in the whole history of a chronic disease, to enable him to discover its fundamental cause, which generally depends on a chronic miasm. In these investigations, the apparent physical constitution of the patient (especially when the disease is chronic), his moral and intellectual character, his occupation, mode of living and habits, his social and domestic relations, his age, sexual functions, etc., are to be taken into consideration."

There are, you will observe, two distinct points made in this aphorism. The first is that the causes of disease, predisposing and exciting, are to be taken into account, not merely that they may be removed where possible, but as guides to the selection of the remedy. Thus, in choosing between *Nux vomica* and *Pulsatilla* in a case of Dyspepsia, the sex, temperament and disposition of the patient, as also the kind of food which most disagrees, go for something in including the balance ; in prescribing for Rheumatic pains, we think of *Aconite* or *Bryonia* if dry cold, of *Rhus* or *Dulcamara* if damp, has been the exciting cause. If a morbid condition is traceable to a fit of anger, we are thereby inclined to give *Chamomilla* for it ; if to a fright,

Aconite or *Opium;* if to long-continued depressing emotions, *Phosphoric acid.* For complaints having origin in an injury, *Arnica* is always useful, not only immediately upon its reception, but long afterwards.

Dr. Drysdale is the only writer—as far as I am aware—who has enquired into the reasonableness of this practice, upon Homœopathic principles. He suggests* that any similarity to the effects of definite exciting causes discoverable in the symptoms of a drug indicates that the latter has acted as a predisposing cause, making the system more susceptible to the morbific agency in question. *Dulcamara* is Homœopathic to Catarrhal Diarrhœa, not because it is a purgative, but because patients under its influence are more liable to have Diarrhœa induced by cold and damp than they are without it. It thus goes deeper than the immediate attack, and not only removes this, but renders the patient less apt to its recurrence. The whole action is just another instance of the use of the totality of the symptoms in selecting the similar remedy.

But Hahnemann speaks further of ascertaining the "fundamental cause" of chronic disease, which (he says) is generally a "chronic miasm"—referring to his doctrine of the origin of a large proportion of such disease in Syphilis, Sycosis or Psora. This we have discussed already, as one of Hahnemann's theories. The question now is, why it is useful to have this causation known? Hahnemann again shall speak for himself. In a note to § 80 of the Fifth Edition of the 'Organon,' he writes concerning "Psoric diseases":—"I spent twelve years in investigating the source of this incredibly large number of chronic affections, in ascertaining and collecting certain proofs of this great truth, ... and in discovering at the same time principal (Antipsoric) remedies, which collectively are nearly a match for this thousand-headed monster of disease, in all its different developments and forms. .... Before I had obtained this knowledge, I could only teach how to treat the whole number of chronic diseases as isolated, individual maladies, with the medicinal substances whose pure effects had been tested on healthy persons up to that period; so that every case of chronic disease was treated by my disciples according to the group of symptoms it presested, just like an idiopathic disease, and it was often so far cured that sick mankind rejoiced at the extensive remedial treasures already amassed by the new healing art. How much greater cause is there now for rejoicing that the desired goal has been so much more nearly attained in as much as the recently discovered and far more specific Homœopathic remedies

* B. J. H., xxvi., 275.

for chronic affections resulting from Psora (properly termed Antipsoric remedies), and the special instructions for their preparation and employment, have been published; and from among them the true physician can now select for his curative-agents those whose medicinal symptoms correspond in the most similar (Homœopathic) manner to the chronic disease he has to cure; and thus, from the employment of (Antipsoric) medicines more suitable to this miasm, he is enabled to render more essential service, and almost invariably to effect perfect cures."

The object of seeking the "fundamental cause" now appears. It is that medicines suitable, not only to the existing symptom-group, but to the "miasm," may be taken into account in the selection of the remedy. Translate the dubious "Psoric" into "Syphilitic," and you have the conception free from prejudice. We know that to trace a malady to a Syphilitic origin is of the utmost importance as regards treatment. It guides us to a class of remedies of which otherwise we might not have thought. It is so no less so, Hahnemann teaches, in Homœopathic practice. He considered it a positive gain when morbid states, hitherto regarded as individuals, could be referred to a common type and treated by remedies chosen from a definite group, instead of being made the subject of an indiscriminate search through the Materia Medica.

Now this is obviously bringing Pathology to the aid of symptomatology, and supplies another instance of its usefulness. Nor does it stand alone in Hahnemann's writings. He ever recognised that there were a certain number of diseases of fixed type, acquiring this by origination from a specific cause; and to these he appropriated one or more specific remedies, as always applicable and usually indispensable.

Let me give a few citations and references in support of this statement.

Hahnemann's earliest and fullest utterance on the subject may be read in his 'Medicine of Experience' (1806).* "We observe," he there writes, "a few diseases that always arise from ONE AND THE SAME CAUSE, e.g., the miasmatic maladies—Hydrophobia, the venereal disease, the Plague of the Levant, Yellow Fever, Small Pox, Cow Pox, the Measles, and some others, which bear upon them the distinctive mark of always remaining diseases of a PECULIAR CHARACTER; and, because they arise from a contagious principle that always remains the same, they also, always retain the same character and pursue the same course, excepting as regards some acci-

---

* P. 502 of Dudgeon's translation of the 'Lesser Writing' of Hahnemann.

dental concommitant circumstances, which however do not alter their essential character."

"Probably some other diseases, which we cannot show to depend on a peculiar miasm, as Gout, Marsh-ague, and several other diseases that occur here and there endemically, besides a few others, also arise either from a single unvarying cause or from the confluence of several definite causes that are liable to be associated and that are always the same, otherwise they would not produce diseases of such a specific kind, and these would not occur so frequently.

"These few diseases, at all events those first-mentioned (the miasmatic), we may therefore term specific, and bestow upon them DISTINCTIVE APPELLATIONS.

"If a remedy have been discovered for one of these, it will always be able to cure it, for such a disease always remains essentially identical, both in its manifestations (the representatives of its internal nature) and its cause."

Turning now to the last edition of the 'Organon' (1833), we find Hahnemann dividing miasmatic diseases into acute and chronic. Among the former he names (§ 73) in one category, Small Pox, Measles, Whooping-cough, Scarlet Fever, Mumps; in another, Plague, Yellow Fever, and Asiatic Cholera, adding to each list an "&c." His chronic miasmatic diseases (§ 78—80) are three. The first is Syphilis; the second is another morbid entity, abstracted by him from the manifestation of the former malady, and named Sycosis; the third is Psora. Under the latter head he ranges (as we have seen) all non-venereal chronic diseases not traceable to bad Hygiene or injurious medications, and so refuses the name of specific to such maladies as Gout, Cancer, Rachitis and Scrofula. On the other hand, he does refer them all to the "Psoric" miasm, and provides a special group of remedies with which they are to be encountered. The "Antipsorics," indeed, are numerous, while the Antisyphilitics and Antisycotics are only three in all. But this Hahnemann explains by the hundreds of generations and millions organisms which Psora has infected, and the consequently various forms its influence has assumed (§ 81). The mass of medicines, nevertheless, are apsoric, and are not to be used save as temporary inter-currents in the treatment of chronic non-venereal disease; just as *Mercury* only is to be given in Syphilis, and *Thuja* and *Nitric acid* are to be our sole reliance in Sycosis.

Another class of specific disease recognised by him here are the epidemic fevers. These are not indeed to be referred to known types, and treated accordingly; for each epidemic has features of its own. Itself, however, is the product of a single cause, and all instances of it are amenable to one and the same specific remedy, which is to be reached by a study of the phenomena of several cases, carried on until the symptom-totality of the epidemic is reached and its SIMILIMUM found (§ 73, 100—102, 235—242).

Again, in his "Examination of the Sources of the Common Materia Medica," prefixed to the Third Volume of his 'Reine Arzneimittellehre' (1816 and 1825), he writes thus:

"From the circumstance that constant remedies have already been discovered for those diseases, few though they be, which have a constant character,* one might infer, that for all diseases of a constant character, constant (specific) remedies might be found. And accordingly, since the only trustworthy way, the Homœopathic, has been pursued with honesty and zeal, the specific remedies for several of the other constant diseases have been discovered." To this (in the Second Edition) he appends a note, giving as instances the use of *Belladonna* in Scarlatina, of *Aconite* and *Coffea* in "Purpura miliaris," of *Spongia* and *Hepar sulphuris* in Croup, of *Drosera* in Whooping-cough, of *Thuja* in Condylomata, and of *Mercurius corrosivus* in autumnal Dysentery.

These extracts must suffice. But if, in addition, you will, in reading Hahnemann's writings, consider his estimate of *Bark* in endemic Malarial fever, *Spongia* in Goitre, and of *Veratrum album* in the Water-colic of Lunenburg; his recommendation of *Aurum* in the propensity to suicide; and his belief in the uniform prophylactic power exerted by *Belladonna* against Scarlatina and by *Copper* against Cholera—I think you will admit that my position is amply supported. It is true that for the multitudinous and diverse forms of disorder which come before the physician, arising from common causes (atmospheric and such like), and having no permanent character, selection by totality of symptoms alone and treatment as individual maladies formed the best mode of proceeding. But it is also evident that he was no mere individualiser; that to him there were morbid species, and specific medicines; and that he counted it real gain to reclaim forms of disease from the desert of symptomatology, to trace them to a common origin and connect them with certain remedies. Modern Pathology must often differ from him as to details: It has at times (as in the "Psoric" diseases) to separate where he has blended, at times (as with Syphilis and Sycosis) to identify where he had distin-

---

* Of these he had previously mentioned *Spongia* for Goitre, *Murcury* for Syphilis, *China* for Ague, and *Arnica* for mechanical injuries.

guished. But the difference is not one of principle. The great work which it has accomplished, in forming so many genera, species, and varieties out of the diverse forms of disease which come before us, has—so far as it is real—his entire concurrence, and becomes directly subservient to his therapeutics.

Hahnemann's ideal Homœopathy was thus to obtain a group of medicine for each morbid species, to be chosen from in each case according to its peculiar features. This was not altogether his earliest conception. In the "Suggestions" of 1796 he expresses himself "convinced that there are as many specifics as there are different state of individual diseases, *i.e.*, that there are peculiar specifics for the pure disease, and others for its varieties;" and again—"we only require to know, on the one hand, the diseases of the human frame accurately, in their essential characteristics and their accidental complications, and, on the other hand, the pure effects of drugs, that is, the essential characteristics of the specific artificial disease they usually excite, together with the accidental symptoms caused by difference of dose, form, etc., and by choosing a remedy for a given natural disease that is capable of producing a very similar artificial disease, we shall be able to cure the most obstinate disorders." In a note to the first quotation, he writes—"The history of diseases is not yet advanced so far that we have been at pains to separate the essential from the accidental, the peculiar from the adventitious—the foreign admixture, owing to idiosyncrasy, mode of life, passions, epidemic constitution, and many other circumstances. When reading the description of one disease, we might often imagine it was a compound admixture of many histories of cases, with suppression of the name, place, time, etc., and not true, abstractedly pure, isolated characteristics of a disease separated from the accidental (which might afterwards be appended to it, as it were). The most recent nosologists have attempted to do this; their genera should be what I call the peculiar characteristics of each disease, their species the accidental circumstances." Later, in the 'Organon,' Hahnemann took a juster view of what is specific and generic in disease. "In the course" he says "of writing down the symptoms of several cases of this kind" *i.e.*, of an epidemic fever "the sketch of the morbid picture becomes ever more and more complete, not more extended, and spun out, but more significant (characteristic) and more comprehensive with respect to the peculiarities of this collective disease; on the one hand, the general symptoms (*e.g.*, loss of appetite, sleeplessness, etc.) become particularly and exactly defined, and on the other, the more marked and special symptoms which are peculiar to but few diseases and of rarer occurrence, at least in the same combination, become prominent, and constitute what is characteristic of this malady." These "general symptoms," which are characteristic of all fevers, should surely be classed as generic; these "marked and special symptoms," which characterise the particular epidemic under observation, as "specific." We shall thus have another category left, answering to the "varieties" of natural history; and in this we can place the "accidental circumstances" of Hahnemann's previous description, which are the peculiarities due to the individual idiosyncrasy.

Similarity between disease and drug-action should thus be generic, specific and individual.

I. Generic similarity is that expressed in the sayings, "NIL PRODEST QUOD NON LOEDIT IDEM" and "MAGIS VENENUM, MAGIS REMEDIUM". To make his case a SIMILE of drug-action at all, a person must be ill; on the other side, if he be ill, his remedy must be one capable of causing illness in the healthy, and the more seriously ill he is, the more potent should be the poison with which he is treated. These are broad generalities, but they are the basis of Homœopathy, and the surer one from such breadth. Then we go a little further, and say that the class of affections from one of which the patient is suffering must be such as the drug is capable of producing. If his illness is febrile, his remedy must be pyreto-genetic; if the one be an inflammation, the other must be an irritant.

II. Specific similarity (I use the word now in its scientific, not its medicinal sense) implies the existence of species. These, in natural history, mean forms capable of reproducing their kind; and such we have in the infectious diseases. But no less entitled to the name are those which, though barren, spring from a common cause, as the Malarious fevers and constitutional Syphilis; those which depend on a definite morbid process taking place in particular organ, as Pneumonia and Cirrhosis of the Liver; or those having a known clinical history, as Diabetes and acute Rheumatism. These are recognised and stable forms of disease; each sufferer from them presents their essential features, though each may have them in his own way. If we had drugs which caused them all, as *Strychnia* causes Tetanus and *Arsenic* chronic Morbus Brightii, we should only have to give these, with preference—when more than one existed—to that which corresponded to the individual peculiarities of the case. But it is rarely so; and indeed, in the nature of things, could hardly be expected. The specific morbid states cannot be convinced of as having been fresh creations, full-blown at first and ever since the same. They are the result—probably the gradual result—of interaction between the organism and its environment: even those which now reproduce their kind may well have been evolved in this way, as Darwin has taught us with regard to the species of plants and animals. In this way the PREDISPOSITIONS DEFINIES of which Tessier speaks have been established, resulting, under the action of common causes, in fixed forms of disease : In this way specific viruses, themselves the seed (and now perhaps the only source) of fresh disease of the same kind, have been slowly distilled in the alembic of the organism, till they have become what they are. I venture to think that this is a truer account of the matter than to suppose all infectious diseases to have been parasitic, according to the now fashionable germ-theory.

Specific maladies having thus originated, then can seldom—I say—be imitated by drugs *ab ovo usque ad mala*. The substances so called are either elements and simple compounds, or are the results of the vital Chemistry at work in organisms themselves evolved by natural selection and other processes. They thus move in no parallel plane with the causes of disease ; and the only point of contact between the two is the living body, in which one and the other effect changes, which may well be like—not to say identical—at points, but can hardly be as wholes to wholes. Specific similarity must generally content itself with such corresdondences here and there, and is more or less perfect according as they are quantitatively or qualitatively considerable. Let us consider some of its elements.

1. The first requisite for specific similarity is that the drug shall have the same seat of action as the disease. I have already shown how provision is made for this necessity in the rule that the totality of the symptoms is to be covered. If the phenomena correspond, so also must the noumena. In this way, moreover, identity of seat is secured alike more certainly and more thoroughly : more certainly, because on any other plan it must be an inference, which may possibly be mistaken, and more thoroughly, because the full range and even primary origin of the malady, may lie beyond the organ obviously at fault. But I have also pointed out that there are cases where symptoms fail us as a guide, and where the "Organopathy" of Paracelsus, Rademacher and Sharp comes in welcome aid. Identity of seat is half the battle ; only half, it is true, but to have conquered so far is fair promise of entire victory, and the promise is often fulfilled.

The "seat" of disease contemplated by Dr. Sharp is, as his name for the method implies, an ORGAN ; but he is careful to postulate that the skin shall for such purposes be accounted an organ. It is really a tissue : And this leads us to see that action upon the tissue involved in the disease is sufficient for specific similarity, though there be no correspondence in the localisation. When de Merriot tells us that "the mucous membranes, ten minutes after the injection of *Atropia*, are red, injected, and dry," he is speaking from those which can be observed, but has no hesitation in inferring the same thing of others who are invisible. That inflammation should have its seat in mucous membrane is therefore, CÆTERIS PARIBUS, and indication for *Belladonna*, and this wherever the membrane may be. Symptomatic correspondence will give us this identity also; but in lack thereof it may often be obtained by analogy. It was, for instance, a long time before we had adequate provings by women; and in the absence of these we had little sure knowledge of the action of drugs on their sexual apparatus. But it was justly argued (as by Dr. Leadam*) the substances which inflamed mucous membrane or provoked hæmorrhage elsewhere should be Homœopathic to Endo-Metritis and Metrorrhagia; and so they proved to be.

Another mode of securing what may be called "tissue-remedies" was initiated by Dr. von Grauvogl, and has been elaborated by Dr. Schussler. As each part selects from the blood the elements it requires for its nutriment, so does it behave with the drugs brought to it by the circulatory current. But there must be a difference according as such drug is or is not an actual constituent of the part, still more if it be altogether foreign to the body. In the two latter cases the drug must be classed as a "function-remedy," *i.e.*, it exalts, depresses, or otherwise modifies vital activity without effecting substantive change. It is different when the part for which it has affinity normally contains the substance in question. If this can act elsewhere as poison in health, as medicine in disease, here would seem to supply pabulum only— to be a food; and such it doubtless is as long as the supply is proportioned to the demand. But what occurs when it is in excess? The reason why each part selects from the blood its proper pabulum seems to be that such nutritive elements act as specific stimuli thereto, evoking its assimilative activity. Excess of such stimulation must cause, either morbid hypertrophy, or—by exhaustion—deficient nutrition in respect of this very element; and the latter seems the more frequent occurrence. On the other hand, in such malnutrition idiopathically induced, the best remedy will consist in small doses of these very substances—not as aliment (which proper food best supplies) but as specific stimuli, raising the depressed vital activity to its normal lines.

This was von Grauvogl's argument; and he called such substances "nutrition-remedies," instancing their usefulness by the employment of *Calcarea phosphorica* in defective ossification of the cranium, leading to chronic Hydrocephalus, and of *Silicea* in Enchondroma of the fingers. Dr. Schussler was so enamoured of

* See B. J. H., x. 59.

medicines of this kind, that he would have had us abandon the whole Materia Medica in favour of a dozen of them—the *Fluoride, Phosphate* and *Sulphate of Calcium,* the *Phosphate of Iron,* this *Chloride, Phosphate* and *Sulphate of Potassium,* the *Phosphate of Sodium,* and *Silica.* I need hardly say that he has found no followers (among the profession) in his exclusiveness; but a large measure of success has been obtained with the new remedies of the kind he has proposed for adoption, and by generally following out the indications he has urged on our notice. *

2. Seat of action is of such value in the endeavour after specific similarity; but KIND of action is of no less importance. By this I mean something more than was spoken of among the elements of generic similarity, *viz.,* that the Pathological process shall be the same—fever, inflammation, ulceration, and so forth. I am thinking of the quality which such processes receive from the diathesis or general disease of which they are the outcome. Sydenham long ago pointed to this as an essential element in specificity. "In overcoming a chronic disease," he wrote, "he has the best and truest claim to the name of physician who is in possession of the medicine that shall destroy the species of the disease; not he who merely substitutes one primary or secondary quality for another. This he can do without extinguishing the species at all; *i.e.,* a gouty patient may be cooled or heated, as the case may be, and his Gout continue unconquered." In like manner we may say, that a medicine may be Homœopathic to simple inflammation of an organ, but not to that peculiar modification impressed upon the process by its occurrence as a result of Scrofula or of Syphilis. Intestinal ulceration, again, is a simple thing in itself; but it varies in character according as it is a part of a Typhoid Fever, the ultimate issue of a Dysentery, or the consequence of Tuberculous deposition in the course of Phthisis. To these differences and variations our medicines must correspond so far as is possible. To reach the most suitable remedies for the QUALITIES of morbid processes is no easy task. It requires symptomatic comparison, Pathological inference, analogy, and clinical experience; but when obtained it is worth all the trouble. The superiority of *Colchicum* in gouty inflammation to the *Bryonia* or *Pulsatilla,* the Arthritis would otherwise demand, is an instance in point.

* See "The Twelve Tissue Remedies of Schussler," by Drs. Bœricke and Dewey. Dr. Schussler evolved his theories out of Homœopathy, carried them out for many years in fellowship with our body, and gave them to the last in Homœopathic form and dose. Latterly he (rather ungratefully) withdrew himself from our ranks, and took an independent position. It is amusing to notice that in the last Edition of his Book on the Subject, issued just before his death in 1898, he omits one of his twelve medicines, on the ground of the doubtfulness of its presence as a constituent of the organism. Yet this *Sodium sulphate* has been in use by Schusslerites for many years, and has not been found less active than its associates.

3. Of another feature of specific similarity I have already spoken. It is that modification of disease which its originating CAUSE impresses upon it. It differs according as it is of physical or mental origin, and these classes have to be further sub-divided. A Rheumatism arising from dry cold is one thing, from damp cold another; a Neuralgia induced by injury to a nerve is different from one brought on by Malaria or by Gout. Jaundice from mental emotion is not the same disorder as that arising from heat or from a too stimulating diet. I might multiply examples; but these are sufficient to show my meaning. Now to these modifications also our remedies must correspond; and here again the correspondence may be arrived at in various ways. *Dulcamara* supplies a good illustration. Carrere, who published in 1789 a treatise on its virtues, states that he had several times noticed in patients under its influence some twitching of the eyelids, lips and hands on exposure to cold damp weather, which readily subsided under the application of dry warmth. The Homœopathic inference therefrom was that *Dulcamara* would be suitable as a medicine to affections thus caused, and so it has proved to be in numerous instances. However arrived at, such casual Homœopathicity (if I may so express it) is of the utmost value, and many a time leads as no other guide would to the specific remedy.

4. Another useful point of comparison between disease and drug-action is the CHARACTER of the pains and other sensations present. There is a reason why one should complain of burning pain, another of tearing, another of gnawing, and so forth; we may not be able to explain it, but the kind of sensation present characterises the suffering and on being found in pathogenesy establishes the specific similarity of the drug which causes it. The burning pain of *Arsenic* is a good example—the more so because it is at present inexplicable. It has been thought to depend on mucous membrane being the seat of its action; but this cannot hold good of its Neuralgia, where it no less obtains.

5. Lastly, I would speak of CONCOMITANCE, that is the coincidence of two or more marked symptoms in the pathogenesis of a drug and in the phenomena of a disease. Its value rests on the mathematical law of combinations, or—as it is technically called—permutations. The number of the possible rearrangements of the figures of a series increases in proportion to their number, but by leaps and bounds exceeding not merely arithmetical but even geometrical progression, so that while for five figures it is 120, for seven it is 5040. In the same ratio increase the probabilities against any one combination occurring by chance. You will see, then, if three distinctive symptoms of a case can be found to have been excited by a medicine, there is already considerable likelihood of its acting on the same parts and in the same manner; and that the odds in its favour increase rapidly as the points of analogy are multiplied.

If you have three legs to your stool, Constantine Hering used to say, you may well sit down upon it; but a four-legged chair is better still. He, however, judging from the shape in which he published most of his provings, did not appreciate the full value of this mode of proceeding. It is a small matter that symptoms should be present, compared with their being present in a certain connection and sequence; and this it is as impossible to discover in the schema of Hering as in that of Hahnemann. Now, with the detailed provings in our hands, we can ascertain order as well as occurrence, and thus enhance many-fold our probability of arriving at genuine results.

Dr. Woodward, of Chicago, and Dr. Ord, and Bournemouth, have of late years urged on us the importance of chronological sequence in respect of organs or tissues affected, and have shewn that many a success may be scored by securing Homœopathicity in this matter between disease and drug-action. *

Seat of action, then, in organ or tissue; kind of action, in diathesis or other quality, in causative modification, in character of sensations, and in concomitance and sequence of symptoms these are the main elements of specific similarity. The more you can secure of them the better your prospect of reaching the "Pathological SIMILE," as Drysdale called it, which is the aim of all your endeavours and the best hope for your patient.

* See Transaction of International Hom. Congresses of 1881 and 1896.

LECTURE VIII.

THE SELECTION OF THE SIMILAR REMEDY (*contd.*)

III. Similarity of drug-action to disease is to be generic, specific, and individual. We have considered some of the elements which go to make up generic and specific likeness and have now to see what can further be done by way of making the similarity individual. That it should so be, if possible, must be evident. Even the essential, typical diseases affect each subject in his own way, so that he presents a variety of the species ; and that which is distinctive in him must be taken into account. Individualisation is as important in therapeutics as it confessedly is in education. Still more decisive are such indications for the choice of the remedy in those anomalous morbid conditions, coming under no definite category, which constantly come before us. I cannot quite go with the saying "il n'y a pas des maladies, il n'y a que des maladies ;" but here it is certainly applicable, and we may go with Dr. Clifford Allbut in viewing as "wholesome" the "tendency to the fall of diseases, as abstract names, and to the rise of the patient." *
Of the mode of dealing with such cases I shall speak further on : At present let us consider individual as complementary to specific similarity.

In pursuit hereof must be taken into account the patient's constitution and temperament, his mental and emotional state, the conditions of aggravation and amelioration presented by his sufferings, the side of the body affected, and the time of day or night at which his symptoms are most pronounced.

1. To almost every medicine of importance in Homœopathic practice has been assigned, as it has become well-known, a type of patient to whom it is suited. *Bryonia* corresponds to brunettes of bilious tendencies and choleric temper, with firm flesh ; *Arsenicum* to worn and exhausted constitution ; *Nux vomica* to vigorous persons of dry habits and tense fibre, addicted, it may be to "high thinking," but not to "plain living" ; *Pulsatilla* to the lymphatic, and *Ignatia* to the nervous temperament, in woman and children ; and so forth. These adaptations have mostly been reached by clinical experience, but

---

* BRITISH MED. JOURN., Oct. 6, 1900.

sometimes the Physiological effects of drugs will lead to them; and Teste has suggested that we may often get useful hints from the results of experimentation on animals—poisons which have most effect on carnivora or harnivora respectively finding most receptivity as medicines in corresponding types of human constitution.

2. The mental and moral state of the patient is often a feature of his general temperament, but it may also supervene in the course of his existing malady. It is a matter on which Hahnemann always laid much stress. "In all cases of disease" he wrote in the 'Organon' (§ 210), "that we are called on to cure, the state of the patient's disposition is to be especially noted, along with the totality of the symptoms, if we would trace an accurate picture of the disease, in order to be able therefrom to treat it Homœopathically with success. This holds good to such an extent, that the state of the disposition of the patient often chiefly determines the selection of the Homœopathic remedy." In this category we have the emotional tension of *Aconite*, with fear of death; the crossness of *Chamomilla*; the Melancholia (often suicidal) of *Aurum*; and the ENTETEE state of *Platina*.

3. Conditions of aggravation and amelioration have always played a large part in Homœopathic therapeutics; and as there must be cause for them, it would be wrong to ignore them. It is certainly on account of some real difference in the pains they cause that those of *Bryonia* aggravated by motion, those of *Rhus* (at any rate after the first) relieved by it; and here it may plausibly be suggested that the difference depends on the more acute and inflammatory-like character of the former. But there are other instances in which no such explanation is available, and yet the fact remains, and is fruitful of practical application. The increase of the head pains of *Belladonna* on lying down and of those of *Spigelia* on stooping; the aggravations of *Lachesis* after sleep and the ameliorations of *Nux vomica* from the same cause; the relief afforded by cold to the pains of *Coffea* and by warmth to those of *Arsenicum* and *Silicea*—the latter in its turn making worse those of *Mercurius* and *Pulsatilla*—are examples of what I mean. The "conditions" of every drug commonly employed in Homœopathic practice are known, having been ascertained either by experiment on the part of the provers (as enjoined by Hahnemann) or from clinical observation; and they are worthy of all attention. They are misused only when they are too widely generalised and when, because the pains of a drug are aggravated by motion, the same is assumed to hold good of all its diverse symptoms. This MAY be, so, indeed, as it seems to be in the case of *Lachesis* and the increase of suffering after sleeping; but it must not be taken for granted A PRIORI.

4. The side of the body which is affected may be thought a thing of no moment save when unilateral organs are concerned. Sometimes, indeed, the determination of the malady thereto may be thus accounted for, as when we find right supra-orbital pain associated with herpetic disorder, and calling for *Chelidonium*, while on the left side it is often traceable to the stomach, and is relieved by *Kali Bichromicum*. But how are we to account for such a fact as that which is established in relation to *Viola odorata*, that it removes Rheumatism of the right wrist only, so that if both joints are affected it leaves the left untouched? There are many similar (though hardly so pronounced) phenomena in our pathogenetics and therapeutics: And they may not be ignored. Teste has contributed a valuable suggestion here, viz., : That the left must be regarded as the weaker side of the body, and so most impressible by lowering causes and depressing drugs; while the disorders and medicines of the right side are rather of the sthenic kind. Whatever be the explanation, the fact of the one-sidedness of the action of many drugs certainly hold good. Dr. Gaston Delaunay, in a thesis presented to the Faculte de Paris in 1874, has shown that in many respects the right and left sides of the body have a separate Physiology and Pathology; and the phenomena of Aphasia point in the same direction.

5. The time of day at which symptoms occur or undergo aggravation is made no small account of by many Homœopathic practitioners. The exacerbations of *Nux vomica* about two and three a. m. and of *Pulsatilla* in the evening were early noted by Hahnemann; and we have since come to fix those of *Lycopodium* for 4 p. m. Dr. Claude has published a very interesting essay, entitled "Sur le rythme de quelques medicaments," in which he illustrates this last bit of periodicity by several cases of Bronchitis and Intermittent Fever: and has also established 8 p. m. as an hour of aggravation calling for *Atropine*

Here, too, we have a suggestion in explanation of the phenomena derived from general Physiology. M. Spring, in observation on the diurnal variations of temperature, pulse, and respiration, has found that from 3 to 9 a. m., and from 1 to 5 pm. are periods of functional increase, while from 9 a. m. to 1 p. m., and from 6 p. m. to 3 a. m. are times of diminished functional activity. Drugs and diseases which induce overstimulation may therefore be expected to show their main influence at the former epochs, and VICE VERSA. Whether any of our observed medicinal periodicities can thus be accounted for I am unable to say; but, whatever be their explanation, they often guide us to the choice of a right remedy. In Ague, especially, the hour at which the paroxysm tends to occur is reckoned of much importance; and Dr. Elias Price, of Baltimore, has published a time-chart expressly to aid in the selection of medicines therefrom.

In the union of specific and individual similarity, secured by as many as possible of these elements, lies -generic correspondence being of course assumed—the ideal Homœopathy. It is well illustrated by Dr. Dunham in his "Homœopathy, the Science of Therapeutics."

"Let us suppose" he writes, "a case of uterine hæmorrhage. As many as forty drugs probably produce uterine hæmorrhage. On the basis of this symptom, they form a group isolated from the three hundred and forty remaining drugs of the Materia Medica. We select this group from the Materia Medica, and now we must select a remedy from the group. It is a tedious task to consider and compare them one by one. But we group them again; ten of them produce dark-coloured and ten florid hæmorrhage; ten limpid and ten clotted discharge. Our case has a dark-coloured discharge. Our choice is now restricted to ten drugs. But of the ten which produce a dark discharge, only five produce simultaneously a congestive Headache. Thus we are limited to five drugs. Thus far, the distinctions on which our grouping has been based (or which have been characteristic of the groups) have had a Pathological significance and importance. We can find no such basis for any further subdivision into groups. But we observe in the case a peculiar subjective symptom. The patient complains, 'as though a living body were moving through the abdomen.' This may seem trivial. It is equally, however, a symptom produced by *Crocus*, which is one of the five remedies to which our choice had been restricted, and it is produced by no other drug in the Materia Medica. It is, then, a characteristic symptom of *Crocus*, enabling us to individualise *Crocus*, and to distinguish it from all the other drugs which in many respects agree with it."

Dr. Dunham here conducts his individualisation by means of a single peculiar symptom—one of those of which we shall have hereafter to speak under the title of "characteristics." But he shows further on that the determining feature is sometimes a condition, which may be of time, or circumstance, or concomitance—thus bringing it into the categories we have just been discussing.

This is ideal Homœopathy, and should always be aimed at. But a very little experience will show that it is not always attainable. The deficiency may be either on the side of specific qualities or on that of individual features, or it may be on both. Clinical experience will here often come to our aid; but, if we Homœopathize it all, we must do it by way of individualisation by itself or by that of generalisation by itself. The first secures likeness in the instance, ignoring the type; the second aims at conformity to the type, and disregards the peculiarities of the instance. Which course shall we follow? The former is that advocated by most Homœopathic writers; but it has great disadvantages. It rests for its basis on a minute symptomatology which is at the best uncertain, which even after the sifting it has received cannot always be relied on as a body of genuine drug-effects. Even if the symptoms, which serve as indications, be trustworthy, there is no knowing what relation they bear to the disorder as a whole. Their own Pathological basis (their proximate cause) may be part of its foundation, and then its removal by the drug given is a real gain; but it may just as well be only an outgrowth, and contribute nothing to the strength of the main building. To vary the simile, the pursuit of such indications is too often a lopping off of boughs and leaves, instead of a cutting at the root of a tree.

There is, again, a better word to be said for the alternative of generalisation than is usually conceded to it. If you conduct a school for boys, it is important, as already said, that you consider the character of each individual committed to your care, and act towards him accordingly. But it is quite as important that you make your general arrangements such as to be suitable to the young of the masculine variety of the genus homo. You may not know much about a given new-comer, but you are safe in treating him as a boy. And so with disease. If you must choose, it is surely of greater consequence to secure similarity to the Pathological process itself than (in Hahnemann's words) to some accidental concomitant circumstances, which do not alter its essential character." By pursuing individualisation you MAY strike your mark; but your weapon's point is so fine that though it pierces deep when it hits, it is very liable to miss. Generalisation gives a blunter point, but a broader one; your impression may be less incisive, but it can hardly fail to be made. Since, then, imperfect similarity is confessedly better than no similarity at all, it may often be wiser to make sure of this than to aim at a mark more dimly seen. That less attenuation of dose is here necessary is no argument against the proceeding; for a similar necessity is admitted even in the sphere of minute symptomatology and the higher infinitesimals.

It will be seen that I am far from advocating generalisation as an habitual practice, still less as the ideal mode of Homœopathizing. Though "so careful of the type" I may seem, I would not be "careless of the single life"; while pleading for due subordination in the hierarchy of symptoms, I would have none despised as playing no part in the whole. But individualisation—valuable as it is—was not to Hahnemann (as I showed in my last lecture), and is not in the nature of the case, the be-all and end-all in the selection of the Homœopathic remedy. It is always the better for having generalisation as its complement ; and the latter may often be preferably followed when we have to choose between the two. Wurmb and Casper saying of *Arsenic,* that "it will often cure" chronic Intermittents "when other remedies selected with the greatest care have failed" ;* Espanet reporting that in the numerous cases of Dysentery treated by him in Algeria, he "never found the least advantage from substituting for *Mercurius corrosivus* another remedy which seemed more Homœopathic to the febrile phenomena or the abdominal symptoms" ;† the general experience vouched for by Homœopathists like Jeanes and Sircar, Jousset, Bahr, and Panelli, ‡ that nearly every recent and uncomplicated Ague can be cured by *Quinine*—these are testimonies to the practical value of judicious SPECIFICKERING (as the Germans call it) which are not to be despised.

There are cases, however—as I have freely admitted—in which all idea of conformity to type must be abandoned and we must commit ourselves to individualisation without reserve. In so doing, may follow one or other of two methods—that by totality of symptoms, or that by characteristics.

1st. The first is Hahnemann's mode of proceeding. It is to write down the symptoms of a case in the order of the schema, and then to find what medicine has caused the whole, or the greatest number, or the most characteristic of them. It is illustrated by the two cases he has related in the Preface to the Second Volume of the 'Materia Medica Pura.'§ One was a Gastralgia made up of six symptoms, the patient's health being otherwise good. *Bryonia* was found to possess all the features of the malady, and in a more marked manner than any other medicine ; it also corresponded to the patient's disposition, which was passionate. This remedy was accordingly chosen, and cured in a single dose. The second case was one of Dyspepsia, and to its seven features, and again to the patient's disposition, the pathogenesis of *Pulsatilla* was found quite parallel ; and it effected a similar cure. His Materia Medica was framed (as I have pointed out) in such a manner as to favour comparisons of this kind. At first memory could hold the symptoms, or a little hunting find them ; but as the remedies which had been submitted to proving increased in number, indices to their effects were required.

* See B. J. H. xiii. 430, note.
† BULL. DE LA SOC. MED. DE FRANCE, xix. 179.
‡ See B. J. H. xxxii. 723; M. H. R., xviii. 522; UNITED STATES MED. INVESTIGATOR, iv. 161.
§ It may be found in Vol. 1, p. 18, of Dudgeon's translation.

Hahnemann early perceived their need, and appended one to his first pathogenetic collection—the 'Fragmenta de Viribus.' As the Materia Medica grew towards its present dimensions, the indices to it had to form distinct volumes wrought by separate hands, and hence the "Repertories"—finding-means— of Muller, Hempel, and others. We in this country have been somewhat later in supplying them; but we have tried to make up for our delay by aiming at a fulness hitherto unattempted. The 'Repertory' of the Hahnemann Publishing Society, as far as it went, presented every symptom in full under every category in which it could be reasonably looked for. It effected this without intolerable bulk by an ingenious system of cypher, which, though it has frightened many away from using the repertory, is admitted by all competent judges to be of inestimable value. That the symptoms should always be presented in their completeness is an obvious advantage, and in no other way could this have been done. At the same time, as has been pointed out, the repertory can be used like other works of the kind, without any employment of the cypher whatever; while those who seek counsels of perfection in this matter can do so by mastering its (very moderate) difficulties.

I am the more desirous of doing honour to this most laborious and praiseworthy undertaking, because I have myself endeavoured to supersede it. I have, at the desire of the colleagues who worked with me at the 'Cyclopædia of Drug Pathogenesy', compiled an index to that work which has also embraced the trustworthy material of Hahnemann's symptom-lists. I have explained in the Introduction why I have departed in many respects from the British repertorians and others. The distinctive features of my compilation, however, is that it is not a repertory to the whole range of drug pathogenesy, but an index to a special collection of such phenomena. This may be by some accounted a deficiency : to others, however, it will give a sense of confidence they have hitherto lacked. They may prefer working with a limited body of well-attested and sifted material to taking their chance over a wider area. At any rate, such is the "Repertory to the Cyclopædia of Drug Pathogenesy,"* which is now before the profession, and whose method is fully described in its Indroduction.

In using repertories, two cautions must be borne in mind. The first is that you must not prescribe FROM them, but be guided by them to the Materia Medica, where only you can find the data on which to base a right selection. The repertory can be nothing but an index, and is not responsible for the value of the elements to which it points : This must always be

London; Gould and Son, 59, Moorgate St.

tested by its employer. Again, a medicine may have produced a symptom which the patient has, but in so different a connexion that no real similarity is thereby established : This a repertory cannot tell us, but the Materia Medica may. The second caution is that while you should seek the totality of your patient's symptoms in a medicine, you should not expect to find all the symptoms of the medicine in your patient. If *Cantharis* is indicated by his renal symptoms, you must not reject it because he has no Dysuria : If *Belladonna* is suited to his Angina Faucium, it requires no delirium to be present to validate its Homœopathicity. These are independent morbid states, each with its own proximate cause, and the drug can extinguish as it can excite them separately.

2nd. The other method of which I have spoken works by what are called "characteristics". Hahnemann, in the 'Organon, taught us the importance of securing resemblance above all things in those symptoms which are peculiar to each drug as an individual. "In the search" he wrote, "for a Homœopathic specific remedy . . . . . the more striking, singular, uncommon and peculiar (characteristic) signs and symptoms of the case of disease are chiefly and almost solely to be kept in view; for it is more particularly with these that very similar ones in the list of symptoms of the selected medicine must correspond, in order to constitute it the most suitable for effecting the cure. . . . If the antitype constructed from the list of symptoms of the most suitable medicine contain those peculiar, uncommon, singular and distinguising (characteristic) symptoms, which are to be met with in the disease to be cured in the greatest number and in the greatest similarity, this medicine is the most appropriate Homœopathic specific remedy for this morbid state' (§ 153, 154). Carroll Dunham expanded the same teaching—"We are so to study Materia Medica" he wrote, "as above all, to bring into strong relief and fix firmly in memory those peculiarities of each drug which are not met with in any other, and which therefore serve to individualise and give character to the drug that produces them, and are called its characteristic symptoms. This term having been much and loosely used of late, it may not be unprofitable to devote a few words to the subject of characteristic symptoms.

"By some writers the leading and most obvious and most frequently recurring symptoms are called characteristic. Thus Bennett calls fever a characteristic of the Exanthemata. By others the pathognomonic symptoms of a class of diseases are called characteristic—by others the Pathologico-Anatomical. Now, the signification of such a word as characteristic is not absolute. It depends on the connection in which you please to use it, and which is determined by the question, 'characteristic of what?" In the instances just adduced, the varieties of symptoms cited may indeed be called characteristic, but—characteristic of what? Of classes (the Exanthemata), of groups (nosological),—but not of individuals. But the only sense in which Homœopathists can use the term is in its application to INDIVIDUALS. Hence a characteristic symptom must mean one which is possessed by none other than the individual drug of which it is predicated, and to which therefore it gives character as an individual. In this sense it corresponds precisely to those features of a man by which his friends are enabled to distinguish him from other persons and to recognise him at a glance.

"It is obvious that these characteristic symptoms so precious to the Therapeutist may seem to be of little or no Pathological value—may even seem accidental to those who forget that there are no accidents in Nature. They would be valueless if we did not need to individualise, but could be content with grouping our diseases and remedies. To the Naturalist whose object it is to group his specimens, it is sufficient to know that John Doe has a vertebral column, is a mammal, has two hands, and is a Caucasian—because this enables him at once to place John Doe in variety Caucasian of the species of man, and his analysis goes no further. From this his whole Physiological status follows. But these items of general knowledge would hardly enable the SHERIFF to recognise John Doe in Broadway. It is of no importance to the naturalist that he has such 'accidental' peculiarities as an aquiline nose, black eyes and hair, and a brown mole on the left ala nasi : but these very peculiarities are all important to the sheriff, for they give him the means of detecting the object of his search upon the crowded street. It must not be forgotten, however, that the points on which the naturalist laid stress are equally important to the sheriff ; for if the latter should bear in mind only the INDIVIDUAL peculiarities of the subject of his quest, and should forget that he is a Caucasian, he might find the former in the person of an Indian, or, if he should forget that he is a bimanous creature, he might arrest a monkey.

"To drop the figure, then, it is evident that we must seek to discover among the symptoms of every drug certain ones that are produced by no other drug, and which shall serve to distinguish it from all other drugs similar in other respects ; and that these symptoms will often be unimportant and trivial in a Physiological point of view."

It was evidently Dunham's idea that these characteristic symptoms should be employed in selecting, from groups of medicines specifically Homœopathic, the one individually so—as illustrated by the example of *Crocus* in Metrorrhagia already cited from him. But they have of late years assumed a much more important place in the minds of a number of our practitioners, of whom Dr. Henry Guernsey, of Philadelphia, was the foremost representative. They have become in their hands the basis of a "keynote system," which dominates their whole practice. If, they say, the characteristics of a drug are present in a patient, the rest of his symptoms will in all probability be found in its pathogenesis, and they identify such characteristics with the peculiar differences which each drug presents as compared with all other. Dr. Guernsey has expounded it, in an essay which you will find in the Third Volume of the HAHNEMANNIAN MONTHLY, and also in the Preface to his treatise on 'Obstetrics.' In the latter he illustrates it by the instance of picking of the nose as an indication for *Cina* in Metrorrhagia. It is well known that the presence of worms in the intestines, has kept up for months, a constant stillicidium of blood from the uterus ; and "here" he writes, "we can readily see the relation between the comparatively trifling symptoms of picking of the nose and the irritation of the bowels, caused by the ASCARIDES and consequent uterine irritation and hæmorrhage. The fact that in many cases it is impossible to trace any Physiological connections between remote symptoms, which still seem to be characteristic, and the disorders themselves, should not therefore induce us to conclude that such connection does not exist."

Such a position is unexceptionable, and only requires testing by facts. But when we examine the "key-notes" affixed to drugs by Drs. Guernsey, Cowperthwaite, Hawkes, and others, we find them far from being identical with their individual characteristics, as explained by Dunham, and by no means always present in their pathogenesis at all. This, however, though it destroys their professed basis, would not make it impossible that they should serve as guide-posts to the remedy which should be found to answer to the totality of the symptoms of a case. But when the practice of the advocates of the method, as reported by themselves, is observed, it is evident that this further enquiry is regarded as of quite secondary importance, and that its negative result does little to outweigh the presence of the characteristic, which thus become not suggestive only, but determining. In the essay already referred to, Dr. Guernsey says of the "keynote"—"it is something peculiar in the case, some prominent feature or marked symptom, that directs to a certain drug, "AND THE TOTALITY AFTERWARDS CONFIRMS OR DISAPPROVES THE CHOICE." But on the next page he relates a case of Dysmenorrhœa to which he was called in consultation. Struck with the "devout, beseeching, earnest, and ceaseless talking" of the patient, he suggested *Stramonium*. The attending physician replied that the other symptoms of the patient were not under the head of that medicine (he might have added that the keynote itself is not to be found there). Dr. Guernsey replied, "that *Stramonium* was undoubtedly the remedy, and if it were properly proven and on every variety of temperament and condition, all of her symptoms would be found in the record of its pathogenesis."

It is obvious that the practice so exemplified, while it may be successful, has no claim to be a following of Hahnemann. It is wholly empirical and hypothetical. The very term used to denote it involves, either a confusion of thought, or a false assumption. It is equivalent, as the late Dr. Madden has argued, to asserting "that two instruments will harmonise if attuned to the same key, on matter whether they play the same tune or not. It seems to us," he goes on, "that the only way of escaping this dilemma is to assert that every drug can cure every disease, provided the drug and the disease agree in the one particular; an assertion which would overthrow all our ideas of specific relationship. Of course, in Dr. Guernsey's analogy, the living body represents the instrument, and the drug and the disease are the players. If, then it is enough to ascertain that the two which are expected to harmonise are playing in the same key, the drug must be capable of playing any tune in that key, otherwise the disease might be playing the Dead March in 'Saul,' while the drug—in the same key—struck up 'Champagne Charley.' Will this constitute one of Nature's harmonies? We trust not.

"Our views of specific relationship, and we think they exactly correspond with those of Hahnemann, would represent medicines as automaton players, whose performances were limited to playing a definite number of tunes in certain fixed keys; and the use of the proving is to determine these two facts; *viz.*, the tunes which each automaton can play, and the key in which each is played. When, therefore, we wish to discover the simile to any disease, we first ascertain the tune which is being played (diagnose the concrete disease), and then compare the remedies known to be capable of playing that tune, so as to determine which agrees in key with the case in point."

Our conclusion must be that these "characteristics" should be somewhat closely scrutinised in themselves, to see if they have any warrant, pathogenetic or clinical; and the best should play the part of suggestions only, their presence not being allowed to outweigh a specific similarity on the part of another drug to which they may not have been affixed. Used in this manner, they may occasionally be of service; but their present predominance in certain fields of practice is, I am convinced, the choice of IGNES FATUI for our guide in place of the steady polestar of SIMILIA SIMILIBUS with the totality of symptoms for its elements of comparison.

In what has now been said there has always been the assumption that the Homœopathist arrives at—or has in the first instance arrived at—his remedies by applying the Law of Similars. This, however, is far from holding good in every instance. Clinical experience, the USUS IN MORBIS as our older writers used to call it, is largely employed amongst us. Hahnemann himself, though deprecating resort to it, and publishing but few cases in its aid, has left enough "therapeutic hints" in his writings to make, in Dr. Dudgeon's compilation, a nice little volume; and his disciples have largely added to this element in our literature. It has found outcome in two ways—the one belonging to the specific, the other to the individual, similarities I have described.

1. We have seen that the species of disease can rarely be reproduced, as wholes, in drug-effects, and that their SIMILIA must rather be sought by correspondences in seat and kind of action, and such-like. But there is another mode of reaching them. Suppose that chance, theory, or any other mental process has led to the discovery of remedial powers in a drug; suppose that this influence is not to be accounted for by any physical or chemical properties it may possess, or by any evacuation on which the effect may indirectly depend, and is not in the same direction with that it exerts in health, we are justified, by the process of exclusion, in assuming it to act Homœopathically, even though no similar phenomena are presented by such pathogenesis as it may have. Sooner or later they are pretty sure to appear; but we need not wait till they rise above the horizon. There are (to vary the figure) breech presentations in Homœopathy as in Obstetrics, Hering wittily says; and though the mode of entrance is abnormal, the child is assuredly born. The power of *Colchicum* over Gout is an instance of this. So many facts have come to light, showing that the irritant properties of *Colchicum* can be exerted on the joints, that the remedy can be claimed for Homœopathy as all specifics have been or may be.* The pains in the joints it cause in the human subject are in animals developed into obvious congestion, so that experimenters upon them are compelled to conclude that it "produces its therapeutic effects by an irritant action," and again that in Gout "it produces a substitutive irritation of the articular surfaces." SUBSTITUTIVEMENT, C'EST A DIRE HOMŒOPATHIQUEMENT, writes Trousseau, and the maxim is never more applicable than in the present example.

2. Here, then, clinical experience re-enforces our attempts at specific similarity: It fills up the groups of remedies for definite types of disease which our treatises on practice present. In another direction, it is employed to supply the gaps in individual similarity which pathogenesy too often displays. Many of the indications of the kind of which I have spoken, derived from the constitution and

---

* See HAHN. MONTHLY for March, 1895, and REVUE, HOM. BELGE, April, 1887.

temperament of the patient, his mental state, the "conditions" of his sufferings, the side of his body affected, the times of day at which he is worse, are derived from the USUS IN MORBIS only, as also are large part of the "characteristics" I have described as so much relied on by a number of our practitioners. One result of this is the development of a new kind of Materia Medica amongst us. Hahnemann applied this name only to "a record of what medicines express concerning their true mode of action in the symptoms they PRODUCE in the human body." In the compilations, however, of Jahr, Bœnninghausen, Hering, Lippe, Cowperthwaite, Gentry, Clarke and others, these pathogenetic effects are mingled (often without note of distinction) with symptoms which have been reported as disappearing under the medicinal use of the drugs. There is no objection to this, so long as they are understood to be what they are, and are not (as too often) quoted in proof of the Homœopathicity of remedies; so long, also, as their use is not held up as a pure following of the method of Hahnemann. It is a supplementing of that method by empirical practice, which, however necessary, in this rough work-a-day world, is not to be vaunted as a matter for pride, but rather to be excused as a concession to the weakness to our nature.

The real justification of such proceedings is, that they lead to the Homœopathic remedy where the ordinary paths thereto are wanting; and in this instance, at least, the end justifies the means. It is for that reason that I have taken so much pains at previous meetings, to characterise these agents in their own essential nature, apart from the mode of reaching them. That we have an assured one in the rule SIMILIA SIMILIBUS; that we are not left to chance for their turning up or to blind experience for their perpetuation, is our claim and our satisfaction. But when they are reached otherwise than by pure inference from pathogenesy—by mixed methods or even by the merest empiricism, they still have features by which we can recognise them; and we feel at home in their employment We are not prescribing Homœopathically; but we may be employing a Homœopathic remedy.

LECTURE IX.

THE ADMINISTRATION OF THE SIMILAR REMEDY

We have now obtained our similar remedy, and have only to consider how to administer it. As we divided its elements of similarity into generic, specific and individual, so let us say that it should be administered, as a rule, singly, rarely, constitutionally and minutely. The first three of these points will occupy our attention today.

1. Hahnemann very early came to entertain a strong aversion to the polypharmacy so prevalent in his day. In the Essay of 1797—"Are the Obstacles to Simplicity and Certainty in Practical Medicine insurmountable?"—one of his main points was the impossibility of obtaining definite results unless remedies were given singly; and of his own practice at this time he writes (in words I have already cited)—"Dare I confess that for many years I have never prescribed anything but a single medicine at once, and have never repeated the dose until the action of the former one had ceased; a venesection alone, a purgative alone, and always a simple, never a compound, remedy, and never a second until I had got a clear notion of the operation of the first?"

In so acting, he was surely before his own time, and even the practitioners of this enlightened day have hardly risen to his level. The Theriaca and Mithridate of our ancestors, with their sixty-five and fifty ingredients respectively, had indeed become obsolete before the beginning of this century. But the PHARMACOLOGIA of Dr. Paris, the leading English treatise on medicines from 1812 to 1843, had for its avowed object (as Dr. Sharp has shown) to expound the "theory and art of medicinal combination," and it opens with the sentence—"It is a truth universally admitted that the arm of physic has derived much additional power and increased energy from the resources which are furnished by the mixture and combination of medicinal bodies."

That polypharmacy is not yet extinct will appear from the

following monstrous prescription for a case of Paraplegia, which I copy from the manuscript of a Glasgow physician:—

R. Strychniæ, gr. 1/6	Sol : Mur : Morph ; 3 j.
Liq : Arsenicalis, gtt. xxxvi.	Sp : Chloroform : 3 iij.
Ammon : carb : 3 iss.	Æth : Sulph : 8 iij.
Ferr : citr : ammon : gr. cxxxii.	Ext : Ergot : liq : 3 viij.
Potass : iodid : 3 ij.	Tinct : Cinch : Co : 3 viij.
Potass : brom : 3 vss.	Glycerin, 3 viij.

Infus : Quassiæ ad 3 vj. I

Ft. Mist. : cujus capiat cochl. magn. ter in die, I may mention in passing that the morbid state, which this charge of grapeshot failed to scatter, was much diminished in force by the single bullet of an attenuation of *Picric acid*.

In contrast to all this, Homœopathy has—like its founder—"dared to confess" that the single remedy has always been the rule in its hand. When we say "single," it must of course be understood that we do not exclude the use of chemical compounds—like the **salts**—or of vegetable products, as *Opium*, which analysis may find of complex constitution. If we know their Physiological effects as simples, then as simples they can be employed. We may even, though cautiously, go further, and administer compounds where we are only acquainted with the action on the healthy of their separate elements. In this way we have made good use of the *Iodide* and *Arseniate of Calcium*, of the *Phosphide of Zinc* and the *Picrate of Iron*. But when we are urged to go further, and to combine in one prescription two drugs of known action, but incapable of entering into chemical combination, we must pause ere we assent. This was the proposal of two of Hahnemann's immediate disciples—Lutze and Ægidi, and almost (it is said) secured the Master's own expressed approval. I am far from saying that such mixtures would be ineffective ; but their use would be fatal to the simplicity of the Homœopathic method, and would embark us once more on the confused and unscientific polypharmacy from which we have so happily escaped. Still more strongly does this apply to the complex blendings of our remedies lately advocated by Drs. Pinella and Conan. All good purpose to be served by such combinations can be better obtained by the successive, or—if need be—the alternate, administration of their component drugs.

This matter of alteration requires some fuller treatment here. In the 'Organon', Hahnemann from the first deprecated it, on the ground of the possible interference of the two drugs one with another. In the last Edition he disallows it on another ground. "If" he writes, (§ 169, 170) "on the first examination of a disease and the first selection of a medicine, we should find that the totality of the symptoms of the disease would not be sufficiently covered by the disease-elements of a single medicine —owing to the insufficient number of known medicines, but that two medicines contend for the preference in point of appropriateness, one of which is more Homœopathically suitable for one part, the other for another part of the symptoms of the disease, it is not advisable, after the employment of the more suitable of the two medicines to administer the other without fresh examination, for the medicine that seemed to be the next best might not, under the change of circumstances that has in the mean time taken place, be suitable for the rest of the symptoms that then remain; in which case consequently, a more appropriate Homœopathic remedy must be selected in place of the second medicine, for the set of symptoms as they appear on a new inspection. Hence, in this as in every case where a change of the morbid state has occurred, the remaining set of symptoms now present must be enquired into, and (without paying any attention to the medicine which at first appeared to be the next in point of suitableness) another Homœopathic medicine, as appropriate as possible to the new state now before us, must be selected. If it should so happen (as it seldom does) that the medicine which at first appeared to be the next best seems still to be well-adapted for the morbid state that remains, so much the more will it merit our confidence, and deserve to be employed in preference to another."

Now, if we had no knowledge of disease but that which consists in the survey of the symptoms of each case as it occurs, there could be no doubt of this being the ideal Homœopathy. But I have already argued that in this region we are CLERI, and not LAICI, and must utilise our special acquaintance with the subject. Hahnemann admits that the second remedy MAY prove to be that which at first seemed almost equally indicated; why should not the skilled physician be able to recognise the cases where it will be so, and prescribe it at once accordingly? Again, all recognise that the alteration is often led to A POSTERIORI—that fresh examinations of the patient's case point now to one, now to another of the two or more remedies which first occurred to us in connection with it. Why may not the physician equally anticipate here, and so provide for cases where frequent inspection is impracticable or unadvisable? It is the existence of real species of disease which enables him to do this; and Hahnemann, who had a full sense of their existence, was practically an alternator, or at any rate an A PRIORI prescriber of successions, in many of them. Thus, in Croup, he tells us always to precede *Spongia* by *Aconite*, and sometimes to follow it up by *Hepar sulphuris*—a practice which one of his most liege disciples, von Bœnninghausen, created into a system, giving to all cases five powders in succession containing respectively *Aconite, Spongia, Hepar, Spongia, Hepar,* in this order. In Purpura miliaris he advised the alternation of *Aconite* and *Coffea,* giving indeed the indications for each, but saying that one or other should be given according to these every twelve, sixteen, or twenty-four hours. Of Cholera, he writes,—"The best Homœopathic practitioners have found *Cuprum* indispensable in the second stage of the fully-developed disease, alternated, if the symptoms indicates this, with *Veratrum album.* I have also advised the alternation of these two substances from week to week as a preventive against the disease." And no less plainly does he say of the Post-choleraic Fever—"in this *Bryonia,* alternately with *Rhus toxicodendron,* proves of eminent service." These are acute diseases; but as regards chronic ones of fixed character, the first three Editions of the 'Organon' recognise the occasional necessity of alternation in these, and the Second and Third speak of the absolute impossibility of doing without it in complicated maladies— instancing, in the Second, the use of *Mercury* and *Sulphur* when Syphilis and Psora coincide, in the Third, the addition of *Thuja* or *Nitric acid* when Sycosis also is present. And in the last Edition, when contemplating the possibility of having to repeat *Sulphur* many times, he advises the occasional interposition of doses of *Hepar sulphuris.*

Dr. Dudgeon has shown us that in this occasional use of the practice of alternation, Hahnemann was followed by many of his foremost disciples, among whom I may mention Hering, Gross, Rummel, Hartmann, Ægidi and Hirsch. It is now largely adopted among Homœopathists; and is defended, by some as an expedient, by others on Philosophical grounds. Of the latter the most prominent are our own Drysdale and Russell, and Drs. Martiny and Bernard of Belgium, who contributed an elaborate essay on the subject to the Transactions of the International Homœopathic Convention of 1881. Dr. Drysdale, after showing that no interference of action need be feared unless the two medicines are (Homœopathic) antidotes, proceeds to argue that an alternate remedy may revive the susceptibility which would otherwise tend to be exhausted, illustrating this by the well-known laws of the re-action of the retina to colours. Dr. Russel, proving that even specific morbid processes—as Typhus and Variola—may concur, suggests that much disease is similarly, though not so palpably, complex and that by judicious alternation we enhance our power for good, and raise the melody of our practice to harmony. Our Belgian colleagues rest their thesis mainly on the practical value of the proceeding, in favour of which they cite many authorities and examples; but they argue that "the medicines alternated act sometimes as useful auxiliaries, sometimes as correctives of each other, sometimes by forming a sort of new remedy, sometimes by drawing out in various ways the re-actions of the organism to make them converge to a cure."

The only formidable opponent of alternation in later times has been Carroll Dunham. In a series of papers (which also you will find in the posthumous volume of his, entitled "Homœopathy, the Science of Therapeutics") he discusses the practice at some length, and disposes—as he thinks—of the arguments alleged in its support. But it is evident that with him every case of disease is an unity, a manifestation of a simple derangement of a central "vital force"; whereas, as Dr. Drysdale has well-shewn, it is by no means always so, several centres of morbid action often co-existing. Dunham, moreover, allows that the A POSTERIORI alternation, which of course is legitimate, may be foreseen and prescribed A PRIORI, as with Bœnninghausen's powders; and this covers a great many of the ordinary instances of its use.

My own views on the subject are, briefly, these:—I earnestly deprecate the slip-shod practice of habitually alternating, so that when you mix medicines in your patients' houses two glasses are brought for you as a matter of course. I further believe that in many cases in which we most of us alternate, a third medicine might be found which should cover the whole case, as we often supersede two opposite half-truths by some deeper whole truth which embraces them both. But I am persuaded that there may be a real "binary Homœopathy"— to use illustrations of Dr. Madden's double stars in the firmament of medicine, compounds which are themselves radicals in therapeutic Chemistry. To arrive at these with certainty, medicines should undoubtedly be proved in alternation; but even in lack of such evidence inferences can be formed as to their relative and joint action. I would further urge that in definite diseases the presence of urgent complications is better met by alternation than by change of remedy—that, *e. g.*, *Mercurius corrosivus* should be continued throughout Dysentery and *Aconite* as long as the fever of Measles lasts, though Colic, Tenesmus, Cough or Ophthalmia should require other medicines concomitantly. Beyond this I have not myself gone at present and the single remedy is entirely the rule in my practice: but I am not indisposed to listen to the suggestions of Drs. Martiny and Bernard in favour of a wider and more methodical use of medicinal groups in the management of complex cases.

II. The second rule for the administration of the similar remedy is that it should be given RARELY. You will remember that Hahnemann, speaking in 1796 of the monopharmacy of his practice for some time then past, adds, "and I have never repeated the dose until the action of the former one had ceased." The single dose, as well as the single medicine, continued to be his ideal for many years thereafter. The two cases I have already related, given by him in 1816 as illustrations of Homœopathic practice, exhibit this feature, and so do all others mentioned in his writings up to 1833. When giving practical instructions, as in the "Medicine of Experience" and the 'Organon,' he lays it down that a second dose should only be given when the action of the first is exhausted. That this point had been reached he at first proposed to determine by ascertaining the duration of each drug's action. But in the First Edition of the 'Organon' he substituted for this rule, as based on an uncertain quantity, another which direct that the manifest effects of the first dose should be allowed to subside ere a second, if necessary, was given. In the recommendations about medicines given in the prefaces and notes of the REINE ARZNEIMITTELLEHRE we find this principle constantly recognised. Suddenly, however, in the 'Organon' of 1833 a complete change appears. The waiting for a dose to exhaust its action is declared needlessly to delay the cure, and more frequent repetitions are counselled, at intervals to be determined A PRIORI and with regard rather to the disease than to the drug.

In this instance Hahnemann's later views have been adopted by the more liberal school of Homœopathists, while those who call themselves peculiarly by his name lean rather to his earlier practice. These, however, do not reject the use of frequently repeated doses in hyper-acute diseases such as Cholera; while, on the other hand, their more advanced colleagues feel the influence of the older mode of practice. There are few of us, I suppose, who do not sometimes, when a medicine has declared its influence, pause for awhile, and allow it to act; and I can myself testify to the value of the plan illustrated especially by the practice of our French colleagues, of intercalating days of repose when a drug has to be taken for a length of time. Professor Hoppe, of Basle, in an ingenious paper which you will find in the Twentieth Volume of the BRITISH JOURNAL OF HOMŒOPATHY, shows how—in recent diseases—a single medicinal impression may well be conceived of as rectifying the disordered balance, and setting going the processes which lead back to health.

I think that the action of single doses in disease has hardly been sufficiently studied,* and that it might derive more light than it has done from the provings of medicines. We know

---

* A good illustration of their value is furnished by Dr. Stens, in a cough of six months' standing, in which, malady and patient calling clearly for *Bryonia* the drug was nevertheless ineffective in both high and low potencies giving in the usual way. A drop of the mother tincture was taken one evening on retiring. By next morning the cough had taken its departure and it did not return. (See HOM. RECORDER, April, 1894).

that there it makes a great difference how we proceed, whether, giving a single full dose, or—which is the same thing—a succession of smaller doses till some effect is produced, we watch the results until their complete subsidence, or whether we keep the subject of experiment under the continual influence of the drug by doses repeated at regular intervals for some space of time. The former plan produces effects which in their regular evolution resemble the course of acute disease: The latter gives rise to the numerous, varied, and apparently incoherent phenomena of chronic disorder. In therapeutics, accordingly, there seems no reason why single doses should not neutralise so much of the disturbance of a recent malady that the remainder might readily undergo resolution. We have an instance of this being done in the use of *Hyoscyamine* in Mania advocated by Dr. Lawson. He gave a grain of the alkaloid once for all, and the artificial mental disorder thus induced dissipated to a large extent the existing one, and left the patient comparatively same.*

In all probability the determining indication for single or repeated dosage is the amount of re-action of which the patient is capable. If this is deficient, you may redouble your medicinal impressions without stint : It it is excessive, you must hold your hand. I am inclined to agree with a recent French writer that we make too little of this—that we ply our patients with medicines till we fret their morbid condition into renewed and accelerated activity. We are not afraid, like our old school friends, of saturating their systems with drug-material, but we do not consider the dynamic disturbance we may set up by repeated drug-action. We are sending an ever-fresh series of vibrations throbbing through the frame, and may shake its delicate machinery out of gear and exhaust its capacity of vital response. I have often been struck by the rapid course taken by cases of hopeless disease, especially of Phthisis, when Homœopathic treatment has been tried as a DERNIER RESSORT. Since it could not save them, there has been little to regret in this; but it would not be justifiable practice if we knew it.

On all these grounds, then, I would emphasize our present rule, and say—whenever the case admits of it, give the similar remedy RARELY.

The foregoing was the advice I gave to my class at the London School of Homœopathy in 1880-3, and it represents my views and practice since. The subject has been re-opened lately by one of our most original therapeutists, Dr. Robert Cooper, in a manner which deserves attention. In a series of

* West Riding Lunatic Asylum Medical Reports, Vol. v. (1875), p. 40.

Articles in journals and separate publications dating from about 1893, he has advocated and illustrated the treatment of chronic disease by what he calls "arbori-vital" medication. This consists in the use of the freshest possible preparations of plants, and the administration of these in material but single doses allowed to act for a length of time. The principle of the selection of the plants is implied to be Homœopathic; though Dr. Cooper employs a number of them hitherto unknown to medicine and certainly unproved on the healthy body, and gives no reason for their choice.

Dr. Cooper's pharmacy is obviously in the right direction; his posology will be grateful to many of us; and his single-dose method is a reversion to Hahnemann's earlier mode of proceeding which I have already urged as worthy of cultivation. His results, in many instances, merit the most respectful attention. I cannot, however, follow him in the theory by which he justifies his practice—comparing, as he does, the effects on the body of the administration of a dose of plant-juice with the germination of plant-seed when sown in the earth. Neither can I see any fruitfulness in the apparent hap-hazard or at best single-symptom similarity by which he selects his medicines. I do not think that he will induce us to use vegetable medicines only, any more than Schussler has persuaded us to employ none but salts of minerals. Few, if any, will be found among the profession to accept arbori-vitalism, as few, if any, have accepted Bio-chemistry, as a dominating working theory; but we shall have to thank the authors of these schemes for many a valuable remedy and mode of procedure.

3. The similar remedy is to be administered singly and rarely; it is also to be given CONSTITUTIONALLY. It is chosen from the correspondence of the totality of its symptoms with those of the patient, that it may embrace his whole malady. It must, therefore, therapeutically as pathogenetically be taken into the system. Its mode of entrance is comparatively unimportant. This may be the olfaction of Hahnemann's practice at one time, or the hypodermic injection advocated for occasional use by Kafka: It may consist in absorption from the cutaneous surface or through the rectal mucous membrane. Ingestion through the mouth into the stomach is ordinarily most convenient, and forms our usual method.

But are local applications never desirable in Homœopathic practice? The answer to this question must occupy us for some little time.

At the British Homœopathic Congress of 1878, Dr. Dyce Brown read a paper "On the Use of External Applications in

Homœopathic Practice." * It grew out of a recommendation of his to the students of London School of Homœopathy, that in obstinate cases of Follicular Pharyngitis they should swab the throat with a solution of *Nitrate of Silver,* which—being printed in the MONTHLY HOMŒOPATHIC REVIEW—had been severely criticised by the stricter practitioners amongst us. He did not succeed in disarming their opposition, and Dr. Fenton Cameron, among others, several times expressed himself very adversely to the employment of such measures. Dr. Gregg, of Buffalo, U.S., had for some time previously been publishing in the HOMŒOPATHIC TIMES a series of articles on the subject, in which he goes still further than Dr. Cameron in condemning all local measures; while in the BULLETIN of the Societe Medicale Homœopathique de France for June, 1878, Dr. Hammelrath makes as decided a departure in the other direction, advocating the direct application of the medicine which is being given internally, whenever this measure is practicable.

You thus have plenty of material from which to build up your own thoughts on the subject. I would aid you by enquiring, regarding local application of remedies, first, "Is it Homœopathic?" "Does it conform to that method of Hahnemann which I am now expounding?" and secondly, 'Whether it is so or not, is the practice necessary, or at any rate advantageous?'

Now, when we have to inquire as to the conformity of any therapeutic procedure to the method of Hahnemann, it is obvious that Hahnemann's own doctrine and practice on the subject—is ascertainable—must have great weight in our determination. It is not decisive, for he like other men was fallible; but it counts for a great deal. I think that Dr. Brown makes too much of the Master's opposition to local applications when he says that he "strongly discouraged, or rather forbade, the use of any external treatment whatever." In the last edition of the 'Organon' (§ 205) he does, indeed, speak to that effect; but only with reference to the manifestation of constitutional infection, whether primary or secondary. His objection to any local interference with these rests on the Pathological ground, that thereby the natural evolution of the malady is checked, and its force either diverted to other and, perhaps, more important organs, or so pent up in the system as to be a source of continued ill-health and recurring complaints. Of course, believing as he did that all chronic disease not traceable to unhealthy living or medicinal poisoning was due either to Psora, to Syphilis, or to Sycosis, his objection to local applications held good for most maladies of long-standing. But it makes nothing in relation to acute diseases, or to non-miasmatic chronic affections;

* See H. H. R., Dec., 1878.

and even admits of exceptions in its own sphere, as we shall see immediately. We must inquire further, therefore, for Hahnemann's general views on this matter.

Dr. Dudgeon, in his Lectures (pp. 516 and 565), mentions two exceptions as made by Hahnemann to his general rejection of topical applications. These were the use of *Arnica*, of *Rhus*, and of *Arsenicum* or heated *Alcohol* for Bruises, Strains, and Burns respectively, and of *Thuja*, for old Condylomata. He shows, indeed, that in earlier times he availed himself more largely of such measures, but these he retained up to the last (1830-5). What, then, is the rationale of the applications now specified?

1. Bruises, Strains and Burns are local injuries, which may occur in an otherwise healthy person. They are PRIMARILY local, only affect the general system—if at all—secondarily and by way of sympathy. It is rational, therefore, to treat them locally, whether by medicinal agents specifically adapted to the changes the parts have undergone or (as with burns) by a Homœopathic application of temperature. The reason, I take it, why Hahnemann was content with topical treatment here, but eschewed it elsewhere, was his persuasion of the necessity of covering the totality of the symptoms, and making the medicinal action correspondent to that of the malady. All true disease, he believed (as distinct from external injury), proceeded from within —from a primary derangement of the "vital force." The Pathogenetic action of medicines was similarly induced when these were introduced into the body; and hence the precept SIMILIA SIMILIBUS CURENTUR could only be fully obeyed when the drug corresponding to the patient's morbid state was internally administered. He says nothing anywhere that I know of in condemnation of a conjoint internal and local use of the Homœopathic remedy, but seems to have been so satisfied with the former that the question of the need of the latter hardly occurred to his mind.

2. The application of *Thuja* to Condylomata seems quite another thing, and Dr. Dudgeon characterises it as a departure on Hahnemann's part from his avowed principles. But let us consider the exact terms of his recommendation. In the introductory essay to his treatise on 'Chronic Diseases' (at p. 106 of the first part of the Second Edition, 1835), after recommending the internal administration of *Thuja* 30 and *Nitric acid* 6 he goes on:—'This will suffice to remove both Gonorrhœa and Condylomata, *i. e.*, the whole Sycosis, without its being necessary to apply anything of an external character, save, in the most ancient and stubborn cases, the touching of the larger Figwarts once a day with the mild pure juice (mixed with equal parts of *Alcohol*) expressed from the green leaves of the arbor vitæ." I

think there can be no doubt of his meaning here being that he regarded these "old and stubborn" Figwarts as well-nigh extra-vital things, remaining behind after the whole internal malady —"the entire Sycosis"—had been cured. They were dead results of a past process, withered fruits of a germination which had ceased to proceed; they had no root in the system, and could not be reached from within, and were, therefore, best dealt with by the local application of the remedy. This, it is important to observe, is to be carried out with the mother-tincture, while for internal use a high attenuation is recommended. The infinite-simal dose was in Hahnemann's eyes most suitable to the dynamic process—the crude drug to its material results. It is ano-ther illustration of the same view when he says (in 1801),* "In cases where, along with a local affection, the general health seems to be good, we must proceed first from the small doses to larger ones." I think that on this principle we can explain how it is that the substantial quantities of *Arsenic* given in the old school cure without much aggravation the many forms of chronic cutaneous disease to which the drug is so perfectly Homœo-pathic. The patients thus affected are generally otherwise in good health. In this case, you cannot—as with Condylomata apply the "larger dose" locally; but you carry out the same thought when you administer it internally, leaving it to reach the skin by elective affinity.

The conclusion seems to be that Hahnemann's only objection to local applications arose from their failing in most cases to cover the totality of the symptoms. When the affection was local from the first, or had become so secondarily, he was entirely in favour of the topical use of the indicated remedy, and this in doses far more substantial than those he recommended for internal administra-tion.

I think that we need hardly go further in our inquiry. Local applications, under certain circumstances, are Homœopathic upon Hahnemann's own showing: We need not ask whether they are so inspite of his contrary judgment, or whether, not being so, they are nevertheless to be employed. The only question that remains is, how far do the local applications in ordinary use among (so-called) Homœopathic practitioners conform to Hahne-mann's canons?

As affections local from the first in which we employ them a good many may be ranked. There are the Bruises, Strains and Burns already mentioned, to which we may add—as of like character—Wounds and Stings. There are then several forms of Conjunctivitis, and especially the various kinds of purulent

Lesser Writings (Dudgeon's transl.) p. 446.

Ophthalmia, all of which seem to be due of the actual contact of virulent matter with the eye. Malignant Pustule is often caused by inoculation at the spot affected, and involves the constitution secondarily : Stomatitis, Œsophagitis and Gastritis set up by irritant poisoning belong to the same category, and several affections of the skin due to external irritations. Whatever we can do in all these instances by the local application of medicines Homœopathic to them, we are doing according to the method of Hahnemann.

A still wider sphere is open to us when we look for lesions which, at first the product of some internal malady, have now become local only. Almost all chronic inflammations of skin and mucous membrane, which are of fixed area and of unvarying persistence, find place here. Such are Granular Ophthalmia, with its Pannus; and other forms of chronic Conjunctivitis ; chronic Otorrhœa : Ozæna ; chronic Laryngitis ; Winter-cough, with dyspnœa (*i.e.*, chronic Bronchitis, with thickening of mucous membrane) : Gleet, Ulceration of the Cervix Uteri and many local Eczemas, as of the ears and scrotum, with other cutaneous affections. These morbid patches have often become as nearly extravital and as purely local as Hahnemann's old Condylomata, and require topical treatment accordingly. Without it, indeed, they will rarely get well. In this same category might sometimes be ranged the Follicular Pharyngitis, the recommendation of *Nitrate of Silver* applications for which by Dr. Brown has caused so much disturbance in certain minds. But here we are on less certain ground, as this lesion is often a symptomatic affection only—the gouty, hæmorrhoidal, or herpetic diathesis lying in the background. It will generally, I think, be our wisdom to treat it mainly by internal medication, even though in obstinate cases we conjoin topical measures.

We are thus led to the question whether, even in local affections having a constitutional root, we do not act wisely in bringing our remedies to bear directly upon them, where practicable, while covering the totality of the symptoms by giving them internally at the same time. Dr. Dudgeon quotes several Homœopathic authorities in favour of a limited use of this method, —among them Gross, who is found recommending *Lachesis*. *Silicea* and *Rhus* as external applicants to Ulcers of the Leg. But this practice has now been advocated and carried out on a very extensive scale by Dr. Hammelrath. In the communication to which I have referred, he has told us how he has brought it to bear wherever available, using always the same remedy locally which, upon Homœopathic principles, was being given internally. He began with affections of the eyes, and was (he says) "astonished at the results which he obtained." He then went on to affections of other parts, as the ears, the nares, the mouth, and the ano-genital region: And had the same markedly increased success as compared with that which he had previously gained from internal treatment alone. He commonly employed the remedies locally in the first trituration or (aqueous) dilution, adding lard or water as required.

I think that such practice deserves further consideration and trial; * and that, although we have not Hahnemann's example or precept in its favour, it is in entire conformity with the spirit of his method. What then shall we say to Dr. Gregg, who denounces all local measures, even to the pulling out of an aching tooth or the poulticing of a Gumboil? I think it is quite possible to agree with him also in substance, though we cannot follow him into all the details through which he would carry us. The arguments and facts he brings forward relate to violent repressive measures—cauterisations and such like, and to morbid states in which the possibility of metastasis exists. In such maladies and by such means topical treatment is indeed to be condemned; and it is one of the great benefits conveyed by Homœopathy that its practitioners have always set their faces against it. How many affection of the brain, eyes and ears have resulted in children from the forcible suppression of eruptions on the head! and from how many have we saved them by our invariable practice of curing such eruptions from within!

But this brings us to the question of the NATURE of our local application. Hitherto those we have had before us have been chiefly such as consist of the drugs internally Homœopathic to the malady present, *i.e.*, capable of producing something like it from within. Such is the relation of *Arnica* to Bruises, of *Rhus* to Strains, of *Arsenicum* to Burns, and of *Thuja* to Condylomata; to the same class belong the topical applications of Gross and of Hammelrath. But Dr. Brown would carry us further. He would embrace in his means of treatment remedies locally Homœopathic to the lesion, *i.e.*, capable of inducing its SIMILE when externally applied, and thus only. He would take up the words of Trousseau (which I have already cited): 'The primary effect of *Nitrate of Silver* and similar agents is analogous to that produced by inflammation, and it was easy to understand that inflammation artificially induced in tissues already the seat of inflammation led to a cure of the original inflammatory attack. When the view was once acquired, there flowed from it the great therapeutical principle of SUBSTITUTION which, at present, reigns supreme in medical practice." Re-

---

* Dr. J. S. Mitchell's result with *Arsenical* triturations, locally applied as well as internally administered, in malignant ulcerations are favourable illustrations of its value (see NEW ENGL. MED. GAZETTE July, 1895).

place (as Trousseau himself warrants us in doing) "substitution" by "Homœopathy," and (Dr. Brown says) we have the justification of any topical treatment of this kind which we may find desirable.

I do not see how his position can be controverted, so long as he deals with lesions primarily or secondarily local only. *Cantharis* is Homœopathic to a Burn or Scald, because its external employment causes similar inflammation and vesication, not because of any symptoms resulting from its internal use. Yet it is Homœopathic, and its curative action is undoubted and most satisfactory. The same drug, employed as a blister, if applied to the thorax of a healthy animal produces a patch of inflammation in the subjacent pleura. Though we had no evidence of its power to cause Pleurisy when taken by the mouth we should not be quite justified in claiming for Homœopathy any benefit which blistering can produce in this malady. Similar reasoning may be used in all cases in which a local irritant is applied to cure a local inflammation.

But I cannot go with Dr. Brown when he attempts to explain the rationale of the process, and upon the basis of the theory propounded to advocate the use of other applications, not provedly Homœopathic to the case. He supposes that irritants act by causing primary contraction and secondary dilatation of the bloodvessels, and that, when applied in moderate strength to an inflamed part, they induce their primary influence only upon it, contracting its vessels, and so reducing its hyperæmia. Any substance or agent, therefore—as temperature or astringent drugs—which can contract the vessel is suitable for the purpose, and is presumably Homœopathic to the mischief; for, if it, can primarily contract, it can secondarily dilate. I have more than once given my reasons for believing that this is a very imperfect account both of inflammation and of the action of irritants; and I cannot think that we are warranted in assuming its truth and acting upon it. I would remind Dr. Brown of what Dr. Drysdale had said about "substitutive" treatment: "The cure also is only partial, and consists most probably in mere constriction of the capillaries without removal of the other elements of the morbid process, for dilatation of the capillaries or mere hyperæmia does not of itself constitute inflammation, as is well shown by Virchow, although it is essential to the manifestation of all the prominent symptoms."*

I cannot, moreover, assent to the explanation which would resolve all the effects of hot and cold applications into similar changes in the calibre of the small vessels. Cold has its own

---

* B. J. H., xxvii, 500.

physical effect in robbing an inflamed part of its preternatural heat, which should be taken into account; and such pleasant warmth as is ordinarily applied in poultices than fomentations rather relaxes the muscular coats of the arteries that contracts them, as any one can see by applying a hot sponge to the surface of his body. It probably does this by raising the whole vital energy of the part, and so inducing a fuller afflux of blood to it. I must urge my esteemed colleague to look a little beyond nerves and blood-vessels in his explanations of Pathological conditions and Pathogenetic effects, if he would satisfy all the requirements of the case.*

These, gentlemen, are the views I would impress upon you on the subject of local applications. They do not, as you will have perceived, involve the advocacy of any indiscriminate use of such measures: They are, indeed, only an extension of the principles laid down by Hahnemann himself, and an application of them to instances beyond the range of his recorded perception. They should not, therefore, I submit, receive the condemnation of the most devoted follower of the Master; and the practice to which they lead should not be stigmatized as any departure from the method he has bequeathed to us.

* Holding the views above expressed as to the superiority of constitutional over local treatment, it may be imagined that I hailed with warm welcome Sir Felix Semon's lectures (BRIT. MED. JOURN., Nov. 2nd and 9th, 1901) on the subject, which appeared while this sheet was going through the press. Sir Felix points to the established treatment of Syphilitic lesions, and the recently introduced serum-therapy of Diphtheria, as shewing how victoriously topical treatment may be superseded by general, and he hopes for a similar change to be wrought by the judicious use of *Tuberculin*—of which in our hands the following pages will show many an example.

LECTURE X.

THE ADMINISTRATION OF THE SIMILAR REMEDY
(*continued*)

We have seen how the remedy arrived at by the Law of Similars is to be administered, as a rule, singly, rarely and constitutionally. We have today to consider the precept that it be given MINUTELY; and in so speaking we raise the whole question—truly a QUÆSTIO VEXATA— of the Homœopathic dose.

I have already touched upon this subject more than once. In defining at the outset what, in its essence, Homœopathy is, I included in the statement the provision that its remedies should be given "in doses too small to excite aggravation or collateral disturbance"; and I endeavoured to shew the reasonableness and advantage of such a requirement. In lecturing on the 'Organon' I went a step further. I shewed that even in its Second Edition, Hahnemann had come to occasionally recommending infinitesimals—thousandths, millionths, and yet higher fractions of a grain; and that from the Third Edition onwards he had propounded a theory (that of dynamisation) to account for their efficacy when prepared according to his directions. I did not disguise my conviction that, whatever be the value of the theory (as propounded by him), the practice was a distinct step in advance, a discovery well-tested and fruitful. I cautioned you, however, against viewing it as of the essence of Homœopathy. The small dose is a logical consequence of the Law of Similars; infinitesimals belong to it historically only.

Historically, however, they do belong to it; and you will justly expect me to give you some information and guidance about them here. I will not go again over the ground traversed in the Lecture (VII) on "Homœopathic Posology" which you will find among the preliminary matter of my "Pharmacodynamics.' But, referring to or summarising this as may be needful, I will endeavour to lay before you the past and present of the subject, and to give you some suggestions for wise thought and action about it.

When Hahnemann first began to prescribe medicines according to the rule SIMILIA SIMILIBUS, he gave them in the usual quantities.

THE ADMINISTRATION OF THE SIMILAR REMEDY 123

It is not surprising that his patients' symptoms, even though ultimately removed, were often in the first instance severely aggravated. It needs no argument to shew that the ordinary doses of *Arsenic*, against which even a healthy stomach needs to be shielded by its administration after meals, would increase the irritation of one already inflamed—for which, nevertheless, the Homœopathic principle would direct its being given. So Hahnemann found, and he reduced his doses accordingly. At what stage of this reduction he found that fractional quantities of a smallness (hitherto undreamt of) exercised a potent influence, we cannot say. If you will read the Article on "Hahnemann's Dosage" which I have reprinted as an Appendix to my 'Pharmacodynamics' you will see that the transition was made, somewhat PER SALTUM, between 1798 and 1799. It only then took him as far as ten-thousandths and millionths, and it is not till 1809 that we find him using higher fractions than these. But from the trillionths and sextillionths arrived at then we see him in 1816 mounting in the case of *Arsenic* to decillionths, in which finally, in 1829, he (for the sake of uniformity) advised all Homœopathic remedies to be given. To make such solutions he devised a graduated attenuation which after some variations, settled down upon a centesimal scale. The first dilution was made to contain one part of the drug in a hundred of vehicle. This was done for dry plants, which were treated with twenty parts of *Alcohol* for a given time, by adding eighty parts more subsequently. The tinctures prepared from fresh plants by mixing their expressed juice with equal parts of *Spirit* were to be considered as of half-strength, so that 2 drops were to be added to 98 of *Alcohol* to make their first dilution. Henceforward, the attenuation was to be carried on through successive phials by adding 1 part of the first to 99 more to make the third, and so on; from which it will be seen that in his final decillionths Hahnemann had reached the 30th degree of the scale adopted. In the case of insolubles like the metals, attenuation was obtained by adding to a grain of the substance 99 grains of Sugar of Milk, and after trituration in a mortar sufficient to ensure thorough admixture adding a grain of the product to 99 more grains of the vehicle. This process might of course be continued indefinitely, but Hahnemann saw reason to believe that after the third degree the substance treated became practically soluble; he accordingly directed the fourth attenuation to be prepared with water, the fifth with equal parts of water and Spirit, and the sixth and upwards with pure Spirit—all in the proportion of one part in a hundred.

With the exception of a suggestion in the Preface to the proving of *Thuja* that such a drug might be with advantage raised even to the 50th, and in a statement in the Fifth Edition of the 'Organon' that the 60th, 150th, and 300th potencies displayed more rapid and penetrating, though shorter, action than the 30th, Hahnemann seems to have kept himself to the latter as an ultimatum. Some of his disciples, however, were not content with this. They pushed on until the exalted region into which the Master had looked but seldom entered, became their habitual dwelling-place, and from thence they mounted higher and even higher. You will find an account of the doings of these "high-potency men" in Dr. Dudgeon's Lectures. They have nearly died out in Germany, and have found very few representatives in France or England. But in America the school has taken a fresh lease of life. With a number of practitioners there the 200th is considered a low potency, suited for common use; while the 1000th forms a new unit from which to start, and we hear of cures being wrought by the millionth.

I must advise you to reject these preparations, not so much upon the grounds of science and reason as upon those of pharmacy. They are simple impossibilities. It has been calculated that to make the millionth potency of a single medicine according to Hahnemann's instructions would require 2,000 gallons of *Alcohol*, and would occupy more than a year in the process. Whenever, accordingly, we are able to learn the manner in which these preparations are made (and the tendency is to keep it a secret), we always find it other than that recognised among us, and illegitimate in itself. Jenichen's, which first broke ground in the new field, are now known to be simply succussions of an ordinary attenuation with only occasional dilution—so many shakes being reckoned as producing a potency one step higher in the scale. Korsakoffs contact potencies need only to be mentioned to be rejected. The preparations which go under the names of Fincke and Swan are made by what is called "fluxion." A stream of water is allowed to flow in and out of a vessel holding a fixed quantity, which is previously filled with a given dilution of a drug. This is supposed to be further attenuated according to the quantity of water which passes through the vessel, or according to the time required for a certain fixed quantity of water to pass. In Dr. Swan's method a "perturbation more violent than succussion" is superadded by letting the water pass through a finely perforated tube into the potentising vessel. The question at once arises—does this continuous "displacement" effect attenuation in the Hahnemannian proportions? Tests with *Eosine* have answered it in the negative; and in Dr. Swan's case a further error has been made in confounding addition with multiplication, so that his millionth comes to equal Hahnemann's tenth! Dr. Fincke's process does not come quite so badly off, but it has been found to give "unesimal" dilutions instead of centesimal, so that his 1000th is Hahnemann's 151st. Dr. Skinner, who has done much in exposing the unreality of his colleagues' preparations, thinks that in his "centesimal fluxion potentiser" he has avoided their errors. But while he believed their potencies genuine, he testified that he found no difference between them and his own. The inference is obvious.*

I am glad that I have not to justify to you these insensate and often dubious proceedings. They are a chapter in the history of Homœopathy which had to be glanced at; but we will trust that it has only been an episode, and will go back to the practice of Hahnemann's method as he left it. Can we sustain even this in the face of science? Is matter divisible into such fractional parts as are denoted by the high figures of even his potencies? Is it still active as far as it goes? And is there any ground for preferring it in this finely-divided state to preparations of a cruder kind?

I. The pharmaceutical question obviously requires a distinct answer according as it is trituration of insolubles or dilution of solubles which is being practised.

1. The Homœopathic triturations were about twenty years ago made the subject of a very thorough microscopical investigation by Drs. Conrad Wesselhœft, Samuel Jones and Edwards Smith in America and Dr. Buchmann in Germany. Of this an account was given in the Thirty-Eighth Volume of the BRITISH JOURNAL OF HOMŒOPATHY (p. 324). The results were there summed up as follows:—

"*a.* It is clear that trituration, to approach anywhere near its ideal, must be conducted upon a better method than that laid down by Hahnemann, and with a rigid scrutiny of its results as it proceeds. With this view the instructions of our own Pharmacopœia † may be called, as of much value. It directs not only that a decimal scale shall be followed instead of the centesimal, but that the first step of this shall be the rubbing-up of the medicinal substance with EQUAL PARTS of Sugar of Milk; and it adds—'as the reducing of the medicines to the finest possible powder is a most essential point in this method of preparation, and as it is very difficult to effect this after a large proportion of Sugar of Milk has been added, a small portion of the trituration should be carefully examined under the microscope at this stage, and if the particles are found to be very unequal in size, the trituration should be continued until the reduction of the

---

* For full development of this subject, see B. J. H., xxxix. 17.

† "British Homœopathic Pharmacopœia." London: Gould and Son. 3rd Ed., 1882.

particles to a uniform degree of fineness is complete.' The remaining eight parts of Saccharum Lactis are then gradually added and incorporated, the whole process lasting an hour. The subsequent attenuations are effected in two stages, taking forty minutes in all. Triturations thus prepared bid fair to be all that can be expected of them.

"*b*. This 'all,' however, is not so much as their theory requires, or as we have hitherto supposed it to be. The concurrence of all observers shews that a large proportion—about one-third—of the drug undergoes nothing but coarse comminution; that much of the finest subdivision is already reached in the first step of the progress; and that at the succeeding stages there is a progressive diminution in the number of particles present. We cannot, therefore, say with any precision that a grain of the third centesimal trituration represents a millionth of a grain of the original substance. All we can affirm is that it contains an indefinite number of more or less minute particles thereof; and those hardly smaller while certainly fewer than would be furnished by a similar proportion of the second potency. It begins to look as if Hahnemann was wisest in his earliest practice with triturations, in which the first was used for provings and the second for medicinal purposes. We hardly seem to gain anything by going beyond this point.

"*c*. The question of the solubility of insoluble can hardly be said to have been decided by these investigations. They certainly do not make anything in favour of substituting trituration for dilution above the third, as was once recommended; for they shew that on this plan few particles of the drug would survive at the sixth. If we would raise the drug further, it must be by means of a liquid medium; and here again our Pharmacopœia seems to speak most wisely. 'At this point'—the third—'experience has shown that even the most insoluble substances have become soluble both in water and in *Alcohol;* OR, IF NOT ACTUALLY SOLUBLE, THEY ARE REDUCED TO SUCH MINUTE PARTICLES THAT THEY ARE CAPABLE OF PERMANENT SUSPENSION THROUGH THE FLUID, so that it retains their medicinal virtues, and answers all the purposes of a perfect solution."

As regards the last point, the "Amethystine fluid" of Faraday is cited. This is Gold dissolved in Aqua Regia, and reduced therefrom with an Etherial solution of *Phosphorus*. There results a fluid in which Gold is present in the proportion of one part of the metal to 760,000 parts of liquid. In this the highest power of the microscope fails to find any particles of Gold; but if it be illuminated by a cone of condensed sunlight the golden gleam in the path of light shews that the Gold is present in suspension, not in solution, and a film of it is left after evaporation. Dr. Wesselhœft found a similar result when he diffused through water finely powdered glass. But as to the solubility, or quasi-solubility of metals, science has made a vast stride in the researches of Nageli. I shall have to cite these immediately in support of the power of infinitesimals to produce Physiological effects. I mention them now as showing that Copper, at least, can be taken up by Distilled Water in sufficient quantity to poison a spirogyra growing in it, though the metal was presented to it in the crude form of coins.

2. This brings us to the other distinctive feature of Homœopathic pharmacy—its dilutions. There can be no question here of the adequacy of the mode of preparation to effect all of which the process is capable. The doubt is how far attenuation can be carried.

This has been expressed from within our ranks as well as from without. Thus we have Essays from Dr. Samuel Cockburn, of Glasgow,* and Dr. S. Whitney, of Boston, U.S.A. † The former argues that succussion of a liquid must result in uniform size of its particles, and hence, that the drop of the first dilution, containing a hundredth part of the drug, cannot be subdivided another hundred times at the second step, as the theory requires. Dr. Whitney points out that to suppose a drop of the juice of a plant to be uniformly diffused through the mass of fluid representing the third attenuation is to make it 640 times more attenuated than it would be in the gaseous form, which he assumes to be the ultimate rarefaction of matter; and maintains that this is impossible.

Now these objections might very well be met on their own ground of theory. To Dr. Cockburn we might reply that he makes no allowance for diffusion, but suppose his drop of the first dilution to live an isolated life among those of the next dilution to which it is introduced; which is absurd. To Dr. Whitney it might be urged that the "radiant matter" of Crookes has already shown us a fourth state in which it can exist, and that it would be most unwise to fix a rigid limit, derived from our present knowledge of it, beyond which we cannot allow it to be separable. But there is a more conclusive answer to either; the doubt SOLVITUR AMBULANDO. Take as Dr. Deschere has done, ‡ a deeply colouring matter like *Eosine*. You will see it with ordinary vision pervading every portion of the second attenuation, where it must exist in the proportion of one ten-thousandth, and the cone of concentrated sunlight will

* ANNALS OF BRIT. HOM. SOCIETY, iii. 21.

† N. ENGL. MED. GAZETTE, DEC. 1879, p. 268.

‡ N. A. J. H. Feb., 1880, p. 417.

show its fluorescence in the fifth, where its attenuation is represented by the ten-thousand millionth.

Here, too, comes in the evidence furnished by chemical analysis, by the microscope, and by the spectroscope. The first has detected Nitrate of Lead and Sulphate of Copper pervading the third attenuation.* The second of course has no place where true solutions are to be examined; but if Mayerhofer's experiments can be relied on, has followed up several suspended metals to dilutions (on a scale of 2 to 98) ranging from the tenth to the fourteenth. The third in Dr. Douglas Hale's hands,† has revealed the presence of Strontium and Barium in the 5th dilution; and Dr. Ozanam's, ‡ of Lithium in the 6th, and of Sodium in the 8th. Dr. Wesselhœft's repetition of experiments with the two last metals failed § to trace the former above the third decimal, the latter above the the 7th of the same scale; but there seems no reason to question the validity of the older observations.

We have, moreover, additional testimonies derived from experiments made to see how far semen, vaccine lymph and septic blood can be attenuated without losing their distinctive properties. I adduce these here, rather than under the head of the proofs of the activity of our potencies. Since the substances used can hardly be ranked as drugs in respect of MODUS OPERANDI. Dr. Arnold has fecundated frogs' eggs by immersing them in the 3rd dilution of their semen, and has successfully vaccinated children from the first (aqueous) dilution of vaccine lymph.** But it is with septic blood that the most astonishing results have been obtained. You will find in the Thirty-First Volume of the BRITISH JOURNAL OF HOMŒOPATHY an account of the experiments made herewith by M. Davaine, who is no Homœopathist, though he has diluted according to the Hahnemannian scale. He found that the blood of rabbits dying of Septicæmia could, in the dose of a ten-trillionth of a drop, induce a similar and fatal disease in other animals of the same species. As this represents a point between our 9th and 10th attenuations, it shows conclusively that matter can be carried by the Homœopathic process to that degree without ceasing to be present, or losing the activity proper to it.

But a far more serious objection has arisen of late years, not indeed to the soundness of the points we have hitherto made, but to the possibility of indefinite attenuation. The conception

* B. J. H., xx. 278.
† ANNALS, iii. 31.
‡ L'ART MEDICAL, Jan. 1862 : see also Vol. xx. of B. J. H., p. 282.
§ HOM. TIMES, Aug., 1880.
** Dudgeon, Lectures, p. 368

of the infinite divisibility of matter current in Hahnemman's day*
has now been exchanged for that of its atomic constitution,
which implies that we must at length arrive at a stage at which
we can divide more. This idea was not disturbing to us at
first, as imagination might suppose the atom as small as it
pleased, and far beyond the reach of any attenuation reasonable
Homœopathists were likely to use. Our confidence was rudely
shaken, however, when physicists began to attack the question
of atomic magnitudes, and agreed that these—minute as they
were—did not carry us into numbers exceeding trillions.
Thompson and Clark Maxwell estimate the number of ultimate
atoms which can be contained in a space $\frac{1}{1000}$ of an inch cube
as between a hundred billions and ten thousand billions; and
supposing these atoms to be of Oxygen and Hydrogen, and to
unite to form water, Sorby calculates that four thousand billions
of molecules of water might occupy such a space. † Drs.
Wesselhœft and Sherman ‡ have shown that, upon such data,
the molecures of a liquid drug would become exhausted at about
the eleventh centesimal dilution, and at the twelfth would cease
to be even probably present.

This startling difficulty is evaded by some by saying that the
atomic constitution of matter is at best only a theory, that it can
never be proved. Others, with more plausibility, affirm that the
size of atoms may hereafter be found more minute than at
present estimated. The late Dr. von Grauvogl attempted to
make a great point of the experiments of Jolly, who found that
a certain amount of contraction accompanied the attenuation of a
solution of Saltpetre. "Since every new attenuation," he
wrote, § "produces, by molecular contraction, a new MINUS of the
volume present before their preparation," "Hahnemann's
decillionths and all other calculations fall to the ground." But
when we come to look at the amount of this contraction, we
find that at the first stage it is only 21 c.c. in 2257, *i.e.*, about one
part in a hundred, and that on further dilution the proportion
diminishes still further. Although, therefore, some allowance
must be made in our calculations in consequence of this discovery,
it cannot make a difference of more than one or two steps of the
centesimal scale.

* He takes it for granted that "a substance divided into ever so many parts must still always contain in its smallest conceivable parts *somewhat* of this substance." (Organon, 5th Ed., § 280, note).

† MONTHLY MICROSCOPICAL JOURNAL, March, 1876.

‡ Transactions of Amer. Institute for 1879; AMERICAN HOMŒOPATHIST, May, 1878.

§ Text-book of Homœopathy, tr. by Shipman, ii. 65.

On the other hand, in support both of the limited divisibility of matter and of the estimates made as to the size of its ultimate particles, we have the negative bearing of the facts already adduced. That vaccine lymph is active at the first dilution and semen at the third; that colour is perceptible in the second and fluorescence in the fifth; that Chemistry can detect substances in the third potency, and spectrum analysis in the eighth; that septic blood retains its virulence even in the ninth—all this has hitherto been urged only as proving the extent of our power of subdivision. But state the facts conversely—that lymph will not vaccinate beyond the first dilution, or semen impregnate beyond the third; that Chemistry and Spectroscopy find decreasing evidence of the presence of drugs as we go on attenuating, and at length lose sight of them altogether; that septic blood at a certain degree of dilution will no longer infect—and they no less forcibly suggest that that power has a limit. It is curious, moreover, that the highest point yet reached—Davaine's ten-trillionth—closely corresponds with the physicists' calculations as to what the limit is.

. Our second question was—Is matter still active as far as it is divisible? Some of the experiments already adduced answer this question in the affirmative as far as animal ferments are concerned: We have yet to establish the same fact as regards drugs. It is to this mainly that I have addressed myself in the lecture referred to in my 'Pharmacodynamics.' I have there shewn, on unimpeachable testimony, the astonishing heights to which poisons like *Arsenic* and *Phosphorus*, alkaloids like *Atropine*, *Strychnine* and *Aconite* can be carried without losing their power to produce their wonted Physiological effects. That lecture stands as it first appeared in 1880. Were I writing it now I could add several pertinent observations of like nature. Let me indicate a few of them.

1. Darwin, in his experiments on the quasi-sensibility of insectivorous plants, was led to try how far dilution and reduction of dose could be carried without re-action failing. The plant chosen was the Sundew (Drosera rotundifolia); the re-agent consisted of Salts of Ammonia. His letters, as published by his son, shew amusingly how surprised he was at the extent to which he was carried, and how much he feared that his results would be accounted incredible. "You will laugh," he first says to a correspondent when telling him that the Drosera leaves detect (and move in consequence of) gr. $\frac{1}{2880}$ of the *Nitrate*; but before he has finished he has ascertained that similar results follow gr. $\frac{1}{20000000}$ of the *Phosphate*.

2. Dr. Blackley, in the course of his well-known researches on Hay-fever, thought of trying how small a quantity of the causative

agent of this trouble—the pollen of plants—could induce its phenomena. "From careful and oft-repeated experiments" he writes, "I am certain that so small a quality as the $\frac{1}{100000}$ of a grain of pollen will give rise to very perceptible symptoms if this is inhaled within a given time.

3. Pollen, you may say, is not exactly a drug; but you will allow that Copper is. Carl von Nageli has recognised a lethal potency in this metal so far exceeding any chemical power that he has coined a new word, "Oligodynamic," to denote it. His experiments had their origin in the observation that water drawn from a brass faucet, or distilled in Copper vessels had a fatal effect on spirogyra. He then began to try how far he could reduce the amount of poison without losing its effects. He distilled one litre of water in glass retorts, suspended four clean Copper coins in such water during four days, and found that this solution killed his plants in a few minutes. When the water was poured away, the glass rinsed and washed carefully and refilled with neutral water, the spirogyra again died in a very short time. This rinsing and refilling could be repeated many times before the walls of the vessels lost the "Copper force" they had acquired, and their power of communicating it to their contents. † If, however, the glass was washed out with dilute *Nitric acid*, and refilled with fresh neutral water, the plants flourished and remained healthy. Nageli attempted to ascertain the amount of Copper dissolved by suspending twelve small Copper coins in twelve quarts of neutral water, during four days. These twelve quarts were slowly evaporated, and the minute residue, supposed to be a hydroxide of the metal, was found to be in the proportion of one part to nearly one hundred million of the vehicle. From this and other experiments he concluded that the "Oligodynamic" effects of Copper result from solutions in the proportion of from 100 to 1000 millionth.

4. Professor Oswald, of Leipzig, published in 1897 some interesting researches on the crystallization of super-saturated solutions. This took place, he found, on the addition of very small quantities of the same or an isomorphous substance in the solid state. Wishing to ascertain how minute the added matter might be, he availed himself of the Homœopathic triturations, and found that crystallization could be effected in the case of Salol and Thymol with traces of the 6th, in that of *Thiosulphate of Soda* with the 9th,

* M. H. R., xxxiv, 604.

† This observation has been thought to give scientific sanction to the "bottle-washing" attenuation practised by Fincke, Swan and others, and to render inexcusable the putting any limit whatever to the extent to which such process may be carried. Though the vessels lose their communicating power "very slowly" however, they do lose it in time; and a thousand millionth is only the 9th dilution of the decimal scale.

and in that of *Chlorate of Soda* with the 10th dilution of the demimal scale.

5. Lastly, let me bring to your notice the facts which Becquard, Curie and Debierne have ascertained relative to the Phosphorescence of certain metals—Uranium to wit, and the more recently discovered Polonium, Radium and Actinium. The luminous emanations they give forth have been conceived of as corpuscular, but the loss of substance hereby induced is so minute that it has been calculated that a flat piece of Radium one centimetre square, shining continuously with an appreciable glow, would diminish in weight by less than a milligramme in 1,000,000,000 years. How infinitesimal is the quantity of luminiferous matter given forth, then ! and yet it suffices to impress the retina with the sensation of light. Debierene's discovery is that such Phosphorescence can be transmitted, as from a metal like Radium, which has it, to one like Barium which by nature has it not; and that even in solution. This would seem to make the luminous energy a dynamic one.

III. The foregoing are facts; but they do not carry us beyond the point at which we reached when considering the subject from the pharmaceutical standpoint. Physiologically we can get as far as we can physically; action corresponds to substance. But after all we have only got as high as the 15th dilution at the utmost; it is a far cry to Hahnemann's 30th's and what shall we say to Dunham's 200th's—which, prepared by himself in legitimate manner he comes to use almost exclusively in his practice, esteeming them of more efficacy, both in acute and chronic disease, than any lower attenuation ? * Bœnninghausen had preceded him, and Tessier and Grauvogl have followed him in the same estimate—positively if not comparatively—of this exalted potency. We cannot ignore such testimony; yet even if Hahnemann's theory of dynamization could be accepted, and would substantiate their experience from the scientific side, we could not get over the lack of evidence that matter is so far divisible, or can transfer its medicinal property to the vehicle in which it is dissolved or suspended. We must act here, if at all, on empirical grounds only, admitting that Logic has nothing to say for us, and that science—which has gone with us so far—is now not only inactive but become our opponent.

The one field in which a real dynamization can be reasonably recognised is that of those substances which are inert in their crude state, but which, when rubbed up with some indifferent vehicle so as to ensure a fine division of their particles, become active enough.

We have a familiar instance in *Mercury*, which as pure

* See his Homœopathy, the Science of Therapeutics, pp. 227-266.

Quicksilver may be swallowed by the pound, but which, when intimately mixed with confection of roses or with chalk, becomes a potent drug. It is now recognised that the amount of oxidation which takes place in the preparation of blue-pill and grey powder is very small, and that minute sub-division is the essence of the process. Hahnemann, as you have been told, largely developed this mode of preparing drugs, introducing the improved method of a graduated trituration with Sugar of Milk. The metals—Gold, Silver, Platinum, Zinc, together with such neutral substances as Charcoal, Flint, and Lycopodium, are awakened to energy by this potent process, and show themselves capable of no little influence upon the organism. But it is obvious that since in this way a real development of power is effected, there must be a certain stage in the process at which the drug, inert in its crude state, begins to be active, and another at which this newly-awakened energy is at its height, after which all further attenuation must have a contrary effect.

Hahnemann indeed thought that an indefinite development of power resulted from the dilution he at first practised to avoid aggravations and collateral effects. When asked to explain how such increased power could be elicited, he replied that the thorough solution and diffusion of the medicine enabled it to present so many more points of contact to the living matter. That is the same thought which has subsequently been expressed by the phrase, that medicines act by their surface, not by their mass, and are therefore effective in proportion as the former is extended. Grauvogl aptly says:—"It is a matter of indifference what quantity of Iron I make red hot, even were it many hundredweights, whose quality of heaviness might crush me; it could burn me, on coming near to it, only so far as it could touch me with its surface." This thought was pushed by Doppler to a calculation of the extent of surface developed by the Hahnemannic trituration, which reached from two square miles in the third trituration to the whole area of the constituents of the solar system in the ninth. But it has been pointed out * that such calculation assumes that the whole original grain is carried on into every successive trituration; whereas we know it to be reduced a hundredfold at each step, so that "even supposing each successive trituration to be thoroughly penetrated with the medicine, the superficies can never exceed that which was presented by the first." Conversely, then, it would seem better that we should dilute without reduction of mass, and this idea Hahnemann at one time countenanced, saying in the "Organon" of 1833. "I dissolved a grain of *Soda* in an ounce of water mixed with *Alcohol* in a phial, which was thereby filled half full, and shook the solution continuously for half an hour, and this was in dynamisation and energy equal to the 30th development of

* Dudgeon, Lectures, p. 366.

potency." In 1839, however, he tells us that it is absolutely necessary to dilute medicines in order to potentise or dynamise them:—"The greatest amount of succussion or trituration of substances in a concentrated form will not enable us to liberate and bring to light the more subtle part of the medicinal power that lies still deeper."

As my penultimate quotation shows, Hahnemann came later to ascribe an occult virtue to the processes of trituration and succussion employed by him, independent of their aid towards effecting a more thorough solution. In this he has been followed by many of his more enthusiastic followers; but I am glad to find the latest of these falling back upon the more rational explanation. I refer to Dr. Skinner, who has written a series of Articles on "The Dynamisation of Medicines" in the Journal edited by him called THE ORGANON. I would call attention to the arguments adduced in the number for January, 1880, as entirely commending themselves, save where he ends by saying that the 30th centesimal of Hahnemann can be made by allowing 3,000 minims of water to pass slowly (through a funnel) in and out of a 100-minim measure containing one minim of motor-tincture. It is not only that the process is quite inadequate to the task, as Dr. Skinner himself admits in the next number of his Journal (p. 194); but is very doubtful whether any SOLUTION D'EMBLEE can be equivalent to the graduated method devised by Hahnemann. Grauvogl made some experiments to determine this. He found that the 30th, 10th and 3rd decimal attenuations of *Arsenic* prepared in the usual way, produced a certain definite effect upon him (the first showing its influence by great thirst). He then made at once a solution corresponding in strength to about the 7th decimal, and not till after taking this for six days did he experience an effect, which at the utmost only amounted to that which the 30th produced on the second day of proving it.

Returning from this digression to our former point, it seems that extension of surface will not account for development of power in the Hahnemann attenuations beyond the first. A later discovery of science, however, comes to our aid; and seems to show that separation of particles may have something to do with it. We refer to the researches of Crsokes on the behaviour of matter in a fourth state—beyond the solid, liquid, or gaseous—which he calls "radiant." If from a closed globe full of air as much as possible be withdrawn by an exhausting pump, the molecules that remain require an astonishing activity, manifesting itself by luminous, thermic, and electric phenomena according to the circumstances. Dr. Garcia Lopez, in the CRITERIO MEDICO,* has fairly turned this fact to account in defending the energy of the Homœopathic infinitesimals : And we truly get far enough when we find that on reducing the pressure to

* Feb., 1880.

the millionth of an atmosphere or less, gases acquire these peculiar properties. It is impossible to say how much further the separation might not be carried without advantage. On the other hand it must be remembered that the energy manifested is rather that of the forces of Nature than of the properties of matter, and that drug-action belongs to the latter category. It would seem to be the greater scope for molecular motion afforded by the wider range given to the particles which enables them to display the phenomena of Light, Heat and Electricity in this enhanced degree ; and it would not be easy to apply such a conception to the reactions of medicinal particles with the living matter of the organism. At the best, suggestions derived from this source must stand or fall with the doctrine of the atomic constitution of matter, and cannot harmonise with the notion of its infinite divisibility. If separation of particles be the cause of their greater activity, the time must come when further distance will outweigh ampler space, and the energy allowed by the latter will be lost in the expenditure required for the former. *

* The above paragraph would be my answer to the ingenious considerations brought before the British Homœopathic Society by Dr. Percy Wilde, and published in the Tenth Volume of its JOURNAL under the title of "Energy, in its relation to Drugs and Drug Action." I cannot think that the power of drugs to induce changes in protoplasm is a result of any potential energy they may possess as physical substances; nor can I admit that even this is INDEFINITELY increased by separation of their particles, that is, fails to diminish and finally disappear as these lessen in number and increase in distance from each other.

LECTURE XI.

HOMŒOPATHIC PRACTICE

We have now surveyed the method of Hahnemann, in all that is essential to it. It is a rule—LET LIKES BE TREATED BY LIKES. The "likes" are—on the one-side the clinical features of disease, with such knowledge of its Ætiology and Pathology as can be had; on the other, the Physiological action of drugs. Their similarity is to be, as far as possible, generic, specific, and individual; and the remedy thus selected is to be given (as a rule) singly, rarely, constitutionally, and minutely. If you have followed with concurrence the reasonings I have set before you, I trust you are satisfied that this method has every claim—scientific and practical—upon our acceptance; that our wisdom as medical men is to carry it out wherever it is applicable.

I have yet to speak to you of some subsidiary matters—of the Philosophy of Homœopathy, the rationale of its curative process; of its history in the world of medicine; and of its claims on the profession. But before passing on to these, I feel bound to dwell on another series of considerations. I am assuming that you accept the method of Hahnemann, that you intend to adopt "Homœopathic practice." What does this involve? What alteration does it make in your relation to the profession and the public? What duties does it lay upon you? What provision must you make, and what course of action must you follow, to carry it out aright? You may well ask such questions; and I am bound to answer them. Let us pass today, then, from the principles of Homœopathy to its practice.

I. When Hahnemann first propounded his method, he did so in the ordinary medical journals, addressing himself to his colleagues. He wrote, as he acted, in the liberty which every qualified physician is supposed to have, of doing what he thinks best for his patients, and of expressing his views among his peers. But this liberty, which had been granted to every systematiser who had preceded him, and has never since been refused, was denied to him. The reform in Therapeutics he proposed was so great, so sweeping; the mode of treatment he would substitute for that then current so put to shame its complexity, its violence, its absence of solid base, that the practitioners of his day could not bear it. They silenced him in their journals; they stirred up the druggists to hinder him dispensing his medicines; they invoked the arm of the State to forbid the new practice. If any man would carry it on, he must do secretly. It was outlawed alike professionally and politically.

Nevertheless, it was believed in: It was adopted. Those who dared to adhere to it, found themselves excluded from all the associations whereby the practitioners of medicine seek to advance themselves in the knowledge of their art. Membership of medical societies, practice in established hospitals, freedom of utterance in professional journals, was denied them: The recognition of truth to which their reason led them, and the application of it for the good of their patients to which their conscience constrained them, were treated as crimes. Their only wish was to practise freely, in their natural position, what their judgment dictated to be best; but this was sternly disallowed. What was the result? As they multiplied, they set up societies, hospitals, journals for themselves, calling these by the name of the method to which they were devoted. As time went on, school and colleges had to be established to teach the new method, whose very mention was tabooed in the existing educational institutions; and Homœopathic pharmacies became necessary, where our medicines could be obtained, and Homœopathic directories, from which the public could learn who were practitioners of the system.

The consequence is, that Homœopathy has acquired an organisation. From a creed it has become a church. The new adherent to it at the present day finds it in this position, and the first question he has to decide is whether he shall join this church or not. Shall he simply embrace the creed, practising it as far as his patients and colleagues permit, and professing it no more than occasion demands? Or shall we avow his faith, affiliate himself to Homœopathic institutions, and allow his name to appear in the HOMŒOPATHIC DIRECTORY, or at least in the annually published list of members of the British Homœopathic Society? Now I am well aware of how much there is to be said for the former alternative. In the abstract, it is the legitimate course to follow. It was the mode of proceeding adopted in every country at the first, until the intolerance of the profession compelled its abandonment; and each new convert must feel strongly induced to attempt it afresh. But, much as I sympathise with the sentiment which actuates him, I can have no hesitation in advising him to prefer the other course. The organisation of Homœopathy was, indeed, forced up on it; but, however acquired, it now belongs to it as a body to its soul. The position it has taken up was not of its seeking; but having been occupied, it cannot be abandoned without fatal misunderstanding. We, who have held the fort for many a days, must continue to hold it until our claims are yielded, and our method receives its legitimate recognition, our mode of practice, its due liberty asd honour. We cannot do so unless from time to time we receive reinforcements to supply the gaps left by age, sickness and death. The greater our numbers, the better our Institutions are manned and our Journals filled, the more respect we shall win for our system, the nearer we shall bring the day when the profession shall be forced to recognise it and to invite us back to free fellowship. Till then, do not weaken the cause by standing aloof from its embodiments. Allow your names to be placed in our published lists, or rather, be proud of it as of an enrolment in a Legion of Honour. Seek service in any Homœopathic hospital or dispensary which may be in your neighbourhood; send cases to the Homœopathic Journals; apply for membership in the British or other Homœopathic Society. Every man who acts thus lends fresh strength to the witness we bear to truth in medicine, and hastens the day of its victory.

I know that in the meantime the course of conduct to which I invite you involves heavy sacrifices. Things are not indeed as bad as they were, when to avow one's belief in Homœopathy meant professional and even social outlawry. But the price is still a heavy one one to pay. Such memberships and appointments as you may have, you will find it hard to retain, and you will get no more. Consultations and assistance will be generally grudged, often refused. By many of your fellows you will be treated as a black sheep; spoken of behind your back as a fool, if not knave: met face to face with significant coldness. Even the more liberal-minded, though they tolerate you, will do it with a pity which is often contemptuous. There are, of course, exceptions to this rule, in individuals, and even in circles—among which Birmingham deserves honourable mention; but as a rule it holds good. You must run the risk of being so treated. But what of that? Are you the first who have have had to suffer to truth—to go, if need be, without the camp, bearing its reproach? Count the cost, indeed, before you make your avowal; but do not let it deter you from making it. To some extent you will find compensation. Another fellowship will welcome you, other places of honour and usefulness will be opened to you. Still, you will be a heavy loser, and can only incur the loss in the firm conviction that you are thereby serving the cause of truth. The conviction is mine; I trust it may also be yours.

II. This, then, is the first thing I have to advise—that you avow your new faith in the most practical way, identify yourself with its body and not merely its soul, join its church as well as profess its creed. And now arises the next question—What are the duties of the new position you have taken up? In what way do they differ from those of every practitioner of medicine?

Do you, in acknowledging the truth of Homœopathy, bind yourselves to its exclusive practice? No; by no means. In becoming (as men will call you) "Homœopaths," you have not ceased to be physicians. "Medicus nomem, Homœopathicus cognomen," we may say after St. Augustine's manner. It is the supreme duty of us all to do what we judge best for our patients, irrespective of any creed or system. We have protested against the tyranny which has ostracised us because we believe this "best", ordinarily to be Homœopathy; and it is not for us to be entangled again with any other yoke of bondage. We must let no one impugn our right of unfettered therapeutic choice. In allaying ourselves to Homœopathic Institutions we manfully recognise a truth which has laid hold of us, but which is at present denied and cast out: We in no way determine how far its practical consequences shall reach. Take up this position from the first. Claim to be priests of the one Catholic Church of Medicine, however much the prevailing majority deny your orders and invalidate your sacraments. They force you into a sectarian position; but let them not inspire you with a sectarian spirit. Assert your inheritance in all the past of medicine, and your share in all its present: Maintain your liberty to avail yourselves of every resource which the wit of man has devised or shall devise for the averting of death and the relief of suffering. This is the only legitimate ground to occupy, and you should make it plain that on this you stand.

But while desirous of impressing this primary truth upon you, I would remind you that you have duties as "Homœopathicus," and not only as "medicus." Duties to your patients, for they will seek your aid as such: Duties to the method itself, under whose name you enlist, and whose advantages you enjoy. The correlative of liberty here, as everywhere else, is loyalty; and without such counterpoise it degenerates into mere haphazard and empiricism. Our special vantage-ground is our practice according to law, instead of in the "unchartered freedom" of which our old-school colleagues boast, but of which the best of them must often tire. Do not readily forsake it. At the outset think even of liberty as little as possible. Children are not the better for being free; and the same may be said of novices in the method of Hahnemann. Your wisdom at the first is to practise it as exclusively as you can. Let experience rather than A PRIORI assumption, teach you where it needs supplementing by other means. You will actually do more good to your patients on the whole, than if you began as eclectics; and you will be acquiring habits of order and precision which will stand you in good stead as you go on.

I am speaking thus, as regards men who are about to commence practice in a new locality as avowed Homœopathists. There are others, of course, who—already in harness—must erect their new building within the walls and under the cover of the old. They will begin by treating selected cases with their novel remedies, leaving unchanged the great bulk of their practice. As they learn confidence and experience, they will push their Homœopathy further on, and let their former expedients drop more and more into the background. At last the latter will have become the exception, and the former the rule of their practice, and the term "Homœopathic" becomes justly applicable to their position and mode of treatment. They will then have reached the ground already occupied by those who have practised Homœopathically from the beginning. But there will be this difference. They will have learnt what are the exceptions to the rule SIMILIA SIMILIBUS CURENTUR, and what are the auxiliaries with which it must be carried out. No man can know these so well as he who has worked out the subject for himself. Nevertheless, Homœopathic practice as a whole is regarded scientifically, a vast experiment towards the decision of the question how far likes cure all diseases without the aid of other means; and the results of that experiment, so far as it has gone, are available for the beginner. Let me briefly indicate them here.

1. First of all, let me remind you again that drug-giving, however important, is not the beginning and end of the physician's duty. He has to adapt to his patient all natural forces and circumstances within his control—heat and cold, light, air and water, rest and exercise, food and stimulus. He has to remove mechanical obstacles, and neutralise chemical or organic infections. You must not call the measures—surgical, regiminal, hydropathic—by which you effect these ends, "auxiliaries"; you must not imply that they lie outside the ordinary path of medicine. Do not enter upon Homœopathic practice with the thought that all your knowledge and command of natural influences may henceforth be laid aside. You must be—as Hahnemann ever was—Hygienists, that you may also be healers.

2. This applies to the fundamental duty of the physician, whatever be his medical creed. He must obey the rule "TOLLE CAUSAM" when practicable, before any other; he must remove the LŒDENTIA and supply the JUVANTIA of Nature at large. But

when, now, the physician practising Homœopathically comes to his own rule, SIMILIA SIMILIBUS CURENTUR, he must bear in mind the limitations of it inherent in its own nature. Likes can only be treated by likes, where likes are to be found. Where your patient's trouble is one which drugs cannot stimulate on the healthy body, you cannot apply your law. You will remember the instances of this which were suggested when we were were on the subject. How can drugs produce anything like the disorder of sensation and function attending the passage of a calculus? How can they supply analogues to neoplasmata? Homœopathic MEDICINES may do something for such conditions, as every now and then they have done; but there is no Homœopathy, strictly speaking, in their selection. The Homœopathic practitioner is not passing by his law, if in the one case he hushes pain or relaxes spasm, if in the other he melts down the morbid growth by a liquefacient.

3. But, over and above such qualifications and limitations, the rule SIMILIA SIMILIBUS may have practical exceptions —exceptions found to be such from experience, not necessary, not such as could be foreseen A PRIORI; in all probability provisional only, but actual, and to be duly regarded. Are there many, or any, such? Well, my proposed teaching expressly contemplates contingencies of this kind. I am to tell you what Homœopathy can do in the various recognised forms of disease. There may be diseases which lie beyond its possible range and still more likely is that there are diseases which have not yet come within its practical range. Accordingly, our first step must be to enquire how much it can effect, as compared with the capabilities of old physic, in each malady that comes before us. If the answer to such enquiry should be its disparagement, we must follow the leading of the facts. Thus:

(*a*.) The use of cold baths in Typhoid Fever seems to give somewhat better statistics as regards recoveries than even our own treatment can boast.*

(*b*.) The recurrence in Relapsing Fever cannot be prevented by Homœopathic remedies; but can be by antiseptics like the *Hyposulphide of Soda.* †

(*c*.) We have nothing to take the place of full doses of *Iodide of Potassium* in Tertiary Syphilis.

(*d*.) In Peritonitis from perforation we must give full doses of *Opium*, as in ordinary practice, if we are to have a chance of saving our patients.

* See Dr. Bakody's Report of the Pesth Hospital (B. J. H., xxxiv. 149).
† See Dr. Dyce Brown in B. J. H., xxxi. 363.

(*e.*) In Cardiac Dropsy we can rarely get the good effects of *Digitalis* and its congeners without the induction of their primary Physiological effect, so raising the arterial tension.

(*f.*) *Nitrite of Amyl* is a better palliative in the paroxysms of Angina Pectoris than any Homœopathically-acting remedy.

(*g.*) The use of *Iodide of Potassium* in Aneurism, seems outside the range of our method and is yet a valuable piece of practice, on which we can hardly improve.

(*h.*) In uræmic Coma, measures for relieving the brain of the "perilous stuff" which is oppressing it—if needful, venesection itself—are of more avail than the best drug-treatment.

These eight are only instances that at present occur to me in which, Homœopathic treatment being applicable in the nature of things, it is at present so excelled as to be displaced by measures of another kind. You will see at once how few they are in proportion to the mass of ills where the balance is just the other way. You will thus be encouraged to commit yourself freely, with such reservations, to the guidance of the Homœopathic law. Let none impugn your liberty, but let all respect your loyalty: So you will witness to the method you profess, and will have the approval of your own best judgment.

III. Such is the counsel I would give you as to the general ordering of your practice. Let us now go more into detail, and see what should be your actual work at the bedside and in the consulting room.

I have spoken of the selection of the Homœopathic remedy. I have shown you that its similarity should be, as far possible, generic, specific, and individual: I have indicated the parts which generalisation and individualisation respectively should play in the process. Descending now from principles to practice, let me advise you to let generalisation predominate in your prescriptions for acute disease. That is, do not let your thoughts range down the whole Materia Medica, from *Aconite* to *Zincum* (as we used to say; now it must be from *Abies* to *Zizia*), in search of your similimum. Fix them rather upon the group of medicines which general consent has associated with the malady before you. They were first arrived at by the rule SIMILIA SIMILIBUS; or, if obtained EX USU IN MORBIS, they have seemed warranted A POSTERIORI by it. They have stood the test of long and wide experience, so that you may be sure of their answering to the species—the essence of the disease. Suit them, as among themselves, to the form and stage of the malady; but do not, without very grave cause, go beyond them in search of a closer similarity, which is too often illusory. Of course no finality is contemplated; new remedies must from time to time be introduced and old ones extend their known range of action. Leave this, however, to men of larger experience; as beginners, you had better keep to the ground already surveyed. In the presence of Pleurisy, the best thing you can do for your patient is to appropriate *Aconite* and *Bryonia, Cantharis* and *Apis, Arsenicum, Sulphur* and *Hepar sulphuris* to the inflammation and effusion. If Pneumonia is before you, *Aconite, Bryonia* and *Sulphur* again, with *Phosphorus, Iodine* and *Tartar emetic,* comprise the whole ordinary Therapeutics of the disease. Some five or six medicines in Variola, seven or eight in Scarlatina, ten in Continued Fever, twelve in chronic Intermittents (in recent ones four will suffice), are as many as are ordinarily required for your choice; and our best comparative results have obtained where — as with Yellow Fever and Cholera—our remedies have been few in number and everywhere the same.

The same rule holds good even in chronic disease, where the disorder conforms to a recognised type. You will rarely get good, in Diabetes, by deserting *Phosphoric acid* and *Uranium;* in Rickets, by going beyond *Calcarea, Phosphoric acid,* again or *Phosphorus,* and *Silicea.* But when your patient's narrative has gone so far as to satisfy you that you have to deal with an anomalous case of no definite character, you will do well to let your mind work freely among the medicines which the symptoms suggest. Go upon the plan of exclusion. Test the remedy which first occur to you by the next symptom mentioned. If you have chosen aright, it will harmonise therewith, if not, it will suggest another, and the symptom next following will decide between these, or supply a third candidate for your acceptance. So, step by step, you will proceed; and when the whole case is before you, you will have obtained as the result of your elimination one, two or three medicines which seem well to cover the case. These you will then prescribe, in succession or alternation as you may determine; and, if you have proceeded carefully, you will find them the fundamental remedies for the disorder. They may be with advantage suspended for a time, or even replaced by others; but you will be driven again and again to them, and ultimately it will be with them—if ever—that you gain the day.

In thus choosing, do not neglect to supplement your memory by reference to the Materia Medica, and to its indices—the Repertories. Do not, indeed, be ashamed of doing so in the presence of your patients, if need so requires: They will not complain of you for taking too much pains. But especially when the day's work is over, when a new case has come before you, or an old one hangs fire—review its symptoms. Look them up one by one in your Repertory; follow the drugs indicated in the Materia Medica, and weigh well what you find. Do not be hasty, or too fondly credulous: Examine into the source of symptoms ere you trust them; but if you can safely do so, essay the medicines to which they point. You will thus frequently gain unexpected successes, and will be ever enriching your armamentarium. In acute and typical diseases, the fewer your remedies the better, but beyond this range, you can hardly have too many. It is here that the more SPECIFICKER, the mere organopathist fails; while the full method of Hahnemann wins victories which are a continual source of delight.

IV. And now a few words about the choice of dose. I think I have spoken with sufficient fulness of the general facts and principles of Homœopathic Posology. Short of actual experience, you are in a position to judge for yourselves what you will do in the matter. I do not wish unduly to bias you on so moot a question. It would, however, be carrying reserve too far, it would be neglecting your obvious interest, if I failed to give you some practical advice—from an experience of over forty years—as to the doses you should commonly employ.

And here, as in the choice of the remedy, I would distinguish two categories into which your cases will fall. We have seen that the object of attenuation is two-fold—to avoid aggravation and collateral disturbances, and to develop the peculiar properties of drugs. Now in the acute, typical disorders—the fevers, inflammations, catarrhs, neuralgias, spasms—which constitute the bulk of daily practice, the first-named object need alone be sought. The medicines with which you combat them are such as are already active in their crude state; your only care need be to protect your patients from their over-activity, to see that their Physiological be wholly absorbed in their Therapeutical action. For this purpose but moderate attenuation suffices. If you carry in your pocket-case the first decimal of *Aconite*, *Baptisia*, *Belladonna*, *Bryonia*, *Gelsemium*, *Ipecacuanha*, *Iris*, *Nux vomica* and *Spongia*; the first centesimal of *Apis*, and *Tartar emetic*; the third of *Mercurius corrosivus*, *Phosphorus*, and *Veratrum album*; the sixth of *Arsenicum*; if you reinforce these with a few medicines of full strength to meet special contingencies —as *Hamamelis* for hæmorrhage, and *Camphor* for shock and collapse—you will have a quiverful of shafts which will rarely need augmenting. By further dilution, if need be, at your patient's house you can exactly proportion the dose to age, sex and susceptibility; and you will rarely do anything but pure good.

It is otherwise when you have to deal with chronic disorder in its almost infinite variety. Your range of medicines here is a wide one, and so also must be that of your dose. Of the drugs among which you will have to choose many are such as only develop active properties after a certain degree of attenuation : such are *Sulphur, Calcarea, Silicea, Lycopodium, Natrum muriaticum, Sepia*. Certain actions, moreover, of the more potent, and even of the feebler drugs, belong to them peculiarly in infinitesimal form. I may cite *Arsenic, Phosphorus,* and *Nux vomica* in the former category, *Chamomilla* and *Coffea* in the latter. In my 'Pharmacodynamics', when speaking of the dosage of each drug, I have noted these points; and they may well lead you, as they have led me, to associate certain potencies with certain medicines, making the two almost as inseparable as the words and tune of a song. *Sulphur 30* is a definite remedy to me, dose and all. I know what I can do with it as I know the powers of *Aconite* 1x. So I can say of *Lycopodium 12* and *Silicea 6,* and of many other drugs. I require here, therefore, a wide range of dosage as regards my remedies; and still more as regards my patients. Their variations in susceptibility are great; they require change of potency from time to time as well as of medicines; the protean transformations of their maladies have to be followed up with corresponding shiftings of the means. I do not know that you need go higher than Hahnemann's 30ths; but, as you have thus already got beyond the estimated divisibility of matter, you will hardly be taking a fresh step if you dip occasionally into Dunham's 200ths.

In such affections, then, while not neglecting the lowest preparations, I advise you to rely largely upon the medium and higher—to use attenuation for developing the finer action of drugs which you desire to bring into play. In prescribing for other than acute disorders, you should always—if possible—do so from a Homœopathic Chemist. There are plenty of such in this country—intelligent, well-informed men; they have an excellent Pharmacopœia for their guidance! You may rely upon them, and should support them. The best way of prescribing is to order a drachm or two of the tincture or trituration, directing the proper number (three is a good average one) of drops or grains to be taken at a dose. The tinctures can be thus measured by being dropped into water from the phial; for the triturations small scoops are provided, holding about three grains by weight, which will best be taken dry on the tongue. Tablets of these are now prepared and are very convenient. Sometimes, when quantity is no consideration, and when the convenience of busy men or the tastes of children are to be consulted, you may give the medicines in the form of pilules, or even of globules; but I confess that I am not fond of these preparations, and do not advise their preferential choice.

V. A practitioner's medicines form his chief apparatus for practice; but next come his books. What works, you may fairly ask me, should you add to your library, and what use should you make of them, to enable you to superadd a literary knowledge of Homœopathic to that of medicine in general?

Well: First of all you should be well grounded in the principles of our system. You should study Hahnemann's 'Organon,' in the light of the introduction to it I gave you in the Second and Third Lectures of this course: And should follow it up by a thoughtful preusal of the volume of essays I have often mentioned, by Carrol Dunham, entitled (from the first of the series) "Homœopathy, the Science of Therapeutics." For an independent study and presentation of the subject, I may commend to you the 'Essays on Medicine' of Dr. Sharp. If you will also read the "Lesser Writings" of Hahnemann which under that name Dr. Dudgeon has collected and translated for us, you will have attained a thorough and scholarly knowledge of the basis of the new method you intend to practise.

Next, you must possess, in some form or other, the Materia Medica of Homœopathy—the collection of the pathogenetic effects of drugs with which it works the rule "let likes be treated by likes." You should procure Hahnemann's own "Materia Medica Pura," which we now have in excellent rendering and shape. Its prefaces and notes alone make it worth possessing; and though you may not learn much A PRIORI from reading its lists of detached symptoms, yet, when a Repertory refers you to them, you will have them in their oriignal and only available form. To this add the "Cyclopædia of Drug Pathogenesy," and—if you feel inclined to range beyond its borders—Dr. Clark's "Dictionary of Practical Materia Medica." Read also as we have no lecturers on Homœopathic Materia Medica in this country, some of the exposition of this kind which have found their way into print, among which I may name Hempel's, Dunham's, and my own as contained in the latter editions of my "Pharmacodynamics."

Of 'Repertories' themselves I have already spoken to you; it only remains that I indicate the best treatises on the Homœopathic practice of physic. By some amongst us these are discountenanced altogether, on the ground of the pure individualisation which is conceived of as governing our Therapeutics. To this I need not tell you that I cannot assent: I hold it on the contrary a great gain that the accredited Homœopathic treatment of the definite types of disease should be set down for the guidance of the beginner. I have worked myself in this field also; but far more elaborate treatises have been given us by Drs. Bahr and Kafka in Germany, Dr. Jousset in France, and Dr. Goodno in America. 'The Science of Therapeutics' of the first and the 'CLINICAL LECTURES' and 'PRACTICE OF MEDICINE' of the third, are available for us in an English dress; and we shall all welcome Dr. Dyce Brown's addition to our store, when he gives to the world the teachings on the subject which were so long valued in the London School of Homœopathy. Read such books through; consult their appropriate sections when you have to treat each form of disease; and you will gain strength and light incalculable for your daily work.

In addition to these, take in as many Homœopathic Journals as you can afford, from England, from America, and from other countries with whose language you may be acquainted. Take them in, AND READ THEM—a consequence which does not always follow. Give those who edit and supply them the support of feeling that their work is appreciated; and reap the utmost benefit of it for yourselves. Dwell in no isolation; indulge in no self-sufficiency. You can only live in the life of the body to which you belong: In its growth alone can you grow. You are cut off at present from the wider fellowship of the profession at large; but you can cultivate the corporate virtues in your narrower circle. The great hindrance to the spread of Homœopathy in the old world has been the lack of ESPIRIT DE CORPS among Homœopathists; had it not, indeed, possessed the vitality which truth alone can give, it had perished long ago in the midst of our dissensions and divisions. I trust that you will not contribute to these, but will rather bring strength to the heart of the body—its centre of the life and unity. You will do this as you think more of the essentials of the method than of its accidents, as you cultivate it for the good of your patients rather than of the filling of your own pockets; as you count all difference of opinion as to means a small thing in comparison with our common end—the promotion of the good cause we have at heart. Practise Homœopathy in this spirit; and you will do your part, small or great as it may be for the reform in medicine which one day will be seen to mark with white the nineteenth century of our era.

LECTURE XII.

THE PHILOSOPHY OF HOMŒOPATHY

Homœopathy, as I have hitherto presented it to you, is a METHOD. It has indeed been framed by scientific processes—reached by inductive generalisation and tested by deductive verification: But the thing framed is not a law of science,—it is a rule of art. It does not say—such and such is: it says—let such and such be—in this case "let likes be treated by likes." My exposition and vindication of it, accordingly, has dealt solely with facts. We have considered the elements of the comparison, the relation between them, and the manner of carrying out the rule, with pure reference to their sufficiency, practicability and advantage; and, if you were to choose to stop here, you would be in full possession of Homœopathy as a a working method.

But the mind of man is not so constituted as to rest content in phenomena only. He must know the "why" and "how," and not merely the "what"; and Homœopathy has been throughout an object of thought as well as of fact. From his first writing on the subject Hahnemann endeavoured to explain how likes were cured by likes, and his followers have never been weary in suggesting further explanations of their own. You may well ask me to tell you something about these, and whether I can commend any of them to you as affording a satisfactory rationale of the process. This accordingly, I shall endeavour to do to-day.

There is, indeed, a special reason why the Homœopathic cure should be accounted for. There is no difficulty in understanding the action of drugs Allœopathically or Antipathically related to the disorder presented for treatment. The former by some evacuation or revulsion, the latter by direct opposition to the seat of the morbid change, can readily be conceived of as restoring the affected part to its normal condition. But it is not so when we come to give drugs which cause in the healthy a similar disorder to that before us. It would seem at first sight, as if nothing but aggravation could ensue; that if one fire can put out another's burning when applied to other parts of the body than that which is the sea of conflagration, if directed to the same part it can but increase the original flame to twofold intensity. Yet it is not so. Even were the general experience of the Homœopathic school put out of sight, there is no doubt that *Arsenic*, which causes Gastritis and Enteritis in the healthy, cures irritative Dyspepsia and chronic Diarrhœa in the sick ; or that it is capable of setting up nearly every form of the cutaneous mischief for which it is so efficient a remedy. Here, if nowhere else, we should have to enquire, IN QUO MODO ? But we Homœopathists know that the field of the problem is co-extensive with specific medication, and are deeply concerned in making what approach we may to its solution.

Now, since medicines whose influence is directly opposed to the tendency of the morbid process operate in cure after a manner easy to be conceived, it is not strange that attempts should have been made to resolve into such an operation the behaviour of similarly acting medicines ; to suppose that, though they seem Homœopathic, and are selected because of such apparent relationship, they are really and within the system antipathic.

1. The first to propound such a theory of cure by SIMILIA SIMILIBUS was Hahnemann himself. He supposed that every drug, whether given in health or disease, produced two series of effects, the secondary being precisely opposite to the primary ; that, if given in morbid states corresponding to its secondary effects, *i.e.*, Antipathically, it acted at first as a palliative, but then its own secondary operation supervening, increased the disease : While, if given when a condition answering to its primary effect was present (Homœopathically), it caused a temporary aggravation indeed, but then by its secondary effects, which were opposite to the disease, a considerable amelioration thereof.

I believe that this was substantially Hahnemann's doctrine from first to last. But as a somewhat different account of it has been given by the historian and exponent of Homœopathy to whom I so constantly refer as an authority—I mean Dr. Dudgeon— it is necessary that I should say somewhat in justification of my statement. Dr. Dudgeon considers that in the "Medicine of Experience" and the "Organon", Hahnemann conceived of Homœopathic action as the substitution we have heard of from Trousseau, that is, as the overpowering and annihilation of the natural disease by an artifical one excited at the same spot, which latter, being but of brief duration, soon subsides, leaving health behind. "At a subsequent period, however," writes our author, *viz.*, in the Preface to the Fourth Volume of the 'Chronic Diseases' (1838), Hahnemann attempted another explanation of the curative process." This is the doctrine that it is the vital force which is always the conqueror of disease; that in our patients, especially those chronically sick, its power is insufficient for this victory; and that by administering a medicine acting in a direction similar to that of the malady, the vital force is, as it were, stirred up to fresh efforts in opposition, "until" (I quote Hahnemann himself) "at length it becomes so much stronger than was the original disease as that it can again become the autocrat in its own organism, can again, take the reins and conduct the system on the way to health." But if you will listen to a short extract from the "Organon" (§ xxix), I think you will agree that the earlier and later thoughts of the Master had very much in common:—

"As every disease," he writes, "(not strictly surgical) depends only on a peculiar morbid derangement of our vital force in sensations and functions, when a Homœopathic cure of the vital force deranged by natural disease is accomplished by the administration of a medicinal agent selected on account of an accurate similarity of symptoms, a somewhat stronger, similar, artificial morbid affection is brought into contact with, and, as it were, pushed into the place of the weaker, similar, natural morbid irritation, AGAINST WHICH THE INSTINCTIVE VITAL FORCE, now merely (though in a stronger degree) medicinally diseased, IS THEN COMPELLED TO DIRECT AN INCREASED AMOUNT OF ENERGY; but, on account of the shorter duration of the action of the medicinal agent that now morbidly affects it, the vital force soon overcomes this, and as it was in the first instance relieved from the natural morbid affection, so it is now at last freed from the substituted artificial (medicinal) one and hence is enabled again to carry on healthily the vital operations of the organism."

Now, though there is certainly a substitution of medicinal for natural disease contemplated here, rather than the reinforcement of the one by the other as suggested in the 'Chronic Disease,' yet the exaltation of the reactive vital force is (in the words I have capitalised) distinctly stated to be the means whereby the ultimate cure is effected, just as it is in the latter putting.

It remains only to connect this view of Hahnemann's with his doctrine as to the primary and secondary actions of medicines which again is hardly done by Dr. Dudgeon.

In the "Essay on a New Principle for ascertaining the Curative Power of Drugs," published in 1796, Hahnemann writes:— *

---

* **Lesser Writings** (Dudgeon's translation), P. 312.

"Most medicines have more than one action; the first a DIRECT ACTION, which gradually changes into the second (which I call the indirect secondary action). The latter is a state exactly the opposite of the former. In this way most vegetable substances act."

After saying that such opposite states are not so discernible in most mineral medicines, he goes on:—

"If, in a case of chronic disease, a medicine be given whose direct primary action corresponds to the disease, the indirect secondary action is sometimes exactly the state of body to be brought about; but sometimes (especially when a wrong dose has been given) there occurs in the secondary action a derangement for some hours, seldom days."

This, however, he says, is a mere transitory affection, and if, troublesome, may readily be suppressed by a dose of some antagonistically acting palliative, as *Opium* when the medicine was *Hyoscyamus*.

Thus the cure, in Homœopathic treatment, is conceived to result from the induction of the secondary action of the drug, which is antagonistic to the morbid condition present. And now, in the "Organon," we find him identifying this secondary action of the medicine with the stirring up of the opposing vital force of which we heard previously.

"Every agent * that acts upon the vitality, every medicine deranges more or less the vital force, and causes a certain alteration in the health of the individual for a longer or shorter period. This is termed PRIMARY ACTION. Although a product of the medicinal and vital powers conjointly, it is principally due to the former power. To its action our vital force endeavours to oppose its own energy. THIS REACTION BELONGS TO OUR PRESERVING VITAL FORCE, OF WHICH IT IS AN AUTOMATIC ACTION, AND IT IS TERMED SECONDARY ACTION OR COUNTER-ACTION.

"During the primary action of the artificial morbific agents (medicines) on our healthy body, our vital force seems to conduct itself merely in a passive (receptive) manner, and appears, so to say, compelled to permit the impressions of the artificial power acting from without to take place in it, and thereby alter its state of health. It then, however, appears to rouse itself again, as it were, and to develop, (*a*) the exact opposite condition of health (COUNTER-ACTION, SECONDARY ACTION) to this effect (PRIMARY ACTION)

---

* Organon (Dudgeon's translation), §§ cxiii, cxiv

produced on it, if there be such an opposite, and that in as great a degree as was the effect (PRIMARY ACTION) of the artificial morbific or medicinal agent on it, and proportionate to its own energy; or, (b) if there be not in Nature a state exactly opposite to the primary action, it appears to endeavour to indifferentiate itself, that is to make its superior power available in the extinction of the change wrought in it from without (by the medicine); in the place of which it substitutes its normal state (SECONDARY ACTION, CURATIVE ACTION)."

He here seems to set down all the effects which follow the administration of a drug to its direct action. Later, when the conception of a vital force had taken hold of his mind, the secondary drug effects were ascribed to its reaction. But the hypothesis remained essentially the same. The disorder was not cured by the primary but by the subsequent and opposite results of the medicinal impression. The process seemed to be Homœopathic, but was really Antipathic; the remedy was chosen as a similar, but acted as a contrary.

This is Hahnemann's rationale of Homœopathic cure. As we study his Works we find it carried on into all its logical consequences. One of these is the 'Homœopathic Aggravation,' on which we know him to have insisted as being in some degree a necessary step in the process of cure. Another is the merely temporarily palliative and ultimately injurious effects of all medicines whose primary action is antagonistic to the disorder present. He makes this point continually in his Prefaces to the pathogeneses of the various medicines in his "Materia Medica Pura." Of what avail is it, he demands, that you induce upon the quickened circulation of a Phthisical subject the retardation which is the first effect of *Digitalis?* Secondary reaction will speedily follow, and your patient will have a more rapid pulse than before. What is the use of forcing sleep on this excited brain by *Opium,* when, as soon as its primary soporific effect has worn off, by the recoil of the organism the sleeplessness will become more complete than ever? On the other hand, he says, give the Homœopathic remedy; and, though a slight and fleeting aggravation will ensure during its first effect, the permanent reaction it will excite is just the healthy condition you desire to restore.

II. Dr. Dudgeon, after criticising Hahnemann's theory of the nature of Homœopathic cure, concludes that it is unbearable. The same, he considers, must be said of those of the later Homœopathists, which he goes on to enumerate. Some of these assume as their basis the reaction or the substitution which we have already described. Others conceive of the similar remedy as hurrying the disease through its stages, and so making a speedy end of it. I know of no facts which warrant such a notion ; and the process seems hardly a desirable one in itself. Dr. Dudgeon's own view, as also Dr. Drysdale's, is that of Fletcher. This eminent Physiologist, though not practising, and therefore never ranked amongst Homœopathists, took great and sympathetic interest in Hahnemann's method, and proposed an explanation of its rationale, which I shall now proceed to expound.

Fletcher's doctrine is, like Hahnemann's, based on the primary and secondary actions of drugs, and the opposition between them ; but it is radically different both in the account it gives of these phenomena, and in the application it makes of them. With Hahnemann, the secondary effects were such as the constipation which follows the action of a purgative, and the sleeplessness which ensues upon the sopor induced by *Opium*. Fletcher has no regard to these, and Dr. Drysdale dismisses them as merely signs of exhaustion and fatigue after excessive vital action. He does not allow them as to be medicinal effects at all, and agrees with Hahnemann in rejecting them from the drug-pathogeneses which we apply to disease according to the rule SIMILIA SIMILIBUS. Fletcher's primaries and secondaries lie within Hahnemann's primaries. He considers that all morbid actions, whether produced as diseases or by drugs, are of the nature, or at least conform to the type, of INFLAMMATION. There is here a primary increase of the vital activity of the part showing itself in a contraction of the capillary vessels ; but this is followed by a secondary depression in which the capillaries are relaxed and dilated. The former stage is mostly latent ; it is the latter which presents the classical features of inflammation—CALOR, RUBOR, TUMOR, DOLOR, and in which we are ordinarily called upon to treat it. Drugs also, like the causes of disease, are primarily stimuli, and contract the vessels of the part on which they act. But here again the action is latent ; and it is the reactive depression which is noted as the condition produced by the drug. When, therefore, a medicine is given upon the rule SIMILIA SIMILIBUS, it is the secondary effects of drug and disease which coincide. But, the disease being already in its second stage, the primary action of the drug finds a condition present which it precisely counteracts, so that unless the dose have been excessive, its secondary influence is never manifested at all. "The first stage of the drug-action," writes Dr. Drysdale, "fits into the second stage of the disease, thereby filling up a want, and not overpowering an exalted diseased action by a still greater medicinal action. The therapeutic action is, therefore, antipathic after all, though the drug be Homœopathic in respect to its Physiological action," I should rather say, "apparently Homœopathic."

* "Elements of General Pathology", Edinb. 1842 : Book III. ch. 2.

Dr. Dudgeon expresses himself to the same effect, as a single extract from his discussion of the subject will show, "I was much gratified," he writes, "to observe in an essay by Dr. Clotar Muller, of Leipzig, that he takes a very similar view of the curative process to that which I have given. He takes the inflammatory process as his theme of illustration, and after showing that inflammation consists in a kind of partial Paralysis of the nerves of the capillaries, he asserts that the medicine cures by the stimulation it applies to these paralysed nerves, by virtue of its primary action; that its action, in fact, is the opposite of the actual condition of the diseased part, and that the principle SIMILIA SIMILIBUS is merely our guide to the selection of a remedy, but that it by no means expresses the part that remedy performs in relation to the disease. APROPOS of this explanation, I may mention a remark of J. Hunter's which is strikingly corroborative of these views. 'If,' says he 'we had medicines which were endowed with the power of making the capillary vessels contract, such, I apprehend, would be the proper medicines in inflammation'; and such undoubtedly, are our Homœopathic remedies in their primary action."

This theory is a fascinating one, and the names of those who advocate it give it weighty recommendation. I will not stay, however, to examine it, but will pass on to the other forms the doctrine has assumed.

III. The doctrines of Hahnemann and of Fletcher both invoke for their purpose the opposite results of the primary and secondary actions of medicines, though differing widely in their conception of these actions, and their application of them to the curative process. I have now to give an account of another set of hypotheses. These likewise declare that when we seem to be practising Homœopathy, it is really Antipathy we are carrying out; that while SIMILIA SIMILIBUS is our principle of drug selection, CONTRARIA CONTRARIIS expresses the facts of drug-action. But they find their contraries, not in the primary and secondary effects of medicines, but in their larger and smaller doses. They aver that small doses—those below a certain line of division special to each substance—have an action precisely the reverse of that of longer quantities; that the pathogenetic phenomena we seek to fit to the symptoms of disease are the effects of large doses; so that, when we give a small dose of a similarly-acting remedy, it will necessarily exert an opposite influence, at the same seat and of the same kind, to the morbid condition present, and hence cure it.

Here, also we have more than one advocate of the hypothesis, and as many conceptions of it as there are expositors. I will endeavour to set forth the views of each.

1. The first, so far as I know to propound any idea of the kind

was Dr. Bayes. In a series of Papers entitled, "Cure-Work," which appeared in the MONTHLY HOMŒOPATHIC REVIEW for 1869, and were subsequently published in his "Applied Homœopathy" (1871), he advanced the view that disease is always a negative state, a condition of debility; that specific restorative stimulation is true indication for its cure; and that such stimulation is best applied by drugs acting upon the tracts, parts, or organs of the body invaded by the disease, such drugs being only to be discovered by proving them upon the healthy body. Further, that in such provings the large doses employed cause a depressed condition of the part affected; ALL DRUGS BEING STIMULANTS IN SMALL DOSES BUT PARALYSERS IN LARGE; but that these very substances, administered in small doses in conditions similar to those which they cause, will excite their specific stimulation therein, and thereby restore the part to its healthy state.

In a later Presidential Address delivered at the British Homœopathic Congress of 1875, Dr. Bayes somewhat modified his theory. He cannot now agree with Dr. Chambers that "diseases, IN ALL CASES, is not a positive existence, but a negative." He thinks that "large classes of disease exist, whose whole phenomena are not satisfactorily explained upon the dynamic or adynamic theory alone"; and that, where it is so, Hahnemann's system fails to apply. He can only "claim for Homœopathic Therapeutics that they best guide us in the cure of all such diseases as arise from a want of balance between the functional action of the various parts and organs of the body, and are characterised by pains and sensations." Within this sphere he maintains his former explanations, adding to his doctrine of disease that the depression he postulates resides in the nervous supply of the part affected—motor, sensory, or sympathetic, and that thereon also must the medicinal stimulation be exerted.

Now this is surely a very serious result to which we are brought. If Dr. Bayes' doctrine be true, "large classes of disease" are excluded from the operation, at any rate the preferable operation of the Homœopathic law; and among these he specifies the infectious, contagious, and Malarious diseases— *i.e.*, (among others) the acute Exanthemata and the Continued and Intermittent Fevers. If, moreover, the fact about inflammation ascertained by modern Pathology are valid, this process also must be excluded from the functional neurotic disorders of which alone he allows Homœopathic Therapeutics to be our best guide. Thus nine-tenths of acute diseases and a fair half of those classed as chronic are excluded by this remorseless theory from the range of the method of Hahnemann. We must scrutinise with some suspicion an hypothesis which brings us to such unwelcome conclusions.

We are told that all drugs are stimulants in small doses, but paralysers in large. What is the evidence for this sweeping proposition? Dr. Bayes' chief instance, in both his utterances, is *Alcohol*. Now I must hold that this substance is a most unfortunate one from which to draw inferences as to the action of drugs. *Alcohol* is not a mere drug; unlike these, it is oxidised and consumed in the body very little of an ordinary dose passing out by the emunctories. This fact the experiments of Anstie and Dupre have conclusively established. It follows that *Alcohol* is a supplier of force; and so far a food and a rapidly acting one. This confusing element accordingly comes in whenever we regard its action, as if it were a mere drug, and vitiates our inferences. I cannot, therefore, think that Dr. Bayes is warranted in assuming, because *Alcohol* increases the arterial tone when lowered by fatigue or other depressing causes, while it diminishes it when given in health, that all drugs act in the same manner upon one or more of the three divisions of the nervous supply of the parts they affect. It is entirely an assumption (I use the word of course in a logical sense) : he makes no attempt to argue it. But let us take such a drug as *Strychnia*. In the moderate quantities in which it is ordinarily used it is what Dr. Bayes would call a stimulant, *i.e.*, an excitant of nervous function. But let it now be given in large, even poisonous lethal doses. Does it depress? Nay; it excites still more potently, till it kills by the violent spasms it sets up. We give it Homœopathically for such conditions of excitement and spasm, so that upon Dr. Bayes' principles—it must be called a stimulant in large doses, but a sedative in small. Or let us take a drug of another kind—*Kali bichromicum*. Throughout the pathogenesis of this Salt, throughout its clinical uses, I find no trace of either excitation or depression of nervous function: Everywhere is displayed the irritation of organic substance which characterises it, and which makes it so valuable a remedy in many conditions of sub-acute and chronic inflammation—such as those, for instance, which the Rheumatic and Syphilitic poisons set up.

I submit, therefore, that there is no evidence that all drugs act dynamically by disordering nervous function, or that those which do so act, are all stimulant in small doses but depressant in large; and hence that such supposed law of drug-operation is inadequate to explain Homœopathic cure, and that we need not exclude more than half our practice from the range of the method of Hahnemann because it does not conform to the theory put forward to account for the success of that method. Dr. Bayes' own practice is the best antidote to his theory; for in the pages of his very useful book occur numerous instances of the beneficial operation of Homœopathic remedies in those very morbid conditions to which he would make them comparatively inapplicable.

2. It will have been observed that the opposite action of large and small doses affirmed by Dr. Bayes belongs to two different regions. All drugs, according to him, are paralysers in large doses when taken in health, stimulants in small doses when administered in diseases. But at the meeting of the British Homœopathic Congress at Leamington in 1873, it was announced from the presidential chair that a number of medicines had been found by experiment to have this reverse action according to dose IN HEALTH: and that here, assuming the same fact to hold good of all medicines, was the explanation of likes being cured by likes.

The occupier of the chair on this occasion, and the propounder of the view thus stated, was the late Dr. Sharp. The Address he delivered, and some subsequent papers from him to the same subject, may be read in the volume of "Essays on Medicine" which he published in 1874. His well-known "Tracts" are contained herein, and many other communications to journal and medical meetings: I again commend the whole to your best consideration.

Dr. Sharp maintains, as I have said, that all medicines have two actions in health, according to the dose in which they are given—the effect of a large dose being the direct opposite to that of a small one. The dividing line is a shifting one, according to the drug used, and the individual experimented upon; but in all cases it is there, and constitutes a real point of transition between the two reverse actions. This (supposed) general fact he denominates ANTIPRAXY. When, accordingly, we give in disease small doses of a drug which in large doses has caused a similar condition to that before us, we are administering an agent whose influence is in direct opposition to the morbid state. He would call the process what it is, ANTIPATHY, reserving the name HOMŒOPATHY for the principle of selection.

It will be seen that Dr. Sharp here avoids what I have ventured to describe as the untenable assumption made by Dr. Bayes, that all medicines are stimulant in small doses, and depressant in large. He affirms nothing as to the direction of action of large or small doses, but simply that they are opposite one to the other. Nor does his theory require (in terms) that all diseases to come within the range of Homœopathic action must be merely functional derangements. So far, he is not open to the objections I have made to the doctrine of his predecesosr. But inferences quite as serious are necessitated by the position he takes up, as I shall now proceed to show.

First, if the power of medicines to cure diseases similar

to those which they cause depends upon the dose in which they are given, no Homœopathic cure is possible save with the minute doses with which Dr. Sharp gets his reverse actions in health, these being, as will be seen, in nearly all instances from one or three drops of the first centesimal dilution. Substantial quantities, such as are used in ordinary practice, could not cure morbid states like those which they cause, as they would be Homœopathic to them, not in appearance only, but in reality; and antipathic action is required for real remedies. If this were, so, there might be a satisfaction in finding our small dose more closely interlocked than ever with our principle, by being the essence of its MODUS OPERANDI. But I would point out that, upon this showing, all arguments in favour of Homœopathy drawn from ordinary practice are invalidated. Hahnemann's collection of cures wrought by similarly acting drugs in the introduction to his 'Organon,' Dr. Dyce Brown's later series appended to Dr. Reith's Pamphlet on "Homœopathy, &c."—these seventy instances in which disease-exciting and disease-curing properties of drugs were seen as coincident, are nearly all put out of court. The same thing would apply to Hahnemann's own cases published before 1800. They could not have been really Homœopathic cures, for they miss the indispensable small dose.

A still more important consequence follows in the sphere of the Physiological action of medicines. As none but small doses can effect Homœopathic cures, so no symptoms of drugs can be used in Homœopathising save those produced by large doses. When, in our existing pathogeneses, opposite effects are ascribed to the same medicine, these must be supposed to have resulted from different doses, and only those belonging to the larger doses to be available for working the Law of Similars. Dr. Sharp perceives and unhesitatingly adopts this conclusion. But he does not seem aware that a very large proportion of our pathogenetic material has been obtained by provings with what he would call small doses, representing indeed the least possible effect producible by the medicines; while, according to him, such symptoms are quite inadmissible for comparison with disease as likes to likes.

We have now to enquire into the basis of a doctrine fraught with such destructive operations. But before doing so, I desire to notice the manner in which the same theory has been brought before us by the Editors of that excellent Journal, the MONTHLY HOMŒOPATHIC REVIEW.

3. From the first enunciation of Dr. Sharp's views on this subject, the REVIEW declared itself in their favour. In an Article entitled, "Similia and Contraria" in its number of April, 1874,

it defended them against one of the objections raised to them by the BRITISH JOURNAL OF HOMŒOPATHY in the previous October. This paper, I imagine, bears traces of the style of Dr. Herbert Nankivell, who was then on the editorial staff. Subsequently, in 1875, the opposite action of large and small doses was affirmed as part of "the scientific basis of Homœopathy"; and in 1876 the Journal went as far as to say, that if it were not a fact, "farewell to the Law of Similars?" The "double action of medicines" was elaborately argued out in that year's volume; and two of the present editors, Dr. Pope and Dr. Dyce Brown, have issued pamphlets on Homœopathy, under their own names, in which the doctrine is maintained.

Substantially, the putting of the MONTHLY REVIEWERS has been the same as that of Dr. Sharp. But they have more lately shown a tendency to affiliate their views to those of the primary and secondary actions of medicines, as expounded by Fletcher. By Dr. Pope this connection has been fully enunciated. All disease is asserted to be a "modification of functional activity," and "every form of functional disturbance, howsoever arising," to be "traceable in its earliest phase to inflammatory action." This process is then described as Fletcher conceived it, *viz.*, as consisting in primary contraction and secondary dilatation of the blood-vessels of a part. Drugs are next affirmed to act similarly to the causes of disease; and like these, while pursuing one course, to have two stages of action, the one reverse of the other; while "the degree to which each stage is developed is contingnt upon the dose in which it is administered." "A small dose of a drug will set up the first or stimulating stage of inflammation," *i.e.*, the contraction of the capillaries, "which will be more or less distinctly marked, while the second, or stage of re-action, will be scarcely, if at all, observable. If, on the other hand, a large dose is given, the first stage is but faintly marked, passes rapidly into the second—that of depression, and this alone it is which attracts the attention of the observer." "In disease, as it is presented to us at the bed-side and in the consulting-room, the primary and stimulated condition of parts have given place to that which is secondary or depressed," and which therefore resembles the effect of large doses of drugs. Give a small dose, accordingly, of the most similar remedy, and you will induce upon this depression a precisely analogous stimulation, and so cure the disease.

Now if this theory were sound, it would supply a missing link in Dr. Sharp's chain; it would show HOW large and small doses of drugs should have an opposite action, which at present is by no means easy to conceive in every case. But it is obviously open to all the objections which might be made to the doctrine of Fletcher. All diseases are not inflammatory, or of the type of inflammation; inflammation itself cannot be set up by mere depression of the vaso-motor nerves; when it does occur, dilatation of the vessels is not necessarily preceded by their contraction, still less is a necessary result thereof. Again, all drugs do not cause inflammation; those which do may act by irritating the extra-vascular tissue rather than by affecting the functions of the vaso-motor nerves; inflammation cannot be directly cured by contracting the blood-vessels of affected part, and it would require strong and repeated doses of any drug to do so. It is the advantage of Dr. Sharp's doctrine that it keeps clear of all these theories of disease and of drug-action; it is, indeed, less complete thereby, but it is also less assailable. If only it had a sufficient basis in fact, it might be accepted in its own sphere.

There is, however, I fear, very insufficient evidence of the alleged opposition. In a lecture on "The Rationale of Homœopathic Cure" which you will find in the MONTHLY HOMŒOPATHIC REVIEW for April, 1877. I have analysed the experiments made by Dr. Sharp, and the observations adduced by the REVIEWERS, and have arrived at the conclusion that the residuum of fact left behind is far too insignificant to be the basis of a general doctrine. Instead of affirming that all drugs have an opposite action, according as they are given in large or small doses, I submitted that we must simply say that under these circumstances some drugs exhibit opposite phenomena. Nor can the instances of contrary working according to quantity brought forward by Dr. Cretin, who communicated a paper supporting this view to the International Congress of 1881, avail to alter this conclusion. They all belong to the extra-pharmaceutical sphere—to Heat, Light, *Alcohol*, etc., and admit of an entirely different explanation.

I have been unable to conceal my lack of satisfaction with the various hypotheses which explain apparent Homœopathic action by maintaining that in the system it becomes antipathic. If, nevertheless, I commend the essential thought to your acceptance, it is because this bids fair to be a common ground on which we and our brethren of the old school may stand together. In 1868, Dr. Reith, of Aberdeen, arrived independently at Fletcher's doctrine of the primary and secondary action of drugs upon the capillary vessels, and began to expound his views in the EDINBURGH MEDICAL JOURNAL. He was at once told that they were merely Homœopathic under another name. At first he repudiated the identification, but, further enquiry convincing him of its truth, he fearlessly acknowledged the fact. He had of course to suffer the penalty of his honesty, and to go without the camp, bearing the reproach of the cause he had espoused. He was however, only a few years too soon. In 1875, Dr. (now Sir Thomas) Laude, Brunton, Lecturer on Materia Medica at St. Bartholomew's delivered himself thus: "The opposite action of large and small doses seems to be the basis of truth on which the doctrine of Homœopathy has been founded. The irrational practice of giving infinitesimal doses has of course nothing to do with the principle of Homœopathy, SIMILIA SIMILIBUS CURANTUR; the only requisite is that mentioned by Hippocrates, when he recommended *Mandrake* in Mania, *viz.*, that the dose be smaller than would be sufficient to produce in a healthy man symptoms similar to those of the disease." * On the death of Dr. Anstie, Dr. Brunton became Editor of the PRACTITIONER. In 1877, articles appeared in that Journal from the pen of Dr. Rabagliati, surgeon to the Bradford Infirmary. They were entitled, "Are there Therapeutic Laws?" and their aim seemed the demonstration that the apparently opposite effects of large and small doses were due to the primary and secondary actions of drugs, and their various developments thereby, these actions themselves being to his mind the most important facts in Thrapeutics. The ingenious author was of course entirely unaware that the same views and reasonings were household words in our own school. In 1878, a better-informed writer, Dr. James Ross, physician to the Royal · Infirmary at Manchester, was allowed to publish in the same Journal an article containing the following sentences: "No one who is competent to form an opinion can deny that one or two of the principles lying at the foundation of this" (the Homœopathic) "system are fundamentally true. These principles are what may be briefly termed the local action of medicines or the elective affinities of tissues, the double action of medicines, and the opposite effects of large and small doses." Finally, the Editor himself, after permitting Dr. Sharp to express his own views in his pages, said in a note to one of them—"As there are many drugs which in small doses will produce an action the contrary of that which they produce in large ones, it is evident that Homœopathy and Antipathy are one and the same thing as regards drugs, and differ only in dose." †

Now I cannot say how far the language of Drs. Brunton, Ross and Rabagliati would be endorsed by their colleagues generally. They seem, however, to be fairly representative men; and no one has come forward to protest against the admissions they have made. What, then, is the situation? On the one side are a body of men, guided by the Homœopathic law of selection, but explaining the effects of remedies so chosen by the actions and reactions of medicines, and the opposing influence of varied dosage, so as to make them really

* "Experimental Investigation of the Actions of Medicines," Part I, p. 12.
† PRACTITIONER, June, 1879.

antipathic to the morbid condition. On the other side we have these doctrines accepted as true in themselves, and as veritable explanations of apparently Homœopathic action. How can those who think thus harmoniously stand much longer in disunion? For such prospect of peace we may well be content to sink merely intellectual differences. If the explanation now current commend our method to those who have hitherto refused it,* render it in their eyes reasonable and admissible, what is it if to some amongst us, as to myself, it seems to give an inadequate account of the facts? We must say so, but we may be wrong; and in the meantime the facts are true, the method no less precious though the theory affixed to it be disputable. I only plead that the method be not so bound up with its explanation that the two must stand or fall together; and then I am quite content to allow the latter as plausible enough for provisional acceptance. If our liberty to practice apparent Homœopathy be acknowledged, we care little about its being considered real Antipathy; and if, because so considering it, our colleagues of the other school will join us in following it, our content will merge into gladness.

This at least is certain, that opposite EFFECTS result from many drugs in health and disease, respectively, and it is a fair inference that opposite ACTIONS also may be exerted. Opposites to concrete states, though not always predictable or producible in health, may be induced in disease. This is well-argued in the Editorial Article in the MONTHLY HOMŒOPATHIC REVIEW for 1874 (p. 195), and by Dr. Sharp in the same Journal for 1880 (p. 531). In the former, it is maintained that there are and must be opposites to the state or states which lie at the bottom of the surface phenomena we call disease : There must also be some reverse direction to that which the abnormal change has travelled, and along which the part may be conducted back to health. Dr. Sharp in like manner writes—"Did we know what the inflammatory process is (which we do not), we should doubtless see that there could be an opposite process, and very probably see small doses of *Belladonna* produced that opposite.

In connection with this point, let me call your attention to two interesting Papers by Dr. Percy Wilde, appearing in the Fortieth Volume of the MONTHLY HOMŒOPATHIC REVIEW. Dr. Wilde thinks that we are not doing justice to SIMILIA SIMILIBUS when we limit it to drug-action. He would extend it to all agents influencing vital substance; and would state the law of their action thus :—

A maximum stimulus abolishes the functions of the vital element either completely or temporarily.

"A medium stimulus excites the functions of the vital element,

---

* It seems to do so to Hueppe also. See M.H.R. xliii, 400,

such stimulation being followed by exhaustion, the result of overstimulation.

"A minimum stimulus increases the function of the vital element, and when this element if previously weak such stimulation restores the normal balance, and is not followed by exhaustion." Drugs, he would say, conform to these laws of action because they are stimuli. He has such respectable authority for the assumption that I do not feel inclined to dispute it, though to my mind it presents grave difficulties. If it could be granted, I should have no difficulty in following Dr. Wilde when he extends his principles to all kinds of stimuli, whether chemical, thermal, mechanical, or electrical. For the present, however, in face of the difficulties to which I have alluded, I have confined my enquiries to drug-action on its own merits, leaving the other fields to be cultivated by those who would work on them.

APPENDIX TO LECTURE XII.

Two good illustrations of the apparently opposite action of large and small doses, as such, have been furnished of late years by the LITERATURE OF TRADITIONAL MEDICINE.

1. In 1880, Dr. Murrell reported in the LANCET (April 27th), the results of treatment of Whooping-cough in an adult. He first took *Bromide of Potassium* for a fortnight without any benefit, whereupon he was given "five drop doses of a 1 in 10 tincture of *Drosera rotundifolia.*" "He took this," says the narrative, "for a week, and then returned, saying that it had made him much worse. It increased the spasm and cough, and made him whoop more; he whooped as many as twelve times in one paroxysm." The dose was then reduced to half a drop of the same tincture, and at the end of a week he came reporting great improvement which in another fortnight resulted in complete cure.

2. In 1896, Dr. Lauder relates in the same Journal (May 30th), his experience with *Opium* in constipation, a pretty enough Homœopathic prescription. Given indiscriminately to his hospital outpatients, it naturally gave only occasional satisfaction; but in a private case the results were interesting. The patient—a lady—was ordered one minim of the ordinary tincture every night. After a week the report was better. He replied, "Double the quantity." In a few days the word came, "Rather worse." He then wrote to say, "Give her half the first dose." Three or four days afterwards he had a letter to say that the last medicine acted well, if anything too violently.

LECTURE XIII.

THE HISTORY OF HOMŒOPATHY

In inviting you to practise Homœopathy, I have urged that you should not adopt a creed but join a church. I have today to tell you what manner of institution this church is; to show you how the method of Hahnemann has organized itself during the nineteenth century, which saw its birth and growth, and in what shape and dimensions it exists at the dawn of the twentieth at which now we stand. The authentic materials for such a history lie ready in our hands. To the International Homœopathic Congresses, held quinquennially since 1786, have been presented reports from all civilised countries in the world dealing with the past annals and present condition of our system; and in the published Transactions of the Congresses we have these reports before us. From them I shall draw the information I now bring under your notice.

The early history of Homœopathy is the genesis of the idea in the originator's own mind, and this we have sufficiently traced. He remained its one advocate, so far as we know, until, in 1810, he settled in Leipzig, and, in 1812, Germany obtained permission to lecture in the University of that capital. He soon gathered round him a band of disciples who learned from his lips, assisted him in his provings, and one by one went forth to carry out in their chosen fields of practice the method he had taught them. This was the beginning of Homœopathy in Germany; and to it belong the well-known names of Stapf, Gross, Franz, Hartmann, Herrman, Lehmann, Ruckert, Wislicenus and Moritz Muller. The first and second of these, in 1821, established the first Homœopathic journal, well-known as the ARCHIV, which continued to appear until 1843. In 1832, another journal was founded, the ALLGEMEINE HOMŒOPATHISCHE ZEITUNG; and this, under various editors, has survived to the present day. In 1830, the adherents of Homœopathy had grown so numerous that they felt the need of regular intercourse and a CENTRAL VEREIN was constituted, to meet annually in some German city, as it has done ever since. The first meeting was held in Leipzig, under the presidency of Muller, and a proposal was set on foot for establishing a hospital in this city, which took form in 1832. After ten years of useful life, it was merged in a Dispensary—a Policlinic as they call it in Germany; and this, mainly under Clotar, the son of Moritz Muller, flourished for thirty-five years, carrying out its operations on a large scale, and forming a practical seminary for the incipient Homœopathists of the country. It played the same part in Germany as that performed by Liverpool in England, and as in that city, the Dispensary was in its turn re-merged in a hospital. This was opened in 1888, with 200 beds, and continues its useful work.

The Homœopathic like other bodies has had its parties, and these are very like those of the French Parliament. There is a Right, to which tradition is dear, and which departs as little as possible from the established ways of medicine; there is a Left, which cuts itself entirely adrift from the past, and lives by its prospects for the future; and each of these has its extreme wing and its centre. Hahnemann's earlier disciples were of the "Left" type, as their master himself increasingly became: but a representative of the "Right" had already appeared in Muller, and he was later reinforced by Griesselich, Rau, Schron, Trinks, Arnold and Paul Wolf. The HYGEA (1834-1848) ably expounded the views of these physicians, and was followed later by the VIERTELIAHRSCHRIFT and the INTERNATIONALE PRESSE of which Clotar Muller was the inspiring soul. These with Hirschel's ZEITSCHRIFT, have disappeared with their editors; and the only living contemporary of the A.H.Z. (as we briefly style it) is the ZEITSCHRIFT DES BERLINER VEREINS HOMŒOPATHISCHER AERZTE, a journal which has appeared monthly since 1882, and is a credit to our school both in form and substance.

Under the influence of the men, the journals and the institutions I have mentioned, Homœopathy has continued to "hold its own" in the land of its nativity. The number of avowed Homœopathists practising there is given as 300 in 1876, 400 in 1896, 500 in 1900. * Besides the hospital in Leipzig already mentioned, there has for many years been one in Munich and in Stuttgart; and another has just been founded in Berlin, Veith Meyer, Hoppe, Rapp, Bahr, Grauvogl, Elb, Sorge, Goullon, Heinigke, Villers and Lohrbacher are names which have added lustre to German Homœopathy; and welcome aid has of late been afforded by Drs. Augo Schulz and Arndt, of the University of Greifswald, who, without identifying themselves with us, have supported our doctrines and practice in a very effective manner. The CENTRAL VEREIN is supported and fed by several local societies of Homœopathic physicians; and a marked

* In 1891 it is estimated at 600; but this is probably a slip either of the reporter or of the press.

feature of our existence in Germany is the number of lay societies for the advancement of the system. "The whole of Germany is dotted over with a network" of these, wrote Dr. Lorbacher in 1891. Several periodicals are issued under their auspices, and serve to keep the flame of Homœopathy burning among the people.

Little provision for the teaching of our method has existed in Germany. Hahnemann's lectureship in the University of Leipzig was continued by Moritz Muller, and Dr. Buchner occupied a similar position in that of Munich; that is all that can be said. It is pleasant to hear, therefore, that since 1898 regular courses of lectures have been delivered at the Berlin Dispensary by physicians of that city, and have had greater success than could have been expected.

As was only natural, Austria was the first-country to catch a spark from the new fire kindled in Germany. Homœopathy had made sufficient advance there in 1819 to be forbidden by Imperial Decree, and had in spite of this so successfully asserted itself by 1837 that in that year the edict was rescinded. Marenzeller, first in Prague, then in Vienna, and Fleischmann in the Capital itself, were the main agents in this progress; and when once the new method had won its liberty, a number of able man flocked to its standard. Arneth, Gerstel, Huber, Mayerhofer, Wachtel, Watzke, Wurmb and Zlatarowich are some of the best-known names among them. They founded a Society, established a journal (the OESTERREICHISCHE ZEITSCHRIFT) and conducted a series of provings and reprovings of the most admirable character. One public and two private hospitals in Vienna were placed in their hands and Fleischmann's results at the Gumpendorff and Wurmb and Caspar's clinical studies at the Leopoldstadt made the men and the institutions famous. The contagion soon spread over the Empire. Hospitals were established at Linz and other places, including Buda-Pesth, in which University two chairs of Homœopathic doctrine and practice were founded, and given to Drs. Haussmann and Bakody respectively.

Austria-Hungary

This rate of progress had hardly been maintained and the later Austrian Homœopathists, with the exception of Kafka, of Prague, have not been of the stature of the earlier groups. They maintained their hospitals, however, and one of their chairs in the Hungarian University; and the method has a large following among the upper classes of both divisions of the Dual Monarchy. Statistics are rarely given; but as far as can be inferred from the data there have not been more than 300 practitioners of our method in this country at any given time.

THE HISTORY OF HOMŒOPATHY

Italy. As Austria received Homœopathy from Germany, it transmitted it to Italy; and thus the three nations which now form the "Tripple Alliance" for military purposes were at an earlier time a TRIPLICE in possessing the new medical truth. An Austrian occupation of Naples took place in 1821; and the commander of the foreign troops, Baron Francis Koller, was a devoted disciple of Hahnemann. He had not been there long when he sent for his physician Dr. Necker, to come and settle in the Italian city. Necker had been a pupil of the master and was a practitioner of distinction. During the four years he remained in Naples he made a most favourable impression with the new practice; and when he left, three of the leading physicians of the city had become converts to it. These were Romani, Mauro and De Horatiis. A full account of their career is given in the Transactions of the Congress of 1876. They translated the 'Organon' and the 'Reine Arzneimittellehre,'; they founded a journal (1892), entitled EFFEMERIDI DI MEDICINA OMIOPATICA; and they made converts all over Italy.

But, as in Austria, this good beginning has hardly fulfilled its promise for the future, Romani, died in 1847, De Horatiis in 1850, Mauro (nearly a centenarian) in 1857. Among their converts and successors the only prominent name is that of Rubini, who lived into our own time, and has earned our gratitude by giving us *Cactus grandiflorus*, and proving (after Hahnemann) what wonders *Camphor*, freely administered, can work in Cholera. Other worthy names in Italian Homœopathy are Centamori, De Rinaldis, Panelli, Ladelci, Dadea, Pompili, Bonino and Cigliano; but they do not attain to the level at first reached. Dr. Pompili founded, and has for many years carried on a small monthly journal—the RIVISTA OMIOPATICA. To Dr. Bonino, mainly, we owe the organisation of the Italian Homœopathists of the present day into the 'Instituto Omiopatico Italiano,' which meets annually; publishes from time to time a fasciculus entitled L'OMIOPATIA IN ITALIA; and sustains a small hospital in Turin and dispensaries in this and other Italian cities.

The number of Homœopathic practitioners in Italy has rarely exceeded 100, and is not above 50.

It was from Italy that both France and England received Homœopathy. The former enjoyed priority in order of time and so must be taken first here.

"In 1828", we are told in the Report of 1876, "Hahnemann or his doctrine was scarcely known in France . . . At this epoch the Comte des Guidi, a Doctor of Medicine and Science and Inspector of the University of Lyons, was in Naples, Unsuccessful in arresting the supposed fatal malady of his wife, who accompanied him to get the benefit of the baths of Pozzuoli, he was induced to consult Dr. Romani. France Her cure by his treatment made a profound impression on des Guidi, and induced him to study the doctrines of Hahnemann." He also followed a clinique which Romani, with De Horatis, was then carrying on at the Ospedale Delia Trintia. In 1830, he returned to Lyons, and devoted himself to the practice and advocacy of Homœopathy. Antonie Petroz, a physician of high-standing in Paris, was one of his earliest converts, and he in turn won many others over: so that when Hahnemann, after his second marriage in 1835, migrated to Paris, he found a body of disciples there to welcome him, organized into a society ("Institut Homœpathique") and represented by two Journals (JOURNAL and ARCHIVES DE LA MEDECINE HOMŒOPATHICQUE). When he died in 1843, he left his system firmly established in France—among its adherents being a professor in the ancient Univeristy of Montpellier, Dr. d'Amador.

Nor have we here, as in the case of Austria and Italy, to lament any subsequent decline. In 1847 Tessier, one of the hospital physicians of Paris, became an avowed convert, and, maintaining his appointments, took advantage of his position to shew by clinical evidence the relative superiority of Homœopathic treatment. He brought with him into our ranks a number of pupils and friends who have since been among their brightest ornaments: I am thinking especially of Timbart, Gabalda, Milcent, Devasse, Fredualt, Ozanam and Jousset—the last of whom still remains to adorn and serve them. Dr. Imbert Gourbeyre, Professor in the School at Clermont-Ferrand, has taken d'Amador's place as our academic representative, and has enriched medical literature by a number of valuable monographs. The literary output of French Homœopathy has indeed been phenomenal, both in quantity and quality, especially considering the paucity of its numbers; which have rarely reached 300 at any epoch, and have often been nearer 200.

The older school of Parisian Homœopathists were at first disposed to look somewhat askance at the new body of adherents, who called Tessier their master rather than Hahnemann, and distinguished between the latter's doctrine and practice. The result was that for a long time the practitioners of the capital were divided into two camps, each having its hospital, its society, and its journal. These feuds are now healed. The "Societe Francaise d'Homœopathie" at this day unites them all; and though L'ART MEDICAL, the journal founded by Tessier, is still carried on by the Joussets, PERE ET FILS (and long may it flourish !), it has no polemical aspect, and the REVIEW HOMOEOPATHIQUE FRANCAISE, the organ of the Society, contains contributions from both sides alike. The two hospitals, the Hospital Hahnemann and St. Jacques respectively (making up about 100 beds between them), continue as separate establishments, but with no antagonism; and to them has recently been added a hospital for children.

In the provinces, French Homœopathy is well, though too sparsely represented. The Hospital St. Luc, at Lyons, founded in 1875, endowed and flourishing, is the only institution of the kind to be found outside Paris; but dispensaries abound everywhere, as (I might have said) they do in the Capital itself.

Several attempts have been made to establish systematic teaching of Homœopathy in Paris; and during 1836-1845, 1863-9, for some years after 1880, and again during 1898-9, regular courses of lectures were delivered, with varying success.

Besides the names I have mentioned, others that have shed lustre upon Homœopathy in France, have been those of the Leon Simons, GRANDPERE PERE ER FILS; the Curies and Molins, PERE ET FILS; Cretin; Meyhoffer; Charge: David Roth; Jahr; Espanet; Teste; Claude and Gonnard.

Among the physicians who, with des Guidi, attended the clinique of Romani and de Horatiis at the TRINITA in 1829 was Frederic Foster Quin. Quin had been graduated at Edinburgh in 1820, and was intending to practise in London; but delicate lungs induced him to spend some years first in Italy. He went as travelling physician to the Duchess of Devonshire, and subsequently settled in Naples to practise amongst the large English Colony there. In 1825, his attention was directed to Homœopathy by Necker, and he saw and read enough to make him feel that the system deserved a serious examination. He went to Leipzig for the purpose, became more and more satisfied of the value of Hahnemann's method, and after some wanderings having settled in London in 1832, determined to advocate and practise it. His good connections and high social qualities, combined with his ability, energy and knowledge, made him an apt apostle of the new practice in the English Metropolis. He soon gathered colleagues around him, and in 1844, with seven others, he founded the British Homœopathic Society, the presidency of which he enjoyed—by repeated re-elections—till his death in 1878.

Meantime something analogous to the accession of Tessier and his disciples in Paris had taken place in Edinburgh. Drysdale and Russell, influenced by the Physiological Professor of whom I have already spoken—Fletcher, has devoted their early post-graduate years to a study of Homœopathy in Germany and Austria. Black, learning from them, had gone to Paris to study and practise under Hahnemann himself. On their return, Drysdale settled at Liverpool, but Black and Russel reverted to the city of their studies, and opened a Homœopathic Dispensary there. In 1844, Henderson, Professor of Pathology in the University, became an avowed convert; and was followed by not a few of his students, amongst whom the most distinguished name is that of Madden. Thus arose the "Edinburgh School" of British Homœopathists, which, while loyally embracing the method of Hahnemann, has formed what I have called the "Right" of our body here, and has found many to hand on its traditions.

In London, Edinburgh and Liverpool, British Homœopathy now had three centres, and from these it steadily widened out over the kingdom. Round Quin came Cameron, Hamilton, Kidd and Yeldham; Edinburgh sent Pope and Ker to join our ranks; Drysdale converted Dudgeon, Chapman and Hilbers. In 1843, the BRITISH JOURNAL OF HOMŒOPATHY was founded, and continued to appear quarterly (or oftener) up till 1884. Its editorial staff had included at different times the names of Drysdale, Black, Russel and Dudgeon, and with these champions of our cause I was myself honoured by association for the last twenty-two years of the Journal's life. In 1856, it was reinforced in its advocacy of the new system by the MONTHLY HOMŒOPATHIC REVIEW, among whose editors the names of Pope and Dyce Brown shine out with the brightest lustre. In 1850, the London Homœopathic Hospital was founded, and dispensaries sprang up wherever converts settled for practice. Among these were numbered a former President of the British Medical Association, Dr. Horner; a Lecturer at St. Bartholomew's, Dr. Conquest; and a F.R.S, Dr. Sharp of Rugby, whose "Tracts" did great things towards propagating the cause. In 1857, it was reckoned that there were upwards of 200 practitioners in the British Islands.

Nor have we to lament in this country a blight on the promise of our spring such as we have seen in Austria and Italy. The forty years and more which have elapsed since the foregoing estimate was made, have seen many changes, but retrogression and decadence have not been amongst them. Our numbers reach 300 rather than 200—the British Homœopathic Soceity alone counting more than the latter on its roll. This body has continued to meet monthly from its formation, and since 1860 has issued its transactions, under the title first of the ANNALS, then of the JOURNAL of the Soceity. The London Homœopathic Hospital has continued to grow, and during the nineties was rebuilt on its foundations at a cost of £45,000 and re-opened with a capacity of 100 beds. It has, since 1891, published an annual volume of REPORTS, embodying much of the experience gained within its walls. It has been gratifying to witness the growth of sister-institutions in many parts of the kingdom, among which I may specify Liverpool, Birmingham, Bath, Plymouth, Bromley and St. Leonards, all of which are doing good work. In journalism we have a new accession in the HOMŒOPATHIC WORLD, a semi-popular monthly, edited successively by Drs. Ruddock, Shuldham, Burnett and Clarke.

The teaching of Homœopathy in England, has not been uncared-for. Besides sporadic courses of lectures at the Hospital in London during 1852-1864, given by Drs. Quin, Leadam, Russell and others, an attempt at systematic instruction was commenced (mainly at the instance and by the efforts of Dr. Bayes) under the auspices of the British Society in 1874, which culminated in the establishment of the London School of Homœopathy in 1877. Its Chair of Practice was from the commencement filled by Dr. Dyce Brown; that of Materia Medica successively by myself, Dr. Pope, Dr. Burnett and Dr. Clarke. After some eight years of existence, it was merged in the Hospital, which has always added "and School of Medicine" to its title; and courses of instruction conducted by members of the staff and others have been continued with varying regularity ever since.

Before leaving our own country, we must say something of the history of Homœopathy in the various colonies and dependencies which make up the British Empire.

The early annals of the system in INDIA are occupied with the occasional sojourns there of foreign Homœopathists—among whom the names of Honigberger, Tonnerre and Berigny may be mentioned—and spasmodic attempts made by native magnates to establish dispensaries and even hospitals for its practice in their domains. Its real history begins with the conversion, in 1867, of Dr. Mahendra Lal Sircar, a graduate of the University of Calcutta, and a man of high-standing in that city. He founded a Dispensary for the poor, and a Periodical— the CALCUTTA JOURNAL OF MEDICINE; both of which he has carried on single-handed to the present day. In 1891 he was able to report that there were thirty qualified Homœopathic practitioners in Calcutta and its suburbs, and as many more in other parts of India. Besides these, there are multitudes of native lay practitioners scattered over the country—the demand for knowledge of the system on whose part has led to the establishment of two Schools of Homœopathy in the metropolis, conducted by Drs. Majumdar and Bose respectively. The INDIAN HOMŒOPATHIC

REVIEW, edited by the former of these gentlemen, and the INDIAN HOMŒOPATHICIAN, of which Mr. Ghose is the conductor and almost the sole writer, represent this section of our following, and the number of Homœopathic pharmacies in Calcutta, which minister to and depend mainly on their practice, is said to be extraordinary.

CANADA first reported in 1881. It seems that Homœopathy was introduced there in 1846 by a Dr. Lancaster. It has made fair progress, and has representatives in most towns of the Dominion. Five of its practitioners have seats on the Ontario Medical Council, which is the licensing as well as governing body of the Canadian profession. From later reports we learn that we have a share in two hospitals, one in Toronto and one in London; and in Montreal possess one of our own which has 25 beds. In 1880 the number of Homœopathists in the Dominion was about 110, and no great accessions seem to have been made since then.

And now as regards AUSTRALASIA. Our system was introduced into Sydney and Melbourne about 1851. In the former city it has, after rising to a certain level, remained pretty stationary; but in Melbourne a hospital has been in existence since 1869, which has done such good work, especially in the treatment of Typhoid, that it has received large support and Government grants, and occupies now a building erected for it making up 60 beds. We have also a place in the hospitals of Adelaide, S.A., and of Bathurst, N.S.W.; while Hobart and Launceston in Tasmania have lately opened institutions of the kind devoted entirely to the practice of our method. New Zealand is not so forward, but Homœopathy is worthily represented in several of its cities. It was introduced there as early as 1853.

From SOUTH AFRICA we are glad to learn that the Boers have at least this good point about them that they appreciate Homœopathy. Their practice of it is mainly domestic; but Capetown long had a capable professional representative of the method in its midst, in the shape of Dr. Kitchen, who died last year.

Homœopathy was first practised in JAMAICA by a Spanish physician from Cuba, Dr. Navarro. We have had no reports from the island since 1876, but a Dr. Reinke writes from it in an American journal of 1883.

Spain

I have next to speak of SPAIN. It would have been strange had no news leaked into this country from France or Italy of the reform in medicine associated with Hahnemann's name; and there are traces of a knowledge of it as early as 1829-30. In 1833, however, a real beginning of Spanish Homœopathy was made in the persons of three physicians—

Pinciano, Hurtado and Querol. How they were made converts does not appear, possibly through literature imported during the former epoch just named : but they did great things to spread the knowledge of the new method, by translations of its publications as well as by their own successful practice. There were then already a number of Homœopathic practitioners in Spain when Numez, who had learnt the method from des Guidi and practised it in Bordeaux, came to Madrid in 1844, and rapidly reached the leading place in the movement. He was appointed physician to then Queen Isabella, and was ennobled by her. He founded the Hahnemannian Society of Madrid, and induced it to issue a periodical BOLETIN which subsequently became EL CRITERIO MEDICO and continued to represent Spanish Homœopathy for many years—doing so, for all I know, to this day. Still more important was his action in promoting the establishment of a hospital and school of medicine. The Hospital (dedicated to St. Joseph) was opened in 1878, containing 50 beds; and the course of teaching in connection with it inaugurated. In 1879, Nunez died, leaving all his fortune to it, and thus in nearly every respect being in Spain what Quin had been in England.

His country, with its colonies, is said to have contained in 1865, as many as 600 Homœopathic practitioners.* Cuba and Puerto Rico, now lost to it, stood first among the colonies; but the other island groups—Balearic, Canary, Philippine—had representatives of the system. We have had little news from Spain since 1881. What has come is chiefly from Barcelona, which publishes a REVISTA HOMŒOPATICA of its own, and has a flourishing local Society.

I would add a word as to what may be called SPANISH AMERICA. We hear of Homœopathy at times from many of the republics embraced within this category, but have definite information concerning Mexico and Uruguay only. In Montevideo, the capital of the latter state, there were seven Homœopathic practitioners in 1875, the one who reports having been such from his graduation in 1847. In Mexico, our system seems to have begun its career in about 1853, when practitioners from Havana and Spain (Navarrete and Cornellas) settled there. It has advanced since with commendable rapidity and steadiness. Two Societies have existed since the early seventies and three journals have been issued—one of which, at any rate, LA HOMŒOPATIA, continues to flourish. In 1880, two wards of a public hospital were made over to us, and a School has been founded,

---

* This estimate must be too liberal, or there must have been a great falling-off, for in 1885 we find the Homœopathists in Spain itself only 241 in number.

the degrees of which are recognised by the government as qualifying for practice.

From Spain we naturally pass to PORTUGAL. We heard nothing from this country till 1896, when a layman—Senhor A Nery de Vasconcellos, of Oporto—kindly collected and sent the necessary information. As early as 1883, we find a Professor in the medical school of Lisbon requesting permission from the government to try practically the Homœopathic method. This was refused him; but, being in 1839 president of the Society for Medical Sciences of that city, he prevailed upon it to make Hahnemann an honorary member of its first class. This was, I believe, the only old-school distinction our Master ever received. In the succeeding years stragglers from Brazil began to practise Homœopathically in Portugal, but in the fifties it first acquired a solid footing there through the favour shewn it by the Duke of Saldanha, the foremost statesman in the country. Lisbon and Oporto soon had a fair complement of practitioners, who have continued to represent our cause to this day, when they are between 20 and 30 in number. At Oporto, they have a ward in the general hospital, and a hospital for children of their own.

Portugal

BRAZIL has been so long connected politically with Portugal that the history of Homœopathy in it seems best recounted here. It begins earlier than in the mother country, dating from about 1837, when a student from Leipzig made the method a subject of his graduation thesis, and induced a physician named Estrado to study and practise it. It made rapid progress, and in 1876—to which belongs its only Report—it had about 75 practitioners, organized in two Societies.

We must now turn northwards again, and first must enquire how Homœopathy has fared in RUSSIA.

In the Second Edition of the Sixth volume of the REINE ARZNEIMITTELLEHRE published in 1827, we find among the provers of *Carbo vegetabilis*—"the Russian physician, Dr. Adam." He seems to have become acquainted with Hahnemann in Germany in 1823 and soon to have begun to practise his method in St. Petersburg. A letter from one of his converts in Stapf's ARCHIV of 1823, shows considerable progress have been already made, and favourable criticisms were written by Sahmen in Dorpat and Marcus in Moscow. An important adhesion was made about this time in the person of Dr. Bigel, physician to the wife of the Grand Duke Constantine, and the cause now rapidly made advance. Its story is related in the detailed reports supplied to the Congress from 1876 to

Russia

1891 inclusive by one of its leading personages—the late Dr. Bojanus. When the infirmities of age rendered him unable to take up the pen, another protagonist of our method assumed it, and the reports of 1896 and 1900 were supplied by Dr. Brasol. It is impossible in this place to summarise the mass of information thus supplied. It shews the usual phenomena—rapid advance among the laity, slow adoption by the profession. All Russia does not contain more than 50 Homœopathic practitioners, 17 of whom are at St. Petersburg. Together with their lay friends, they have formed 12 Societies, most of which support pharmacies and dispensaries. A hospital has been erected in the capital, making up 50 beds; and it was opened in 1898.

Besides the names already specified, those of Deriker, Villers Sen, Hermann, Dahl and Dittmann may be mentioned as prominent in Russian Homœopathy. In Poland, Wieniawski attained some eminence, and did a good stroke of work in converting, before his own decease, a Professor at the Hospital of the Holy Ghost in Warsaw, Dr. Drzwiecki.

Of the three Scandinavian countries, SWEDEN and NORWAY were reported of in 1876 by Dr. Liedbeck of Stockholm. He told of several Swedish practitioners of our method in the past, but of one only living colleague. In Norway also he Scandinavia knew of only two. We heard nothing more from Sweden till 1896, when Dr. Hagemark presented himself at our Congress, telling us how he and a Dr. Grundal alone occupied the place at Stockholm which Dr. Liedbeck had vacated by death in 1876. Of Norway he could say nothing.

We did not hear from DENMARK till 1886, but then Dr. Hansen of Copenhagen, gave us an unexpectedly far-reaching history of Homœopathy in that country. Lund having begun its practice there as early as 1821. The succession of its representatives has never been broken, and when Dr. Hansen wrote, he had eight like-minded colleagues in the kingdom. Little change is noted in his subsequent Reports of 1896 and 1900, but it is pleasant to learn that they have 450,000 Francs in their hands for a hospital in Copenhagen.

Of HOLLAND we only heard in 1896. Dr. Von dem Borne, of Amsterdam, who came to our Congress that year, sent us also an account of the present state of Homœopathy in his country, but gave no details or dates as to its past. There Holland were only six physicians practising it when he wrote, a number sadly disproportionate to the wants of the thousands of its lay adherents. "There are regions," he writes, "as in the province of Zeeland, where the totality of the inhabitants are partisans of our method of treatment, where physicians of the other school cannot earn their livelihood, and where yet it is quite impossible to find a Homœopathic doctor." Our four representatives have formed a Society, and issue a monthly journal—the HOM. MAANBLAD.

The other division of the Netherlands had begun to appreciate the blessings of Homœopathy before it became an independent kingdom. Dr. de Moor of Alost, described as "titular Surgeon" of the Civil Hospital of that city, embraced it in 1829; Belgium and though too old to do much towards its propagation, gave us in his son, Dr. Charles de Moor, a worthy inheritor of his name and convictions. In 1831, Dr. Carlier and in 1832 Dr. Varlez began its practice in Brussels; and, with the adherents who accrued in 1837 founded a society and a dispensary.

Thus inaugurated, Homœopathy went on prosperously up to 1896, when Dr. Schepenes could report to the London Congress that there were about 100 avowed practitioners of the method, as well as many practising it partially or secretly; that as a rule, all were doing large and lucrative practices; and that there were specialists—surgeons, oculists, &c.—who openly professed to be Homœopathic in their convictions. He reported two Societies, and two Journals issued under their respective auspices. He related, moreover, the triumph obtained in Antwerp, where the Bureau de Bienfaisance of the city had placed one of its Dispensaries under Homœopathic control.

Either, however, Dr. Schepens saw things too much EN COULEUR DE ROSE, or his successor has taken too gloomy a view, for Dr. Mersch reports to the Congress of 1900 the number of practitioners as fallen to 30, one of the Journals (the REVUE HOMŒOPATHIQUE BELGE) discontinued, and the Antwerp Dispensary—though the poor flock to it in rapidly increasing numbers—hardly able to carry on its medical service. There is no doubt that here, as almost everywhere else, the need is MEN; and could we only manufacture Homœopathic practitioners, as America can, our system would be sure of an ample following.

Besides the names already given, I may mention Mouremans, Bernard, Martiny, Gaudy, Stockman and Gaillard as prominent among Belgian Homœopathists. The last-named was an intrepid controversialist, and the Journal he long sustained, L'HOMŒOPATHIC MILITANTE, well represents his energy and his learning.

The last European country I have to include in this sketch is SWITZERLAND. There are no historical notices of Homœopathy in it; but in 1876, Dr. Bruckner reckons 33 practitioners of

Switzerland.

the method, and a small hospital in Basle. In 1886, however, when the Congress met in that city, we heard nothing about its hospital; and Switzerland sent us only nine representatives. In 1891, Dr. Bruckner again reports, with the old story; abundance of popular favour and success of lay practitioners, but hardly conversions enough to make up our death-losses.

United States.

And now we must cross the Atlantic again landing this time not at Quebec, but at New York; must view the method of Hahnemann, not as it just maintains its foothold in Canada, but as it counts its practitioners by the thousand, its institutions by the hundred, in the UNITED STATES OF AMERICA. Here alone in all the world it has been seen what Homœopathy can do on a fair field with no favour, but on the other hand with no prejudice to obstruct and officialism to stifle its natural growth. The results have been most satisfactory. In 1825, the system had but one representative in the States: in 1900, the most moderate computation reckons its practitioners there as 9,369 in number. It has nine national societies (one, the American Institute of Homœopathy, having 1,900 members); 34 State and 116 local societies; 70 general hospitals making up between them some 4,829 beds, and 32 special ones with 6,592. There are 20 Medical Schools, which either on their own account or by the co-operation of a University to which they are affiliated, graduate medical students and qualify them for practice. They turn out between 400 and 500 alumni each year, and so not only fill gaps in our ranks but augment their members continually.

To trace the history of American Homœopathy would require a lecture to itself. It has spread from several centres, and gathered around many men. The one representative, I have said it had in 1825, was Dr. Gram, a Dane by family, but born in Boston (in 1786). After practising with distinction in Copenhagen, and there becoming a convert to Hahnemann's method, he returned to his native country to carry it out and propagate it. He soon obtained disciples in New York, where he settled, among these the names of Gray, Hull, Channing and Curtis being best known. He died in 1840. Seven years before his decease Constantine Hering (born in 1800) had settled in Philadelphia. He came from Germany, where he had become a disciple of Hahnemann; and he brought with him a vigorous and original mind, a vast store of knowledge, and an indefatigable energy. Under his auspices Philadelphia became a second centre of Homœopathy in America; a college was founded to teach it, provings were made to supply materials for its practice, and in 1844 the "American Institute" organized to bind together its scattered practitioners. Round Hering gathered Jeanes, Gardiner, Williamson, Kitchen, Neidhard—all honoured names; Reichelm set up the banner in Pittsburg and Detwiller at Euston. And now new centres began to form. Gregg and Flagg led the way in Boston, and were succeeded by the Wesselhœfts, de Gersdorff and Talbot—to the last of whom the flourishing state of our system in Massachusetts, and its splendid "institutions" are mainly due. Illinois soon followed, with David Smith, Temple and Lord. Chicago naturally took the lead among its cities, and found in Ludlam and Small, chief corner-stones on whom its present Homœopathic edifices could be erected. And so progress went on. The first published list of the members of the American Institute (1846) shewed 137 names, but in ten years more these had become 327, and in 1866 they were 535. The pioneers, I have mentioned, were succeeded by scores of others rivalling them in ability and emulating them in zeal. I can only specify Carrol Dunham, J. P. Dake, Farrington, Lippe, Guernsey, Hempel, McClelland, T. F. Allen, Raue and Holcombe, to whom must be added the surgeons who, with Helmuth at their head, have repaid Homœopathy by their credit for the aid it has brought them in their art. These pioneers also have mostly gone to their rest; but if sublunary things are known to them now, and they have their pristine interest, they must be warmly gratified to see the present flourishing state of the new Therapeutics which in their life-time they did so much to advance.

LECTURE XIV.

THE PHILOSOPHY OF HOMŒOPATHY.

I have now sketched for you, in the bare outline which time would allow, the manner in which Homœopathy has become organized in the several countries of the civilised world in which from a creed it has become a church. Before we go on, let me point the moral of this story.

It was in 1796 that Hahnemann first published his "New Principle for ascertaining the Curative Powers of Drugs." In 1801 he began to speak of the power of minute doses; and in 1805 the "Fragmenta de Viribus Medicamentorum Positivis" appeared. Homœopathy may thus be said to have lived for just upon a century. This has been ample time for it, if it be a delusion, to sprout up and die down again; or if it be a truth, to grow to a maturity which shall be some test of its value. Well, our survey of the present status of Homœopathy shews that it has at the present time no less than 12,000 avowed practitioners in the world,—there being some 10,000 in America and 2,000 in Europe. In nearly all countries where it is represented, there are Homœopathic journals —quarterly, monthly, fortnightly or weekly, and also medical schools. Whatever the most unfavourable criticism may find to object to in these men, these publications, these institutions, at least their number is of indubitable significance. They have sprung up from the seed which Hahnemann cast into the ground a hundred years ago; hence comes all their independent life. How could they exist were not that seed the receptacle of mighty forces, the germ of luxuriant growth?

And then consider that this host of medical men implies a corresponding CLIENTELE, that if there are thousands of doctors there must be millions of patients, The testimony of a large body of skilled practitioners is worth much; but perhaps the testimony of the still larger body of suffering subjects is worth more. The laity are indeed incapable of deciding between rival medical theories. But they are after all the best judges of what cures their complaints most safely, most quickly and most pleasantly. As Dr. Garth Wilkinson once said—We may not understand cobbling, but we know when our boots fit. I think it must be admitted that, so far as their verdict has been given, it is in favour of Homœopathy. It is reasonable to suppose that the great majority of those who now adopt it have also had experience of the other system; while, on the other hand, it is probable that by far the greater number of people have never tried Homœopathic treatment at all. Hence the testimony in its favour of its adherents far outweighs that of its non-adherents against it; for in the former case only has there commonly been opportunity of comparison and choice.

There is an obvious objection to this argument from the large adhesion of the laity. It may be cited (it will be said) in favour of every medical quackery and delusion. But there is this difference in kind between the lay support of Homœopathy, and that which has been and is accorded to panaceas and wonder-workers. In the latter case, when anything more than the habitual *DOMESTIC* use of certain secret remedies (which may have their virtues), it is the resort of persons labouring under chronic or inveterate complaints to some new pretender to their cure. The orthodox medicine of the day has failed to relieve their sufferings; and they can hardly be blamed for seeking elsewhere for aid. But with Homœopathy it is quite different. Here the patient selects for his habitual adviser a medical man who, while indeed holding himself at perfect liberty to treat his patients as he may think best, nearly always thinks it best to do so according to the Hahnemannian method. With no other professional help scores of thousands of families now live and die; and this among the educated as largely as among the working classes. These are not the features, nor is the past of Homœopathy the history of a delusion. They tell rather of a successful practice swiftly working its way in spite of inertia and prejudice.

In such numbers, with such features, Homœopathy has become an organized body. I must ask you to believe that its followers have not sought such a separatist attitude; that they have been forced into it by the intolerance, hostility and persecution everywhere shown towards it by the profession at large, as I have described in my Lecture XI. A large part of its history, as related in the Transactions from which I have drawn it, is taken up with the narrative of the attacks made upon its practitioners. But I think we may say with the poet—

"Now hath descended a serener hour."

The recent utterances, say from 1881, on the subject of Homœopathy have breathed a far milder spirit than those of the thirty years beginning with 1851; the medical journals notice our doings with good-humoured badinage instead of the truculent animosity to which we were accustomed; and most of us have of late years found in professional intercourse an amenity which was as welcome as it was unexpected. I think the time has come for serious endeavours to heal the breaches and terminate the schism; and to all, on either side, whom these words may reach I would re-state the causes which hold us apart, and the claims on the part of Homœopathy the frank allowance of which would justify, indeed would compel, our re-absorption into the general body of the profession.

First of all, let us recall what is the doctrine which constitutes our creed and has formed us into a church. Doctrine, I say; for Homœopathy is this, and nothing more. Like every other doctrine, it has practical corollaries; and one of these, the small dose, has caught the common eye as the prominent distinction of our method. But as every one who will look into our literature may satisfy himself, we are not globulists, or even necessarily infinitesimalists: we are not characterized essentially by any of the theories or practices which may have marked the school of Hahnemann. We are simply HOMŒOPATHISTS; i.e., adherents of the relation of similarity between disease and drug-action as the cardinal principle of Therapeutics.

Let me explain.

Dr. Hughes Bennet, in the Introduction to his "Principles and Practice of Medicine," after showing that the difference between the exact and the inexact sciences is the possession by the former of a "primitive fact," writes thus:—

"Medicine, then, in its present state possesses no primitive fact, but is it not very possible that it may do so at some future time? During the many ages that existed before Newton, Physical Science was as inexact as that of Physiology is now. Before the time of Lavoisior, Chemistry, like Physiology, consisted of nothing but groups of phenomena. These sciences went on gradually advancing, however, and accumulating facts, until at length Philosophers appeared who united these together under one law. So medicine, we trust, is destined to advance; and one day another Newton, another Lavoisier, may arise whose genius will furnish our science with ITS primitive fact, and stamp upon it the character of precision and exactitude.

Now Homœopathy is nothing more than one of the many attempts which have been made from time to time to supply this missing "primitive fact." Like Brown and Broussais, Hahnemann propounded his doctrine from within the ranks of traditional medicine, and indeed, from no undistinguished position there. One would have thought that its reception might also have had the same course as theirs. That there should have been Hahnemannists would not have been strange any more than that there should be Broussaists and Brownists. But the task of the profession at large was to examine the New Doctrine, to estimate the worth of the arguments alleged in its support, to test it in practice, and ultimately to assign its place in the resources of Therapeutic art.

Had this been done, there would not have been at the present day a number of medical men known as "Homœopathists," and occupying a separate position. No other doctrine, not even that of Rademacher, has led to a schism and formed a sect. How has it come about in the case of Homœopathy? I will not re-open the question. History must one day pronounce upon it, and we may well leave the decision to her impartial verdict. We have a strong conviction that though there were doubtless faults on both sides, in the main we were not to blame. But however it may have been in the past, there can be no doubt of the cause of our combined separateness now. It is because we are denied the liberty to which every qualified medical man has a right, and which he is bound to vindicate for himself—the liberty to practise according to the best of his judgment. When I say that we are denied of this, I do not mean that Physical force is put upon us, or that attempt is made to restrain us by an action of the law. But Pericles has spoken,* and Mill written,† in vain, if these are to be esteemed the only fetters whereby man's freedom can be abridged by his fellows. Practise as you think best, it is said; but if your best thinking leads you to the system called Homœopathy, we shall send you to Coventry. You shall enjoy no membership in the Societies we have formed for mutual intercourse and improvement. If you are on the staff of any hospital, we will resign EN MASSE rather than act with you. You shall not have an article published or your books advertised in our Journals. If any patient you attend requires our diagnostic or mechanical aid, you must stand out of the way, temporarily or altogether, ere we will render it. All public appointments and the service of the Army and Navy, shall be closed to you; for we will not associate professionally with you. Call you this liberty? It is not liberty; it is terrorism.

I think it very important that we should insist upon this one cause of our isolation to the ignoring of all other considerations. An attempt is often made by our opponents to evade the real issue, and to represent us as excluded because of the irrational nature of our doctrine or the sectarian character of our pro-

---

* See Grote's History of Greece, ch. xlviii.   † "On Liberty."

ceedings. Our reply on the first count is that it is entirely irrelevent to the question. We claim freedom, as qualified medical men, to do what commends itself to OUR judgement, not to yours. You may think our principles absurd; to us they are as reasonable as they are fruitful, and we demand the liberty we concede to all others—the liberty of putting them in practice without prejudice to professional fellowship. To say, you are free to do everything save what we consider irrational,—this is not to open our prison: it is but to lengthen the tether of our chain. We protest against all such interference with freedom, as injury to science: we should protest were we not ourselves the sufferers, we should (as Montalembert said under similar circumstances) feel the gag in our own throats. And as to sectarianism,—of course there have been INTRANSIGENTS and even black sheep amongst us, as there have been also amongst you; but such fault cannot be found with our main body and for its conduct you have no one but yourselves to thank. You have thrust us into separateness, and kept us there; we have only done what in such a position was befitting to men who knew the value of free discussion and full experiment, who desired to promulgate their method and to practise it. If we are a sect, it is you who have made us one. There is nothing in our spirit which has led us into schism; and nothing in our doctrine and practice which keeps us there. Open your doors; make us free of the organization of the profession at large; and if we do anything sectarian, then condemn us and degrade us if you will.

Accordingly, our position is this:—We are ready to admit that in the past there have been faults of temper and errors in judgment on the one side as on the other. But as regards the ground taken up by the leading maintainers of Homœopathy—as represented, for instance, in this country by the British Homœopathic Society, the BRITISH JOURNAL OF HOMŒOPATHY and the MONTHLY HOMŒOPATHIC REVIEW—we have no foot to stir and no pardon to ask. We earnestly desire reconciliation and reunion, but these can only come about by a frank recognition on the part of our colleagues of the soundness of our contentions. They are already, as we have seen, here and there admitting them; we ask them only to do it generally, officially, and without ARRIERE PENSEE.

What, then, are these claims for which we do not so much crave a hearing, as demand acknowledgement?

The first is this—that the treatment of disease by medicines selected for the similarity of their effects to the symptoms present, is a legitimate Therapeutic method, one which may be avowedly practised and which requires investigation. We do not parade it as universal and exclusive. We do not claim credence for even its partial value without trial. We only ask that no prejudice should operate against its fair consideration, The profession is confessedly not so armed at every point against its foe as to be able to slight an additional weapon offered to its hand. Let every physician in the presence of disease feel himself free—aye more, BOUND—to consider whether this is a case in a which a similarly-acting remedy promises to do more than one of contrary properties, or one operating only indirectly upon the morbid process. That is, let his choice lie between Homœopathy, Enantiopathy and Allœopathy, as we have seen these defined by Hahnemann. At present the second and third only are thought of; or, if the first be allowed a place, it is in slience—as when, noting the 'intense desquamation of the skin" occuring in Myxœdematous patients 'under treatment with Thyroid extract, Dr. Byrom Bramwell was led to test the remedy in Psoriasis, where he found it very effective, with apology; or under another name such as Trousseau's "substitution." As long as prejudice thus operates to exclude the trial of similarly-acting medicines by the profession at large, so long we must appear singular in admitting them, and must, perhaps, be partial in preferring them. If our brethren wish us to be impartial, they must be impartial too. They blame us for basing our practice on an "exclusive" theory; but it is they who make it such by excluding it from their own. We urge upon them to let it be thus no longer. Let them test the principle in their own way, if they please—with such rough pathogenetic knowledge as they have, with such limited range of dose as they are accustomed to use. We are sure that the results will lead to further enquiry, and will support the claim of the further principles we maintain.

Secondly : The rule SIMILIA SIMILIBUS can obviously be carried out only in proportion as the effects of drugs on the healthy body are ascertained. We therefore place, as the second plank of our platform, the necessity of the proving of medicines. We hail with gratification the attempts of the kind made in various quarters. We ask only that they be carried on systematically and thoroughly, and that the contributions of Homœopathists towards the knowledge of Pathogenetics be not ignored or rejected without trial. The effects of poisons on animals, the symptoms caused in main by large and single doses, must not be assumed to suffice for our need : if true similarity is to be ascertained, the symptomatology of drugs must be not less exhaustively and minutely studied than that of disease. Our interminable SYMPTOMEN-CODICES are derided. By all means let better ones be given us ; but at least let it be admitted that the attempt was in the right direction. The results of such long and painful labours may show more grains of Gold than might be supposed to careful sifting. But however this may be, we make no claim for our practice; we assert it only for the principle.

And now our third demand is this—that the question of DOSE be thrown open, and all judgment upon it reserved till further experiment has been made. Let our brethren remember that their associations on this subject are derived from practising with a view to oppose the direction of disease (Enantiopathy), or to act on healthy parts (Allœopathy). They cannot A PRIORI say what reduction of dose may be required for medicines acting on the diseased parts similar to the morbific cause (Homœopathy). It is obvious that some reduction is required; that *Strychnia* in quantities suitable to excite the cord in Paralysis, would aggravate its trouble in Tetanus. Ringer had to go to sixtieths of a grain before he could get good without harm in Athetosis. And it is evident that, when similarly-acting remedies have been applied with admitted advantage, it has always been in minute dose, like the drops of *Ipecacuanha* wine in Vomiting. But it may be said from the other school—This is all very well; it is when you get among your infinitesimals that we cannot follow you. Good; we should be thankful to you if you could prove their needlessness. We have no pleasure in dealing with these impalpable points, these inconceivable fractions. We would (most of us) gladly abandon them, if we could apply the Law of Similars without them. And so we are farthest from the wish to impose them upon others. Our claim is not for the recognition of certain doses, but for freedom in the use of all doses. It is absurd, in these days of continued demonstration by science, of the activity of the infinitely little, to draw a hard and fast line of medicinal quantity, and say —Thus far shalt thou go, and no further. If we have gone too far, prove it by experiment : ridicule has here no place, and incredulity must not be allowed to debar enquiry.

This is all. The word "Homœopathy" often suggests to the minds of its opponents the many fancies and follies which have been connected with it—Psora and dynamization theories, globule-sniffings, provings of inert and loathsome substances, and the like. Well: we have read in the annals of traditional medicine of hypotheses as baseless, of practices as objectionable. We have no more to do with the inanities of our school than the present race of physicians with those of their own in former times. Homœopathy proper is responsible only for the Law of Similars, for the proved medicines, for the reduced dose. There is surely nothing in these which required a separate organization for working it out, nothing which justifies exclusion of its supporters from the main body of the profession. If medicine is not wide enough to embrace us, the fault is medicine's not ours; and it is a fault easily remediable. The profession has only to say—"There has been misunderstanding; we have been provoked by some extravagances from amongst you, and have allowed ourselves to be prejudiced against your real position. Resume your place in our ranks, from which it is our fault that you were ever expelled. If you have doctrines to propound and practices to recommend, our journals, our societies our hospitals and dispensaries, are as open to you as to any other qualified men." Do our brethren know what would be the result of such generous policy? We should at once cease to exist as a separate body. Our name would remain only as a technical term to designate our doctrine; while "Homœopathic" journals, societies, hospitals, dispensaries, pharmacopœas, directories, UNDER SUCH TITLE, would loose their RAISON D'ETRE, and cease to be. The rivalry between "Homœopathic" and "Allopathic" practitioners would no longer embitter doctors and perplex patients. If (as is now generally admitted) we have hit upon some good things, they would become the general property of the profession; and we on our part should be even readier than we are to avail ourselves of all that is useful in the ordinary practice. You can only kill Homœopathy by recognising it. Allow it to be legitimate and valid as far as it goes; and then the part will be, and will rejoice to be, amalgamated with the whole, and will lose its independent and troublesome identity. How far it will leaven the whole, time only can decide. We have our thoughts on the subject; but at least whatever happens in this direction will be the just result of the comparison of practice.

Do our brethren shrink from making such advances? Very well, then, we must wait. But let us assure them that to this, sooner or later, they must come. It is not possible to escape it. It is admitted on all hands that there is a Homœopathic action of medicines. Then this method of using them must be discussed exactly in the same way and with the same freedom as any other theory in medicine or in the arts and sciences generally. We claim for it (as I have said) no position or predominance other than what may be found to be its due after proper testing. We assert, and have asserted from the beginning, that we do not know what that position is. We are quite prepared to abandon the attempt to apply it to any particular diseased conditions so soon as it is demonstrated to be inapplicable to them, or inferior to other methods of treating them. And in such cases we are prepared to use, and in fact have all along used, other means, either as substitutes or as auxiliaries. As far as our experience goes, these cases are comparatively few. But if wider experience in the hands of competent men shows them to be more numerous, we are prepared to accept the inference. Again, the necessity of proving on the healthy is acknowledged. When this has been properly carried out, it must be determined after what manner the results are to be applied—whether solely according to their primary action, as giving *Opiates* for Sleep and Purgatives for Constipation, or upon the Homœopathic specific plan. This can only be decided by the ordinary rules of scientific experiment, and in no other way; and, whatever the result, it must be accepted. This is precisely our position; this, and nothing more than this. The dose likewise must be settled in the same fashion. The medicine of the future must, therefore, perforce follow our methods; there is no third way.

To our position, we say, sooner or later all must come. The accidents of our separate existence are but temporary; but we claim for our essential standpoint that it is the only tenable one. We are the assertors of liberty in medicine. We call ourselves, our literature, and our associations "Homœopathic," not as implying an exclusive devotion to this creed, but simply as meaning that here it is recognised and its proper value allowed. If any one of its opponents have anything worth saying against it, the pages of our journals are open to him; and we are sure that there are none of our societies but would give him a patient hearing and a candid discussion. How little liberty of this kind exists on the other side has been already seen. Which course of conduct implies most confidence in principles and desire of progress? If our brethren would satisfy their own conscience, and approve themselves in the public eye, let them be at least as ready AUDIRE ALTERAM PARTEM in Homœopathy's favour as we are when the argument is against it. Let the mistakes and errors, the strifes and bitterness of the last hundred years be buried by common consent; and then we shall find ourselves, as it were, at Hahnemann's original starting-post when he propounded the rule "Similia Similibus," and began to prove medicines and experiment upon the dose. Could any honest and enlightened physician of the old school allow himself now in the blind opposition which greeted the German Reformer then, and which has perpetuated itself towards all his adherents since? If not, the opportunity is offered of showing how much the present generation has advanced in liberality. I have set forth once again (as has often been set forth before) what is our essential doctrine. I think I speak for my colleagues when I say that we shall be more than willing to forget its reception in the past, if we can secure a hearing and a testing for it now.

But one word more. If any of the highly-trained hospital physicians of this day should read these words, and should look into the little world we inhabit apart, he must not expect to find it TOTUS TERES ATQUE ROTUNDUS. He will not indeed be offended by anything which he (and we no less) resents as "quackery". We have no secrets or mysteries,* no pompous pretensions, no panaceas. But he will find in us much weakness and imperfection. Our central principle remains a phenomenal, not to say empirical, rule. Our provings of medicines are mostly fragmentary, and the records of many of them wellnigh useless through mal-arrangement. We are widely, and to present seeming, hopelessly, divided on the question of dose; and many other practical matters—as repetition and alternation —remain unsettled. But let him not despise this day of small things; rather let him ask how it is that it has not waxed greater. And the answer is simple. It is because the profession at large has refused us any help in our task. It is because no one has been allowed to cultivate this field or practice except at the price of ostracism from his brethren and loss of position and prospects. The treatment of Henderson did not serve POUR ENCOURAGER LES AUTRES; and it is not strange that we have but few men of note amongst us. Persecution is bracing air, as a rule; but sometimes it proves stifling. In this case it has hindered all but a few hundreds in the several countries of the Old World from devoting themselves to the despised doctrine. No wonder then that, overwhelmed by the demands of the public upon our time, we have been able to do so little towards deepening and widening our foundation, towards investigating the significance of our provings. The marvel is that so much has been accompanied. What we say to our brethren is—come and help us. Bring to our inquiries and experiments your numbers, your wealth, your leisure, your trained observers, your ample materials. There is probably much that is partial and extreme of which you may cure us. If only with this motive, take, we beg of you, our Homœopathy, and throw it into your crucible. We know what wealth of Gold will come out; and then we hope for it to go on accumulating, far faster than in our feeble hands. What medicine might become in ten years, if only the profession at large would test Homœopathy as it deserves, is a dream almost too bright to dwell upon.

So far I have been addressing myself to the general profession. But I pray my own colleagues of the Homœopathic body to observe the consequence of the position thus taken up. It

---

*How little is really known of us may be inferred from a fact like this. An eminent Practitioner of the old school wrote a short time ago to a Homœopathic friend:—"What is really wanted is some common ground on which various hypotheses of the mode in which matter and materials act on the human or animal frame can be tested. THIS CAN NEVER BE DONE UNTIL YOUR PHARMACOPŒA IS AS OPEN AND PUBLIC AS OURS, and with every one who practises on his fellow creatures knows exactly and can prepare what he is ordering, on any system". Now, our mode of preparing our medicines has never been any mystery; and since the publication of the BRITISH HOMŒOPATHIC PHARMACOPŒA in 1870, he who runs may read it.

is that should our claims be allowed, and the liberty we demand be granted us, we must renounce our separateness, and resume the place in the body of the profession from which we should never have been extruded. I cannot say that the signs of the times indicate such a consummation as never than when I forecasted it at the British Congress of 1879. But ever and anon they do unexpectedly shine out; and be it near or far, it must come one day, and we should be prepared for it. It would be a change not to be effected without difficulties and perhaps some painfulnesses. We have lived so long shut up in our prison that its walls have seemed our natural limits, and its habits have grown part of our nature. Some of us, perhaps, like captives of whom history tells, may decline to go forth, and prefer to end their days in their accustomed seclusion. But we should be inconsistent with our principles if, as a body, we refuse to avail ourselves of the rights we have demanded, when they were yielded to us. Once made free of the City of Medicine, it will behove us to play our part in its civic life.

I go further, and maintain that we should be untrue to our cause if we did otherwise. I believe that the greatest hindrance to the consideration of Homœopathy on the part of our old-school colleagues is the existence of the Homœopathic body. Its rival institutions, its competing practitioners, prejudice the system itself in their eyes, and keep up a bitterness against it which is quite out of place in a question of science. Our desire must be that it should leaven to the uttermost the practice of medicine, and acquire the confidence of the greatest possible number of medical men. With this view we must heartily welcome the obliteration of distinctions which keep men apart from one another, and too often cause the subject to be viewed in that LUMEN MADIDUM of passion which Bacon deprecated, instead of the LUMEN SICCUM of unclouded reason. If our cause can best be served by our individual extinction, or rather absorption into the common mass, let us not shrink from any self-abnegation that may be required.

Nor need we doubt that here, as elsewhere, to lose our life may be to gain it. Though we are not the cause of the schism which isolates us, we are the sufferers from it. The dangers which haunt all small societies, gathered round a special principle, and withdrawn from the main current of the life of the body from which they are separated, do press sorely upon us. We all know how among men so situated, narrowness of sentiment and exclusiveness of view are almost inevitable; how rife are personalities, rivalries, jealousies, how vehement controversies about the details of the common faith. In such associations, those disproportions come to prevail which have given rise to the figure of the triton among the minnows, and the proverb

"Parmi les aveugles le borrne est goi." And when, as here, there is bread-winning connected with the questions at issue, there is the additional peril that the standard may be joined for the sake of gain, that men may trade on the distinctive name and position taken up, I am sure that we Homœopathists cannot claim to have been exempt from the evils thus incident to our situation. See with what bitterness discussion has been conducted between the two sections into which such a body must needs fall—the COTE GAUCHE and COTE DROIT of which I have spoken, those who cultivate exclusively and to the uttermost the method of Hahnemann and those who seek rather to harmonize him with general medicine. Such a division has existed amongst us in every country, and it has involved us in continual internecine strife. See how difficult it is for us to unite in any common course of action. The storms which in this country have raged round the cradle of the British Homœopathic Society, the London Homœopathic Hospital and the London School of Homœopathy, have been paralleled in many other parts of the world, and have sadly wasted our time and strength and resources. I am afraid, too, that we are not altogether free from narrowness. Indeed, to hear some amongst us talk, it would seem as if Homœopathy (at any rate in their hands) could cure everything, and no other way of proceeding could cure anything. To deliver us from these faults, we need the freer air and less dense aggregation we should obtain by being transferred from our little encampment into the general array of the profession.

It will require, indeed, much wise deliberation to accomplish the transition without rude harm. There must be due regard paid to vested interests, and much tenderness exercised in dealing with existing ties and expectations. It may be that no very great changes will be required, at any rate at first. It will be a long time before Homœopathy becomes to all the guiding-star of Therapeutics; for many years it is likely to be followed, as a dominant rule, by the few only. There may still be place then for some "Hahnemann Society" where under a name which could repel none who love the art of healing, his method might receive adequate cultivation and criticism. Some "Journal of Specific Therapeutics" may still be required, in which there shall be secured due space for the essays and records illustrative of our system. The most difficult question is that of our hospitals and dispensaries. In maintaining them in existence, however—should we decide so to do—we should have the precedent of the Temperance Hospital. This has been established at the instance of those who believe Alcoholic stimulants to be at least unnecessary in the treatment of disease, and for the benefit of the poor who may elect to be so treated. Its physicians and surgeons, in accepting office there (and no one has challenged them for so doing), pledge themselves to nothing beyond a general acceptance of the principle; they do not bind their hands to any abstention from *Alcohol*, if in their judgment it should become necessary. The staff of a Homœopathic hospital takes up a precisely parallel position; and these should not, any more than those do, incur odium thereby. We have here, moreover, to consider the interests of the public as well as of the profession, and especially of its proper position. It will be easy enough for the well-to-do to find practitioners who will treat them Homœopathically, especially as the peculiarities of our pharmacy will probably always require the existence of distinctively Homœopathic chemists. But how are the multitudes of the poor who prefer our treatment to obtain it, unless there are charitable institutions devoted to its practice? For them, therefore, if for nothing else, it would seem that our hospitals and dispensaries must be maintained; though the example of the Hahnemann Hospital of Liverpool shews that they do not necessarily require an even apparently sectarian name,

For such changes, I say, we ought to be prepared; but till there come the great changes on the part of others which will necessitate them, let us loyally support our institutions as we have them. Let there be no individual secessions, no abstention because one is in a minority, Let us all stand firmly in our ranks, doing our duty where Providence has placed us until the time comes when as a body we can reconsider our position, and make what changes are necessary in our organization. And one further caution I must add, and that is that it is not for us to take the first step towards the reconciliation we nevertheless invite, and devoutly desire, We cannot do so without misunderstanding. There must be no excuse for saying that we have "hauled down our flag": when we evacuate the fort we have so long held, it must be with all the honours of war, with drums beating and colours flying. A true note was struck by the late Dr. Hayle, of Rochdale, when at the British Congress of 1876 he compared our attitude to that of St. Paul in the dungeon of Philippi. "Let them come themselves and fetch us out". It was from no pride that the Apostle spoke thus, no unwillingness to overlook the wrong done him: but the rights and immunities of Roman citizenship had been violated in his person; and he owed it to them, and to those who shared with him in them, not to condone the offence. We too, for like reasons, having expressed our readiness to receive overtures of peace, and laid down the grounds on which alone we can make it, must wait the action of the other side. I can hardly now say, as I did twenty years ago, that I hope my generation will see 'it. The next, however, it will assuredly visit. For our children we may safely anticipate the time when the name of Homœopathy shall no longer denote a prosecuted sect, but a faith and practice recognised universally as legitimate and largely as true; when the antagonisms of to-day shall have ceased to separate between brethren, and all shall be united in generous emulation as to who shall do most good to the objects of their care.

LECTURE XV.

GENERAL DISEASES.

––o––

THE ACUTE INFECTIOUS DISORDERS

We have now spent some time together in considering the principles of Homœopathy, including its history and the position and claims of the body of practitioners designated by its name. I will ask you to carry in your mind what we have thus ascertained while I proceed to apply to special Therapeutics, the method I have been describing. I will ask you also to posses yourselves of, or secure ready access to, my "Manual of Pharmacodynamics" in one of its later editions. I have there gone fully into the actions of drugs, both pathogenetic and curative, and do not want to spend time in traversing the ground anew on our present journey. I wish to take up the subject from the side of disease to tell you, as I have said, what Homœopathy can do for its various forms, and how it does it.

You may ask why I do not refer you for this purpose to the treatises on the 'Practice of Medicine' which already exist in the school of Hahnemann (I have mentioned some of them in my Lecture XI.), and which aim at superseding, for Homœopathic students and practitioners, the ordinary text-books. I do not mean indeed those of the last generation, as Hartmann's,* Laurie's, † or Marcy and Hunt's. ‡ Whatever their measure of usefulness in their time, they are to us alike imperfect and obsolete. But in the works of Bahr § and of Jousset ‖ (and, if you read German, I would add that of Kafka ¶) you will find nothing to repel you and much, very much, that will interest and instruct. I SHOULD content myself with referring you to these excellent treatises, but for one defect they all possess. Each

---

* "Acute and Chronic Diseases and their Homœopathic Treatment," by F. Hartmann. Tr. Hempel.

† "Elements of the Homœopathic Practice of Physic." 1850. (See B. J. H., vi., 227).

‡ "Homœopathic Theory and Practice of Medicine." 1865. (See IBID., xxiii., 475.)

§ "Science of Therapeutics according to Principles of Homœopathy." Tr. by Hempel. 1869. (See IBID,, xxviii., 607.)

‖ ELEMENTS DE MEDICINE PRATIQUE. 1868. (See IBID., xxvii., 123.)

¶ DIE HOMOOPATHISCHE THERAPIE AUF GRUNDLAGE DER PHYSIOLOGISCHEN SCHULE 1865-9, (See IBID., xxvii., 333.)

author is limited in his Therapeutics by the experience of himself and his compatriots. Bahr and Kafka know nothing of French Homœopathic literature and Jousset as little of German; while (with rare exceptions) both display entire unacquaintance with the writings in the English tongue which have come from this country and from America. The same may be said of the otherwise excellent 'Treatise' which I have commended to you from the pen of Dr. Goodno of Philadelphia;* and still more of a volume I shall often quote—the "Forty Years' Practice" of the well-known Jahr, which is, as its title implies, a purely personal record. The result is that in none are the means and the possibilities of Homœopathy in the treatment of disease fully set forth. I strongly recommend you to procure and study as many of these books as you can; but I cannot feel that by such advice I am meeting your whole need.

In the lack, accordingly, of other works fitted for the object, I proceed myself to discourse to you on special as I have done on general Homœopathic Therapeutics. In so doing, I shall make no attempt to follow most of the authors I have mentoined in constructing a complete Practice of Physic. It is quite unnecessary for your purpose. You know disease as well as I do. I can tell you nothing about the history, the diagnosis, or the Pathology of its various forms but what you know already, or at any rate may acquaint yourselves with, by consulting the authorities on your bookshelves. You will meet me halfway here; and I may spare myself the travel over the familiar road. What you want to know is this. Here is a recognised malady, you have learnt or have been accustomed to treat it in such and such a way, and with such and such success. Has Homœopathy discovered how to treat it as well, or better? How far shall you be justified in any given case in dispensing with measures which, however rude, are TRIED, and trusting unreservedly to the action of specific medicines? The question is a fair, and indeed an imperative one for you to put. The Law of Similars, relating as it does solely to the dynamic action of medicines, has obviously limitations inherent in its own nature. It is further only capable of application to practice when similarly-acting medicines have been discovered. There may be diseases, therefore, which lie beyond its possible range; and still more likely is it that there are diseases which have not yet come within its practical range. Accordingly, our first step must be to inquire what Homœopathy can do—as compared with the capabilities of Old Physic—in each malady that comes before us. And next you will require to know what are the specific remedies with which success has hitherto been obtained and how far they need supplementing by auxiliary means.

* "The Practice of Medicine." Philad., 1894.

To answer these questions, from a survey of Homœopathic literature, and from my own experience, will be my only and sufficient task. I shall say no more upon the nature of the various diseases than is necessary for their identification, that we may know we are thinking of the same thing. Confining ourselves thus to their prognosis and treatment, we shall have an infinity of time and space, and shall be devoting our energies to what are really the only points on which your adoption of Homœopathy will require you to have fresh knowledge and modified views.

The literature on which I shall draw consists of the clinical records scattered throughout Homœopathic Periodicals, or brought together in the collections of Ruckert* and Beauvais; † and of the Monographs we have on special forms of diseases. To these I shall make copius reference as I go on. I shall also glean all I can from the text-books, and refer you to them when their teatment of any subject is especially instructive. My lecture will thus serve as an index to our Therapeutic literature at large; so that under their guidance you will be able to read up most of what has been written on any malady which is demanding your special attention.

In choosing a classification of diseases for my purpose, I shall adopt, as in duty bound, the Nomenclature drawn up by the Royal College of Physicians, and furnished to us officially by our government (3rd Ed., 1896). I shall not, however, deny myself the liberty of making occasional transferences of order and shiftings of place—still less of supplying ommisions—when such alterations seem to subserve the practical ends I have in view.

Concerning all these forms of disease I shall have to tell you, as I have said, the actual results Homœopathy has obtained in their treatment, and the means it has employed. But ever and anon, I shall come upon a malady which has never fallen under my own notice, and regarding whose specific Therapeutics we have no recorded experience. What am I to do then? Well, I shall consider the features of the disorder as described by those who have seen it; and shall specify what medicines seem to be Homœopathically indicated for it in its several varieties and stages. But, besides this, you yourselves will continually be meeting in practice with cases which do not readily fall into the categories of the best classification, to which indeed you

---

* KLINISCHE ERFAHRUNGEN IN DER HOMOOPATHIC, 1852, &c. (See also BRITISV JOURN. OF HOM., xx., 491.)

† CLINIOUE HOMOEOPATHIQUE. 1850.

can hardly give a name, but which are not less true cases of disease. What are YOU to do? for my lectures will hardly help you here. The answer is obvious: you in your turn must draw upon your knowledge of Pharmacodynamics, and select the medicine most appropriate to the phenomena before you.

But here another consideration comes in. The appropriateness of a remedy in Homœopathic practice depends upon the similariry of its pathogenetic effects to the symptoms of the disease; and the closer the similarity the more perfect the appropriateness. Now these cases of which I speak consist ordinarily of a good many symptoms. Your aim must be to "cover" all or as many as possible of these with the corresponding medicine, so that you may get no rough SIMILE merely, but a SIMILLIMUM, to the morbid state before you. Can any 'Manual of Pharmacodynamics' picture all the pathogenetic effects of all drugs, or can any study of the 'Materia Medica' itself enable you to retain them all in your mind? It is evidently impossible. You must, under these circumstances, adopt unreservedly Hahnemann's original mode of Homœopathizing, as he has described and illustrated it in the Preface to the Second Volume of the later editions of his REINE ARZNEIMITTELLEHRE.* You must note the symptoms of the case before you; and then turn to the 'Materia Medica' itself and not your mere recollection of it, to find the medicine which most closely corresponds.

But the 'Materia Medica' of Homœopathy is at the present day a most voluminous collection. Are you to wade through it every time you prescribe for such cases in search of your SIMILLIMUM? Nay, you must have an index; and such indices exsist (as I have told you) in no small number in Homœopathic literature, under the title of 'Repertories'. A Repertory, as its name implies, is a means of FINDING that to which it belongs. The subject matter of a Homœopathic Repertory is the Symptomen-Codex, and its object is to save us the turning over every page of that collection in search of what we want. But an index may be a good or a bad one. It is good in proportion as it is copious—as by repeating each topic in every element of which it consists it ensures immidiate success in consulting it. I have told you where you may best find such guides, and can only urge that you possess yourselves of one or other of them, as indispensable to the practice you have in view.

Nor is it in these anomalous cases only that you should, with the aid of your 'Repertory,' consult the 'Materia Medica.' You will ever and anon, have to do so in the treatment even of the

* Vol. I., p. 20, of Dudgeon's translation.

ordinary forms of disease. Lectures on Therapeutics can only deal with species and their recognised varieties: but the practitioner has to care for individuals. Such individuals MAY be undistinguished members of the species, or variety of the species, to which they belong; and then you have nothing but the disease to consider, and its standard remedies to apply. But sometimes, especially in lingering or chronic maladies, the peculiar tendencies of the patient will imprint a character of their own on the morbid process, and will make him, in fact, a "variety" by himself.* Now here you must know how to make the right choice among the several medicines which correspond to the disease present; and you can only do this by comparing the patient's special symptoms with theirs, as they are recorded in the 'Materia Medica.' Nay, more. You may have to go beyond their range. If there is anything very distinctive about the case before you, and you find similar peculiarities to have been produced by a drug, you will do well (especially if the ordinary remedies are not telling) to try that drug even though it has not produced the lesion present in the patient. Sometimes, indeed, it will fail to do more than extinguish the symptom which had indicated it: it has cut (as Dr. Madden expresses it) at a branch, and not at the root. † But sometimes, on the other hand, the disappearance of the disease does prove the proximate cause of the symptom which you remove, to be the root of the whole malady; or, as is more probable, it establishes the true Homœopathicity of the medicine to it, although its proving has not been carried sufficiently far or wide to effect the change in question. It is an encouragement so to act when we learn that it was in this way that Hahnemann discovered the virtues of *Aconite* in Inflammatory Fever.‡

There are some of our American brethren, indeed, who would make such practice the rule instead of the exception; who

---

* "Chronic diseases, forming themselves slowly in us, and arising most frequently from original or acquired vitiations of our constitution, are, if we may so speak, much more personal, much more idio-syncratic, than acute diseases. In acute diseases the physician should consider the malady much more than the sick person, while it is generally the other way in chronic diseases. But if, in virtue of internal conditions little known, an acute disease—a Typhoid Fever for example—is imperfectly developed, evolves itself badly, or is prolonged in any one beyond the usual period of the malady, the general principles of the treatment give place to those which we have established for chronic diseases" (Trousseau and Pidoux, Introduction to TRAITE DE THERAPEUTIQUE).

† I am referring to his valuable Essay, "On the true place of Repertories in Homœopathic Practice," in Vol. xxviii, of the BRITISH JOURNAL OF HOMŒOPATHY. His conclusion, that we should use them when the symptoms of a case are characteristic of the patient rather than of the disease, is identical with the advice I have given above.

‡ See B. J. H. V., 387.

would bid us banish Nosology and Pathology altogether from our minds when the question of medicinal treatment comes up, using our knowledge about them solely for purposes of prognosis and of general management. They would have us regard each patient, for therapeutic purposes, as a new bundle of symptoms, the like of which we never saw before, and for whose case we must find AB INITIO a similar picture in the Materia Medica. They consistently wish to keep the Materia Medica in the same state of a mere symptom-list, that the one set of phenomena may correspond with the other.

I cannot agree with this doctrine. The progress of Pathology has established the existence of a number of morbid species which are as truly entitled to the name as those which Natural History identifies in the animal and vegetable kingdom. When capable of reproduction (as in the case of infectious fevers), they invariably reproduce their kind ; and, when sterile, they prove their individual unity by springing from a common cause (as do the Malarious Fevers), or consisting in a certain process taking place in a certain organ (as does Pneumonia). Now these specific forms of diseases are acknowledged as realities, for when diagnosis perceives their presence, prognosis speaks accordingly. I maintain that our knowledge of morbid species should be used for therapeutic purposes also, and to this end would strive to raise Pharmacodynamics to the level of Pathology. While the latter was in its merely phenomenal stage : while Jaundice and Dropsy were regarded as morbid entities, and "Gastric," "Bilious," "Mucous," and "Nervous" Fevers as seperate forms of disease, the pathogenesy of drugs could only be a like series of appearances. Hahnemann, seeing the baseless character of most of the Pathology of his day, wisely rejected it for the symptomatic observation of disease, and conformed his registration of drug effects thereto. But the advance of Physiology, the cultivation of morbid Anatomy, and the refinement of our means of diagnosing internal changes during life, have raised Pathology to a° much higher level, and built it on a sure foundation. The interpretation of the observed facts of disease has now become to a large extent possible. Those whom I am controverting admit the validity of such interpretations by using them for prognosis ; so that they cannot take up Hahnemann's position as against the Pathology of to-day. Why, then, should we not carry the same well-substantiated principles of interpretation into the phenomena of drug-action ? If fever, pain in the side, hurried respiration and cough with rusty sputa mean Pneumonia in a patient, do they not mean the same thing in the subject of a proving or poisoning? And am I forbidden to Homœopathize by means of the interpretation, while I may do so freely with the phenomena ? Are we not, indeed, treading on surer ground when we oppose to a Pneumonia, a drug capable of causing Pneumonia than when we choose the remedy on the ground merely of the resemblance of the effects to certain outward symptoms present? The latter comparison may err; the former cannot. Of course, *to* make our SIMILE a SIMILIMUM we should endeavour, if possible, to cover those outward symptoms also,—from the remedies which correspond to the morbid species choosing those which suit the variety present, and from these the one which meets the individual case before us, For such selection we must use all the materials which pure symptomatology supplies; all conditions and concomitants; all circumstances of amelioration and aggravation; all mental states and subjective sensations. But it is quite another thing to say that these and the external symptoms of the case are to be our only consideration in the choice of a medicine. Such a doctrine seems to me mistaking the means for the end. Our object in seeking symptomatic resemblance is that we may secure Pathological resemblance; for it is the disease itself, and not its outward manifestation, which we have to cure.

I quite admit that there is many a TERRA INCOGNITA as yet in disease, and many a case which as yet we can only treat symptomatically. I am most thankful that the Law of Similars enables us to fit drug to disease, even when we are unable to say what the phenomena of either mean. But when we are able, I hold it a sin to neglect to use our knowledge for therapeutic as well as for prognostic purposes. In my lectures on 'Pharmacodynamics' I have endeavoured, wherever possible to study what may be called the Physiological as distinct from the merely semeiogenetic action of drugs. In my present lectures on Therapeutics I shall make the same attempt in the field of disease dealing with its recognised species as realities and not mere names, and endeavouring to fit to them medicines having true specific relationship with them. I believe that a scientific Pharmacology, linked to a scientific Pathology by the bond of the Homœopathic method, will constitute the Therapeutics of the future; and I design my work as an humble contribution thereto.

There is only one class of disease which, although Pathologically recognised and defined, we must for some time to come (if not always) be content to treat symptomatically. These are such as involve grave organic changes—Cancer, Mollities ossium. Degenerations of the Nerve-Centres, and such like. We have not yet pushed, and we shall not readily push, our drug-provings to the extent of producing these changes; and hence direct pathological resemblance is hardly to be expected. But it nearly always happens that, ere they are actually set up, the organism gives out signs of the imminence of the morbid process. These signs are of the nature of objective phenomena or of subjective sensations and in either case are of such kind that similarly-acting remedies can be adapted to them. Thus, Sir William Jenner has shown that the clinical history of Rickets reveals an unhealthy state of the system preceding for several weeks or months the lesion of the bones. Some of the symptoms of this state are common to other disorders of early life, as feverishness with thirst, altered intestinal secretions, and the like; but some of them, which are usually later in occurrence, are pathognomonic of the disease, viz.,: profuse perspiration of the head and neck, desire for coolness of the surface, and general tenderness of the body. Our best chance of curing Rickets must be by taking it in this early stage, ere yet its organic changes are developed; and we know that we have in such medicines as *Calcarea, Silicea* and *Phosphoric acid* remedies truly similar to the special phenomena before us. The same thing has been shown by Sander of Barlin and others with reference to Progressive Paralysis of the Insane. For years, they say, before the disease becomes developed, the patient suffers from peculiar rheumatoid pains and headaches, sometimes from colour-blindness, oftener from sleeplessness, vertigo, irritability, loss of memory, etc. Dr. Lilienthal has done well in bringing these observations before us,* that (as he says) we may "see whether we cannot by our rich armamentarium prevent what we cannot cure when at last it is fully developed."

There is only one caution to be given in selecting our remedies upon these principles. We should choose such remedies as, from our knowledge of their sphere and kind of action, might conceivably cause these morbid changes if pushed far enough, rather than others to which no such likelihood belongs. The Rheumatoid pains described by Sander as premonitory of Dementia Paralytica are not unlike those which *Chamomilla* causes and cures; and it is not impossible that even here it might remove them for a time. But it would not check the impending mischief of which they were a sign, having no specific relationship thereto; whereas a medicine might do this whose similarity to the phenomena present was not so manifest, but which we know to have capacities in it which might establish its Homœopathicity to the entire disease. The "totality of symptoms" which we seek must embrace the future, when this can be foreseen, as well as the present and the past.

I have spoken thus far that you may recognise with me the limitations of my present task. Without further preface, I will now address myself to it, and will endeavour within my sphere to teach you to apply the method of Hahnemann.

* See Hahnemannian Monthly, xii., 161.

Our Nomenclature begins with "GENERAL DISEASES," and takes first THE ACUTE INFECTIOUS DISORDERS—a group marked by this common characteristic that they are communicable, and always reproduce their kind. They include the pestilences which from time to time visit us, like Cholera and Influenza; the Continued Fevers—Typhus, Typhoid, and so forth; the Exanthemata—Variola, Scarlatina, Measles; the primarily local infections, such as Diphtheria and Erysipelas. They are those which have hitherto been classed as "zymotic," from some analogy in their development to the process of fermentation: they are now, like that process itself, explained by the reception of a CONTAGIUM VIVUM, to whose life-history their course of symptoms is supposed to be due.

The first question which arises is: Does not this view of tneir nature put them outside the proper range of Homœopathic medication? They are parasitic in origin: should not their treatment be parasiticidal? Should we not deal with germs inside the body as we do with those outside, and attack the cause with Antiseptics rather than the effect with similar medicines? We have frankly admitted the propriety and necessity of such proceedings in the instances of Helminthiasis, of Beri-beri, and of Scabies; why should we refuse assent thereto when as logically demanded here?

These questions were very properly brought before us by Dr. Galley Blackley at our British Congress in 1878, and he said all that could fairly be alleged in favour of treating blood-infections with drugs addressed to their supposed CAUSÆ ANIMATÆ. You will see, however, if you read the discussion which followed his Paper, that he failed to carry the meeting with him; and at the Congress of 1884, after six years' further consideration, Dr. Hayward from the chair expressed what I think is the mind of nearly all Homœopathists—that we have no call to alter our treatment here because of the new views. To attack acari on the surface and worms in the intestine with their appropriate poisons; to guard breaches of surface against intruding spores, or cleanse them when infected, by local sporicides,—this is rational and harmless enough. But when you have—as upon the theory you have here—the whole mass of blood in the body swarming with these organisms, you will want large doses of poison to kill them; and can you expect that the host will remain immune while your toxic agents are destroying his guests? Even in the instances where such measures have been allowed, they may easily be carried too far. Hahnemann is not the only writer who has shown the harm done by suppressing, with strong parasiticides, any extensive Itch; *Santonine* and (as is now recognised) *Filix mas* have been the agents of many a poisoning; Keith has declared that in his Laparotomies he has seen as much harm result from *Carbolic*-dressings as from the operation itself, and Asepsis rather than Antisepsis is now the aim of most wise surgeons and obstetricians. The practice I am criticising would do, on a large scale and of malice prepense, the evil here occurring occasionally and incidentally only. It offends against the rule of PRIMO NON NOCERE; and, even were its results more encouraging than they are, could not be commended. If Dr. Dyce Brown's experience be confirmed, that the relapse which gives the "Famine Fever," its distinctive name can be prevented by five-grain doses of the *Hyposulphide of Soda* (as it cannot be by Homœopathic remedies), this would be a justifiable occasion for its employment; but as a rule, we can show a more excellent way.

This way is that which Nature herself seems to follow, in limiting the development of, and so promoting recovery from, the infectious diseases. Were She quite passive in their presence, there seems no reason why their ravages should ever cease, save with the death of the patient. The spores once introduced must fulfil their destiny of indefinite multiplication, until the whole body becomes the seat of their operations and the prey of their requirements. To defend Herself against such fate, Nature goes upon the principle, that for germination, two factors are needed—the seed and the soil. To kill the seed, when it has once sprouted, would be a wasteful exertion of Her power. She addresses Herself rather to making the soil such as will forbid its further development. Some process, it is evident, goes on in the tissues of an infected subject—some production of defensive phagocytes, some exhaustion of combustible or alimentary material, some establishment of callousness to provocation—which at length disallows the life of the foreign invader, and brings its history to a close. Immunity is secured, and that not only for the nonce, but in the future—always for a time, often for a life-time; so that the subject of a specific infection is proof against it henceforward. Now the part played by Homœopathic remedies in such diseases is to favour the introduction of this immunity. Chosen on account of the similarity of their effects to those of the CONTAGIUM in question, they must evidently act on the same parts and in a similar manner. Such action—explain it how you will—is provedly incompatible with the idiopathic morbid process; it neutralises, obliterates, extinguishes it. The bacteria present find no scope for their activities: they languish and die, while the disorders they have induced are rapidly subdued to order again. The immunity of course is temporary; drugs are not self-multiplying in the body. But this lack is supplied by repetition of doses, and the defensive change can be sustained until all the present need for it has passed away.

We are then, on rational ground; we are MINISTRY ET INTERPRETES NATURÆ, if we treat the infectious diseases on ordinary Homœopathic principles, regardless of their presumed causation by the reception and development of animated germs. There is, too, in so directing our Therapeutics this further advantage, that we provide for that prevention which is, proverbially and confessedly, better than cure. If to occupy the invaded soil our specifics dislodge the intruders, to preoccupy it they may obviate their intrusion altogether. This field of medicinal prophylaxis has been but slightly cultivated; but we have two products of it which indicate its probable fruitfulness. I do not at present include *Quinine* for Malaria among them; for there is here a moot questionn as to Homœopathicity, and a rival alternative as to MODUS OPERANDI. On these I propose to touch when the Malarious diseases come under our notice. Nor will I mention the "Mithridatism" (so-called from the endeavour of the celebrated adversary of Rome to make himself proof against poisons) now increasingly in vogue, though it has included confessedly Homœopathic medications as *Tansy* in Rabies* and *Strychnia* in Tetanus;† or the success on one occasion of inoculation with *Antimonial*-ointment in the absence of Vaccine lymph as a preventive of Small-pox.† At present, I am thinking of *Belladonna* in Scarlatina and of *Cuprum* in Cholera. Of the success of the former practice I will not here produce the detailed evidence, but will content myself by referring you to that adduced by Dr. Dudgeon in his Lectures and Dr. Stille in his "Therapeutics and Materia Medica." It has made the latter—no favourable judge, for he has just spoken of "the impudent heresy of Homœopathy"—express his "conviction that the virtues of *Belladonna* as a preventive to Scarlatina are so far proven, that it becomes the duty of practitioners to invoke their aid whenever the disease break out in a locality where there are persons liable to the contagion, particularly in boarding-schools, orphans' asylums, and similar institutions, and among the families of the poor." Now it was the similarity of the effects of *Belladonna* to the symptoms of Scarlatina which led Hahnemann to employ it in this malady, first as curative and then as preventive—as you may read in his Treatise on the subject contained in his "Lesser Writings"; nor can any one who thinks over the fever, the rapid pulse, the scarlet rash and the sore-throat of the drug deny the parallelism. There is no question of germicidal action here, so that SIMILIA SIMILIBUS must have all the credit. The case for *Cuprum* in Cholera is not quite so obvious, but it is well-sustained. The immunity of workers with the metal, first observed and communicated by

* See BULL. DE LA SOC. MED. HOM. DE FRANCE xxix., 570.
† See M. H. R., xxxix, 552.

Burq in 1849, has been substantiated in later epidemics; and those who at his advice have worn a plate of it next the skin when Cholera was about them have always (I believe) had reason to congratulate themselves upon the precaution. The Homœopathicity here is not so precise and complete; but it was sufficient to induce Hahnemann, in the epidemic of 1831, to advise reliance on *Cuprum* as the specific remedy in the second stage of the malady, when its "spasmodic" character was well-marked. When recommending it (as he did) for prophylactic purposes, also to cover the symptoms of the entire disease he gave it in alternation with *Veratrum album*; but he evidently relied most upon the *Cuprum*.*

I must defer the further consideration of this subject till next meeting.

* Lesser Writings tr. Dudgeon, p. 848.

LECTURE XVI.

GENERAL DISEASES

THE ACUTE INFECTIOUS DISORDERS.-THE EXANTHEMATA

VARIOLA

We have seen that Homœopathy enables us, not only to fortify the tissues invaded by CONTAGIA VIVA but to predispose them against their invasion. Can it do more? Can it shorten the duration of the seige as well as sustain the beleaguered during its progress? In other words, can it jugulate, blight, nip in the bud these maladies of definite history and ascertained process, so that they shall not go on to their full development? Can it do for the infectious diseases in general, what Vaccination (when still effective) does for Small-pox, averting the stage of suppuration and secondary fever and reducing Variola to Varioloid? Well: its doing so would only be an extension of the lines on which we have already seen its remedies moving, and it was from the apparent effect of *Belladona* in aborting an incipient Scarlatina that Hahnemann was led to employ it as a prophylactic of that disease. As evidence of the possibilities of similar medicines here we may cite the action of *Camphor* in Cholera and of *Baptisia* in Common Continued Fever.

1. On the first appearance of Cholera in Europe in 1831, Hahnemann, before he had seen a single case of the disorder, declared that *Camphor* should be its initial remedy. He did so, believing—as Trousseau and Pidoux—that its primary action in health is refrigerant and depressant, and that therefore it is Homœopathic to the first stage of Cholera, marked by sinking of strength, coldness, and anxietas, ere yet the vomiting, purging and cramps have fully set in. Wherever his advice has been followed it has been found that when *Camphor* is given in time, it cures the attack then and there, so that no second or third stage is reached; the patient warms up, *becomes quiet, goes to

---

* This effect of *Camphor* was specially noted by an old-school observer in the "frightful epidemic during the Bohemian Campaign of 1866." Here the spirit proved very effective. Various persons who recovered stated that they could not sufficiently praise the extraordinarily warming and enlivening action of the *Camphor;* whereas 'schnapps' in no way lessened the frightful algidity and dread of death, but rather increased the nausea and consciousness of danger. After an hour the Camphor produced a comfortable sense of warmth, and after a day it enabled them to urinate." THERAPEUTIC GAZETTE, Sept., 1892.

sleep, and wakes free from the malady. It is abortive, and it seems also preventive, in Cholera. Encouraged by the success of Dr. Rubini in the Epidemics of 1854 and 1865, in which he treated hundreds of cases by this drug alone without a single death, the Homœopathic physicians of Naples, when revisited by the pestilence in 1894, advised all their patients to take as a prophylactic a drop of a saturated solution twice or three times a day. They had not a single case in their CLIENTELE—embracing, they calculate, some 2,000 families.

2. The question about *Baptisia* is a more complex one. I have discussed it at length in my "Pharmacodynamics,' and shall not do so here. The conclusion, however, to which I have been brought, and which I think you will acknowledge to be warranted by the facts adduced, is this. There is, over and above the four types of idiopathic fever generally recognised—Typhus, Typhoid, Relapsing, and Febricula, a common Continued Fever, the "Gastric" of popular nomenclature, the "Synoque" of the French nosologists. It is sometimes epidemic, often severe, and under ordinary remedies—*Aconite, Bryonia, Rhus*—always runs a prolonged course, and may end fatally. If this Fever be taken early, and treated with repeated doses of a low dilution of *Baptisia tinctoria*, it can be aborted, and it departs in a few days with copious perspiration. The moot point is whether this Fever is Typhoid, or has a specific character of its own. For myself, too many cases of undoubted Enteric Fever have been recorded, and have come under my own care, which have pursued their wonted course unchecked by the medicine, to allow of any illusions as to the possibility of its—at least habitual—jugulation by the drug; and I must adopt the latter alternative. I am bound to say, however, that so excellent a clinician as Dr. Dyce Brown still cherishes the belief that true Typhoid may sometimes be cut short by *Baptisia*, when the symptoms indicate it; and has related three cases which certainly, as far as they go, bear out his contention.* They will encourage us to persevere in the use of the remedy, when appropriate, even in the genuine disease,—so taking advantage of the natural tendency to resolution noted by observers about the middle of the second week, and doing something to tranquillise the brain and cleanse the digestive mucous membrane. But my point here is that in the Common Continued Fever whose distinctiveness I have maintained, *Baptisia* is as true an abortive as *Camphor* is in Cholera, and can be depended on unfailingly.

I have mentioned Vaccination as the type of such abortives. To put it in line with medicines acting in this way we must

* M. H. R., xxvi, 202.

think of it in terms of the matter it employs—Vaccine Lymph, or let us call it *"Vaccinine."* Is this a Homœopathic medicine? Does it act upon the principle of similarity? If we were to claim it as such, we had the support of one of the leaders of the old school, Sir George Humphry. In an Address reported in the LANCET of October 24th, 1895, he is represented as saying,—"I often wondered that the advocates of the 'Similia Similibus' doctrine, in their vain efforts to find some reasonable ground for their theory, did not alight upon, or make more of the practice and results of Vaccination coupled with those of inoculation. Here was to hand the unmistakable evidence of a disease being hindered or prevented or stopped by modification of the like, that is to say, of that which caused it. By inoculation—the introduction, that is, direct of the poison of Small-pox—the disease was produced; by Vaccination—the introduction of the like of that poison—the disease was prevented. Prevention and cure are near allies; and was it not possible, even probable, that cure might be effected by means like those which staved off disease?" Sir George is not very lucid, and betrays a somewhat imperfect grasp of what the "Similia" of our formula are; but that may pass. We welcome him as crediting to Homœopathy the actual benefits of and prospective inferences to be drawn from Vaccination; and we can assure him that Homœopathists have not been blind to the support apparently brought to them from this quarter. They are aware that the accepted doctrine is that the Vaccinia of cows is their Variola; and hence that in vaccinating we are really inoculating Small-pox, and that the immunity of the vaccinated arises from their having already had a mild but effectual attack of the disease itself. But they have urged that the Cow-pox, whether spontaneous or produced by *Vaccinine*, is similar to, by no means the same as, Small-pox; and have argued that what happens when Vaccination is practised after exposure to Variolous infection seems to make strongly against the identity of the two poisons. You know that if within a certain time after such exposure the patient is vaccinated, the disease will not be developed; and if it is done one day later, although the Pox will appear, it will be modified as we ordinarily see it in vaccinated subjects—it will be Varioloid rather than Variola. The relation of the two CONTAGIA here looks like one of similarity rather than identity. Again, *Vaccinine* has been amongst us (as we shall see) attenuated after our fashion (generally to the third degree), and administered as an internal remedy in Small-pox. So given, it has been found either exerting its recognised abortive power, and that more rapidly than when inoculated in the usual manner; or if too late for this, it has behaved as our remedies ordinarily do, and has conducted the case through to our entire satisfaction.

Nevertheless I must venture to think Hahnemann, who

refrained from claiming Vaccination (even where he might naturally have done so—Organon, § 46*) as an illustration of the Law of Similars, was wiser than some of his disciples have been; and that the true account of the prophylaxis it effects is that ordinarily given. It has perhaps been forgotten that Jenner's practice was introduced as a substitute for the inoculation of Small-pox itself, which was (to say the least) quite an effective for prevention, and was only objectionable as occasionally violent in its effects, and always setting up fresh foci of infection. At the other end of the scale we have the experience of men like Trinks and Dudgeon showing that attenuated Small-pox matter itself (Varioline, as we call it) has the same "alterative, shortening and curative power" as *Vaccinine* in the treatment of the idiopathic disease.† Does not all this look like difference of degree rather than of kind between the two viruses? Does it seem as if the virtues of *Vaccinine* depended in any way of its acting as a SIMILE instead of an IDEM? The apparent antogonism, moreover, manifested when Vaccination is practised after Variolous infection, proves on examination to be apparent only; for it obtains equally when *Vaccinine* is used against itself. If lymph is inserted after the formation of the secondary areola, it will not "take". There is no possible antagonism here: there is at work only the law of exhaustion of susceptibility on which the whole value of the practice depends.

That this is the true account of the matter appears from the direction in which its planes of action extend when prolonged. The great scientist, the world has lately lost, called the preventive inoculations (against Charbon and Chicken-Cholera) which have immortalised him, "vaccinations." The term would have been inappropriate if used etymologically, but its analogical force was evident. And what were the lymphs he inserted? They were not SIMILIA, but EADEM—the identical poison or poisoned parts of the diseases he sought to combat, only tempered and mitigated in virulence by the "cultivation" they had undergone. I am not now discussing the value of Pasteur's methods,—although, however doubtful they may be in respect of Hydrophobia, as regards Charbon and Chicken-Cholera I suppose there can be no

---

* Herein I must differ from Dr. Edward Madden, who in his Presidential Address at our Congress of 1895 speaks of Hahnemann as "clearly claiming Vaccination as an example of SIMILIA SIMILIBUS." He does so in respect of the modification exerted by Cow-pox over Small-pox, if induced in time; but not (I think) as regards its protective power.

† See B. J. H., ix. 473, x. 262. Drs. Winterburn and Bishop have more lately reported similar experience,—the former giving the 30th dil., the latter the 3rd trit. (J. B. H. S., ii. 369, iv. 352).

question of their merits. I am only shewing that when he sought to apply elsewhere the principle involved in Vaccination, it was identity, not similarity, with which he had worked.

The same thing appears when we prolong the other plane, and enquire what analogues exist to the treatment of Small-pox by *Vaccinine* and *Varioline*. It is *Varioline* which forms the type of such remedies. We are brought into the sphere of Isopathy—that is, the treatment of diseases by their own morbid products. The history of this practice, whether as carried out in the East, or as revived during the last century in our own school (it may be read at length in Dr. Dudgeon's Sixth Lecture), presents many follies and much nastiness; and is on the whole rather humiliating than encouraging. There are, however, a few grains of wheat to be gathered from its dunghill, and for what they are worth must be credited to Homœopathists, though not to Homœopathy. When I say "not to Homœopathy." I mean that the principle of selection is other than that contemplated by the rule SIMILIA SIMILIBUS. That a substance chosen Isopathically may act Homœopathically in the system, it would be rash to deny: we can hardly follow Hahnemann (organon, § 56, note) in maintaining that it does so because "dynamized" and so altered, but there is a theory of the MODUS OPERANDI of similar remedies to which these would lend themselves, so as to make it different whether the medicinal agent was an $\hat{o}\mu oιov$ or an $ιov$.* Waiving this, my point is that the treatment of Small-pox by *Vaccinine* as well as by *Varioline* is to be referred to the Isopathic category; it finds its analogue in our use of morbid products for their own mother disease. Such use we have made, with much success, of what we call *"Anthracine"* in Charbon—here anticipating Pasteur, save that we have given it curatively, not prophylactically, and have robbed it of its virulence by dilution instead of cultivation. Similarly good results have followed the administration of attenuated Lymph derived from the "Rot" of sheep—which is just "Variola ovina."‡ I shall have more to say on this subject another day, when the subject of "Nosodes" must be handled in connexion with Koch's *Tuberculin*.

The result of what has now been said is that we can hardly ascribe to Homœopathy (strictly so called) the immunity conferred by Vaccination. A FORTIORI must we refrain from claiming for it, the practice with Antitoxic serums, which has followed on the discovery that such immunity can be (temporarily at least) transferred by inoculation with the immune blood. Here I am

---

* See Dudgeon, op. CIT., p. 164.
† IBID., p. 167; and B. J. H., xxxi. 624.

glad to have Dr. Madden's concurrence. "It has been," he says, "suggested by some that these injections of Serum taken from immunised subjects act curatively, because they contain attenuated doses of the original Toxin and not in virtue of any Anti-toxic element the Lymph is supposed to contain, and that they are thus examples of unconscious Homœopathic (I should have said, Isopathic) practice". Such a conclusion, however, gratifying as it might be to us, I fear cannot be maintained, as it has been shewn that the Anti-toxin Serum destroys the vitality and morbific power in the bacilli which are introduced into it, outside the body as well as within, so that it is no longer possible to doubt that a real Anti-toxic element does exist in such Serum. The question for us, then, in Diphtheria—for it is mainly in this disease that the Serum Treatment has been adopted—is, Can we do better ? The testimony to reduction of mortality effected by it in old-school treatment was, at the Meeting of the British Medical Association in London in 1895, so general from all countries represented, that Mr. Lennox Browne's different results (which I shall mention immediately) may fairly be held in suspense for the present. But what does the reduction amount to ? From an average of 40 to 50 the per-centage of deaths has fallen to about 17. This is well ; and some careful observations by one of our own colleagues, Dr. W. C. Cutler, *illustrate the undoubted power of the treatment. In a series of 31 hospital cases, four deaths only occured, of which but one—he considers—was part of the ordinary course of the disease, and this case was not injected with the Serum till the fifth day. He notes that the mode of disappearance of the membrane under the influence 'of the Serum is that it rolls up at its edges, and so peels off: whereas under drug treatment it rather softens and breaks away piecemeal. But now 'let us turn to Homœopathic Statistics. I will take 'the results obtained with one drug only, though others find well-defined place in certain forms and stages of the disease : I speak of the *Cyanide of Mercury*. I will ask the candid enquirer first to read the provings and poisonings with this drug, as recorded in the Cyclopædia of Drug Pathogenesy (iii. 260). Let him then read the Essay of Dr. Villers, senr., translated in Vol. xli, of the BRITISH JOURNAL OF HOMŒOPATHY. He will see how the inference—whose validity he cannot doubt—was made from such poisonings that it was applied accordingly ; and that in the course of the next five years Dr. Villers treated with (at St. Petersburg) some 200 cases of the disease, of all sorts of severity, without a single death—giving the dilutions from the 6th to the 30th, Dr. Neusehafer, giving the drug from the 15th to 5th dilution

---

* NEW ENGLAND MED. GAZETTE, May, 1895.

hypodermically, has treated 85 cases with only 3 deaths.* If these infinitesimals stagger him, I may refer him to the similar results reported by Dr. Burt, of Chicago, who has treated many scores of cases with only a single failure, using the 3rd dec. trituration. † Or, if he will have evidence from his own side, let him hear the Swedish practitioner Dr. H. Sellden ‡ His formula is—*Cyanide of Mercury,* two centigrammes : tincture of *Aconite,* two grammes ; Honey, fifty grammes : mix, and give a teaspoonful every 15-60 minutes, according to the patient's age. (This, according to my reckoning, makes each such dose contain 1/43 of a grain.) He also orders a gargle of the strength of 1 in 10,000. Under this treatment he and his colleagues had, in 1,400 cases occurring during a term of years, a mortality of 5 per cent. only ; whereas under ordinary treatment this assumed frightful proportions. The figures here were not quite so good —the dosage being probably too large ; but they bear out the still better ones of the Homœopathic reporters. Really, therefore, with all due respect to the Serum Treatment, we do not want it. Our results are already better than it can shew, and we are not fond of injecting foreign matter into our patients' circulation, incurring consequences which already have sometimes proved unpleasant, and may be worse. Mr. Lennox Browne indeed, § "questions whether we are justified in continuing to pursue a treatment, in which there is such a marked increase in some of the recognised complications of Diphtheria, and the occurrence of several new ones of undesirable, if not actually of fatal significance." He himself doubts the real reduction of mortality by it, shewing that in 100 well-marked cases submitted to the Serum Treatment in a London fever hospital, the mortality was identical (27 per cent.) with that of the last 100 cases treated in the ordinary way.

Some of my hearers, perhaps, who are unacquainted with Homœopathic literature, may be surprised at such statistics as I have brought forward. They may have thought the method of Hahnemann possibly available where there is plenty of time and no danger ; but in the presence of these menacing toxications they would deem its employment mere trifling. I can assure them, however, that it is just the pestilential epidemics, like Cholera and Yellow Fever, and the hardly less fatal endemics like Diphtheria and Typhoid, which have made the fortune of Homœopathy by its comparative success. Take the last-named disease. Would not any hospital be well-satisfied, if during a term of 23 years its average mortality in Typhoid cases was 7 per cent ? Well: that is the rate ascertained to have prevailed in our Hospital St. Jacques at Paris. Or, to get comparative

---

* M. H. R., xxxviii. 250. † AMER. HOMOEOPATHIST, ii. 22. ‡ See LANCET. April 24, 1888. § "Diphtheria and its Associates," 1895.

statistics in a small compass, let us go to the antipodes, and see how such patients fare in the three hospitals of Melbourne respectively. During the five years 1889-94. the mortality from Enteric Fever in the Hospital named from the city was 19·49 per cent.; in the Alfred Hospital it was 10·54 : is the Homœopathic it was only 7.22. Nor is the advantage gained by the number of cases being fewer. Our institution is indeed a smaller one ; but it makes up by quickness of recovery for deficiency in beds,* and its number of cases of this Fever treated during the five years falls short of that of the Alfred Hospital by only 4, and of the large Melbourne Hospital by but 126.

Again, Cholera and Yellow Fever are disorders fairly trying the mettle of any method of treatment. Homœopathy 'has never blenched before them, formidable as they are ; and has always come off the field comparatively, if not positively, victorious. As regards Cholera :—Naples in 1884, Hamburg in 1892, showed that no advance had been made since the past by the old-school treatment ; the deaths averaging 53 per cent. in the former, 40-45 per cent. in the latter Epidemic. Our mortality has never risen to such heights. Dr. Hesse in Hamburg lost 20 per cent. only of his cases ; and our latest experience of the pestilence in England, when Dr. Proctor encountered it at Liverpool in 1866, gave out of 99 fully-developed cases, 85 recoveries. Of Yellow Fever it will suffice that I recall the statements made to us by the late Dr. J. P. Dake at our International Congress of 1881. He told us of the Yellow Fever Commission appointed by the President of the American Institute of Homœopathy after the Epidemic of 1878—the severest they had known in America. He and his colleagues followed on its heels, as it were, gaining information while memory was fresh. They had 6,569 cases reported to them from Homœopathic physicians, with 360 deaths,—that is a percentage of 5·4. "The moratlity of the old-school treatment ranged all the way from 15 to 60 per cent., and the general average would come up to 20 per cent." It is easy to calculate that had it not been for Homœopathy, a thousand of the survivors of the band treated thereby would have succumbed to the Plague.

Another gratifying feature in the Report of this Commission was the near approach to unanimity ascertained to have prevailed as regards the medicines used. It was especially shown in this, that in the second stage—that of Hæmatic Jaundice and Hæmorrhages—all Homœopathic practitioners employed one or other of the *Snake-poisons.* The use of these substances is

---

* The same thing was noted in Tessier's experience at the Hospital St. Marguerite in Paris.

a DIFFERENTIA of our practice, and has given us some of our most potent agents. For *Lachesis*—the venom of the lance-headed viper, the "Churukuku," of Surinam—we are indebted to Constantine Hering; for *Naja*—that of the Cobra to Rutherford Russell; but for *Crotalus*—that of the Rattle-snake—we owe mainly to Dr. Hayward of Liverpool, whose Monograph upon it, in the "Materia Medica, Physiological and Applied" (Vol. I.) is a mine of information on the whole subject. Many years ago * I endeavoured (basing myself on the phenomena of snake-bite) to formulate the main action of these substances thus : that they were indicated "when a local affection assumes a malignant character, and from thence proceed poisoning of the blood and prostration of the nervous energies." I was then inclined to doubt their applicability to primary Toxæmiæ; but Dr. Drysdale in 1872 called my attention to the occurrence of cases in which the bite was not at all inflamed, yet the paitent died fast enough—showing that the venom might be fatal without any secondary Septicæmic infection. † Wider knowledge has confirmed this inference; and in the later editions of my 'Manual' I have given a notable list of morbid hæmatic conditions in which the *Snake-venoms* have proved curative. They thus play an important part in the treatment of the Specific Infectious Fevers which have been under our notice to-day, coming in when Jaundice with hæmorrhages occurs, whether primarily or as in Yellow-Fever itself : when a purpuric condition supervenes upon Typhus or Variola, constituting their hæmorrhagic varieties; when epidemic Cerebro-spinal Meningitis appears in the form known as "Malignant purpuric" or "Spotted" Fever; in Plague; and in the invasion of malignant Scarlatina. In two cases of the latter kind, occurring in his own family, which Dr. Hayward has recorded in his Monograph, the curative action of *Crotalus* was very marked. But after all it is in malignant inflammations, with secondary blood-poisoning and prostration—often out of proportion to the local mischief that *Snake-venom* finds its chief place. Traumatic Gangrene, Septicæmia from dissecting-wound, Malignant Pustule and Carbuncle, Pyæmia from Phlebitis. Diphtheria—these are the formidable conditions in which it has come to our aid, and enabled us to triumph in almost hopeless circumstances. That it is still ready to do similar service appears from the cases of Pyæmia from suppurative Periostitis and of commencing constitutional infection from a poisoned wound reported within the last few years to the British Homœopathic Society. ‡ Of the former, the reporter (Dr. C. W. Hayward) says, "The terrible

---

* Manual of Pharmacodynamics, 1st Ed., 1867.

† M. H. R., xvi., 636.

‡ See J. B. H. S., iii. 383, and M. H. R., xxxvi. 212 (In the former, at line 8, "May, 28" should be "May 20.").

condition to which the patient was reduced at the time of operation, and the undoubted Pyæmia from which he suffered, would, I am sure, under Sergery alone have been fatal. The effect of *Crotalus* was most marked." In the latter, Dr. Madden speaks of the rapid and unmistakable effect produced by *Lachesis,* which in a few hours transformed the case from one of the gravest danger and anxiety into one of a simple skin wound, which only required to be kept clean and quiet to be certain to heel speedily and well.

I think I have now said enough, generally, of Homœopathy in the ACUTE INFECTIOUS DISEASES. I am glad that the first class of maladies we have had to consider have been such as from their severity might seem beyond the range of our method, and from the hypothesis of their nature now accepted might be supposed to require least doses of germicides rather than small ones of specifics. In neither way is the presumption against Homœopathy borne out by the facts : it exhibits itself effectively all along the line. We shall thus be encouraged to depend upon it with confidence in the less acute and more purely dynamic disorders which will subsequently come before us.

We will proceed to the consideration of the treatment of the several maladies included in the group now before us, and will take first the EXANTHEMATA. At the head of these stands SMALL-POX.

VARIOLA.—Let me begin by saying that as regards Vaccination we are, as a body, entirely at one with our brethren of the old school, though we have individual dissidents in our ranks as they have in theirs. Statistics at large demonstrate the extensive immunity from the disease secured by this invaluable prophylactic ; and no one who has had the opportunity of comparing the unmodified Small-Pox with that form of it which ordinarily appears in vaccinated subjects can do otherwise than bless the name of Jenner. If I cannot now, as I once did,* argue that the efficacy of Vaccination is probably an illustration of the Law of Similars ; if I have had to give good reasons for believing it to be an inoculation in a milder form, it is none the less a successful practice, and demands a loyal adhesion on our part.

I must first speak of the treatment of VARIOLOID—that is, of Small-Pox as modified by Vaccination or by a previous attack. The distinctive feature of this form of the disease is that the pustules do not mature, so that the suppurative stage and its accompanying fever are abolished, and the duration of the illness proportionately shortened. Almost the only thing you will have to do here is to mitigate the severity of the initial fever

---

* See paper, "On the Present Doctrine of Vaccination" in B. J. H., xxvi, 223.

and its concomitant symptoms, which is often considerable. I must agree with Bahr that **Belladonna** is more appropriate, Homœopathically, than *Aconite* to this fever, and I have seen better results from it. Occasionally, however, the condition of the patient may indicate other Antipyretics, as *Gelsemium, Baptisia*, or *Veratrum viride*, according to the characteristics of each as pointed out in my 'Pharmacodynamics.' The last named would be specially called for, if other symptoms concurred, when the pain in the back was severe. If the vomiting is troublesome. **Tartar emetic** (of whose relation to Variola I shall have more to say subsequently) will prove your best aid; and you can hardly do better than continue the administration of this medicine when the eruption has appeared and the temperature fallen. It will carry your patient on to a satisfactory convalescence.

It is altogether different when the subject of Small-Pox is unprotected, and you have to deal with Variola Vera. If you see the case early enough, an attempt should be made even yet to convert the disease into Varioloid. This can hardly indeed be done by Vaccination; for Mr. Marson has shown * that this operation, to be effective, must be performed not later than the third day after the patient has been exposed to contagion, which is eight or nine days before he begins to be ill. But you may get a much more rapid effect by giving your Cow-Pox Lymph internally as a medicine. You may smile at this idea. But let me ask you to read the experiments of Severin, Schneider, Norman Johnson, Kaczkowski, Landell and Collet regarding this matter. † You will see that Vaccine Lymph, even in infinitesimal doses will, when taken into stomach, develop the Cow-Pox vesicles with their concomitant fever, and vesicles so true that Vaccination from them has succeeded perfectly. You will also note that the effect is often much more rapid than when the Lymph is introduced into the arm, the fever and rash sometimes appearing as early as the third day. When given to persons actually suffering from Small-Pox, the action of the Lymph is still more rapid. Within twenty-four hours the pocks begin to feel its influence, and shrink, shrivel, and dry up. This is the experience alike of Dr. Landell, who gave about a third of a drop of the pure Lymph, and of Dr. Kaczkowski, who administered it in the third Homœopathic attenuation; only the latter seemed to act with greater rapidity. Thus Vaccininum has become an accredited medicine amongst us in the treatment of Small-Pox. Drs. Rummel, Pulte, Bayes and Goodno concur in testifying to its great value.

---

* See his Article on Small-Pox in Russell Reynolds' "System of Medicine."
† B. J. H., xxiv., 171; xxv., 340; xxxi., 905; xxxii., 720.

I have no personal experience of this medication; and have always, in the treatment of Variola, relied (after *Belladonna* at the outset) upon **Tartar emetic**. I have, when writing upon this medicine, shown its close Homœopathicity to our present disease; and I can quite go with Drs. Leidbeck * and Ludlam, † when they claim for it a real abortive control over the Variolous process, analogous to that exerted by prior Vaccination. I cannot better illustrate this than by citing a case of the disease treated by the latter physician.

"Frank——,aged six years, a fine healthy boy, the child of German parents. had never been vaccinated. I had promised to vaccinate him as soon as it was possible to procure a little good virus. Meanwhile he contracted the Small-Pox. The papular stage was well-defined. One could not mistake the shot-like pimples beneath the skin. The vesicles were formed, and in due time most of them became umbilicated. The eruption was thick, but yet distinct in its location, suggesting to an experienced eye that, when the pustular stage should set in, the case would assume the confluent form. All the attendant symptoms, the odour of the breath and the exhalations, the swollen eyelids and features, the sore-throat and salivary symptoms, were equally pronounced. The little fellow was really ill with genuine Small-Pox. We prescribed *Tartar emetic*. 3rd dec. trituration, of which he was to have a dose every three hours.

When the period arrived at which the serous fluid contained in the vesicles should have become turbid and purulent, it was remarked that no such change took place. Some of the vesicles burst, but the majority of them disappeared by desiccation and desquamation. Pus was not formed, and the third stage was not developed. The CUTIS VERA was not seriously implicated, and did not slough away; consequently even upon the most exposed portion of the face and extremities there was no 'pitting' at all. The child recovered without any of the ordinary sequelæ of severe Small-Pox, as Ophthalmia, Chronic Diarrhœa, &c. During the whole course of the disease he took no other medicine than *Tartar emetic*."

If you have not had the opportunity, or have failed to modify the disease in these earlier stages by *Vaccinine* or *Tartar emetic*, you must treat the fully developed pock according to the symptoms. When maturation is impending, and the suppurative fever rising, general consent points to **Mercurious** as the most effective—as I have already shown it to be the most Homœopathic—remedy. Hartmann, Rapou and Bahr are its especial panegyrists. Where the swelling is great, or when itching is troublesome, **Apis** is a useful adjunct.

---

* B. J. H., vii., 475.

† NORTH AMER. JOURN. OF HOM., xii., 567. To these I may add the experience of an old-school physician, who reports himself "highly gratified with the results of treating 33 cases during an epidemic with doses of gr. 1/100 each" (J.B. H. S., vii., 324).

All the complications and SEQUELÆ of Variola Vera (except the early Bronchitis, which is controlled by *Tartar emetic*) are results of the suppurative condition of the system induced during the maturation of the pustules, and are best averted or moderated by the *Mercurius* you are giving in this stage. But there is a frightful modification of the disease which may manifest itself from the first, or may be induced at any point of its progress. In the former case we call the whole malady Purpura Variolosa : in the latter we say that the Small-Pox has become hæmorrhagic. Some serious change has taken place in the blood or its vessels or both, which leads to its extravasation throughout the body; and the result is almost inevitably fatal. Can we do anything for this casualty? Dr. Hale records a case in which purpuric symptoms supervened during Varioloid, and yielded pretty speedily to *Hamamelis*. Teste writes :—"When the disease pursues an irregular course ; when the eruption exhibits a tendency to disappear from the surface ; when the pustules, in stead of being transparent or yellow, are green, purple or black; when the blood with which they are filled announces a decomposition of this fluid and threatens the approach of putrid symptoms, it is not to *Arsenicum* that we should have recourse, but to *Sulphur*." These are the only practical hints I can find on the subject in Homœopathic writings. I have myself suggested the *Snake-poisons* as the most Homœopathic remedies for this condition ; and though Dr. Galley Blackley says that in three cases of the kind occurring in an epidemic in Liverpool, he found *Crotalus* useless, I must still entertain a hope that with it or *Lachesis* we shall learn to control them in the future. Perhaps, too, *Phosphorus* might come in usefully here, as in primary Purpura. Dr. Jousset has reported a case of success with it (Lecons Cliniques, 1st Sers., L. 28). It is true that the patient had been vaccinated, and that the modifying influence of the prophylactic duly shewed itself in the abortion of the second stage of the disease. But even under such circumstances Variola Hæmorrhagica is apt to be fatal.

I have now sketched for you the ordinary Homœopathic treatment of Small-Pox, and with it you may expect to gain, as others have gained before you, a very fair measure of success. But I must mention briefly certain other remedial means which have been used by individual Homœopathists, and from which they claim more than ordinary good results.

1. Dr. Garth Wilkinson * thought **Hydrastis** a specific antidote to Small-Pox, capable of arresting the disease at its outset,

---

* "On the Cure, Arrest and Isolation of Small-Pox by a New Method," &c. 1864.

of extinguishing the infection by its local application, and of securing immunity to the healthy by its prophylactic use. Dr. Wilkinson should have, I think, adduced more evidence than he did to establish these positions. But those who have, at his recommendation, dabbed the swollen faces of their Variolous patients with an infusion of the plant, have testified to much relief of itching and reduction of œdema having been thereby obtained.

2. Dr. von Bœnninghausen was led to use **Thuja,** in Small-Pox on the strength of some Variola-like pustules having appeared on the knee in one of Hahnemann's provers, and (a better reason) because it had proved the specific remedy for the "Grease" of horses, which seems to be the same thing in them as Vaccinia in the cow. He states that it causes the early drying up of the pocks without pitting, and also acts as a temporary prophylactic like *Belladonna* in Scarlatina. Here again corroboration is required.

3. I need not reproduce what I have written elsewhere about the history of **Sarracenia purpurea** as an Anti-variolous remedy." That it has claims upon our notice is undoubted; but it has hardly yet established a superior efficacy on its part over the ordinary treatment.

4. Much more satisfactory evidence exists as to the virtue of the last remedy I have to mention to you, the **Baptisia tinctoria.** Dr. Eubulus Williams is physician to a large Children's Home in Bristol. As epidemic of Small-Pox occurred there in 1872, nearly 300 children being attacked. All had been vaccinated in infancy, but none re-vaccinated. The result was that no child under three took the disease; that between the ages of three and eleven forty-three only were affected, and none died; while those from eleven to eighteen (the extreme limit of age in the Home) furnished all the remaining cases out of the 300. Now, of 185 of these treated with ordinary remedies (*Tartar emetic, Vaccinine, Thuja*) nineteen died; of seventy-two treated with *Baptisia* alone, none. Yet these (Dr. Williams says) were as severe in their character at the outset as the others; some more so. Three of them had hæmorrhages, two from the vagina and one from the nose, but they recovered without an untoward symptom; whereas under other treatment such losses of blood had always been followed by death. Dr. Williams is satisfied that the *Baptisia* often aborted the disease; and it always averted prostration, improved appetite, obviated decomposition (as shown by the absence of the usual offensive effluvia), and prevented pitting. "In two cases only, of those treated by

---

* To the references given in my 'Pharmacodynamics' add J. B. H. S., ii., 100.

Baptisia, were there any evident scars two months after recovery." You may read Dr. Williams' valuable communication in the Thirty-First Volume of the BRITISH JOURNAL of HOMŒOPATHY.

I have already mentioned *Baptisia* as one of the possible remedies for the initial fever of Variola. The results now related would point to a still more intimate connection between the drug and the disease, and would encourage us, when we find the medicine indicated at the outset, to persevere with it throughout the malady.

Dr. Williams' Statistics are the only ones we have on a large scale for testing the comparative success of Homœopathic treatment in Small-pox. Under ordinary treatment the mortality among the vaccinated ranges from ½ to 8 per cent. Among the unvaccinated it averages 37 per cent. These are the results obtained at the London Small-Pox Hospital. Dr. Williams lost no case at all during the time when primary Vaccination continues effective—*i.e.*, from the age of three to that of eleven. After that period, when the course of the disease showed that the subjects of it were no longer protected, his mortality was 19 out of 257—about 7½ per cent. I think you will agree with me that it is high time that a ward of the above-named Hospital was handed over to Homœopathic treatment.

---

* In the INDIAN HOMŒOPATHIC REVIEW of May, 1895, Dr. Bhaduri writes that quite a virulent epidemic of Small-Pox had raged at Calcutta, and that great success had been gained by Homœopathic treatment. 'We have been able to check hæmorrhages in the pocks by medicines like *Arsenic, Crotalus, Rhus tox.* etc., and we have made the disease take a milder type by the use of *Vaccinine*. The last medicine has helped us more than any other, and even beyond our expectation, in this epidemic.'

LECTURE XVII.

GENERAL DISEASES

THE EXANTHEMATA (*Continued*).

VACCINIA—VARICELLA—MORBILLI—RUBELLA—SCARLATINA—DENGUE—MILIARIA.

After Variola the next disease on our list is Cow-Pox itself—

VACCINIA.—You may think that its interest in us is purely Pathological, as it is not communicable by contagion to the human subject. No: but it is by inoculation, and in this way it is set up in millions of human beings every year. Ordinarily, indeed, the indisposition occasioned by Vaccination is so slight as to demand no treatment, save for a little **Aconite** if the patient is feverish, or some **Belladonna** when the areola is more inflamed than usual. But ever and anon—at any rate in the days when we took lymph from children's arms, and were not always sufficiently particular about securing it before it had become purulent—unpleasent after-effects, local or general, have followed upon Jenner's prophylactic method. These generally take the form of ulcers or pustular eruptions, and when thus occurring are well-controlled by **Silicea**—which, Constantine Hering having been the first to recommend it, I have always given in the 30th.

Some of our colleagues would go further. In 1860 Dr. C. W. Wolf, of Berlin, published a Treatise* in which he maintained that the virus introduced by Vaccination was really that of Hahnemann's "Sycosis"; that many more chronic affections than Hahnemann dreamed of were caused thereby, and that his chief Anti-sycotic, **Thuja**, was their all-sufficient remedy. In 1884, our own Dr. Burnett (of whose sudden death I regretted to hear as I wrote these lines) published a small volume entitled "Vaccinosis and its cure by *Thuja*," and propounding a similar thesis. He had not, he tells us, heard of Wolf; but the ideas of the latter would seem, to have filtered into his mind through the German authors to whom he acknowledges his indebtedness—Drs, Kunkel and H. Goullon. They appear in his pages,

---

* See an account of it in B. J. H., xviii., 459.

however, in a much more restrained and rational form. He does not speculate about "Sycosis," nor does he follow Goullon in requiring Grauvogl's "Hydrogenoid" constitution to characterize the subjects fitted for his medication. His contention is that the modern practice of repeated Vaccination is, whether the Lymph "takes" or not, and indeed especially when it does not take, the frequent cause of a morbid habit of the body which he would call "Vaccinosis." It manifests itself in pustular eruption, chronic Headaches and Neuralgias, diseased finger-nails, and a variety of other phenomena; and whenever occurring is more or less amenable to the influence of *Thuja*—generally given in highest dilution. The cases he gives are often very striking and they certainly bear out his recommendation of the remedy—whatever may be thought of his theory.*

Still shorter may be my notice of the following malady—

VARICELLA—the "CHICKEN-POX" of common parlance. You will naturally give mild doses of **Aconite** while the temperature is elevated; and I think you will find **Apis** useful if, as often happens, there is much itching with the eruption.

Of much greater importance than Vaccinia or Varicella is the Exanthem next coming before us, MEASLES—

MORBILLI—The Homœopathic treatment of this disorder is very simple and very successful. "The most important thing in the Therapeutics of Measles," writes Thomas in Ziemssen's Cyclopædia, "is the suppression of immoderate fever in the prodromal, and especially in the eruptive stage." For this purpose he advises a complicated and most troublesome course of cold baths, packings and compresses.† We, without neglecting any comfort and refreshment which can be derived from

---

* An illustrative case is recorded in the MEDICAL CENTURY, for June 15, 1895. A general Psoriasis, of four years' standing in a girl of ten, was traced to Vaccination, with aggravation by overdosing with *Arsenic*. *Thuja* in the 3rd and 2nd dilutions caused an almost complete recovery. (See also J. B. H. S., iv. 341).

† With what success may be inferred from the fact that Statistics show a hospital mortality of 10 to 40 per cent. In our Hospital St. Jacques, in Paris, where the ward of six beds reserved for cases of this malady is often full, no death from it has been registered for thirty years. This statement includes the Broncho-Pneumonic cases, (L' ART MEDICAL, May, 1900; p. 342).

cold water without or within, rely for antipyretic purposes on one medicine, **Aconite**. We give it from the commencement, and we do not suspend its use till complete defervescence has occurred. Dr. Ozanne, who has given in the Sixth Volume of the BRITISH JOURNAL OF HOMŒOPATHY an interesting account of an Epidemic of Measles observed by him in Guernsey, writes thus on the last-named point:—'I remarked that after giving the *Aconitum* either for twenty-four or forty-eight hours, and producing a fall of 30 or 40 pulsations per minute, on replacing it with *Pulsatilla* the pulse frequently rose again from 80 pulsations per minute to 90 or 100, its strength and fulness gaining in proportion, whilst the heat of the skin and the restlessness at night, together with the peculiar harsh and troublesome cough, continued or increased." To this corresponds that which is noted by all writers on the fever of Measles, that, unlike that of Small-Pox, it does not subside on the occurrence of the eruption, but rather increases; and also, which thermometric investigation has since established, that the MAXIMA of fever and eruption coincide. He, therefore, gave *Aconite* more persistently, and with the happiest results.

Fever being thus a continuous feature in Measles, and its type being quite that of *Aconite*, you will employ this medicine throughout its course; and (if comparative observation on my own children with the 1st decimal and the 12th centesimal may be trusted) preferably in the lower dilutions. But I am persuaded that much benefit is obtained from alternating with it medicines suitable to the local catarrhal disorder present. When this is chiefly conjunctival and nasal, **Euphrasia** is invaluable. Dr. Pope, who has communicated to the Sixteenth Volume of the MONTHLY HOMŒOPATHIC REVIEW a very practical Essay on Measles, recommends also bathing the eyes, when they are much affected, with an infusion of the plant. The catarrh of the digestive canal, which occurs later, calls for **Pulsatilla**, which is a medicine of high repute in Measles, and will generally control the Diarrhœa to your satisfaction. If the Cough is very troublesome and the larynx evidently much affected, I agree with Dr. Lippe in thinking **Kali bichromicum** the most Homœopathic as well as the most effective remedy; but Jousset recommends *Viola-odorata*. Nor is the first-named of less avail if simple Bronchitis should supervene, *Aconite* being continued or resumed as the case may have happened.

There are other graver complications and SEQUELÆ of Measles —Laryngitis, Diphtheria, Broncho-Pneumonia, Ophthalmic and Aural troubles, Gangrenous processes in mouth or genitals. But these constitute substantive diseases, and will be discussed in their proper places. I will only speak here of the danger into which the patient is occasionally thrown by the imperfect development or retrocession of the eruption. When the effect of this casualty is of a general character—coldness, prostration and so forth—I have seen the best results from repeated doses of **Camphor**. When the chest is especially affected thereby, **Ammonium carbonicum** (in the first dilution) has served me well; but Hartmann and Teste concur in commending **Bryonia**. When the brain is oppressed, there is a general agreement—here as in Scarlatina—as to the virtues of **Cuprum aceticum**; and here also **Zincum** may be a possible alternative.*

When the embers of the Morbillous fire seem unwilling to go out, their extinguishment may often be greatly promoted (especially in strumous subjects) by a course of **Sulphur**. If however, the conjunctiva be the part affected, Bahr supports Dr. Pope in commending **Arsenicum** as the best medicine. In a severe epidemic occurring at Antwerp, where Dr. Lambreghts had fifty cases under his care, he found this drug the one best able to remove all SEQUELÆ. I agree with Dr. Jousset in advising reliance on the same remedy if Measles ever assume a malignant form.

RUBELLA is the next name on our official list and it designates what is popularly known as "GERMAN MEASLES,' and which I have in my 'Manual of Therapeutics' called by its German name, "ROTHELN." It seems to combine the Morbillous skin and mucous membrane with the Scarlatinal mouth and throat. The German writer on it, in Ziemssen's work, makes it a much higher disease than it is known here — as described, for instance, in Copelands "Dictionary" or Aitken's "Science and Practice of Medicine". According to him it is ordinarily feverless. I much suspect that confusion has arisen from identifying this malady with "Epidemic Roseola"—Rose-Rash as we used to call it, that simulates Scarlatina, while Rubella is much more like Measles; and (the former) is slight indeed.

An account of an epidemic of Rubella occurring in a school, given by Mr. Harmar Smith in the Sixteenth Volume of the MONTHLY HOMŒOPATHIC REVIEW shows that it may assume diverse forms and degrees of severity according to the patient attacked. You must treat these as you would Measles and Scarlatina, according to the condition present.

SCARLATINA is unquestionably one of the most important diseases with which we have to deal. Its great frequency where

---

* See a case in J. B. H. S., iv. 170.

sanitary considerations are neglected, its high mortality and the variety of its forms, complications and sequelæ invest it alike with practical and scientific interest. You will be eager to know what Homœopathy can do in its treatment, and how its work is done.

I have mentioned the prophylactic virtues, in this disease, of **Belladonna**. If you will consider the evidence I have adduced or referred you to, you will see that these are amply attested. That results of an opposite kind have been obtained I know well; but two considerations must be borne in mind in estimating their weight in the question. First, what was the dose used? Hahnemann recommended one or two drops of a solution of the extract equivalent to about the third centesimal dilution, every third or fourth day. Those who have confirmed his results have approximated more or less closely to his dose: while the reporters from the opposite side (notably in Mr. Benjamin Bell's experiments in George Watson's Hospital) seem generally to have given the drug in quantities large enough to excite its Physiological effects. The second question is still more important — what was the form of the epidemic present? Hahnemann long ago pointed out that there were two distinct forms of Scarlatina,—the eruption in the one being smooth, shining, bright and scarlet, in the other dusky, sometimes purplish, patchy and rough, in the form of very minute vesicles. The constitutional concomitants and the suitable medicines vary in these two forms of the disease. The distinction thus drawn has since been verified by Dr. Bayes in an Epidemic observed by him at Cambridge, of which he has given an account in the Fourth Volume of the ANNALS. Now Hahnemann expressly limits the prophylatic virtues of *Belladonna* to the former of these varieties. To demonstrate its failure, therefore, it is necessary that the kind of Exanthem present in the epidemic in question be distinctly identified; which has not been done. I conclude accordingly that the weight of evidence is in favour of the power of *Belladonna* to protect against, or to render milder, a threatened attack of Scarlatina; and I recommend you always to give it where the disorder is prevalent or has already appeared in a house.

And now as to treatment—
We must begin by eliminating the miliary variety which is rarely met with in the present day. Dr. Bayes confirms Hahnemann's observation that *Belladonna* is as useless here to modify, as it is to prevent and that the specific remedies are **Aconite** and **Coffea**, in medium dilution. I have myself seen this form of Scarlatina in one family only; and I was led to these medicines by the symptoms before I had clearly identified the disorder before me. The complications and sequelæ of the miliary variety require the same treatment as those of the more ordinary form of the disease.

The true smooth Scarlatina of Sydenham is, as you know, styled "Simplex," "Anginosa," or 'Maligna" according to its severity. These divisions afford a sound practical basis for my sketch of its treatment.

"SCARLATINA SIMPLEX," we are told, "proves fatal only through the officiousness of the doctor;" and hence we are advised to leave it to Nature and nursing. I think you will find, however, that great relief may be given during its progress by Homœopathic medicines,—especially **Aconite** and **Belladonna**. This is one of the few instances in which I find alternation necessary. I have sometimes tried *Belladonna* alone but the fever has been far more persistent. In Scarlatina, like Measles and unlike Small-Pox, the fever keeps up after the rash has appeared; and hence the necessity of *Aconite* throughout. This is also the experience of Drs. Ozanne and Pope.

It is right to mention that some physicians prefer **Gelsemium** for the Scarlatinal fever, considering it hardly sthenic enough for *Aconite*.

In the "SCARLATINA ANGINOSA" you will have begun with *Aconite* and perhaps *Belladonna*; but very soon you will find that the state of the throat demands special remedies. You will generally have either swelling or ulceration as the prominent symptom present; and your remedies must be selected accordingly. For the former condition I have been disappointed in *Baryta carbonica,* which I was led to use from its value in Quinsy; but it is now generally agreed that we have a capital medicine for it in **Apis**. For the ulceration, often so destructive, which obtains in Scarlatina, we have an excellent and most Homœopathic remedy in **Mercurius**. Dr. Pope thinks the *Biniodide* its best form; but I am inclined to prefer, for the reasons given when lecturing upon the drug, a more purely Mercurial preparation. The *Biniodide*, on the other hand, has often served me well in the Quasi-Diphtheretic condition which sometimes complicates Scarlatina.

Symptomatic affections of the neck accompany all forms of Scarlatina Anginosa. If they consist of swelling of the glands only, the *Mercurius* we shall be giving for the internal trouble will be all that is required. But if the areolar tissue become impliacted grave trouble is threatened, and we need to direct our main energies on this point. Dr. P. P. Wells, who has lately given us in a completed form some previous valuable commentaries on the Therapeutics of Scarlatina,* recommends **Rhus** in the incipience of such cases, **Lachesis** when they are more advanced.

And now of that frightful disease which we call "SCARLATINA MALIGNA." We usually first recognise it in the general nervous toxication which characterizes its primary invasion. The

---

* See AMAB. HOM. REVIEW, VOL. iv., NORTH AMER. JOURN. of HOM., Vol. xxiv.

obvious indication here is to get the poison to the skin; for which purpose, you may well call in the aid of Hydropathy, in the form either of the wet pack, or the cold affusion with subsequent wrapping in blankets. At the same time you will administer medicines suitable to the condition present. **Camphor**, in repeated doses, is commended by Hartmann, and would be indicated where the symptoms were rather those of general collapse with coldness, the mental functions continuing unimpeded. But when (as often happens) the oppression of the brain is the most prominent symptom, we have two medicines in high repute, **Cuprum aceticum** and **Zincum**. The evidence in favour of the former is adduced by Dr. G. Schmid in the First Volume of the BRITISH JOURNAL OF HOMŒOPATHY; the latter is advocated by Dr. Elb in the Seventh Volume of the same Journal. It is not easy to distinguish between the two; but Dr. Pope thinks the *Cuprum* preferable the more intense the prostration and the more violent the Convulsions.

Dr. Wells suggests as additional remedies for consideration in the primary invasion of Malignant Scarlatina. *Hydrocyanic acid, Tabacum, Lachesis* and the *Ailanthus glandulosa*. Striking results have followed his mention of **Ailanthus**. I have told the story in my 'Pharmacodynamics.' The facts justify the conclusion that we have in this medicine a most potent antidote to Scarlatina Maligna. When the disease sets in with angry symptoms, the throat livid and rapidly swelling, the eruption patchy and dark-coloured, the pulse very quick and feeble, and the brain oppressed, *Ailanthus* seems to do all that medicine can do. It quite supersedes *Arsenicum* and *Lachesis*, and probably renders even *Cuprum* and *Zincum* unnecessary here though they would be the remedies were the cerebral symptoms consequent on the retrocession of an otherwise normal Rash. *Ailanthus* should be given alone, in about the first decimal dilution. An alternative to it would be **Baptisia**, with which Dr. H. Macdonald communicates to the CLINIQUE of August 1895, a lengthened favourable experience.

Sometimes however, when the general condition of the patient has been greatly improved by these means, the throat-symptoms continue malignant and may even set up fresh constitutional disturbance, the system being, as it were, re-inoculated from the ulcerated and gangrenous fauces. I have been accustomed to rely upon **Lachesis** here as truly indicated, and it has not disappointed me. From America, however, the **Arum triphyllum** is highly commended, especially when the nose and mouth are sore and the discharges acrid. With regard to *Lachesis*, I may mention that Dr. Jousset esteems it the principal remedy in Malignant Scarlatina; "it has procured us," he says, "unhoped-for successes." Dr. Spranger says that in his early medical life he saw so many cases "go to the bad" under *Belladonna*—Septicæmia, as he thinks, complicating the Scarlatina proper—that he began to give *Lachesis* from the first. Under this treatment for the last fifteen years he has never had a troublesome case, and Scarlatina brings no more terrors to him.*

Dr. Wells (as also Dr. Jousset) speaks of "inflammation of the brain and its membranes" as not unfrequently occurring in Scarlatina, and describes the characteristics of its remedies, notably *Belladonna* and *Sulphur*. I suspect that the complication is a very rare one. Laryngitis, also, is happily unfrequent: *Spongia* and *Bromine* might touch it when occurring.

The "Post-scarlatinal Dropsy" forms a connecting link between the complications and the sequelæ of Scarlatina. I mean that it seems now ascertained that renal implication, as shown by Albuminuria, is no accident of this Exanthem, but of its essence, and constant. This requires no treatment; but it is otherwise when it results subsequently in acute desquamative Nephritis and Dropsy. Several medicines are in repute for this malady. I was glad to see that Dr. Yeldham had softened the recommendation of *Terebinthina* to be once made.† I have been woefully disappointed in it. **Arsenicum, Cantharis, Helleborus** and **Apis** have been most frequently used. The second would seem most truly Homœopathic to the lesion present; but I have best reason to be satisfied with *Arsenicum*. Dr. Ozanne, in an epidemic occurring at Guernsey, relied on *Helleborus* with the best results; and the same medicine is also praised by an old school physician ‡ *Apis* is reported to have acted well in American epidemics: I have myself given it occasionally without manifest effect. *Apocynum, Colchicum,* and *Hepar sulphuris* also are only theoretical. I shall return to this subject when I come to speak of renal disease.

I may dismiss briefly the other sequelæ of Scarlatina. The sore and bleeding nose, and the Otorrhœa and Deafness, which often remain behind, are singularly under the control of **Muriatic acid**, sometimes, in the ear cases, reinforced by *Hepar sulphuris*. Bahr recommends also *Aurum muriaticum* for the nose, and Pope, *Silicea* for the ear. But when these troubles occur as parts of a general bursting forth of the scrofulous diathesis resultant upon the disease, **Sulphur** must be administered.

I think I have now pretty well prepared you for the treatment of Scarlet Fever; nor do I doubt but that you will be abundantly satisfied with your comparative measure of success. For fuller information I may refer you to our systematic Treatises in general; to the accounts of Epidemics of the disease by Dr. Ozanne in the Third Volume of the BRITISH JOURNAL OF HOMŒOPATHY, by Dr. Wilde and Dr. Bayes in the Fourth

---

* PACIFIC COAST JOURN. OF HOMŒOPATHY, Feb., 1896.
† See ANNALS i., 390; iv. 71.   ‡ See B. J. H., iv., 6.

Volume of the ANNALS, and by Mr. Nankivell in the Seventh Volume of the MONTHLY HOMŒOPATHIC REVIEW in Acute Diseases," and by Dr. Laurie in the Second Volume of the BRITISH JOURNAL. I must also mention an able series of papers by Dr. Pope (to which I have made frequent reference) in the Fourteenth Volume of the MONTHLY HOMŒOPATHIC REVIEW. Our Therapeutics of the disease have been so well-established by these and similar treatises, that few communications regarding it have appeared in our later literature. A "Symposium" devoted to it appeared in the MEDICAL CENTURY of May 1st and 15th, 1895. The remedies I have mentioned seem, in the hands of the contributors, to have sustained their reputation. Dr. George Royal praises **Bryonia** in repercussion of the eruption, or *Stramonium* when the urine is suppressed. Dr. Fisher says that *Carbolic acid* (4th dil.) has rendered him excellent service in confirmed blood-poisoning types, with coma, fœtor oris, besotted countenance, Otorrhœa—profuse and offensive, glandular involvement —destructive; and our own Dr. Vawdrey regards the specific action of *Cantharis* (1_x—3_x) in the acute Nephritis "one of the few certainties of medicine."

I would add that Scarlatina, like Small-Pox, may show malignancy by taking on the hæmorrhagic form. What **Phosphorus** may do in such cases, I cannot say; but we have an alternative in **Crotalus** which Hayward's experience seems to establish as being as effective here as it is Homœopathic. You will find his record of it in the "Materia Medica, Physiological and Applied," VOL. I., p. 362.

I conclude my remarks on the treatment of the Exanthemata with a mention of two affections not ordinarily so accounted, "DENGUE" and "MILIARIA."

DENGUE is classed in our official Nomenclature among the pestilences, with Typhus, Plague and Influenza. The definition given of it in Quain's Dictionary, "an eruptive fever, considered by many to be infectious," places it rather in our present category. It seems to be a sort of relapsing febricula, made up of two short paroxysms separated by an interval. The first paroxysm consists of high continuous fever, with severe pain in head, limbs and joints, and swelling of the latter; with which occurs a Scarlatinoid Rash. The second has a less intense fever, with a Rubeoloid or Urticarious exanthem, often with itching and implication of the mucous membrane of the nose, mouth and throat.

Judging from these symptoms, I think there can be no doubt of the suitableness of **Aconite** in the first paroxysm, as the fundamental remedy. Remembering, however, that when Dengue invaded America in 1827 it was known as the "Break-bone Fever," and that the **Eupatorium perfoliatum** was found most beneficial in relieving the pains indicated by this title, we may wisely give it in alternation with the Anti-pyretic. In the second paroxysm **Gelsemium** would take the place of *Aconite*; and the symptoms of skin and mucous membrane would call for **Rhus**—preferably, I think, in the "Venenata" variety.

Thus, in substance, I wrote in my "Therapeutics" of 1877. In January, 1898, Dr. Bliem, of San Antonio, Texas, gives an account of a severe Epidemic. "The remedies," he writes, "narrowed themselves down to *Gelsemium, Bryonia* and *Eupatorium*, with now and then a call for *Belladonna*. Nothing seemed to beat down the temperature until it had run its course." I would venture to suggest that this was for lack of *Aconite* in the first paroxysm.

Sir Joseph Fayrer, in Quain's Dictionary, commends *Belladonna* as often conferring great relief.

The other exanthematous affection altogether omitted in the Nomenclature of the College of Physicians is—

MILIARIA.—This seems to be the modern representative of the mediæval "Sweating Sickness," and, according to Zuelzer (whose Article on the disease in Ziemssen's 'Cyclopædia' is very full and instructive), has not unfrequently, even in later times, manifested the malignant character of that terrible scourge. Dr. Aitken has described it from his personal observation among the Turks at Scutari during the Crimean war. He characterizes it as "a disease in which there is an eruption of innumerable minute pimples, with white summits, occurring in successive crops upon the skin of the trunk and extremities, preceded and accompanied with fever, anxieties, oppression of respiration, and copious sweats of a rank, sour, fœtid odour peculiar to the disease." Zuelzer lays greater stress upon the anxieties and oppression here noted. "In many cases," he says, ',the patients experience, together with a violent and tumultuous palpitation and abdominal pulsation, a feeling of constriction in the chest and epigastrium (BARRE EPIGASTRIQUE), and præcordial pain. The symptoms increase not unfrequently to a frightful degree, although neither in the heart nor in the lungs is any Anatomical lesion to be "discovered". They disappear, suddenly or gradually, after the outbreak of the eruption.

There is everything in this picture to encourage us to use **Aconite** as the fundamental remedy for Miliaria also and to expect the best results from its use. But if ever **Cactus** is to replace it when fever is present, it is when the above-mentioned oppression and anxietas, with præcordial Pain, are a marked feature of the case. The sense of constriction experienced is generally recognised as characteristic of this drug.* I think. moreover, that when the sweating is very profuse, we might give the patient the benefit of the exquisitely Homœopathic **Jaborandi**. Lastly, the 30th of the poisonings by **Arsenic** contained in the "Cylopædia of drug Pathogenesy" bears so striking a resemblance to Miliary fever, that the drug ought to find a leading place among its remedies.

We come now to the various forms of CONTINUED FEVER. But as these constitute too large a subject to be taken up at the fag end of a lecture, I will defer their consideration till our next meeting.

---

* See, for instance, B. J. H. xxxiv., 690.

LECTURE XVIII.

GENERAL DISEASES.
—o—
THE CONTINUED FEVERS.
—o—
TYPHUS—TYPHOID FEVER.

I begin (as I promised) to take up in this Lecture the Therapeutics of the CONTINUED FEVERS. I will discuss TYPHUS and TYPHOID on the present occasion, reserving the less important varieties for another lecture.

First, then, we will take the Jail, Hospital, and Camp Fever of old, the Petechial or Exanthematous TYPHUS of German Nomenclature, which we now in this country call simply—

TYPHUS.—Of this disease I cannot speak from personal experince. It has never appeared, I believe, in Brighton. Nor have those of our practitioners who inhabit the great towns which it chiefly visits given us their experience in its treatment. The only exception is Dr. Russell (in this, as in so many ways, much lamented), whose Volume of "Clinical Lectures" contains two on Fever, giving an account of thirty cases treated at the London Homœopathic Hospital in 1864, nearly all of which were true Typhus. Bahr, Trinks,* Wurmb and Caspar † have discussed our Typhous medicines with much fulness; but as they unfortunately blend Typhus and Typhoid together, it is sometimes difficult to utilise their recommendations in the fevers of this country. I propose to give here the best account I can, of the treatment of the two disorders, as we are accustomed to see them; and then to present the indications for remedies in Typhoid conditions as such, according to the views of our Therapeutists.

1. If, placed in the midst of an Epidemic of Typhus, you have an opportunity of seeing a case within the first few days, I would strongly advise you to try what **Baptisia** will do. The statements I have had to make about it in Variola and Scarlatina, and shall make relative to its action in Common Continued Fever and in Typhoid, seem to warrant its more extended application to similar conditions; and the first week of Typhus is one of these.

---

* "On Typhus abdominalis," B. J. H., xxix., 286.
† "Clinical Studies," IBID., xii.

2. Supposing that *Baptisia* is not telling, or that you begin the treatment at a more advanced stage, what are you to do? You will have one of the three conditions present, which will call for suitable treatment accordingly.

(*a*) If the Headache is a marked symptom; if it does not subside when (at about the eighth day) Delirium supervenes ; if signs of cerebral congestion are present—**Belladonna** is a remedy of obvious Homœopathicity and tried power. **Hyoscyamus** may occasionally take its place when the cerebral symptoms are more adynamic, as when Wine relieves the Headache (Typhomania) or **Stramonium** when the Derilium (d. ferox) is so excessive as to threaten the patient's exhaustion. **Opium** supplements either if torpor has supervened. This is the "Cerebral Typhus" of the old writers ; and the medicines I have named give us great power over it.

Drs. Drysdale and Simmons have recorded some experience leading us to think that **Agaricus** may occasionally play an important part in this form of Typhus. It is when general Ataxia is present—as shown by great restlessness, twitching, and tremor—that they find it so beneficial.*

(*b*) In a second class of cases the symptoms are those of great nervous depression with but slight febrile excitement or signs of blood-poisoning. Here you will give **Phosphoric acid**, which Wurmb, Bahr, Jousset and Trinks unite with observers of the old school in commending. A lower grade of this nervous prostration calls for the still more potent **Phosphorus**, which may save life at the utmost extremity.

(*c*) Thirdly, the phenomena of ferbile Toxæmia may predominate from the first. **Muriatic acid, Rhus** and **Arsenicum** correspond to this condition in the direct order of intensity.

I think that these are the leading forms of Typhus which you are likely to have to treat. If exceptional varieties occur, run down the list of medicines whose indications I shall summarise presently. But a word first upon local complications. The Pulmonary affections of Typhus call for **Phosphorus**, which would also oppose the Typhous softening of the heart, this being an acute Fatty Degeneration. This medicine has the same relation to the other parenchymatous degenerations which occur in both Typhus and Typhoid, and constitute so much of the danger and destruction they involve.† Convulsions occurring in the course of Typhus are, I suppose, invariably uræmic, and require the treatment of that affection. If the blood can be relieved

---

* See also another testimony to the same thing in B.J.H., xxxiii., 569.

† "These changes are not specifically different from the degenerations which occur in consequence of many poisonings, AS WITH *Phosphorus*, &c." Liebermeister, in Zimssen's CYCLOPÆDIA).

of its perilous stuff," it will probably be wise to direct your medicinal treatment to the kidneys, after the manner I shall indicate when discussing renal disease. I may just say here that the *Arsenic* I have already indicated as one of the chief remedies for the Typhoid condition will generally be your medicine for the kidney mischief. A no less serious phenomenon is inflammatory swelling of the salivary glands and the areolar tissue about the neck. Dr. Russel had two instances of this in the Hospital. One died, *Belladonna* having been given in vain; in the other the swelling was immediately checked by the first trituration of the *Biniodide of Mercury.*

Whether we can hasten the defervescence of Typhus is a question which further and more precise observation must determine. But we have every reason to believe that, under good general management, our remedies do much to favour the patient's recovery. Of the thirty cases treated in the London Homœopathic Hospital in 1864, two only died, one from the Glandular Swellings just mentioned, and one from Convulsions. No uncomplicated case was lost. Dr. Murchison, making a very moderate estimate, reckons the average mortality of Typhus to be ten per cent. This is a satisfactory result.

In a later outbreak of Typhus in London, out of 17 cases reported, 9 were treated at our Hospital, 8 elsewhere. Of the latter, 2 died; of the former none. The medicines used were those mentioned above.*

I pass now to TYPHOID, or—as our Nomenclature better calls it—

ENTERIC FEVER.—This is the "Abdominal Typhus" of German writers, the "Dothien Enterite" of Bretonneau and Trousseau, the "Fievre Typhoid" of Louis and of our own French writers. It is defined as "Continued Fever, characterized by the presence of rose-coloured spots, chiefly on the abdomen, and a tendency to Diarrhœa, with specific lesion of the bowels." I wish to limit it by this definition. Of course it will occur with Typhoid as with other specific diseases, that mild or abortive cases are seen which fall short of its distinctive characters. But if these occur in the course of an epidemic of the true disorder, or are in any way traceable to its infection, they are instances of Enteric Fever, and of nothing else. On the other hand, if we have sporadic cases or even epidemics of a Continued Fever, which—

---

*See L. H. H. R., ii., 91

being neither Typhus nor Relapsing—does not conform to the Enteric Type, does not exhibit its well-established features, that fever must not be reckoned as Typhoid in our estimate of the efficacy of treatment.

I make these remarks with reference to the value of **Baptisia** in our present disease. My former colleague in practice, the elder Dr. Madden, taught me to rely upon *Bryonia*, followed, if necessary, by *Rhus* and *Arsenicum*, in the Continued Fever we were in the habit of meeting with in Brighton. In 1862, we were led to test the newly introduced *Baptisia tinctoria* in this disease; and he the veteran, not less than I the novice, was much impressed with the power it displayed. Unlike the remedies previously named, it seemed not to control or mitigate only, but actually to break up the disease. Since that time I have used the drug as my primary and fundamental remedy for every case of the kind which has come under my care, and have frequently expressed my entire satisfaction with its efficacy : I have lost but one patient, and advanced age had in that case much to do with the fatal result.

I have always assumed that this Continued Fever was Typhoid—diarrhœa, abdominal tenderness and distension and dry brown tongue, used often to follow the previous "Gastric" stage when we treated it with the ordinary remedies, and to appear in neglected cases. I had not learnt from my teachers to recognise any endemic fever but Febricula and Typhoid ; and as the malady I saw was certainly not the one, I concluded it to be the other. I could not therefore but believe that *Baptisia* exerted an abortive as well as a controlling power over Enteric Fever, and I expressed myself accordingly. I was not shaken by the negative results obtained by Dr. Yeldham and Dr. Edward Blake.* or by the occasional occurrence in my own practice of cases which escaped from the influence of the drug and ran a protracted course. When I read at our York Congress in 1872, a Paper "On the Place and Value of *Baptisia* in Typhoid Fever," embodying the above view, † my belief was confirmed by the testimony of good men and true from many parts of England, and I was naturally strengthened in it.

Subsequent observation, however, has forced upon me the conviction that there is a "Common Continued Fever" which does not own the Typhoid poison for its cause, and has not the distinctive characters of the fever induced by that miasm, Examining, in the light of this thought, the evidence in favour of *Baptisia* adduced and elicited at the Congress, and also my own experience and those recently recorded by others with the drug, I have been unable to resist the conclusion that the fever which *Baptisia* aborts is not true Typhoid. When the real disease appears, either

---

* B. J. H., xxx., 746.   † See M. H. R., xvi., 658.

sporadically or epidemically, it runs its typical course in spite of this or any other medicine. As regards abortive power I must relinquish the claims I have hither-to made for the remedy : I must acknowledge the correctness of Dr. Kidd's and Jousset's objection, that the fever I had broken up with *Baptisia* was not Typhoid but Gastric.

But is *Baptisia,* therefore, to be abandoned as a remedy for Enteric Fever ? By no means. The facts of its pathogenesis which I have alleged when lecturing on the drug show it to be a true Homœopathic remedy for the first stage of Tiphoid, before the full development of the intestinal mischief ; and the favourable testimony of many, who have no doubt that they are speaking of the genuine disease, * proves that at all stages of its progress the medicine may be useful. It may be still more valuable, perhaps, in cases where special "characteristics" of the drug are present, as that noted by Dr. James Bell—"The patient cannot go to sleep, because she cannot get herself together ; her head feels as though scattered about, and she tosses about the bed to get the pieces together." The soreness on lying displayed in the pathogenesis of the drug is another of such indications. Dr. Charge adds "softness of the pulse in the first stage and fœtidity later on", Jahr † gives "despair of cure and certainty of death". Again, Mr. Harmer Smith notes (and my own experience is the same) its "tranquillising effect upon the brain", and Dr. Bayes its detergent power upon the alimentary mucous membrane, enabling the fevered stomach to receive, to retain, and to digest food" ‡

We have thus in *Baptisia*—in many, if not in all circumstances —a most useful medicine in the treatment of Typhoid Fever. Its administration in the early stage is additionally expedient, in that (unless you are in the midst of an Epidemic) you can hardly tell at that time whether it is Enteric or Common Continued Fever with which you have to do. But throughout the progress of the malady I advise you to give it as the best means of keeping

---

* See M. H. R., xvi., 632.3. In Vol. xxvi., at p. 203. Dr. Dyce Brown relates three cases of unmistakable Typhoid, in which, under *Baptisia,* the temperature became normal between the 8th and 13th day. In two, a relapse, readily accounted for, occured, and then the fever ran its course ; but in the third there was no subsequent elevation of temperature.

/ See REVUE HOMŒOPATHIQUE BELGE, ii., 8.

‡ Dr. Nimier writes in L' ART MEDICAL of January, 1898, that in the last epidemic he had seen he treated 13 cases, some of them grave, mainly with *Baptisia;* and all recovered. Surgeon-Major Deane, moreover, in his account of 47 cases treated by him in India, writes, "I have had no experience of the abortive effect of *Baptisia*, though I have thought at times it had such a tendency, but the cases have progressed more comfortably under that drug than under any treatment I have seen" (J. B. H. S., vii., 364).

down the high temperature in which so much of the peril consists, and only to supplement or supplant it when certain special manifestations of Typhoid poisoning become prominent. Some of these are common to it with the Typhous, as the cerebral and pulmonary symptoms, the nervous prostration, and the Toxæmia; and require the same treatment. The special feature of Typhoid, however, is the morbid process which goes on in the intestinal glands; and it is to these that our special remedies will most often have to be directed.

Under ordinary circumstances, all that is required to promote the resolution or other termination of the "Dothien-Enterite" is the moderation of the fever with **Muriatic acid** or **Arsenicum** to to subdue the intestinal hyperæmia and consequent diarhœa. This they will do, however severe the symptoms may be. But when the Typhoid deposit in Peyer's patches is giving trouble in its elimination—when active ulceration is showing itself by re-accession of the febrile phenomena, with abdominal pains and tenderness and glazed tongue, or when sloughing of the diseased patches is involving hæmorrhage, more direct remedies seem to be required. I cannot think *Arsenic* perfectly Homœopathic to these conditions, though intestinal lesions like those of Typhoid have not unfrequently been found after death from *Arsenical* poisoning. But in the idiopathic disease Peyer's patches and the solitary glands are affected in concert, with the other parts of the blood-making system—the mesenteric glands and the spleen; and not merely irritated in sympathy with the intestinal surface. The two medicines I think most of here are **Mercurius** and **Iodium**. In favour of the former is its general glandular action and control over ulceration, and the experience of Drs. Petroz and von Tunzelmann with the black *Sulphide*, to which I have referred in my 'Pharmacodynamics.' Dr. Jousset also places *Mercurius* among the principal remedies for the second period of Typhoid, and says that it is indicated by the predominance of the abdominal affection. *Iodine* has yet stronger Physiological evidence in its favour. In a case of slow poisoning of an animal, conducted by Dr. Cogswell, the following appearances were presented POST MORTEM: "The lining membrane of the intestines, for about three feet from their origin was remarkably vascular, oval spots, about the size of a chestnut, then began to occur at every three inches, ON THE SIDE OPPOSITE THE MESENTERY; a similar spot at the junction with the colon was two or three inches in length and was expanded at its lower termination over the whole circuit of the gut. These spots were not injected, and were composed of little aggregated eminences with black points in the centre, separated from one another by white cellular bands. THEY APPEARED TO CONSIST OF THE AGMINATED GLANDS ENLARGED, AS SOMETIMES NOTICED IN THE EARLY PROGRESS OF FEVER." To this must be added its undoubted action upon the mesenteric glands. It is remarkable that

Liebermeister, in his Essay on Typhoid Fever contributed to Ziemssen's Cyclopædia, records his experience on a large scale, showing that the administration of *Iodine* or *Calomel* (especially the latter) notably reduces the duration and mortality of the disease.— Should hæmorrhage from the bowels take place, **Terebinthina** has as much repute amongst us as in the ordinary practice.*

If Peritonitis should occur WITHOUT PERFORATION, its ordinary remedies—especially *Mercurius corrosivus*—would probably suffice. But if that serious accident be its cause, it is probable that our patient's only safety lies in paralyzing his intestines with full doses of *Opium*, according to the usual method.

I must now, as I promised, give you the experience of our therapeutists generally in the treatment of what they call "Typhus," which includes both the fever properly so named, and Typhoid. In citing Dr. Jousset, however, you must understand that it is the latter fever only which he had in view. I must also say something of the classification of fevers generally accepted in the times of our earlier writers, as contrasted with that of the present day. It was that which I have placed on the board behind me, thus:

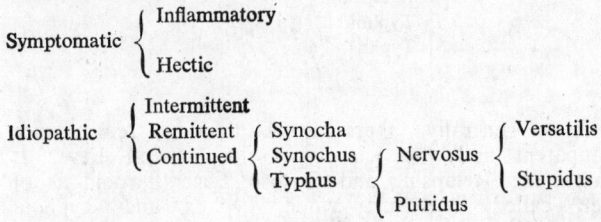

"Symptomatic" fever was that obviously depending on some local inflammation; and, if Continuous, was known simply as "Inflammatory," while, if it occured in a succession of daily paroxysms, it was called "Hectic." "Idiopathic" fevers were those apparently of primary origin; and these too were divided according as their phenomena were Intermittent, Remittent, or Continued. Continued fevers were further subdivided on the basis of the character of their symptoms. If these were of the simple and sthenic kind familiar in Inflammatory Fever, the term Synocha was used to designate the patient's illness. If of a somewhat lower type, "Synochus" was substituted as their designation, leaving "Typhus" for the well-known "Low Fever," and adding "Nervosus" or "Putridus" as the stress of the disease seemed to fall on the nervous centres or on the blood. The "Versatilis" and "Stupidus" further qualifying the Typhus Nervosus need no explanation.

---

* Dr. Searle records a case in which this symptom was checked by *Nitric acid*, while an early gangrene of mouth and labia also complicating it yielded to *Crotalus* (Hahn. Monthly, March, 1896).

Such a classification is obviously unsuited for Nosology, when once the essential nature of certain fevers and their dependence upon definite miasms or contagions is recognised. The distinction of Symptomatic and Idiopathic Pyrexia still indeed holds good, and Pyæmia and Septicæmia find appropriate place as varieties of Hectic. But Intermittent and Remittents are now classed together as Malarious, while Continued Fevers are recognised as occurring under the four forms of Ephemera or febricula, Relapsing Fever, Typhus and Typhoid, to which some, like myself, would add a "Common Continued Fever"—the FIEVERE SYNOQUE of the French, the "Gastric Fever" of popular English speech. Thus we get a second schema :

Symptomatic { Inflammatory / Hectic / Pyæmic / Septicæmic

Idiopathic { Malarious / Continued { Ephemera / Gastric / Relapsing / Typhoid / Typhus

Now, speaking generally, there is a tolerable coincidence between the apparent and the real types. Ephemeral Fever is Synochal in character; Relapsing and Gastric Fevers would as of old have been called Synochus; while Typhus and Typhoid commonly present the character of the Typhus Putridus and Nervosus respectively. But while this is so, we must not let the ancient distinctions be swallowed up in the modern, as though wholly obsolete. While the latter are all-important for prognosis of the course and probable termination of fevers, and for their general management, the former stillo hold good for Therapeutic purposes. They are Symptomatic, and therefore lend themselves with great appopriateness to a method of drug-selection like ours which uses symptoms as its materials. They also enable us, when studying anti-pyertics, to embrace such fevers as the Catarrhal and Rheumatic, and that accompanying the contagious exanthemata, which, though not finding place in the usual classifications, are not less genuine clinical facts. The same may be said of those recognised varieties of the Continued Fevers which are now referred to the "Typhoid" or "Gastric" category. Trousseau gives them as "Mucous," "Bilious," "Inflammatory," "Adynamic," "Putrid," "Ataxic" and "Malignant." Our own Trinks, to whom as I have said we owe a valuable study of "Abdominal Typhus" (i.e., Typhoid) in its drug-relations, describes it as occurring under the forms "Simplex," "Biliosus," "Pituitosus," "Putridus,"

"Nervosus Versatilis" and Nervosus Stupidus." While the essential fever thus manifesting itself may be one and indivisible, the various forms under which it appears are no less realities, and require a suitable adjustment of our drug-remedies, as they do of those of a more general kind.

This, then, being premised, let us see what are the medicines which our writers commend to our confidence in dealing with the Continued Fevers.

Fleischmann, who was fond of single remedies, treated all his fever cases* with *Arsenicum* alone and with fair success. Wurmb and Caspar gave *Phosphoric acid* or *Carbo vegetabilis*, according to the intensity of the symptoms, in the torpid form; and *Rhus* or *Arsenicum*, correspondingly proportioned, when the condition was more erethistic. Bahr considers that "the real Typhus-remedies corresponding with the whole course of the disease are *Bryonia, Rhus, Arsenicum, Phosphorus, Acidum Phosphoricum* and *Muriaticum.*" Jahr gives the same list of "essential Anti-typhous remedies," omitting *Muriatic acid.* Trinks has more or less to say in favour of *Phosphoric* and *Muriatic acids, Belladonnas, Bryonia, Phosphorus, Stramonium, Rhus,* and *Arsenicum.* Russel places *Belladonna, Bryonia, Rhus* and *Arsenicum* in the forefront of his remedies; and Jousset *Muriatic* and *Phosphoric acids, Arsenicum* and *Belladonna.*

So general an agreement is visible here that we cannot but rely with confidence upon the indications given for the several medicines.

Bryonia takes the place I have assigned to *Baptisia*, even abortive power being claimed for it by Trinks. It is the remedy throughout in ordinary cases of moderately severe character (Bahr); in the erethistic stage, before the vitality is greatly lowered (Trinks, Jahr and Goodno); and in Rheumatic and (mild) Bronchitic complications (Trinks). The hyper-oxidation which constitutes its fever consumes the more lowly-organized tissues—the fibrous, serous and muscular; the blood and nervous systems are less involved. That such fever is primary and essential appears from Dr. Jousset's experiments on animals, recorded in L'ART MEDICAL for June, 1896.

Rhus is said to be indicated by a more intense character of the disease, "by excessive reactive endeavours with insufficiency of reactive power, and a great irritability of the nervous system" (Bahr, Wurmb and Caspar). The first supervention of Diarrhœa upon Constipation, of a red upon a coated tongue, calls for it in Gastric Fevers; and in true Typhoid may often indicate it from the first (Jahr, Trinks, Bayes).† A red triangle at the tip

---

* See the Report of his hospital in B. J. H., Vols. iii,-v.
† M. H. R., xvi., 727.

of the tongue is said to be "characteristic" for it here. Trinks commends it in "Cerebral Typhus," with stupor and sopor.

Arsenicum succeeds or replaces *Rhus* when the adynamic erethism which indicates that drug is too severe for it. This is the place assigned to it by all observers, and their testimony to its value is warm. Trinks also commends it when sub-cutaneous and intestinal hæmorrhages occur in Typhus Putridus. The seat of the increased heat production of its fever is the blood. It is, above everything, TOXÆMIA which indicates it here. In proportion as

" . . . the life of all the blood
Is touched corruptibly."

is its control exerted.

Belladonna is rather slighted by Bahr and by Wurmb and Caspar; but Trinks, Jahr, Russell and Hempel praise it highly in the active stages of "Cerebral Typhus." Its fever, indeed, is due to hyper-oxidation of the nervous centres, and in proportion as they are involved is it indicated. Trinks also commends it in severe EARLY BRONCHITIS complicating the fevers, especially in children. This latter use of it Bahr also allows.

Acidum Phosphoricum is unanimously allowed to be the main remedy in lentescent forms of Typhus (the "Mucous" variety of Trousseau). Jousset thinks it an Anti-typhoid of great importance.

Acidum Muriaticum supersedes it in this form if "Putrid" symptoms show themselves ((Bahr). The patient is so weak that he "settles down in the bed in a heap" (Jahr). Trinks thinks it rather applicable to erethistic conditions, too severe for *Bryonia*, too sthenic for *Rhus*, and not cerebral enough for *Belladonna*.

Phosphorus is to *Phosphoric acid* what *Arsenicum* is to *Rhus*; it supplements it in severer cases or stages (Trinks). Wurmb and Caspar give this place to *Carbo vegetabilis*. *Phosphorus* is also the grand remedy in "Pneumo-Typhus" (Bahr).

The minor remedies must be dismissed more briefly. **Aconite** is not generally allowed a place among Typhous medicines; but Trinks, Jousset and Kafka think it useful in the first three or four days of the fever. *Calcarea* is said by Goullon and Jahr to be intercurrently useful in "Exanthematic Typhus" when the rash does not come out properly. **Camphor** is said by Trinks to rally the patient from threatened sinking when coldness is present, **Moschus** being preferable if heat predominates. **Hellebore** has proved curative, in the hands of the same physician in fully-developed "Typhus Nervosus Studpidus;" and **Kreasote** for profuse passive hæmorrhages. **Laurocerasus** is recommended by him when clonic convulsions of the limbs occur; and **Mercurius** to dissect out a "bilious" condition when present. **Tartar emetic** counteracts its special bronchial disorder in Typhus as elsewhere (Trinks and Russell). **Stramonium** is invaluable in the higher degrees of Delirium (Trinks and Jahr); and **Valerian** has succeeded where even this has failed.* Goodno gives an alternative in the *Hyoscine hydrobromate,* of the 3x trituration of which he gives grain doses every hour.†

As regards the dose of these medicines, the names of the observers will suggest whether the higher or lower dilutions were given. The agreement, however, of practioners like Jhar (who always gave 30ths) and Wurmb and Caspar (at the time using only the 15th) with the rest as to the value of the leading remedies indicates that dose is of less consequence here than selection. As to *Baptisia,* it is given by all its advocates in the mother or the 1st decimal tincture.

The only remaining question is the comparative success of Homœopathic treatment in Typhoid. Liebermeister states that in the hospital at Basle the mortality under ordinary treatment —indifferent, expectant, or symptomatic—was twenty-seven per cent., but that by systematic Antipyretic treatment, principally consisting of Cold Baths, it has been reduced to eight per cent. We have already seen, from hospital experience at Paris and Melbourne, that we can do even a shade better than this; and that our Statistics are decidedly more favourable than those furnished before cold water was pressed into service shews that our remedies have at least as potent an influence.

---

* See a case in the PHILADELPHIA JOURNAL OF HOMŒOPATHY ii., 715.
† See also J. B. H. S., vi., 400.

LECTURE XIX.

GENERAL DISEASES.

THE CONTINUED FEVERS (*concluded*)—THE MALARIAL FEVERS.

FEBRICULA—SIMPLE CONTINUED FEVER—RELAPSING FEVER—YEL. LOW FEVER—CEREBRO-SPINAL FEVER—MEDITERANNEAN FEVER PLAGUE-AGUE-REMITTENT FEVER—BILIOUS REMITTENT.

Having now, in Typhus and Typhoid, discussed the two great types of Continued Fever, I turn to its lesser varieties. The first of these is EPHEMERA, or—

FEBRICULA.—This, though an essential fever is "Simple" in every sense of the word. There is no known morbid poison present as its cause, and no blood-tainting as an effect. I agree with Russell and Jousset that we want one medicine only for this malady, and that is Aconite. I believe that it both mitigates the severity and shortens the course of the fever, so as to make it (if taken at once) EPHEMERAL in the strictest sense of the word.

This is no trifling advantage, even in Febricula as we have it in our temperate regions. But still more important does it become to be able to control the malady when we encounter it as the "Ardent Continued Fever" of India. Here even life is threatened, and the heroic antiphlogistic apparatus of forty years ago is still in vogue. I think that Drs. Sircar and Salzer, and others who have practised Homœopathically in our Eastern Empire, could tell us in their hands *Aconite* supersedes lancet, leeches, ET HOC OMNE GENUS, and ensures a successful and speedy termination to every case.

Besides Febricula, the Nomenclature we are employing used to give another, "Simple Continued Fever" (so styling it), which it defined as "Continued Fever having no specific character"— separating it by this word "Continued" from the equally non-specific Febricula, which has a duration of only three or four days. It now identifies the two, thus adding, as I venture to think, to the confusion; and Quain's Dictionary denies the specificity of Febricula and Common Continued Fever alike. Whether such a distinct type of fever, excluding Febricula, exists is still a moot question; and it has considerable importance (as I have said) in its bearing on the claims which I and others have set up *Baptisia*, as having an abortive power over true Typhoid. If there be another Continued Fever resembling the Enteric, but not originating from its specific cause, having, therefore, no fixed type and definite duration, it may be that it is here that *Baptisia* has won its laurels, and that the power of remedies to abort real Typhoid is still unproved.

Now when at the British Homœopathic Congress of 1872, I read the Paper I have mentioned, I was disposed to maintain the negative of this question. I found no evidence on record sufficient to outweigh the opinion of Jenner, of Watson and of Trousseau, that the "Gastric Fever" of common parlance was the "Typhoid" of modern nosology. But the possibility of the opposite alternative having been since made vividly present to my mind, I have scrutinized my own experience and that put forward by others during the succeeding years, with special reference to the question, and have found myself reluctantly driven to the opposite conclusion regarding it.

I must, therefore, speak here of—

SIMPLE CONTINUED FEVER as distinct from Typhoid on the one hand and from Febricula on the other. Bahr also differentiates such a fever as Gastric, Bilious or Mucous, according to its phenomena; and Jousset does the same, calling it "Fever Synoque." The former corroborates my own observation in stating that in Protracted cases the tongue gets brown and dry, the abdomen swells, and Diarrhœa replaces the previous Constipation. This is what English writers mean when they speak of "Gastric Fever running into Typhoid."

It is in this Fever that (according to my present belief) **Baptisia** has shown itself such a true specific. Defervescence and crisis will follow its use in a very short time, far shorter than that which would obtain in the natural course of the disease; the tongue will rapidly clean, and capacity for taking and digesting food return. "Gastric fever" will never, I believe, "run into Typhoid" when treated early with the medicine. If, however, you first meet with the case when the Typhoid symptoms have set in, the suitable remedy will nearly always be **Arsenicum**.

You will find in Bahr and Jousset* indications for several other medicines in this Fever. I cannot advise you however, to

---

* Also in some "Observations on the Treatment of Fevers," by Dr. Anderson, in the M. H. R., viii., 331.

substitute them for the two mentioned above. None of them lay hold of the essence of the disease in the way these do. Some of them may occasionally find a place in alternation with *Baptisia* when the indications for them are very strong; but my own impression is that the latter works just as well without them.

RELAPSING FEVER, which needs no definition on my part. We have a special interest in it, as Medicine owes its differentiation to our own Henderson. Of its Homœopathic treatment we have three special sources of information. The first is an account given by Hahnemann himself of the fever he treated in Leipzig in 1814, which I must agree with Dr. Russel in considering to be of this variety. His main remedies were *Bryonia* and *Rhus*, each in the twelfth dilution; one or the other being given according as the pains were relieved by rest or by motion. He treated 183 cases without a single death, while the mortality under the ordinary heroic treatment was considerable.* The second is Dr. Kidd's experience of the Fever which desolated Ireland in the year 1847.† He treated at Bantry 111 cases, of which he considers 24 to have been instances of Typhus, and 87 of Relapsing Fever. He lost two cases only, which were presumably among the sufferers from Typhus; so that his mortality also was NIL. His chief remedy was *Bryonia*; and, taking up the subject again in 1865, he is satisfied that no medicine can be recommended with so much confidence. Our third authority is Dr. Dyce Brown, who treated 50 cases in an Epidemic occuring in Aberdeen in 1871.‡ He gave nearly all his patients *Baptisia* 1; and found it, by comparison with the natural history of the disease, materially to expedite the crisis. He also lost no case.

It appears, therefore, that Relapsing Fever need never prove fatal under Homœopathic treatment; and that **Bryonia, Rhus** and **Baptisia** (the last being preferred when gastric symptoms predominate) are its chief remedies. I should have thought, from the height and synochal character of the fever, that *Aconite* would have been serviceable; but Dr. Brown says that it was not of the slightest use. I do not think that we can prevent the relapse by Homœopathic remedies;* but we ought to relieve the pains which are such a characteristic feature of this Fever. *Bryonia* or *Rhus*, given according to Hahnemann's indication, and after his manner—*i.e.*, a single dose of the 12th dilution in

---

* See Russell's Lectures, p. 369.
† See B. J. H., vi., 85; and ANNALS, iv., 136.
‡ See B. J. H., xxxi., 355.

the morning, without repetition—may do this; but if not, I should suggest the trial of **Eupatorium perfoliatum**, as in the very similar pains of Dengue and (as we shall see) of Influenza.

We have now finished the British types of fever; but there are four closely allied, though specially 'distinct varieties which are encountered in other countries. These are YELLOW FEVER, CEREBRO-SPINAL FEVER, MEDITERRANEAN FEVER and PLAGUE.

Of the first,—

YELLOW FEVER, we have good deal of experience on record from those who practise Homœopathy in the Southern States of the American Union. In the Third Volume of the NORTH AMERICAN JOURNAL OF HOMŒOPATHY, Dr. Holcombe gave us an account of an Epidemic in which he and an associate treated 1,016 cases. The treatment was general and symptomatic. *Camphor* was given when the primary chill was so severe as to remind the observer of the Choleraic collapse (this is the "algid form" of Dr. Lyons). *Aconite* and *Belladonna* were used to control the reaction; after which *Ipecacuanha* and *Bryonia* were generally required by the gastric symptoms. If the case ran on into the Typhus condition, *Arsenicum* and *Lachesis* were given; and if "black vomit" supervened *Argentum nitricum*. Sometimes *Cantharis* was called for by the condition of the urinary organs, which it speedily modified for the better. Under such treatment they lost only 55 patients—the mortality being thus 5.4: per cent., instead of, as usual from 15 to 25 per cent.

In 1867, Dr. Holcombe had to encounter another epidemic of Yellow Fever, and reported his results to the American Institute of Homœopathy, in whose transactions for 1868 you may read his story. He treated 300 cases with only seven deaths; but the general mortality was also less than usual. Dr. Holcombe had by this time come to the conclusion that the *Serpent poisons* were the most truly Homœopathic remedies for Yellow Fever that we possessed; and he gave them accordingly—in the thirtieth attenuation — in every case. He considered "*Lachesis* especially adapted to the nervous, and *Crotalus* to the vascular elements of the disease—*Lachesis* to the nerve poisoning, *Crotalus* to the blood poisoning"; and accordingly gave *Lachesis* in the

---

* Dr. Brown (as I have said) found the *Hyposulphite of Soda*, in five-grain doses, effective for this purpose.

first stage, and *Crotalus* in the second—that of exhaustion, hæmorrhage and Jaundice. With these he often alternated his old remedies as they were symptomatically indicated. He strongly recommends *Argentum nitricum* for the vomiting of the second stage, but seems to prefer *Arsenicum* when it is sanguineous—*i.e.*, when "black vomit" is present or approaching.*

We have also accounts of epidemics from Dr. Neidhard of Philadelphia,† and Dr. Morse of Memphis. ‡ The former was able to rely almost exclusively upon *Crotalus*. The latter treated his cases symptomatically; but he and his colleagues lost only 12 per cent., while the mortality under old-school treatment was 40 per cent. at least.

These results show that, should you ever encounter Yellow Fever, you may rely with the utmost confidence upon Homœopathic remedies. The facts I have brought forward when speaking of the *Serpent poisons* show how entirely I agree with Drs. Holcombe and Neidhard as to **Lachesis** and **Crotalus** being the true Pathological SIMILIA to this terrible disease. The only candidate for equal honour is **Phosphorus**. The resemblance of poisoning by this substance, with its Jaundice and hæmorrhages, to Yellow Fever is obvious. The only question is whether it affects the blood through the liver, or primarily. It the former be the true account of the matter, I must agree with Dr. Holcombe that the drug is not really Homœopathic to the disease; as in the latter the blood is directly affected, and the Jaundice itself is hæmatic rather than hepatic. But if Hænisch's statements § are correct (they differ somewhat from Frerichs') the condition of liver and kidneys found after death from Yellow Fever show precisely that acute fatty degeneration which *Phosphorus* sets up. *Phosphorus* is said to have proved of much value in the disease during an epidemic occurring at Rio de Janerio. ¶

The next of these Continued Fevers I shall mention is the epidemic Cerebro-Spinal Meningitis, which in the new Nomenclature is styled—

---

* This experience with *Arsenic*, and its general effectiveness in Yellow-Fever, both as prophylactic and curative, has been attested by old-school physicians (J. B. H. S., vii. 324; viii. 76).
† "On *Crotalus horridus* in Yellow Fever," 1868.
‡ N. A. J. H., xxii, 425.
§ Ziemssen's Cyclopædia, Vol. i.
§ B. J. H., xxiii., 130.

CEREBRO-SPINAL FEVER.—In a Paper in the Twenty-Third Volume of the BRITISH JOURNAL OF HOMOEOPATHY I have gathered together all that was then known of the Homœopathic treatment of this malady. You will see that it has always had large comparative success. Thus, in an epidemic occurring at Avignon in 1846-47, Dr. Bechet lost only 22 per cent. as contrasted with a 72 per cent. mortality in the military hospitals. His fundamental remedy was a curious one, *Ipecacuanha*. It was given in the mother tincture, and nearly always alternated with some remedy demanded by special symptoms, of which *Hyoscyamus* was the most frequently used.

Our principal experience, however, in the treatment of Cerebro-Spinal Fever has been obtained in America. The disease there presents itself under two forms. The first is inflammatory and sthenic, and here *Aconite*, *Verarum viride* or *Gelsemium*, with *Belladonna*, have been the remedies. The second and far more common, is of a Typhoid type; and is characterised by petechiæ, so as to give it the name of "Spotted Fever."* Here the Typhous medicines, *Bryonia*, *Rhus* and *Arsenicum*, have been brought into play; and the prostration combated by deodorised absolute *Alcohol*. Where the spasms have continued after the acute symptoms have subsided, Dr. Searle and others have found *Actæa racemosa* very useful.

I think one cannot help feeling that, with the exception of **Aconite** in the frankly inflammatory cases, we have not yet come upon the true Pathological SIMILE of Cerebro-. Spinal Meningitis But I hope that it has been found in **Cicuta**. Dr. Barker of Batavia, has communicated to the New York State Homœopathic Society † a series of sixty consecutive cases of the disease, of all degrees of severity, treated by this medicine alone without a single death. The phenomena of poisoning by *Cicuta* are very Homœopathic to those of the malady, even to the petechiæ and autopsies of animals killed by it show much hyperæmia of the cerebro-spinal meninges. As regards *Aconite*, besides the obvious indications for it (and I may say that the pulse is always, if altered at all, full and tense), we have the recent observations of Harley, who concludes that *Aconite* affects the cranio-spinal axis from the centres of the third nerves to the origin of the phrenics just as *Strychnia* does the whole. ‡ It is in this region that the symptoms of Cerebro-Spinal Meningitis show themselves most severely.

---

* The same symptoms characterised it on a recent appearance in Great Britain; and the name first proposed for it here was "Malignant Purpuric Fever."
† See its Transactions for 1872, p. 60.
‡ DUBLIN JOURNAL OF MEDICAL SCIENCE, No. 45.

I should not forget the *Serpent poisons,* especially *Crotalus* where the petechial phenomena were very prominent. I may also mention that Dr. Searle has recorded some experience in the Deafness so often left behind by the present malay. * He has had much success in its treatment—generally accounted futile—with *Silicea* and *Sulphur.*

MEDITERRANEAN FEVER is a new species defined of late by the labours of our Army Medical Officers, last but by no means least of whom is (alas ! I must say "was," for he was killed while attending to the wounded in the disastrous fight at Colenso, S. A.) a nephew of my own, Surgeon-Captain Louis Hughes. His 'Treatise' on the disease I lay before you. † It is a mine of information regarding its clinical history and Pathology, and so abounds with practical hints as to its general management that no one likely to see such a fever in his practice should be without it. Its one deficiency—lamented by author as well as reader—is in respect of definite medication answering to the treatment of Malarious Fever by *Quinine* and *Arsenic.* If we could supply this, we should be conferring a boon indeed, for, apart from its no slight mortality and unusual amount of suffering, the duration of this malady often extends over a hundred days or more.

"Mediterranean Fever," as its name implies, haunts especially the coasts and islands of the great inland sea which divides Europe from Africa, but is by no means limited hereto. It is defined as "an endemic pyrexial disease, occasionally prevailing as an epedemic, having a long and indefinite duration, and an irregular course with an almost invariable tendency to undulatory pyrexial relapses. It is usually characterized by constipation and profuse perspirations, and accompanied or followed by symptoms of a neuralgic character. It is often accompanied by swelling of and effusion into the joints, and other Rheumatoid phenomena. After death, the spleen is found to be enlarged and often softened, and many of the organs congested; but Peyer's glands are neither enlarged nor ulcerated, nor is ulceration present in other parts of the small intestine,"

---

* See Transactions mentioned above, p. 188.
† "Mediterranean, Malta, or Undulant Fever." Macmillan, 1897.

"Painful inflammatory conditions of certain fibrous structures, of a localised nature," and swelling of the testicles, are also mentioned. The sweats have a distinctive odour, quite different from those of acute Rheumatism. Delirium is rare, but Neuritis to some extent is almost constant. The heart and lungs are rarely affected, and Diarrhœa is only seen in malignant cases. There is no exanthem.

In this picture the symptoms which mainly strike me are those of a Rheumatic character, and I think that the medicines which are most likely to lay hold of Mediterranean Fever are those which act on the vegetative tissues rather than on the nervous substance or the blood, and are most appropriate accordingly to febrile Rheumatism. Such are *Bryonia*, *Rhus* and *Mercurius*, but perhaps better than all would be *Colchicum* Captain Hughes indeed says that this drug "does no good"; but as he goes on to describe it as a gastric irritant and respiratory depressant, it is evident that he has given it in substantial doses only. In minute dosage, perhaps alternated with *Gelsemium* or *Baptisia* as an Anti-pyretic, I should expect much good from it.

"Of the last of the Continued Fevers," I wrote in my 'Therapeutics', "of the

PLAGUE *Kar' εgoXnv*, I have little to say. It appears to be a Typhus characterized by Carbuncles and engorgements of the lymphatic glands. Homœopathy has no practical knowledge of its Therapeutics; and, happily, none of us are likely to have any occasion to treat it. If we had, *Arsenicum* and *Lachesis* are the two medicines on which I should feel disposed to rely."

We are, alas! no longer thus blissfully ignorant of what the ancient "Plague" can do. It had always smouldered in the East; and since, in 1894, it was imported into Hong Kong and thence into Bombay and its neighbourhood, it has become a veritable scourge to our possessions in that quarter of the world. Unfortunately, too, the chief scene of its ravages in India has been one where Homœopathy is but scarcely represented, so that its victims have not had the advantage of what our medication can do for them, and little experience has been gained by which others can profit. What has been reported, however, I will here set down.

1. Plague has visited, though comparatively lightly, the great city of Calcutta, where Homœopathy has a good number of practitioners. Among these Dr. Majumdar writes that his experience with the cases that have come under his notice has been eminently satisfactory. He has had to make no new departure in the way of medicines or attenuations, and has found *Rhus* most frequently indicated. * Dr. B. K. Baptist relates his experience with the Epidemic of 1900. He treated

---

* INDIAN HOM. REVIEW, June, 1899.

26 genuine cases with only 4 deaths—two of the latter occurring within three and eight hours respectively of his undertaking the cases. *Lachesis* 7 was his principal remedy, *Belladonna* helping in the glandular swellings and the delirium. "Almost all Pneumonic cases," he writes, "I have cured by repeated doses of *Phosphorus* alone; sometimes *Ant. tart.* is required for profuse accumulation of mucus."*

2. Dr. Sircar has published a small Brochure on the Therapeutics of Plague. His own recommendations as to remedies are theoretical only; but he cites the experience of a Dr. Honigberger gained in Constantinople in 1836, which indicates that *Ignatia* in somewhat crude dosage, will counteract the premonitory symptoms.

3. Dr. Sircar himself would place the *Serpent-poisons*, with *Arsenicum* and *Phosphorus*, at the head of likely remedies for Plague. This prevision has been borne out by the results obtained by the distinguished representative of Homœopathy we have in the Army Medical Corps, Major H. E. Deane, now Health Officer at Calcutta. † Major Deane had some experience in Bombay in 1897 in a native hospital. He treated 50 cases, mainly with *Lachesis* in the usual dosage and mode of administration, with 22 deaths; but after his departure his successor, probably (he thinks) continuing the same treatment, was able to report a mortality of only 31 per cent. in 158 cases. He had been transferred to Bangalore, where he encountered an epidemic in which he treated 568 cases. At first, his percentage of deaths was 50; but by substituting *Cobra poison* (our "*Naja*") for *Lachesis*, using solutions of one in 500 or 1,000 (of Glycerine), and administering this hypodermically, he acquired so much more power over the disease that in his last 19 consecutive cases he only had 6 deaths. This is a mortality of about 30 per cent. in a disease where 60 per cent. and upwards has been the average in the present epidemic.

Still following our chosen Nosological table, we have now to consider the Therapeutics of the MALARIAL FEVERS which include both the Intermittents (Agues) and the Remittents of which it speaks, and also the condition known as Malarious cachexia. The "masked" or "irregular" forms of Malarial poisoning, such as "Brow-ague" and other Neuralgiæ, I shall discuss when I come to the disorders they simulate.

We will first speak of INTERMITTENT FEVER or
AGUE; and under this heading all general considerations relating to the subject must find place. Such generalities are of great importance in regard to the present disease. They have been largely entered into by Hahnemann himself in his 'Organon,'‡ and by Drs. Wurmb and Caspar, in their 'KLINISCHE

---

* H. W., July, 1900.   † See M. H. R., xliv., 586.
‡§§ ccxxxiii.—ccxliv. of 5th Ed.

STUDIEN.'* Begging you to read for yourselves the pregnant remarks of these authorities, I shall proceed to have my own say upon the matter.

What is it we have to treat in Ague ? Many would reply—a paroxysm of chill, heat and sweat recurring at periodic intervals, which enlarges the patient's spleen and otherwise disorders his health. This description would undoubtedly be true (at least phenomenally) of such Agues as occur sporadically or epidemically in Non-malarious regions, or such as attack a stranger on first entering into places where they are endemic. In the residents in these districts, however, a prodromal stage of longer or shorter duration is nearly always observed, and out of this—suddenly or gradually—the febrile paroxysms develope themselves, the premonitory symptoms remaining during the apyrexia. In these subjects, moreover, a Malarial intoxication often presents itself of which febrile paroxysms are only an incidental or unimportant feature : and this condition may be either primary, or secondary upon an untreated or ill-treated Ague. When primary, the first symptom of the mischief is very frequently Anæmia. "I have seen," writes Dr. Sircar, of Calcutta (whose valuable contribution to the literature of this subject I shall mention hereafter), "healthy, robust men, with no lack of red blood in their system, blanched after a few days residence in a Malarious district, before even the symtoms of the Fever had been quite developed, and long before either the liver or the spleen become enlarged."

From these facts it seems evident that true Ague is no more vaso-motor neurosis, but an infection of the blood and blood-making organs, of which the paroxysm of chill, heat and sweat is but one expression. If, then, the Homœopathic method is to be employed in its treatment, it is obvious that the paroxysm itself can only be our guide to the choice of a remedy when this is the primary or the sole symptom of the disease. Then, indeed, a medicine which covers its features may fairly be presumed to correspond also to the deeper changes which produce it, and so to be its Pathological SIMILE. When I say its features, it is necessary to specify which of these most deserves our regard. Chiefest of all must be named the succession of chill, heat and sweat itself which occurs in varying sequence ; and next the predominance of one or other of these, or the occurrence in either of special conditions or concomitants. "The remedy," Hahnemann says, "must either be able to produce in the healthy body two (or all three) similar alternating states, or else must correspond by similarity of symptoms to the strongest, best marked, and most peculiar alternating state, either to the cold stage with its accessory symptoms, or to the hot or sweating stage with theirs, according as the one or the other is the

---

* Translated in Vols. xii. and xiii. of BRIT. JOURN., OF HOM., and (more fully) in Vol. ii. of the UNITED STATES MEDICAL INVESTIGATOR.

strongest and most peculiar." Next comes the time of day at which the paroxysm, if strictly periodic, occurs; and last of all, and probably of no importance whatever as regards Homœopathic applicability, we have its "type"—Quotidian, Tertian, Quartan, or otherwise. Hahnemann anticipated the recognised practice of to-day in recommending a single dose of the appropriate remedy to be given immediately after a paroxysm, or—where the apyrexia was short or imperfect—during its decline.

But when the Aguish attacks are only one feature of a general Malarial intoxication, then that becomes true which the 'Organon' goes on to lay down, that "the symptoms of the patient's health during the intervals of freedom must be the chief guide to the most appropriate Homœopathic remedy." On this point Drs. Wurmb and Caspar insist with much urgency, and maintain that the rule is of general rather than exceptional application, pointing out that the form of the paroxysms is in the majority of cases very changeable, while the constitutional conditions are fixed. They lay down, therefore, the rule that "if, during the employment of a remedy, the cachectic state should remain unchanged, while the paroxysm decreases in force, the medicine, after being continued for some time, should be exchanged for another, even if the paroxysms should by this time have been entirely subdued by it. On the other hand, the diminution of the cachectic state is a certain sign that the suitable remedy has been chosen; and its use should not be discontinued, even if there should be a more frequent recurrence of the paroxysms: the cure is certain if the medicine be not changed." At the same time they argue that a remedy to be truly applicable to Intermittent Fever must correspond both to the nervous phenomena of the paroxysm and to the disorder of the vegetative life manifested in the apyrexia. If it merely influenced the former, it can suit mild and recent cases only; if the latter be its sole sphere it cannot be a true Antipyretic. The greatest fever medicines accordingly are those which, like *Arsenic,* occupy the whole ground : in the second rank stand such purely nervous remedies as *Ignatia,* and such purely vegetative ones as *Pulsatilla.*

There needs no argument to demonstrate the soundness, upon Homœopathic principles, of these canons for the treatment of Intermittent Fever. But before I go on to their application to practice, you will naturally be desirous of knowing what has been the success of such treatment both positively, and as compared with the ordinary method of administering *Quinine* in substantial doses to every patient suffering from the malady.

Now, as regards CHRONIC Intermittents—cases that have been lingering on for months and years the paroxysms suppressed for a time by *Bark,* but relapsing again and again till it ceases to influence them any more—the testimony in favour of Homœopathic medication (and that of the most Hahnemannian kind as regards individualisation and attenuation) is general and strong.

You have only to look through any of our Journals published in America, where the disease abounds, to satisfy yourself on this point. Nor does the treatment seem less successful when, as sometimes occurs, an epidemic of Ague breaks out in a place ordinarily free from it. Here general experience seems to have confirmed Hahnemann's dictum on the point, "that each epidemic is of a peculiar, uniform character, and that when once this character is found from the totality of symptoms common to all, it guides to the discovery of the Homœopathic specific remedy suitable to all the cases, which is almost universally serviceable in those patients who enjoyed tolerable health before the occurrence of the epidemic."

The experience of Drs. Wurmb and Casper may fairly be cited here, as their cases, were mostly of the chronic class. An account of their results which I am compelled to call very unfair has been given by Dr. Rogers, in his tractate entitled, "The Present State of Therapeutics." He states that "these physicians considered they made rapid cures when not more than seven paroxysms occured alter the commencement of the treatment." He then mentions that one of their patients had 26 paroxysms, a second 25 and a third 21 before the disease was cured. Finally, he quotes them as saying that Homœopathists have every reason to congratulate themselves on their treatment of Intermittent Fever, and that "it is evident, FROM THESE FIGURES, that we may most satisfactorily enter the lists with our rivals"—leaving it to be supposed that the figures are those which he has just summarised. Whereas their actual results on this point, as given by themselves,* in answer to the question whether Homœopathists are able to effect a rapid cure of Intermittents, are that in 77 cases treated by them, after the administration of the Homœopathic remedy there appeared no paroxysm in 11 cases, one only in 12, two in 9 and three in 8. Thus in 40 cases out of 77 the CITO of the cure admitted of no question. Of the remainder, 15 had from 5 to 7 attacks, and the rest from 8 to 26. Of these last, Drs. Wurmb and Casper remark that they would not have shown so high a figure had the right remedy been chosen from the first; for after the last and curative selection had been made, no paroxysm occurred in 19 cases, one only in 16, two in 14 and three in 13—rapid success being thus obtained in 62 out of 77 cases. Remembering, then, that the aim of these physicians was not so much to stop the paroxysms as to cure the whole disease, and that all these 77 patients did leave the hospital well, and remained so, I think they were justified in saying that their results prove the sufficiency of Homœopathy in Ague—at any rate of such Homœopathy as they practised, and in such Agues as come under their care.

Another writer on Intermittent Fever who has expressed and substantiated his confidence in the results of Homœopathic

---

* See B. J. H., xii., 391.

treatment, is Dr. I. S. P, Lord. An account of his work on the subject is given in the Thirtieth Volume of the BRITISH JOURNAL OF HOMŒOPATHY; and I think you will be induced by the review to procure and read the book itself.

As regards the treatment of RECENT Agues occurring in Malarious districts, I do not find the same expression of general confidence. Dr. Bayes, indeed, in an account of his experience of the disease as it occurs in the fen lands about Cambridge,* expressed himself well-satisfied with the results he obtained. But he does not tell us how many of the seventy-five cases he tabulated were recent ones treated by him AB INTIO: nor does he mention the time required for their cure. His best result is, I think, that he can say, "I have not had a single acute case become chronic in my hands, a result" (as he truly adds) "frequently following the SUPPRESSION of Ague by large doses of *Quinine.*" When however, we turn to the statements of those who practise in the thick of Malaria in the United States and in India, we find that the ordinary treatment by symptomatic resemblance and minute dosage gives little satisfaction. The general experience of the American practitioners is fairly given by Dr. Vincent in the Second Volume of the UNITED STATES MEDICAL INVESTIGATOR.

"Intermittent Fever," he writes, "to me has proved an exceptional disease. I have SELDOM been able to cure a RECENT case of Ague with high attenuations nor (I might add) with any other attenuation. Even the best selected remedies fail me in a majority of cases. . . . My own experience in Ague is the experience of nineteen out of every twenty physicians of our school; † and so thoroughly is this matter understood, that it has become proverbial in Malarious districts that 'Homœopathic physicians cannot cure Ague.' Many persons, ardent Homœopathists, will resort to *Quinine* or an Allopath if they or their families take Intermittent Fever, rather than take the chances of a run of the disease for several days and probably have to resort to it at the end."

To the same effect writes Dr. Sircar : ‡
"The fact is, practioners flushed with their unexpected success in chronic cases with infinitesimals alone, and absolutely without *Quinine,* were deluded into the belief that they could dispense with *Quinine* altogether, at least in its massive doses; but when the hour of THEIR trial came, when people began to confide them with cases from the beginning, they began to be disappointed, though unfortunately they could not see their

---

* ANNALS, i., 441.

† The late Dr. Allison Clokey wrote to the same effect in 1897 (see J. B. H. S., v., 290). He gave grain doses; and Dr. Bliem, who writes from Texas to support him, quotes Osler as representing such dosage as sufficient to prevent the paroxysms (IB., vi., 104).

‡ M. H. R., xviii., 522.

mistake. In spite of greater diligence in the search after the appropriate remedy, in spite of renewed endeavours to hunt after symptoms of the patient and symptoms in the Materia Medica, the real remedy seemed always to elude the search and mock the struggle, till the cases were made over to the Allopaths, who, with a few doses of *Quinine*, effected the cure."

I quite agree with Dr. Sircar when he goes on (he was addressing our Congress of 1874):—"Gentlemen, I verily tell you that it is *Bark* and its *alkaloid* which have kept up the vitality of the old school, and it is our disloyalty to them which has stood seriously in the way of the progress of our own school, and which not unfrequently brings unmerited ridicule and abuse upon our doctrines." I have already* demonstrated the full Homœopathicity of *Quinine* to the Aguish paroxysm, and argued that in all cases where the paroxysm is the disease we can follow no better treatment than its administration. Dr. Sircar concludes by saying,—"In our anxiety to be Homœopaths we must not forget to be physicians; in our zeal to worship Hahnemann we must not cease to worship Truth wherever found." But the curious thing is that the treatment of recent Ague by *Bark* alone in otherwise healthy persons residing in Malarious districts is Hahnemann's own recommendation. "The Intermittent Fever endemic there," he writes in the Organon, "would, at the most, only attack such a person on his first arrival; but one or two very small doses of a highly potentised solution of *Cinchona* bark would, conjointly with a well-regulated mode of living, speedily free him from the disease." If such result do not follow the patient must be treated with "Antipsoric" (*i.e.* constitutional) remedies; there is latent disease in him which is only taking an accidentally Aguish form.

The practical conclusion from all that has been said is obvious. It was the power of *Bark* over the Intermittent paroxysm which led Hahnemann to Homœopathy. He never abandoned its use in real Marsh Fever (as he called them); nor, I maintain, should we. He came indeed, AFTER HE HAD CEASED TO PRACTISE IN MALARIOUS DIRTRICTS, to recommend its use in a highly potentised, that is, attenuated form. But if those who now encounter the disease in its HABITAT find such "potentisation" best attained by substantial, or even massive doses, they are acting in the spirit though not according to the letter of his instructions: they are following him in "the medicine of experience." I believe, therefore, that in all recent and uncomplicated Agues you will find it your best practice to give **Quinine** in the apyrexia; a single full dose at its commencement, as ordinarily practised, and as recommended by Jousset, or repeated smaller quantities during its continuance. In the few Intermittents I have myself seen, I have adopted the latter plan; and have found two or three grains of the first decimal trituration, taken every three

---

* **Manual of Pharmacodynamics.** sub voce *Cinchona*.

or four hours, act very satisfactorily. Bahr (who says that, "as a rule, *Bark* cures every case of Ague originating in Malaria, and of recent origin") finds the first centesimal trituration sufficient; and Dr. Panelli, from his Italian experience, says the same thing.* You will also remember the still prevailing tendency of Ague to recur on its appointed days, and will anticipate its advent by an occasional dose of the remedy till a fortnight or so has elapsed. While thus preventing the recurrence of the paroxysms, you may relieve their sufferings and mitigate their severity by drawing upon the rich treasury of Homœopathic remedies and giving them during their continuance. *Aconite,* if there is great thirst, restlessness, and anxiety; *Belladonna* if in the hot stage the head aches badly; *Ipecacuanha,* if vomitting be distressing; *Veratrum album,* if the chill be excessive and simulate the Choleraic collapse—all these have proved helpful according to their indications; and Dr. Sircar gives practical evidence of the value of many other remedies of the same kind. In the "congestive chills," which are the American form of the "Pernicious Fever" of the Roman and other districts, Dr Morse of Memphis, reports † very satisfactory results from *Veratrum viride.* In these Pernicious Fevers, I may say, even so strict a Homœopathist as Dr. Charge admitted that we must fall back upon *Quinine,* and must not shrink from such quantities as may be required for the speedy arrest of the paroxysms.‡

But it is confessed by the most ardent admirers of *Quinine,* that it does not always succeed in checking even recent Agues. If, therefore, the paroxysms are not speedily arrested by its use (and it cures very quickly when it does so at all), you will do well at once to abandon it in favour of other remedies. In Chronic Intermittents, moreover, and in Malarious cachexia, *Quinine* can never be recommended; though its native *Bark* may sometimes find place in virtue of general similarity between its effects and the patients' condition. There is a general agreement between our Therapeutists as to the medicines from which in such cases the choice should be made. *Arsenicum, Nuxvomica, Pulsatilla, Veratrum album, Ignatia,* and *Ipecacuanha* are Wurmb and Caspar's primary list; Bahr gives *Arsenicum, Nux, Veratrum, Ipecacuanha, Natrum muriaticum* and *Arnica*: Jousset recommends, under various circumstances, *Ipecacuanha, Capsicum, Nux* and *Arsenicum.* If to those are added *Aranea,* § *Cedron,* ‖ the *Eupatoriums, Phosphoric acid* and

---

* See United States Med. Investigator, iv., 161.

† United States Med. Investigator, ii., 359.

‡ See his communication to the Transactions of the World's Convention of 1876.

§ See J. B. H. S., iii., 97, 200 ‖ Ibid., v. 391; vi. 99; viii. 156.

Sulpher, I think that I shall have mentioned every medicine on which, save in very exceptional cases, you are likely to have to rely for help. As regards their indications, it is needless that I should repeat here what I have already said when speaking of each drug. The only one I have neglected in reference to this disease is *Pulsatilla*. Both Wurmb and Caspar, and Dr. Lord, esteem it highly. The former cured with it alone seventeen cases out of twenty-seven in which they prescribed it, and speak of it as specially useful when a condition of Chlorosis and Hydræmia has been induced by the marsh-poison. Sometimes—as it acts little on the nervous system—*Ignatia* has to follow it to remove the paroxysms.

In aid of our choice of a remedy for these cases—and we cannot individualise them too strictly—Dr. von Bœnninghausen long ago published a laborius 'Repertory,' which received the honour of favourable notice from Hahnemann himself. A Second Edition, published after an interval of thirty years, has recently been translated for us by Dr. Korndœrfer. I wish I could speak more favourably of this Volume than I have been obliged to do in the BRITISH JOURNAL OF HOMŒOPATHY; † but I cannot. In the Report of the discussion on Dr. Bayes' Paper, there are some useful remarks by Dr. Quin on the medicines indicated in Ague by the presence or absence of thirst in the different stages of the paroxysm; and in the Fourth Volume of the UNITED STATES INVESTIGATOR (p. 141) you will find a "Time-table" indicating the hour at which the paroxysm is apt to begin when this is characteristic of some particular medicine. All these are helps, and not to be despised. But if you wish to be successful in treating Chronic Intermittents, let me especially commend to your repeated perusal the "Study" of Wurmb and Casper on the disease to which I have so often referred.

The Malarious Cachexia is to be met (as you will see from my remarks on the respective drugs) by *Arsenicum, Calcaria arsenica, Chininum arsenicosum,‡ Natrum muriaticum*, or *Sulphur* —the first especially when the symptoms are those of Phthisis Florida, the four latter when they are of a more torpid and degenerative type.

---

* I have spoken of *Sulphur* in connexion only with Chronic Ague. Dr. Cooper, however, has now adduced evidence from India and Turkey of its power over recent fevers of this kind. (See M. H. R., xxxiii., 127, 643). He uses pilules saturated with the *Tincture fortissima*.

† Vol. xxxii., p. 531. ‡ See J. B. H. S., ii., 93; ix., 177,

REMITTENT FEVER, of Malarious origin, is just a severe Ague whose intermission is so perfect as to cause it to be designated a "remission" instead. I know it only from the description given of it in Books; *and in the absence of any Homœopathic literature bearing upon it, must content myself with suggesting the remedies most likely to avail.

Of even more importance than in Intermittents must be the treatment adopted during the attack. "The first and most immediate object of treatment," writes Aitken, "is to reduce the force and frequency of arterial action during the paroxysm." We know too well the power of **Aconite** to effect this end to need the spoliative venesections advised by the Indian writers. With the rule to begin **Quinine** as soon as remission shows itself, I have no quarrel. Dr. Goodno gives two grains of the 1_x trituration of the *Bi-sulphate* every two hours. I would only suggest that in the asthenic form of the Fever, **Arsenic** might not unfrequently be preferable; and that the remarkable power of **Gelsemium** over Remittent feverish state observed in cooler climates makes it worth a trial in the Fevers we are now studying, where the symptoms do not run high enough to require *Aconite*. If the gastric irritability be very marked, a few doses of **Ipecacuanha** may do good service.

BILIOUS REMITTENT appears to differ from simple Remittent only in the implication of the liver in the attack. It is sometimes called "Malarious Yellow Fever," from the resemblance of its symptoms to the contagious Toxæmia properly so named. When this is so, Dr. Neidhard finds **Crotalus** as useful in this Fever as in the true Typhus Icterodes (OP. CIT.). He gives it in the 1st, 2nd and 3rd triturations. This (and that in milder cases, the **Eupatorium perfoliatum** has proved effective) is all I have to tell you about the Homœopathic treatment of the disorder in question.

I have adduced the foregoing considerations as they stand in my 'Therapeutics' of 1877. They are all, I believe, clinically and phenomenally true; and were the best that could be (at any rate that I could) put forward from the Homœopathic stand-point at that time. Since then, however, research has thrown a new light on the Pathology of the MALARIAL FEVERS. It seems to have demonstrated that their phenomena are due to the reception (mainly through mosquito-bites) of an amœboid parasite into the blood; that these grow at the expense of the red corpuscles they inhabit, form black and yellow pigments in their own interior, and then break up, each into from ten to fifteen segments (spores). The corpuscles now burst, and let out the spores and pigments into the liquor sanguinis Therewith occurs the rigor of the fever paroxysm, followed by its heat and sweat; while the destruction of the corpuscles

---

* I speak especially of the articles on it in Aitken's, 'Science and Practice of Medicine', and in the 'System of Medicine' edited by Dr. Russell Reynolds.

accounts for the Anæmia associated with the disease. The spores develope into fresh parasites, which invade new corpuscles; and the morbid cycle would go on indefinitely were not a substance like *Quinine* ingested, which prevents the development of the spores and so arrests the whole process.

I have no exception to take to these doctrines. We have already seen, in other cases where a CONTAGIUM VIVUM has been (presumably) proved to exist, that there is no need on that account for departure from our ordinary medication, which acts by fortifying and defending the tissues against their invaders. But in this instance a special inference is drawn from the hypothesis, which affects us seriously. The similarity of the effects of *Bark* on the healthy to the symptoms of Intermittent Fever was (as I have said elsewhere) the Newton's apple which suggested Homœopathy to Hahnemann. When this similarity has been challenged, we have vindicated it by copious evidence;* and the treatment of Ague by *Quinine* has long stood in our literature as the prerogative instance of cure by specifics, and of the way in which SIMILIA SIMILIBUS enables such remedies to be discovered. Now, however, the advocates of a plasmodial origin for the Malarial Fever claim that our supposed specific is really a germicide; that its efficacy has nothing to do with its action in health, but depends upon its being a poison to protoplasm, and so a destroyer of the low organisms on which Intermittent Fever depends. If this be true, it robs us of a weighty witness to the Homœopathic law; and if it be false, supposition of its truth is unfortunate for patients, as it leads to their being dosed with the drug much more heavily than they would be were its constitutional action alone desired. The question deserves, therefore, a strict investigation.

In my 'Pharmacodynamics,' I have adduced three reasons against the theory now stated. One is that the dose of *Quinine* which suffices to cure an Intermittent is often far too small to affect the vitality of the supposed microzymes—two grains, for instance, sufficing when administered by subcutaneous injection. Another is that when the drug is introduced in the fullest proportion the animal body can bear in its blood, it suspends only, it does not annihilate, bacterial activity. The third lies in the absence, when other substances are considered, of any parallel between their microbicide and their anti-Malarial properties. *Corrosive sublimate* heads the list of agents of the former class, and *Arsenic* is confessedly second only to the *Quinine* among those of the latter; but were we to treat Ague with the sublimate, or attempt to avert sepsis in a wound with an Arsenical solution, we should find that the two were hardly interchangeable.

So far I have written there; but here I would add some

---

* As in my 'Pharmacodynamics,' Lewin, in his "Collateral Actions of Medicines," accepts the testimony there collected, and attests the validity of Hahnemann's experiment. (See M. H. R., xli., 286).

further considerations. The first is that *Quinine,* like the Homœopathic specifics which have already passed before us, is prophylactic as well as curative; and is so in doses far too small to exert any germicide influence. Dr. Maclean states that three grains taken every morning fasting, fully suffice for such preventive action. Does not this look like pre-occupying the ground rather than killing its invaders?* Again, the similarity between Malaria and *Quinine,* as pathogenetic agents, has received a striking confirmation from the recent provings with the *Muriate* conducted by Dr. Schulz.† Nearly every experimenter suffered more or less from supra-orbital Neuralgia; and I need not remind you that the affinity of the marsh-poison for this region is so great as to give the term "Brow-Ague" to the pain it there sets up. Thirdly, the parallel afforded by *Arsenic* has of late received its completing touch. As curative of Ague, its repute is well-known and unquestioned; and that this repute obtains in Homœopathic as well as ordinary circles shews that substantial dosage is no necessary element in its efficacy. Its similarity to Malaria is yet better attested, as regards the febrile paroxysm, than that of *Quinine;* and it extends beyond that of its sister drug, as it kills the red blood-corpuscles, and sets up an Anæmia very like that of the Malarious Cachexia, in which accordingly ‡ it is—in both schools the leading remedy. But it has been ascertained to act as a prophylactic also, even in the fever-haunted Campagna, so that Railway EMPLOYEES and labourers can work there with impunity.§ A similar, a prevenaive and a curative,, having no particular germicidal power, and active in too small doses to exert this if it had it,—*Arsenic* presents in relation to Intermittent Fever a most instructive picture, and, suggesting a corresponding interpretation of the facts regarding *Quinine,* aids the re-instatement of that remedy in Homœopathic Therapeutics.

I hope that such vindication may be useful, moreover, not only for apologetic purposes, but to encourage our own practitioners to a larger use of the remedy, as one acting upon strictly Homœopathic principles. With this view I hail the testimony given to our International Congress of 1896 by Drs. Vincent Leon Simon and P. C. Majumdar. The former told us that we could not cut short the paroxysm of Malarial Fever with anything but *Quinine* in ponderable doses (by which he explained himself as meaning the 1st-3rd trituration): and that

---

* The advocates of the sporicide theory of the curative action of *Quinine* perceive this consequence; and allow themselves to go against all experience by denying its prophylactic powers. So Dr. Fielding Ould, in the BRITISH MEDICAL JOURNAL of Sep., 1st 1900, p. 531.

† See Cyclopædia of Drug Pathogenesy, ii., 738.

‡ This "accordingly" plainly belongs only to the school of Hahnemann. On what ground those of the other can justify its employment we must leave them to say.

§ See the results of Crudeli and others in B. J. H., xliv., 34.

he has never seen such a fever cured whose attacks were of the ordinary form, unless the work was begun by so cutting short the paroxysms. Dr. Majumdar did not go so far; but he was far more kindly disposed towards *Quinine* then when he contributed a tentative Paper on the same subject to the Congress of 1881. "In suitable cases," he wrote, "it does wonders." And these "suitable cases" he defines as those "in which the paroxysm is sudden and the apyrexia complete." The experience of these two physicians thus coincides, and is also identical with the views on the subject I have re-iterated in my writings for these many years past.

Returning from this digression, I would say the present-day theory of Ague need in no way impugn our principles or alter our practice with regard to it. *Quinine* and *Arsenic* are with us as in traditional medicine the two great febrifuges in recent cases,—not as germicides, but as specific remedies, like all those conforming to the Law of Similars. They are thus no mere alternatives, one to be given when the other fails or the system is saturated with it. *Quinine* is most suitable in such Agues as attack a stranger on first entering places where they are endemic, or those which occur sometime after he has ceased to be exposed to the noxious influennce. *Arsenic,* on the other hand, is preferable when the general paludal poisoning is primary and the febrile paroxysms develope out of it. That we have a variety of medicines beyond these two, by apportioning which we can in chronic cases make thorough and permanent cures, and that with quite innfinitesimal doses, is explained by there being in such cases no longer any plasmodia present, the febrile phenomena in them being rather those of a morbid habit acquired by the nervous system. In recent Agues, the case being otherwise, the lower triturations of *Quinine* and *Arsenic* seem required. I can conceive it possible, moving further on such lines, that in very Malarious districts the germicidal powers which *Quinine* undoubtedly possesses MIGHT have to be called into play and the dosage become large accordingly. It may be here as after operations and accouchements. In fairly pure surroundings asepsis is all that is necessary; but in old hospitals, whose atmosphere is laden with germs, antisepsis is really required, and the *Carbolic*-spray or the *Sublimate*-wash must be employed, even at the risk of injuring the patient in other ways. Here I allow the force of Dr. Hayward's plea, who has done so much to popularise the new doctrines about Malaria and to urge action being taken on them on our part as well as on the other side. But while I put this possibility for the sake of fairness, I would lay chief stress on its being an exception, and not the rule—the latter making *Quinine* a truly Homœopathic remedy, to be administered in non-perturbative quantities.

LECTURE XX.

GENERAL DISEASES.
—o—
CHOLERA—DIPHTHERIA—INFLUENZA

On the present occasion I shall have to consider the treatment of three diseases, each "GENERAL" in its invasion of the whole organism, but each localised specially in a particular part thereof which in the first is the bowels, in the second the throat, in the third the air passages. I shall have to speak of CHOLERA, of DIPHTHERIA, and of INFLUENZA.

By
CHOLERA, I mean the Asiatic pestilence, which, endemic in the delta of the Ganges, travels from time to time in a desolating course over the Western World. I do not include the ordinary autumnal vomiting and Diarrhœa, which is sometimes called "Cholera Nostras," and which, as occurring in young children, is sadly familiar (in America especially) as "Cholera Infantum." These will come before us subsequently; the former among the disease of the intestines, the latter among the maladies of childhood. It is the Asiatic Cholera of which I have here to speak.

I have already told you something about the success we have had with this disease. Indeed, the history of its Homœopathic treatment is one of the brightest pages in our records. From Russia, Germany and Hungary in 1831-2; from Liverpool and Edinburgh in this country, and from France and America abroad in 1849; and from Barbadoes and London in 1854, and again from Liverpool in 1866, we have abundant evidence of the comparative value of our Method in the treatment of this terrible scourge. Let me indicate before I go any further where you can find the narratives which bear out this statement.

For the Epidemic of 1831-2 our main source of information is Dr. Quin's 'TRAITEMENT HOMŒOPATHIQUE DE CHOLERA,' his own experience having been gained in Moravia. That of 1848-9 was carefully observed by Tessier at Paris, and in this country by Dr. Russell at Edinburgh and Dr. Drysdale at Liverpool, all of whom had large opportunities of treating the disease. Tessier's account is given in his RECHERCHES CLINIQUES SUR LE TRAITEMENT DE LA PNEUMONIE ET DU CHOLERA, SUIVANT LA METHODE DE HAHNEMANN, which has been translated into English by Dr. Hempel.

Dr. Russell has given his narrative in the Seventh and Dr. Drysdale his in the Eighth Volume of the BRITISH JOURNAL OF HOMŒO-PATHY,—the former having subsequently expanded his Essay into a "Treatise on Epidemic Cholera" (Headland, 1849). The results obtained in London and (by Dr. Goding and others) in Barbadoes during the Epidemic of 1853-4 are narrated in the Thirteenth Volume of the BRITISH JOURNAL' and in a lecture by Dr. Russell —"On Cholera: and historical sketch, with a practical application," published in the Fourth Volume of the ANNALS. The experience gained in Liverpool in the last epidemic has been put on record by Dr. P. Proctor in the Twenty-Fifth Volume of the BRITISH JOURNAL; and the American observations up to 1853 are gathered up by Dr. Joslin in his "Homœopathic Treatment of Cholera," &c. (Walker, 1863).

Three things, I think, will strike you, as you read these observations.

First, you will see that our Statistics are more favourable than those of the old school. While their death-rate rarely falls below fifty per cent., ours rarely reaches thirty. The only notable exception consists of Tessier's cases, treated at the Hospital St. Marguerite in Paris. Even here his losses were ten per cent. less than those of his old-school colleagues in the same Hospital; and their high rate may be accounted for both by the unusually large proportion of cases of the "ataxic" and "black" varieties of the disease, and by his own comparative inexperience at the time in Homœopathic Therapeutics. He made, for instance, no use of *Cuprum*, and a very inadequate one of *Camphor*. The impression which our comparative success has made may be estimated by two facts. The practice of Homœopathy had been, since 1819, forbidden in the Austrian Empire by law. The results of Dr. Fleischmann's practice in the Vienna Epidemic of 1836 were such that the prohibition was repealed. It could hardly have been otherwise; for he saved two-thirds of his patients (he treated 732 cases), while the ordinary practitioners lost two-thirds of theirs. Again, in the London Epidemic of 1857, the returns of the Homœopathic Hospital were excluded from the Report furnished to the Parliament by the College of Physicians. The compliment was paid them because they showed a mortality of 16.4 per cent. only whereas in no other hospital in London was it below 36 per cent.

Secondly, you will notice that the practitioners of our school have acquired a confidence in treating Cholera which is entirely absent from the minds of those who follow the old practice. Lebert sums up the experience of the latter by affirming that the physician at the bedside must painfully reconcile himself to the scientific fact that Indian Cholera, in its well-pronounced, typical, and perfectly developed form, slays the half of all persons attacked, and that there is an entire absence of any certain and specific means of cure. On the other hand (in the words of Dr. Russell), "there reigns in the minds of those who have put the Homœopathic method to the test of personal experience, a firm conviction that it furnishes certain remedies which if properly applied, arrest the disease in its first stage; and other remedies which, although they fail to cure all cases, yet manifestly reduce the mortality of the pestilence."

Thirdly, you will observe with satisfaction the substantial identity of the treatment pursued in every epidemic and in every country. Hahnemann, before he had seen a single case of the disease, indicated *Camphor* as its specific antidote, suggesting *Veratrum* and *Cuprum* also as likely to be beneficial. To these later experience, more specially in Great Britain, has been added *Arsenicum;* and with the four medicines now named nearly all the Homœopathic treatment of Cholera has been carried on. Let me endeavour to lay down their distinctive spheres of action.

1. In speaking of **Camphor** in my lectures I have argued that its Physiological action is that of (in the words of Trousseau and Pidoux) a refrigerant and sedative, producing in its full poisonous effects a state of collapse with chill. It is thus perfectly Homœopathic to Cholera in the stage of invasion; and Dr. Russell justly says that "there is the most perfect unanimity amongst all Homœopathic practitioners as to its efficacy in curing Cholera in the first stage." He relates a striking case, as illustrating its "instantaneous and almost magical effects." He "once saw a little girl actually TAKE Cholera. It was in a room where there were several bad cases; and this child suddenly presented the strange, unnatural look which characterizes the disease, and seemed to shrink in size, becoming cold and of a livid hue. He immediately gave her five or six drops of the tincture of *Camphor*, and in the course of ten minutes the anxious frigid expression of the face gave way: it was succeeded by a glow of warmth; and the pulse, which had become very small, rapid, and irregular, resumed its normal volume and rate. She recovered, but for some days suffered from Diarrhœa."

Whether we should depend upon *Camphor* in later stages of the disease is as yet a moot point. It is not, indeed, directly Homœopathic to the Cramps, Diarrhœa, or Vomiting. But since the condition of algidity and Cyannosis to which it does correspond persists when these have set in, and constitutes the real peril of the case, there is nothinng in our principles which forbids its use at any stage of the attack. I have related the results obtained from its continued use by Dr. Rubini, of Naples, in the Epidemic of 1854-5. In a publication, dated 1866, * he adds his experience in the invasion of the pestilence which took place in 1865—6, which was equally satisfactory; again no death

---

* STATISTICA DEI COLERICI CURATI COLLA SOLA CANFORA IN NAPOLI NEGLI ANNI, 1854, 1855, 1856. 3rd Edizione, ampliata, Napoli, 1866.

occurring in his practice, though he treated 123 patients. He relates some of his cases, whose severity is unquestionable.

2. ***Veratrum album*** stands next to *Camphor* in the certainty of its action in Cholera, when restricted to its proper sphere. This is by general consent, the cases marked by profuse vomiting and purging, with coldness indeed, but without deadly collapse and lividity. To such a condition its Physiological action precisely corresponds : and, it being capable of speedy amelioration, there is here a field in which the medicine has displayed brilliant effects, even in high dilutions.

3. ***Cuprum*** is confessedly the best remedy for the Choleraic cramps, and for the vomitting also, when this is a prominent feature. Its undoubted prophylactic power against the disease, shown mainly by the immunity of workers with the metal suggests a still more intimate relationship to the whole morbid process. I have mentioned in my 'Pharmacodynamics' how Hahnemann originally suggested it as superior even to *Veratrum* for the developed disease, and how Dr. Proctor, in the Epidemic at Liverpool in 1866, "found himself gradually trusting mainly to it in the stage of collapse," with the impression very strong in his mind that herein it is the most reliable of our remedies.

4. This, however, is not the general experience : the medicine most trusted in collapse being ***Arsenicum***. Dr. Drysdale and Dr. Russel* concur in regarding this remedy as the greatest we have, when the time for the administration of *Camphor* is past, and when the danger is less from the discharges than from the general depression of vitality. In this judgement Tessier coincides. I have shown that *Arsenic* is a true Pathological SIMILE to the Choleraic process, though the minute symptomatology of disease and drug may not completely coincide. The burning at the epigastrium, however, so often complained of, should lead symptomatic prescribers to think well of it ; and those who attach more importance to Pathological relationship will especially value it for its power to cause, and to remedy, that condition of the kidneys which leads in Cholera to suppression of urine.

Valuable, however, as *Cuprum* and *Arsenicum* are in the collapse of Cholera, I think that we want a remedy for it still more energetic and effective ; and this I have suggested we may find in ***Aconite***. Let a few cases of poisoning with this plant be read with the thought of Cholera in the mind, and the resemblance will be seen to be striking.† We have the intense

---

* The elder Bakody, who seems to have been the first to employ *Arsenic* largely in Cholera, in 1831 saved 148 patients out of 154 treated mainly by it (JOURN. BELGE D' HOMŒOPATHIC, March-April, 1897).

† See those cited by Dr. Hempel in his 'MATERIA MEDICA,' and in his translation of Bahr (ii. 622). (Cases 2, 3 and 4 in the Cyclopædia of Drug Pathogenesy are some of them.) In all these the resemblance to Cholera is noted by the observers.

chill, even the cold tongue, the blueness, the difficult respiration, the almost imperceptible pulse and the cramps. After death the arterial system is found empty and the venous full. It is to Dr. Hempel that the credit is due of being the first to perceive this analogy, to which he drew attention nearly fifty years ago. Dr. Cramoisy, of Paris, is the only one who (to my knowledge) has put it in practice; and his success has been very encouraging to future employment of the remedy.

If now by some of these means you have brought your Cholera patient out of the cold stage of his Ague fit (for such I maintain it to be), he has two perils before him. The first is that his urine will continue suppressed, and that uræmic intoxication will ensue. It has been ascertained that an acute hyperæmia of the kidneys is present in such cases, analogous to that of Post-Scarlatinal Dropsy. It is obvious that, theoretically and practically alike, there can be no better medicine than *Arsenicum* here; and, unless it has been already freely given, you will do well to rely upon it. Should its action, however, have been already exhausted we have **Terebinthina** and **Cantharis** on which to call, and also **Kali bichromicum**. The latter was used by Dr. Drysdale (in the second trituration) in twelve cases in which Ischuria continued after the use of *Arsenic;* and in eleven the urine returned. The second danger is from the consecutive fever, which is generally of a Typhoid type. It seems to be of comparatively rare occurrence under Homœopathic treatment, probably from the absence of Opiates and stimulants in the previous medication. When it does appear, it must be treated with one or other of our recognised antipyretics, according to its symptoms. Dr. Drysdale found **Phosphoric acid** most frequently indicated.

I must say a few words upon some other medicines which have occasionally filled gaps in the treatment of Cholera.

Acidum hydrocyanicum was found of at least temporary service by Dr. Russell in some cases where there were great oppression of the lungs or heart. Dr. Sircar, from his Indian experience, speaks still more highly of it. *"Hydrocyanic acid,"* he writes, "is useful, in fact, is the only remedy when, along with pulselessness, the respiration is slow, deep, gasping, or difficult and spasmodic, taking place at long intervals, the patient appearing dead in the intermediate time. If any remedy is entitled to be spoken of as a charm, it is this. It would seem at times to restore animation to a corpse."*

Secale is commended highly, both, by Drysdale and Russell, when large watery, painless motions need a remedy of their own; it seems to work well with *Arsenicum.* Dr. Proctor found

---

* Dr. Majumdar, of Calcutta, communicates similar experience with *Naja.* "Many a fatal case," he writes, "has been rescued by it from the jaws of death." (INDIAN HOM. REVIEW Jan. 1896: see also M. H. R., xli., 71).

Phosphorus of great use in a similar condition when persisting after the symptoms were removed.

Cicuta has proved of service in spasmodic Hiccough or belching occurring in Cholera.

Carbo vegetabilis was much used by Tessier to meet the later prostration of Cholera, and Dr. Sircar seems to think it of value. But I am at a loss to perceive its appropriateness to the condition present; and British experience is against its efficacy.

In all that has preceded it will be understood that I have been speaking of true Cholera i.e., where in addition to rice-water vomiting and purging, cramps, and suppressing of urine, there is some amount of algidity and Cyanosis. But it is well-known that the same poison may produce minor forms of disease, which are called Choleraic Diarrhœa and Cholerine. For the former, *Camphor* is the best domestic and routine remedy though the physician will often be led to prefer *Veratrum* or **Croton.** "Cholerine" seems to me to be Cholera Nostras, modified by the epidemic influence: for, unlike Choleraic Diarrhœa, it rarely proves the precursor of the fully-developed disease. **Ipecacuanha** and *Phosphoric acid* have generally been its favourite remedies; but I would commend **Iris** to your notice, with *Veratrum* in reserve should the symptoms assume the Asiatic form.

As regards dosage in Cholera—*Camphor* is always administered in the primary solution, which Dr. Rubini makes a saturated one. *Aconite* also has been used by its commenders in the mother tincture; but *Arsenic, Veratrum* and *Cuprum* have been given in high (6-30) as well as in the lowest attenuations, and with success in either case. *Arsenic* has been also given by Dr. Drysdale in the form of inhalations of *Arseniuretted Hydrogen*. His direction for the preparation and use of this Gas may be found in the Seventh Volume of the BRITISH JOURNAL OF HOMŒOPATHY (p. 559).

I have next to speak of—

DIPHTHERIA.—I think it is quite right to place this malady among general diseases rather than among the diseases of the throat. It is unquestionably a specific Toxæmia, distinct from Scarlatina and (I think) from Croup; and its virus is capable of entering the system at other doors than the throat, as well as of manifesting itself elsewhere when once introduced.

The treatment of Diphtheria illustrates well the conditions necessary for the successful application of the Homœopathic Law. When Cholera first appeared in Europe, Hahnemann (as I have shown) was able, from his profound knowledge of Pathogenesy, to indicate *Camphor, Veratrum* and *Cuprum* as its specific remedies. We have only added *Arsenicum* since; and nearly every Homœopathist throughout the world treats Cholera with these medicines, and with a comparative success which is abundantly satisfactory. It is very different with Diphtheria. If you will look through our Journals from 1859 onwards, you will find for sometime an endless variety of medicines in use, and no great success to boast of with them all. It has not been, in my experience, a disease which it has afforded one much satisfaction to have to treat. Nevertheless, amid the floating mass of records which have now accumulated, there seem certain patches of firm ground on which we can take our stand laying down, provisionally, the best Homœopathic treatment of the malady. I think, too, that by a more single and persistent use of remedies which have come to be known as specially adapted for our Therapeutics of Diphtheria have of late years been increasingly satisfactory.*

For the Homœopathic literature of Diphtheria I may refer you, besides the numerous articles upon it in the Journals of all countries, to the three American Monographs of Drs. Helmuth, Ludlam and Neidhard. My own experience in the disease is recorded in a Paper entitled, "An Account of Fifty cases of Diphtheria," read before the British Homœopathic Society in 1870 and published in the Twenty-Eighth Volume of the BRITISH JOURNAL OF HOMŒOPATHY. Since Brighton has been effectively drained, Diphtheria has rarely appeared in the town; but what little I have seen of late has confirmed the conclusions at which I had then arrived.

The old division of Diphtheria was into Simple, Croupal and Malignant varieties. Oertel, whose Article in Ziemssen's 'Cyclopœdia' is of great excellence, means much the same thing by his Catarrhal, Croupous and Septic forms. Of the Therapeutics of each of these I will speak separately.

---

* Dr. Oehme has recently given us a "Complication and Critical Review" of the German and American literature on the subject, which is well-executed and very useful for reference.

1. In the treatment of SIMPLE DIPHTHERIA, where **Catarrhal Angina** is the sole mischief set up by the poison, *Belladonna* and *Phytolacca* seem to me to be the only medicines required.

Belladonna deserves, I think, a freer use than it has yet received. It is precisely Homœopathic to the Pathological condition of the throat as Oertal describes it, and to the general febrile state. I always commence the treatment with this medicine in the first dilution, and have seen mild symptoms almost immediately, and pretty severe ones rapidly disappear under its use. If, however, decided improvement has not resulted within forty-eight hours of commencing its employment, there is no advantage in persevering with it. If, moreover (as sometimes happens), the deposit disappears at first under the influence of the remedy, but subsequently returns, it should not be continued.

Phytolacca is an addition of real value from the indigenous flora of America to our Anti-Diphtheritic remedies. In considering this drug in my 'Pharmacodynamics' I have endeavoured to establish its true place in the treatment of the disease. It is indicated when the local inflammation is not so acute as in the *Belladonna* cases, but when the general fever is higher, and accompanied with severe aching in the head, back and limbs. Under these circumstances it will act in a truly specific manner.*

2. The term "CROUPAL" was given to the second variety of Diphtheria to signify its invasion of the larynx. Oertel, however, means by "Croupous" a more intense inflammation of the throat than obtains in the Catarrhal form,—the fibrinous exudation of which may and often does invade the air-passages, but even without doing so is a morbid condition of very serious moment. The medicines for this variety of Diphtheria are *Apis, Cantharis*, certain *Mercurial* preparations, *Kali bichromicum*, and *Bromine*.

a. A lower type of inflammation (as shown by a more purple colour of the parts) and much greater œdema are the first signs of the supervention of the Croupous upon the Catarrhal form of Diphtheria, or of its primary onset. **Apis** thus naturally takes the place of *Belladonna* in its treatment; and evidence has come from all sources since 1870 to its great efficacy. I have myself seen striking results from it, and commend it highly.

b. Bretonneau's comparison of Diphtheria to the effects of poisoning by the Spanish fly naturally led Homœopathic practitioners to use it as a remedy for the disease, the Albuminuria of both making the resemblance still more perfect. It hardly rewarded expectation, though Drs. Drysdale, Neidhard and Okie have had some success with it; and Drs. Ludlam and

---

* Another promising medicine for this form of Diphtheria is the *Tarentula cubensis*, of which I shall have to speak when I come to Erysipelas. Dr. W. T. Martin describes it as quite specific. He gives the potencies from 6 to 30 (HAHNEMANNIN MONTHLY, Sept., 1892).

Lawrence Newton have spoken highly of it for the subsequent prostration. I had never used it till 1876, when I had two successive cases in which the throat looked exactly as if it had been dabbed with blistering fluid, and the pain on swallowing was excessive. Here I conceived **Cantharis** to be indicated, and it served me well.

c. It was but natural, on the first glance being taken at the phenomena of Diphtheria, to treat it with **Mercury** in some form. With the ordinary preparations, however—*Mercurius solubilis* and *corrosivus,* and the *Red oxide,*—no advantage was gained. But a different story began to be told as the **Iodides** came into play. In this country Dr. Black with the *proto-iodide,* and Dr. Madden with the *bin-iodide,* obtained very encouraging results ; and our Transatlantic colleagues have followed suit. With one or other of these, in the lowest triturations, perhaps the majority of British and American Homœopathists treat Diphtheria. I have myself, like Drs. Meyhoffer, Drysdale and Neidhard, failed to see any decisive benefit from their action ; but I cannot ignore the results obtained by my colleagues. To obtain the full effect of the *Mercurial iodides* the triturations should have been recently prepared, and the dose should be placed dry in the mouth. The presence of much glandular swellings would of course be the most significant indication for them.

A still more important preparation of *Mercury* has later been introduced into the treatment of Diphtheria in **cyanide**. It was Dr. Beck, of Monthey-en-Valais, in Switzerland, who first inferred its Homœopathicity to the disease. He recommended it to Dr. Villers, of St. Petersburg, whose own son (now our colleague Dr. A. Villers, of Dresden) was lying hopelessly sick of Diphtheria. I have told you of the astonishing success which followed in this case, and in the immense majority of those treated with the drug in subsequent years, from his happy inference.

Mercurius cyanatus stands now at the head of Anti-Diphtheritic remedies in our school ; and has received no small commendation in the other.* I should tell you that Dr. Villers began with the 6th dilution, but has ended by preferring the 30th ; he thinks that where it has caused disappointment it has been by the lower potencies having been employed. Drs. Midgley Cash and Grubenman, who have published formidable cases saved by the remedy, obtained their success with similar dosage.

d. It is the presence of fibrinous exudation which call for **Kali bichromicum** here as elsewhere ; and where the thickness and tenacity of the false membrane are prominent symptoms it

---

* See HAHNEMANNIAN MONFHLY for May, 1877; J. B. H. S., iv., 383; vi. 301; and M. H. R..' xxviii., 377, xxxiii., 313.

† See Trans. of Intern. Hom. Congress of 1886, p. 191, and J. B. H., S., iii., 208.

acts exceedingly well. Drs. Dowling and Joslin of New York* esteem it highly when the throat itself is thus affected; but its great importance is that it follows the disease into the nose and the larynx, where it escapes other remedies. In Nasal Diphtheria I find it specific; in Laryngeal Diphtheria it does all that medicine can do, which unhappily is not much. Dr. Lord obtained good results here by administering inhalations of a weak solution of it, "whenever the cough became dry and respiration whistling and suffocation seemed imminent.

e. **Bromine** is the only rival of *Kali bichromicum,* unless *Hepar sulphuris* † is to be so accounted, when Diphtheria invades the larynx. I have told, when writing upon this drug, how highly Drs. Ozanam and Meyhoffer, two excellent authorities, esteem it as an Anti-Diphtheretic generaly. Its local action upon the exudate is considerable; so that, whether swallowed or inhaled, it may do good in this way also. Dr. Neidhard's experience with it in Laryngeal Diphtheria has not been favourable, and I may say the same of my own. Perhaps **Spongia** might supplement it here, as in Membranous Croup. Dr. Jousset narrates a well-marked case making a good recovery under the 1_x trituration. ‡

I think it an important suggestion of Dr. Neidhard's, that it is necessary to attack the poison in the blood even while, by the medicines specifically affecting the air-passages, you are combating its dangerous local manifestation. He usually administers the first trituration of the *Bichromate of Potash* alternately with his *Chloride of Lime*, and has recorded two instances in which this treatment proved successful. Similarly you might give the *Permanganate of Potash* with *Bromine.*

3. I have now to speak of MALIGNANT or SEPTIC DIPHTHERIA, that in which life is threatened from blood-poisoning. None of the remedies hitherto mentioned are applicable here, unless it be the *Cyanide of Mercury.* Looking beyond these, we have among the old stock of medicines *Muriatic acid* and *Lachesis,* and, as new and special Anti-Diphtheretics, *Carbolic acid,* the *Permanganate of Potash* and *Chlorinated Lime.*

a. **Muriatic acid** has, as I have mentioned when treating of that drug, much analogy and many testimonies § in its favour.

---

* See AMERICAN OBSERVER, xiii., 234, and UNITED STATES MED. INVESTIGATOR, iv., 120.

† See J. B. H. S., iv. 346.   ‡ L'ART MEDICAL, Sept., 1822.

§ To those mentioned in my 'Pharmacodynamies' I may add that of Dr. Neidhard, who citing a commendation of it from Dr. Borchers, of Bremen, writes : This corresponds with my own experience. Next to *Calc. chlor.* and *Kali bichrom.,* I have seen more beneficial effects from *Ac. mariat. del.* than from any other remedy."...I may also refer to a case of poisoning by the *acid* extracted in L'ART MEDICAL of August, 1900, which precisely simulated Diphtheria, even to its paretic SEQUELÆ.

I have found it of undoubted efficacy in the lesser degree of Toxæmia with which we sometimes meet.

b. **Lachesis** is indicated when the general prostration is quite out of proportion to the local mischief, and the subjective symptoms to the objective. The fauces are pale or livid. I have cited Dr. Carroll Dunham's favourable experience with the drug in such cases, and Dr. Oehme's collection will show you that he does not stand alone in this experience.

But quite a new ARMAMENTARIUM against Diphtheria was given us when the Antiseptics began to be used, not as local applications, but as internal medicines. The first to be employed was the *Permanganate of Potash.*

c. **Kali manganicum.**—I have told how Dr. H. C. Allen's heroic proving of this drug showed its elective affinity for the throat, and with what success he used it—in about 1-12th grain doses—in the malignant cases which subsequently came under his care. Other practitioners, as shown by Dr. Neidhard, have had similar success.* As it is also a solvent of the false membrane, and destructive of its odour, it promises well as a remedy for septic forms of the disease.

d. **Calcaraea chlorinata** we owe as a remedy here—a purely empirical one, indeed, at present—to Dr. Neidhard. His Treatise tells us how he was led to use it. His reasoning is not very conclusive to my mind, but his results are amply satisfactory. He states that he has "made almost exclusive use of it in Diphtheria during the last five years † in at least 300 cases," and that during this time he has had only two deaths from the disease. He puts from five to fifteen drops of the liquor *Calcis chlorinata* into half a tumblerful of water, and gives teaspoonful doses as frequently as the urgency of the symptoms demands.

e. **Carbolic acid** is highly commended (as Dr. Oehme shows) by Devidson and Bahr. The latter had for two years used nothing but this medicine, and out of twenty-eight cases (all having Fœtor Oris) had lost none.

So much for the specific medication of Diphtheria. But I need hardly say that with this, as with the cruder treatment of the old school, the general management of the patient is of immense importance. Amongst other things I have often verified the recommendation I first had from the late Dr. Hilbers to remove the patient from the house where the disease was incurred; and Dr. Bryce, of Edinburgh, has also borne testimony to the value of this practice. ‡ For adults and older children ice is very useful, but to young children the extreme

---

* See also UNITED STATES MED. INVESTIGATOR, ii., 18.
† His book was published in 1867.
‡ See M. H. R., xix., 992.

cold is repulsive. As to local applications, I have gone through three stages of opinion. At first I used them in every instance, but when I found all the very bad cases dying in spite of them and observed how much they added to the patient's distress, I abandoned them entirely. Now I adopt a middle course. In the *Belladonna* cases they are unnecessary. In those calling for *Phytolacca*, a gargle of the same drug is useful when there is much exudation; but only, I think, to clear it away the sooner. In Laryngeal Diphtheria gargling or pencilling the fauces is of course futile; but the *Bromine* or *Kali bichromicum* we are administering may advantageously be applied to the laryngo-tracheal membrane by inhalation or (better) spray. The only unquestionable value of local applications seems to me to appear when the false membrane is very foetid, especially if it is also abundant in quantity. Here it is likely that the system becomes secondarily re-infected by the throat deposit and it is undoubted that great temporary relief follows its removal. You may effect this, if you like, by a solvent of the membrane, as Lime-water or Glycerine; or you may follow Oertel's plan of imitating Nature's way of detaching the exudation, and promote suppuration beneath it by the frequent inhalation of hot steam. But seeing that there are no more powerful solvents and deodorisers of the Diphtheretic deposit than the three Antiseptics I have named, I would recommend that in all cases in which they are indicated as constitutional remedies they should also be used as gargles, or applied in the form of spray to the throat.* Dr. Oehme is inclined to explain by their local action the greater part of the benefit they have produced, for they have always been given in the lowest attenuations.

The Post-Diphtheritic Paralysis generally tends towards spontaneous recovery in pure air and with generous diet. I think, however, that I have seen **Gelsemium** of decided use in promoting it. In a long-standing and progressive case of General Spinal Paralysis and anæsthesia thus brought about, **Cocculus** proved in Dr. Trinks hands the curative medicine.†

In the foregoing suggestions as to the treatment of Cholera and Diphtheria, I have done little more than reduce what I had written in my 'Therapeutics' twenty-four years ago, only bringing down some of the items to the present day. Nor have I, in the case of Cholera, anything to add beyond what I have mentioned in my introductory remarks upon this whole class of disorders (Lecture XVI.). As regards Diphtheria, however, I must once more touch on the question already discussed there,—

---

* Dr. Goodno prefers blowing the Antiseptic in a dry form into the throat and nostrils. He uses a grain to the cunce trituration of the *Permanganate*.

† See B. J. H., xix., 312.—A paper on the Subject read before the British Homœopathic Society by Dr. Henry Bodman, with the discussion following, may be consulted with advantage (J. B. H. S., vii., 368).

are we justified in holding our hands from the now generally employed and much-vaunted Antitoxin?

And once more I must give the same answer: I think that, as a rule, we are. I say "as a rule," for I would make an exception in the case of Laryngeal Diphtheria. The power of the injected serum over the exudation is so decided, when it is employed early enough;* the need of preventing the larynx filling with false membrane is so great and urgent, that I would of the two risks run in preference to that of temporarily poisoning my patient's blood with Antitoxion. I have too vivid recollections of what Asphyxia means here to leave any stone unturned to prevent it. But with this exception, I say again with regard to Antitoxion, that we do not want it; and if it be unnecessary, it is hardly justifiable. Venesection undoubtedly diminishes congestion of the lungs; but if you can solicit (as by *Aconite*) the morbidly-determined blood into safer channels, the use of the lancet is forbidden to you. By the remedies I have described, you can do such gentle yet effectual work for the throat invaded with the Diphtheritic membrane; and should not, I submit, look to more violent and perturbing measures for help.

I am aware that in so speaking I am going against the judgment of valued colleagues, I have little doubt, moreover, that to those who hear me it will seem hard to be urged to refrain from a medication which has conquered—it is supposed —the whole medical world. I venture to think, however that with the former the glamour of rapid results has had a bewitching but illegitimate influence; and that the latter are hardly aware of the weight of evidence, testimony and reasoning on the other sides. The counter-case has been presented by Dr. R. N. Tooker of Chicago, and in the "summary" affixed to the JOURNAL of the British Homœopathic Society for the last five years (Art. "Antitoxin"). By reference to these sources you will see that the reduction in mortality effected by the use of the Serum has to be discounted at two ends: first, it is obtained by classing (for the sake of early treatment) a variety of Anginæ as Diphtheritic, which formerly would not have been so rockoned and secondly, the gain has nearly always been upon a previous rate which can only be termed monstrous—running to 50 and even 60 per cent. That this should be reduced to 40 or even less, tells not so much in favour of the new treatment as in derogation of the old—which must have been simply murderous. When, as in Mr. Lennox Browne's cases, the mortality was moderate before, it was little influenced by the change. The figure it remained at was 26 per cent. Dr. Tooker collected

---

* See statistics in J. B. H. S., v., 390; L. H. H. R., vi., 93.

† "The Present Status of Diphtheria Antitoxin at home and abroad", Chicago, 1896.

the experience of Homœopathists over a given area, and obtained reports of 315 cases treated (in 1895) purely Homœopathically with a mortality of 7.3 per cent.

I have last to speak of

INFLUENZA.—In my 'Therapeutics' I discussed this malady among those of the respiratory organs, assuming that it was present when a severe fluent Coryza was accompanied by Headache, pains in the limbs and great prostration, and advised *Arsenicum* and *Eupatorium perfoliatum* in its treatment. I expressed my suspicion, however, that such a condition was to true epidemic Influenza what English is to Asiatic Cholera, and advised consultation of the older Homœopathic writers for their experience in the visitations of the thirties and forties.

My suspicion was well-founded, and do not now speak as one to whom epidemic Influenza is unknown. The waves of it which since 1890 have passed over the world with almost unvarying annual persistency have made all practitioners familiar with its features, and have taught us much as to its nature and various manifestations. It is evidently an essential fever, as much so as Typhoid and Dengue, to which last it presents many points of resemblance, especially in its characteristic pains of head and limbs. Catarrh, nasal and bronchial, is (contrary to our former notions) a secondary and incidental occurrence only. When it does set in, however, it is very apt to run down the air tubes into the cells, and to set up a low diffuse Broncho-Pneumonia, which in aged persons and broken constitutions readily proves fatal.

As regards treatment, Homœopathy has nothing to blush for. While our old-school friends were deafening their patients with *Quinine* or overpowering their vitality with *Antipyrin*, and yet the effect on the death rate was (as in former epidemics) greater than that of Cholera, our mortality has been very small. At the British Congress of 1891 Mr. Harris produced statistical returns from 82 of our practitioners, which showed a total of some 15,000 cases with 73 deaths, *i.e.*, hardly five in the thousand. You will wish to know (as the malady is still with us) how such success has been obtained.

The Influenzal pyrexia is, as I have said, a primary one, as essential as that of Measles and Typhoid. It is not symptomatic of a local inflammation; nor is it a mere disturbance of heat-formation and heat-loss such as chill can produce. It may unquestionably be communicated from person to person (though I doubt whether this is its invariable, or even its ordinary mode of propagation); and, with whatever individual difference, it "breeds true," producing its like and nothing else. It must thus be no longer classed among the diseases of the respiratory organs, but must take rank as a specific infectious fever. And this is no matter of Nosology only. The kind of remedies we employ for the latter group of maladies differs from those suitable for the former; we shall think less readily of *Aconite* and *Arsenicum*, and more so of *Gelsemium*, *Belladonna* and *Baptisia*. According to the form the fever assumes we should administer one or other of our well-tried Antipyretics—*Aconite, Gelsemium, Belladonna* or *Baptisia*.

Aconite is, as I have said, less suitable in such fever than in one resulting from cold; nevertheless, when it is indicated by the symptoms it will do good service as it does for instance, in Measles. The sthenic character of the pyrexia, the fulness with quickness of the pulse, and the presence of thirst, restlessness and distress, are the well-known indications for it, and may be trustfully followed. This only must be said, that it is not to be expected of *Aconite* that it shall act here as it does in a fever from a chill, breaking it up in a few hours. We have a blood affection to deal with, which will have a certain course; and as in Measles, we must give the remedy persistently for two or three days, awaiting the resolution of the pyrexia, which, however, it is all the while moderating and soothing.

Gelsemium takes the place of *Aconite* when the fever is less sthenic and chills mingle frequently with the heat; when the pulse, though it may be full, is less tense and rapid; when there is little thirst; and when the patient's general condition is one rather of tropor and apathy.

Belladonna, standing at the head of our remedies for the infectious fevers, plays its part well here when the symptoms demand it. These include a pulse smaller but even more rapid than that of *Aconite,* and a dry hot skin; but they are chiefly to be found in the head and tongue. Dryness of the latter, heat and pain (with flushed face) of the former, call unmistakably for it; and when they are present we need hardly look further for our remedy.

Baptisia, coming here crowned with its laurels in the "Gastric" type of Continued Fevers, just fills the vacant niche when such symptoms characterise the Influenzal pyrexia. A gastro-intestinal form of the disorder was noted by the early observers, and has recurred in the present epidemic, as may be seen in the Article upon Influenza in the New Edition of Quain's 'DICTIONARY OF MEDICINE.' When the tongue is thickly coated: when there is nausea and vomiting; and when the stools tend to be Diarrhœic —especially if also fœtid, *Baptisia,* already suited to the pyrexia, becomes so to the whole condition, and will change it for the better more rapidly than any other medicine.

The Homœopathicity of the above indications I have thought it unnecessary to argue; it is pretty obvious. They are given, however, from experience, and I can vouch for them practically. It has seemed to me that when they led me to *Gelsemium, Belladonna* or *Baptisia,* the response to the remedy was more prompt and decided, than when *Aconite* was called for. That is the only reservation I would make about their efficacy as a whole. I have always, I should say, given these drugs in the lowest (1x and 2x) dilutions.

In the steady use of the suitable antipyretic, with proper nursing and dieting, the treatment of Influenza mainly consists. I must say something, however, as regards its local manifestations, occasional complications and sequelæ.

1. More or less pain of Rheumatoid character, in head, back and limbs, nearly always accompanies the Influenzal fever. When *Belladonna* is indicated for the latter, it is sufficient for the headache, and when *Gelsemium* or *Baptisia* is given they are so suitable for the general pains that it is hardly necessary to think of any other medicine. In *Aconite* cases, however, and where the local distress is unusually severe, I have found **Bryonia** very helpful to the head* and **Eupatorium perfoliatum** to the back and limbs.

2. The catarrh of Influenza is sometimes sufficiently severe to demand an intercurrent remedy. When it is a simple Coryza, **Euphrasia** if the discharge is bland, and **Arsenicum** if it is acrid, served me well in the first, fluent stage; and **Pulsatilla** after it has become thick and opaque. When the catarrh is laryngo-tracheal, and shown mainly by a cough, **Spongia** I have found the most trustworthy drug. *Rumex* and *Sticta* have hardly

---

* When the tongue has the bluish-white appearance sometimes seen in this malady, *Gymnocladus*—which has caused something like it—will act well on the headache. (See L. H. S., iv., 334; viii., 253; iv., 100).

sustained their previous credit in my estimation when the cough which seemed to indicate them was of Influenza origin; and when this lingers on after the fever is over, and the patient otherwise convalescent, it needs careful individualisation to find its effective remedy. Sometimes this is found in **Senega**, sometimes in **Nitric acid**, sometimes in **Coccus cacti**. In one case I could do nothing for the cough, which was hard and dry, until I had softened it with *Aconite* (3x),—*Belladonna* having been the Antipyretic. It then speedily subsided.

3. The Bronchitis and Pneumonia of the present malady are —the latter especially—more serious matters. Bronchitis has not been frequent in the cases I have had to treat; when it has appeared, **Kali bichromicum** in the first stage, and **Antimonium tartaricum** in that of profuse and thick secretion which soon follows, have done good service in my hands. The Pneumonia I have often seen, and have good cause to dread it. In old and broken constitutions, as I have said, it threatens life; and in more favourable subjects it is apt to drag on a tedious course, little influenced by remedies. It is, I think, a just remark of the writer of the Article "Influenza" in Quain's DICTIONARY, that its Pneumonia, "though lobar in distribution, is probably always catarrhal in type"; and this is an important indication for treatment. In the acute and menacing form, *Bryonia* and *Iodine* have little place, while **Phosphorus** stands supreme. If any medicine can subdue the inflammation of the pulmonary tissue, it is this. It should only be replaced by **Antimonium tartaricum** when pain, dulness on percussion and bronchial breathing have subsided; when pulse, respiration and temperature have fallen; but when yet the chest is full of moist sounds and the patient is oppressed and distressed. In the sub-acute form, the physical condition suggests the term œdema of the lung rather than inflammation. There is little fever or pain, and but slight evidence (if any) of consolidation; and though crepitation is pronounced, the sputum is not rust-coloured. I wish I could speak decidedly of remedial results obtained here; but truth compels me to say that though the patients have got well, I cannot claim that it is owing to anything I have given them. I have not tried the *Iodide of Arsenic*, so warmly commended by some of our collegues.*

4. The debility remaining behind after the acute attack is over, demands medicinal, as well as hygienic and dietetic help. The great "tonic" for it I find to be **Phosphorus**.† The nervous system is its main seat; and there has not been such a drain of fluid as should call for *China*, nor is there evidence of the

---

* See J. B. H. S., vi., 230, 240-1.

† I am bound to notice, however, the commendation bestowed by Dr. Cortier on *Avena sativa* here (L'ART MEDICAL, Oct., 1896). Dr. Proctor finds *Iberis* valuable when the debility most affects the heart (H. W., Nov., 1900).

destruction of red corpuscles which needs *Arsenicum*. A further indication for the remedy is that which is mentioned in the Article from which I have already quoted:—"The morbid changes found after death, and due to Influenza itself, are of a character due to all forms of acute infective disease—namely, parenchymatous degeneration of the liver, kidneys and spleen, of the muscular substance of the heart, and of the minute blood-vessels." A minor degree of such degeneration may fairly be conceived as present in the often extreme debility of convalescents from from the disease. *Phosphorus* is the chief poison whose POST-MORTEM appearances belong to the category: the Law of Similars therefore guides us to it, as the chief medicine to aid in repairing the destruction which has been wrought.

In so speaking, I have confined myself to my own personal experience, which has been fairly extensive. I find, however, similar remedies in use at the hands of those who have written on the subject both at home and abroad. Dr. Grundal, of Stockholm, prefers **Rhus** as the constitutional remedy, deeming it as specific as *Mercury* in Syphilis. He gives the 2 dilution.*

---

* HAHN. MONTHLY, Aug., 1894, p. 543

LECTURE XXI.

GENERAL DISEASES

---o---

THE BLOOD-INFECTIONS & ARTHRITIC AFFECTIONS

---o---

ERYSIPELAS—PHAGEDÆNA—MALIGNANT PUSTULE—
GLANDERS—PYÆMIA—SEPTICÆMIA—ACTINO-MYCOSIS.
GOUT—RHEUMATISM—RHEUMATIC GOUT—GONNOR-
RHŒAL RHEUMATISM

Hitherto I have followed, with but slight variation, the order of our official Nosology. But I am unable to do so with the remainder of the eighty titles it now ranks under the heading of "General Diseases." Most of them are so local in situation, or so limited to particular occasions or stages of life, that I think I shall consult your convenience as well as my own by considering them in other relations than the present. To-day I shall take first the BLOOD-INFECTIONS—ERYSIPELAS; PHAGEDÆNA; MALIGNANT PUSTULES; PYÆMIA and SEPTICÆMIA; ACTINO-MYCOUSIS; and GLANDERS, with FARCY and GREASE.

ERYSIPELAS used to be reckoned, in our Nomenclature, as including phlegmonous inflammation of the integument as well as superficial, and also diffuse Cellulitis. The former inclusion is I think, Pathologically justifiable, and has been maintained; the latter is wisely dropped. We shall speak, then, of simple and of Phlegmonous Erysipelas.

1. The treatment of SIMPLE ERYSIPELAS is one of the most defined and most successful things we have in Homœopathy. It resolves itself into the discriminate use of three medicines—*Belladonna, Apis* and *Rhus*.

The pathogenetic power of **Belladonna** to inflame the skin is unquestionable; you may see it illustrated in numerous symptoms of the "FACE AND SKIN categories of my arrangement of the drug in Part III of the Hahnemann Materia Medica." Of its curative power I cannot speak better than in the words of one who must have had abundant opportunity of comparing its effects with the treatment of Erysipelas by other measures; I mean the distinguished surgeon, Mr. Liston. After detailing some cases of the disease, cured mainly with fractional doses of the extract of *Belladonna*, he said to his students,* "Of course we cannot pretend to say positively in what way this effect is produced, but it seems almost to act by magic. You know that this medicine is recommended by Homœopathists in this affection, because it produces on the skin a fiery eruption or efflorescence, accompanied by inflammatory fever. SIMILIA SIMILIBUS CURANTUR, say they . . . . The medicines in the above cases were certainly given in much smaller doses than have hitherto ever been prescribed; the beneficial effects; as you witnessed, were unquestionable. I have, however, seen similar good effects from the *Belladonna* prepared according to the Homœopathic Pharmacopœia, in a case of very severe Erysipelas of the head and face, under the care of my friend Dr. Quin. The inflammatory symptoms and local signs disappeared with very great rapidity." All Homœopathists are unanimous in parising *Belladonna* where the Dermatitis is intense; nor should the presence of a few vesicles or of some amount of swelling be supposed to render other medicines preferable, as long as the colour of the affected part is bright red and the general fever high. But should œdema become the prominent feature of the local inflammation, or should phlyctenæ form in abundance and the skin be purplish, it is generally allowed that **Apis** or **Rhus** must become its substitute respectively. Of the efficacy of *Apis* you may read some good examples from Dr. Yeldham's pen in the Twelfth Volume of the BRITISH JOURNAL OF HOMOEOPATHY.

2. In PHLEGMONOUS ERYSIPELAS our first reliance must be on **Aconite**. Here, too, we can quote old school authority in support of our practice. "Administered at the commencement," says Dr. Ringer, "it often at once cuts short the attack; and even when the disease continues in spite of it, it will reduce the swelling and hardness, lessen the redness, and prevent the inflammation from speading." Should the cutaneous inflammation be considerable, *Belladonna*, or perhaps *Ferrum phosphoricum*,† may be alternated with it. If, in spite of these remedies, the Cellulitis threatens suppuration, it is—as Bahr says—useless to try to check the process by *Mercurius;* it is better to promote it with **Hepar sulphuris**, holding **Silicea** in reserve to limit it if excessive. I need not say that Surgical measures must be employed as far as may be necessary. Should Gangrene occur, **Lachesis** is the specific remedy; but *Arsenicum* may be required for the Typhoid condition which will ensue.

Thus far I have spoken of Erysipelas as it ordinarily occurs; but I have now to mention some special varieties, complications and squelæ which belong to it.

---

* See LANCET, April 13, 1836.
† See J. B. H. S., v., 195. Another alternative would be the *Tarentula cubensis*, the bite of which spider causes a phlegmonous inflammation, and which has been used with good effect in Carbuncle.

When Erysipelas of the head invades the brain, the **Belladonna** we shall probably be giving for the cutaneous eruption will ordinarily answer every purpose. If, however, *Rhus* should be the remedy for the condition of the surface, **Stramonium** may better suit the delirium; as in a case recorded in the REVUE HOMOEOPATHIQUE BELGE for December, 1876. If the cerebral symptoms are those of oppression, especially when the hyperæmia of the skin has diminished, *Cuprum*—as recommended by Jahr—should be preferred. For Erysipelatous angina, with its threatenings of Œdema Glottidis, *Apis* is an excellent medicine. There is a wandering Erysipelas in which the Dermatitis springs from place to place discontinuously. Bahr and Jahr agree in praising **Graphites** here; the latter adds **Arsenicum** where there is much prostration of strength. Bahr speaks of "Erysipelatous attacks without fever," and says that *Lycopodium* and *Hepar sulphuris* take the place of *Belladonna* and *Rhus* when they occur. He praises the same remedies for the œdema which is sometimes left behind by the disease, when this is often painful; giving *Graphites, Sulphur,* and *Aurum* when it is not so. Recurrent Erysipelas is generally amenable to *Rhus*.

As regards local applications designed to check the progress of the Dermatitis, I can say nothing about the *Nitrate of Silver* and *Sulphate of Iron* in use in ordinary practice; but I may mention that Dr. Garth Wilkinson speaks of obtaining excellent results, from the application of the tincture of *Veratrum viride*, and that Dr. Bays testifies to the same success with a strong lotion of this drug.

PHAGEDÆNA is said to embrace two varieties—"SLOUGH-PHAGEDÆNA" and "HOSPITAL GANGRENE." It may be defined as a morbid change, probably of constitutional origin, occurring in an ulcer or a wound whereby destructive process are set up threatening the death of the part and often of the patient. It was most familiar of old in its nosocomial form; now it chiefly comes before us as an incident of Soft Chancre. In the latter case anti-Syphilitics are sometimes required, and we must leave the question of its treatment till we come to Venereal Disease. But when sloughing sets in upon a non-venereal ulcer, or when the so-called "Traumatic Gangrene" supervenes upon an injury let me recommend you to rely for medication upon **Lachesis**. The references given in my 'Pharmcodynamics' will shew you that in the treatment of the latter trouble it has proved an invaluable ally.*

MALIGNANT PUSTULE, when communicated by direct inoculation, doubtless demands the early excision or cauterization of the affected part. The success attendant upon this measure is too great and constant to justify its neglect. But if the virus has been otherwise introduced into the system, or if the patient is seen too late for local measures to be of any avail, the symptoms are so like those of the Traumatic Gangrene and other blood-poisonings from infected spots in which **Lachesis** has proved the specific remedy, that its administration would be strongly indicated. Indeed, Dr. Carrol Dunham has already used it with the utmost success in an American outburst of the disease, as he thus relates† : —

"In the year 1853 there prevailed quite extensively in Brooklyn an epidemic of what was called 'Malignant Pustule.' A furuncular formation appeared, generally upon the lower lip, attended with severe pain, and frequently surrounded by an Erysipelatous areola. The most marked constitutional symptom was a very rapid and excessive loss of strength, the patient being reduced from vigor to absolute prostration within the space of twenty-four to thirty-six hours. Allopathic physicians at first resorted to the local application of *Nitrate of Silver* to the Pustule. In those cases, thus treated, which came under my personal observation, death followed cauterization within twenty-four hours.

"In eight cases treated by myself, *Lachesis* was the only remedy used. It relieved the pain within a few hours after the first dose was given, and the patients all recovered very speedily."

GALENDERS, "EQUINIA," when occurring in its acute form in the human subject, is so constantly fatal that to cure it would be a triumph indeed. I do not know, that such success has ever been claimed for Homœopathy. Bahr and Jahr do not mention the disease, and Jousset speaks of its remedies theoretically only. He recommends *Aconite* and *Arsenicum*. My own study of the disease, as described in books (for I have no practical knowledge of it), would lead me to suggest **Kali bichromicum, Mercurius** and **Crotalus** as its most promising remedies. The first-named is exquisitely Homœopathic to the respiratory—especially the nasal—affections of the desease, and hardly less so to its cutaneous phenomena, as may be seen on reading the "Skin" section of

---

* Four cases of "Gangrene" various in origin, are reported by Dr. Lambreghts in the JOURNAL BELGE D' HOMŒOPATHIC for July-August, 1897. In all *Lachesis* 6 was markedly curative.
† AMERICAN HOM. REVIEW, iv., 110.

Dr. Drysdale's arrangement of the drug in the "Materia Medica, Physiological and Applied." Mr. Moore speaks of having effected unequivocal cures of Glanders in the horse mainly by its use. *Mercurius* would be preferable when the purulent tendency was more pronounced, and the lymphatic glands were primarily affected—forming the "Farcy-buds" of the veterinarian. But I should be disposed to supplement either of these medicines with one more capable of dealing with the septic condition of the blood which is always present; and this, for the reasons assigned when speaking of the *Serpent-poisons*, I should hope to find in *Crotalus*. This medicine, or *Lachesis*, would be indicated as the sole remedy where malignant symptoms—as black bullæ and tendency to Gangrene—appeared.

The "GREASE" of horses, as occasionally communicated to man, used to be mentioned in our nosology as a distinctive disease, under the name of "Equinia Mitis." It seems to be analogous, if not identical, with the Vaccinia of cows. **Thuja** has proved specific for it in the horse, and might be equally useful in the human subject. The "foot-and-mouth disease," of which at one time we heard so much, is also undoubtedly communicable to man, even through drinking the (unboiled) milk of infected cows. It seems to be an Aphthous Stomatitis, conjoined with a vesicular eruption on the hands and feet, and accompanied by some fever. **Mercurius,** with or without *Aconite*, would seem its most suitable remedy.

In dealing with—
PYÆMIA, I have hitherto been in the habit of basing my suggestions on the conclusions arrived at by Dr. Bristow, in his Article upon it in Russel Reyonlds' "SYSTEM OF MEDICINE.": —

"1. Pyæmia is almost invariable, if not ayways, preceded by some local suppuration, and this of an Erysipelatous, Gangrenous, or otherwise unhealthy sort.

"2. The link between the local mischief and the constitutional infection is most frequently the inflammation of the veins of the part affected, but may be simply absorption of unhealthy ichor.

"3. The local lesicns which characterize Pyæmia are congestions, extravasations of blood, inflammatory deposits, Abscesses, and Necrosis. These are generally, if not always, the result of blocking up of small arteries either by 'cmboli' detached from the veins primarily affected, or by 'thrombi' formed within the artery by the unhealthy blood. To the 'Ichorrhœmia' itself are due certain diffused inflammatory procasses (as inflammation of the joints and of serous surfaces) for which arterial obstruction will not account.

"4. The constitutional symptoms of purulent infection are rigors followed by sweating, a Typhoid condition, quick and weak pulse, Jaundice, early prostration, and generally death. The Jaundice is not dependent on any appreciable affection of the liver. When the disease takes a more chronic course the symptoms are those of hectic."

I gave there details to show the warrant I had for saying that *Lachesis* is the most promising remedy we possess for this condition also. The phenomena, local and general, which follow the serpent's bite lead us to expect that when a local affection assumes a malignant character, and from thence proceed poisoning of the blood and prostration of the nervous energies, there *Lachesis* will be Homœopathic and curative. Now this is just what we have in Pyæmia, if Pyæmia is to be taken as including all the phenomena Dr. Bristowe has enumerated. The tendency of later Pathology, however, as endorsed by our official Nosology, is to divide such non-specific blood-infections into two classes, SEPTICAEMIA and PYAEMIA, including under the first head that which Dr. Bristowe calls "Ichorrhæmia." A valuable paper on the two maladies, from the pen of Dr. Helmuth, may be found in the Transactions of the American Institute for 1884. Septicæmia, he argues, may be set up by any virulent matter however introduced into the system; it is the ordinary "Blood-Poisoning": while Pyæmia always results from the absorption of decomposing pus. The virus of the former, if of local origin, is carried by the lymphatics; that of the latter by the veins. The one has a single chill, and the other many; the fever of the one is irregular, that of the other recurs in periodical paroxysms. Septicæmia has not the infractions, the multiple Abscesses, the Jaundice, or the sweet odour of the breath, characteristic of Pyæmia.

When we thus isolate Pyæmia from its allied conditions, the *Serpent-poisons* seem less applicable to it, unless it be *Crotalus* which has its icteric phenomena.* **Quinine,** is highly esteemed in the old-school treatment of this affection, and Dr. Jousset (who invokes a "purulent diathesis" to account for its features) gives the same medicine and doses, a gramme after each paroxysm, when chills return regularly,—in the absence of this indication relying on *Aconite* and *Arsenicum.* Kafka likewise commends *Quinine* for true Pyæmia; but finds the I_x trituration sufficient. If the prostration is great, he substitutes the **Chininum arsenicosum,** of equal strength.

These are our only authors who handled the subject from a Homœopatnic standpoint, Dr. Helmuth, though praising *Arsenicum* and *Muriatic acid* for subsequent prostration, gives *Phenic acid* in full doses as an Antiseptic. Dr. Gilchrist, while distinguishing Pyæmia from Septicæmia, and justly criticising my recommendation of *Lachesis* in the former, has little to say as to its true remedies. Jahr, after narrating two fatal cases among the wounded during the Insurrection of 1832 in Paris writes:—"In the meantime we became acquainted with Thorer's report on the curative virtues of *Calendula,* and by using this drug we prevented suppuration, and saved all our

---

* Dr. Charles Hayward has reported a case in which *Crotalus* was of marked service (J. B. H. S., iii., 379).

wounded." Grauvogl points in the same direction when, reviving former traditions, he extols the power of *Arnica* to promote the rapid healing of wounds, and to obviate any tendency to purulent infection.* Dr. T. G. Stonham, however, thinks we have a truly Homœopathic medicine for Pyæmia in *Mercurius cyanatus,* which he gives here (as in Diphtheria) in the 30th dilution. He relates two good cases in point.†

In CHRONIC PYAEMIA, with Hectic, the place of *Quinine* would be taken by **China**; and therewith might be conjoined **Silicea,** whose great constitutional power over suppuration would then come into play.

And now for
SEPTICAEMIA as a distinct malady. It is here that my argument from the effects of a serpent's bite acquires validity, and **Lachesis** stands out as pre-eminent among our medicines for the condition. I have already spoken of the proved value of the remedy in Malignant Pustule and Traumatic Gangrene, and these are just the kind of local affection which induces Septicæmia. It is especially effectual when this results from dissecting-wound. Dr. Dunham relates a case occurring in his own person, where the 12th dilution was employed with rapid effect, though both the local and the general symptoms were severe. This was in 1850, and forty-two years later Dr. Edward Madden (as I have mentioned) recorded ‡ a similar case, where the action of *Lachesis* 4 in checking the morbid process was equally striking. How many lives it has saved in the interval, who shall say?

Rhus is an alternative medicine, and one which may be found sufficient in less pronounced cases. Dr. Helmuth, in the Fourth Edition of his System of Surgery (1879), relates an instance of *Rhus*-poisoning coming under his notice where the symptoms were distinctly Septicæmic, and recommends it accordingly as a remedy. Dr. George Royal has verified this suggestion in two cases, one showing the prophylactic, one the curative powers of the drug; and Dr. C. W. Eaton follows with a case of Laparotomy in which septic Peritonitis seemed inevitable, but under *Rhus* all went on in perfectly normal order.§

Two new candidates for notice as remedies for Septic Fevers have appeared of late years in *Pyrogenium* and *Echinacea.*

Pyrogenium was introduced by Dr. Drysdale as far back as 1880. He was struck by the fever-exciting power exerted by the "Sepsin" of Panum, the "Pyrogen" of Burdon-Sanderson, which was the toxin formed by the bacteria of putrefaction.

---

* See B. J. H., xxxiv., 731. In his Textbook (i., 332) he advises *Arsenicum* to be given in conjunction with *Arnica.*
† J. B. H. S., ii., 263.   ‡ M. H. R., xx::vi., 211.   § J. B. H. S., iii., 200, 330,

He inferred that it must also be febrifuge, if only we would define the pyrexiæ to which it was suitable; and, reasoning somewhat isopathically, concluded that this was such as obtained in Septicæmia after wounds, and in the Toxæmic Fevers generally. "The most summary indication for *Pyrogen* would be," he wrote, "to term it the *Aconite* of Typhous or Typhoid quality of pyrexia." He proceeded to act on this inference, and published a Paper embodying his views and results in the BRITISH JOURNAL OF HOMOEOPATHY of that year (p. 140).

Partly from the spoiling of one of his preparations, and partly perhaps from giving the remedy in too low dilution, he was discouraged from proceeding further; but in 1855 his thought was taken up by Dr. Burnett. In his Pamphlet on "Fevers and Blood-Poisoning and their Treatment, with special reference to the use of *Pyrogenium*" (1888) he tells us how he was led to test the remedy, preparing it after Drysdale's fashion, but giving it in the 6th dilution. The result of his experience (some of which he relates) was to assure him that *Pyrogenium* indeed fills the vacant place of a remedy which acts on the Toxæmic Fevers as effectively as *Aconite* on those of the "Inflammatory" type.

Dr. Drysdale now returned to the subject, and shewed by cases that his experience had not been so unsatisfactory as appearances suggested, while he acknowledged that Dr. Burnett's success with the 6th dilution had gone beyond anything he had attained with the 1st. In his Paper (which appeared in the MONTHLY HOMOEOPATHIC REVIEW of, July 1888) he gave a case of Typhoid by Dr. Hayward, in which the drug had acted well. Dr. Burnett, in his Pamphlet, had published some confirmatory experience from Dr. Shuldham; and in the INDIAN HOMOEOPATHIC REVIEW of November—December, 1896, Dr. Majumdar relates two cases of Puerperal Fever in which Burnett's preparation had proved very effiacious.

Echinacea angustifolia is the "narrow-leafed cone flower" or "Black Samson." In the NORTH AMERICAN JOURNAL OF HOMOEOPATHY for December, 1896, Dr. C. F. Otis wrote to commend it as remedial in Malignant Scarlatina and Diphtheria, especially where black coating of the tongue is present. He gives the mother-tincture. In the number for the next May, Dr. Swormsted confirmed the experience, extending the sphere of the drug to septic conditions generally. It was then proved, and found to cause great prostration, erythema of the face and neck, a marked Trigeminal Neuralgia, and general febrile symptoms. [*] There is something here which bids fair to reward further testing.

---

[*] J. B. H. S., v., 195, 286; vii., 84, 414; viii., 78.

ACTINO-MYCOSIS.—That it is of parasitic origin need not hinder our expecting benefit from dynamic medication. That it yields to such treatment is witnessed from other school itself. "*Iodide of Potassium,*" writes Mr. Malcolm Morris,* "is almost as certain a specific here as in Tertiary Syphilis. Its mode of action," he says, "is not clearly understood ; but it does not seem to kill or even injure the Actino-myces. Netter believes that the remedy has a specific action on the Anatomical elements, increasing their power of resistance. It causes rapid subsidence of the Tumours and Nodosities." Now it is just such nodular and tuberous masses which Mr. Hutchinson and others have observed as a result of the over-use of the *Iodide* in Syphilis. If you will read the records adduced by Mr. Knox Shaw, in Volume XXXV, of the MONTHLY HOMOEOPATHIC REVIEW, you will find a number of them. But above all, if you will compare the plate by which Mr. Morris illustrates Actino-Mycosis of the lower jaw with those which Mr. Hutchinson, in the First Volume of his ARCHIVES OF SURGER, gives to exhibit the cutaneous effects of *Iodide of Potassium,* you can hardly fail to be struck with the resemblance. SIMILIA SIMILIBUS here takes outward shape, and appeals to all.†

I pass now to another group of General Diseases—to one which consists of affections very unlike those I have lately been discussing, in that they are largely chronic and not at all infectious. I speak of the ARTHRITIC AFFECTIONS, viz., : the various forms of GOUT and RHEUMATISM.

GOUT has had, so far as I am aware, until quite lately, no special Homœopathic Literature whatever. You will feel with me that this is somewhat ominous as respect our means of dealing with it. I must say that my own experience of the malady confirms this unfavourable impression, at least as regards the acute attack. I have tried all the remedies which seemed indicated or have been recommended—*Aconite, Ledum, Pulsatilla, Arnica, Bryonia, Sabina,* in various dilutions ; but have never been able to trace any decided effect to their use. The attack has seemed to subside in the usual time, or to run its protracted course of remissions and relapses, much as if Nature had been left to take Her course. If the author of "The Nullity of Homœopathy" had taken Gout for his theme, I fear that no answer could have been given to his charge. No response has been made to the challenge I sounded in 1869, ‡ urging my

---

* LANCET, June 6, 1896.

† Hallopeau, describing the skin-tumours caused by *Iodide of Potassium,* notes their resemblance to those of Mycosis; and another writer asks whether it is not possible that many supposed instances of Mycosis may be due to Iodism (J. B. H. S., v., 92).

‡ Manual of Therapeutics, 1st Ed.

colleagues, if they had had better success, to come forward and tell us how they had obtained it. A writer in an American Journal, indeed, found much fault with me for my contempt of our common remedies, but he hardly substantiated his confidence in them. Bahr seems to speak theoretically and at second-hand only, and admits that "the treatment of a single attack is always somewhat precarious." Jousset mentions some remedies—*China, Sabina, Arnica, Bryonia*—as indicated, but says nothing of their efficacy. An evening devoted to the subject at the British Homœopathic Society, moreover, gave very instructive results.* Dr. Vaughan-Hughes, the reader of the paper was enthusiastic about the value of "Homœopathic Treatment" in Gout; but the only case he brought forward seemed quite to justify Dr. Madden's criticism :—"He believed that the auxiliaries alone might be safely credited with all the improvement which took place while the patient was under observation. When we hear of carefully regulated diet, excluding the use of meat, of local applications of a solution of *Iodide of Potassium*, of hot baths with half a pound of pearl-ash in solution, &c., it is not difficult to account for the changes which took place in the patient's condition." Dr. Yeldham stated that he treats his cases of acute Gout with five-drop doses of the mother-tincture of *Colchicum* every four hours or oftener; and though Drs. Drury and Hale thought this a little too "Allopathic," yet they allowed the value of the drug, and had nothing better to recommend. Of the same purport is the therapeutic portion of Dr. Drysdale's most Philosophical discussion of Gout.† I shall refer to this anon : at present I will but quote a sentence:— "The proper clinical study of the disease can hardly be said to be begun; but we have merely the remedies supposed to be useful from the resemblance of a few symptoms copied from one handbook into another without sufficient verification, much in the style of the old-fashioned 'Materia Medica' which the Homœopathic school blames so much."

Under these circumstances I must recommend you to adhere to your *Colchicum*, whose power of giving relief is unquestionable. Moreover, although the associations of the medicine are Allopathic, its character is far more of the Homœopathic order. It is admitted now that its evacuant operation is needless to the obtaining of its soothing effects. Watson, indeed, calls it "an *Anodyne*"; but he must be speaking of the result of its administration, not of its MODUS OPERANDI. It has confessedly no stupefying power over the brain, or benumbing action on the nerves. It seems, therefore, to be one of those remedies which are classed as "specific," and I claim all such remedies for the school which inscribes "$o\mu oios$" as opposed to "$a\gamma\gamma oios$" on its portals.

---

* B. J. H., xxviii., 537,   † I bid., xxvi., 292

For so writing, as I did in 1877, I have been taken to task by Dr. Searle, of Brooklyn, in the HAHNEMANNIAN MONTHLY of June, 1894. In a reply I published in the No. of March, 1895, explained the exact tenor of my statement, which my friend had somewhat misquoted; but went on to adduce evidence in proof of the Homœopathicity of *Colchicum*. The question was does it inflame joints as the Gouty poison inflames them? When I first examined it, in the original issue of my 'Pharmacodynamics' (1867), I knew of no facts that supported an affirmative answer, and was compelled to the conclusion that *Colchicum* acted upon the affected joints "as a specific, indeed, but antipathic remedy, just as *Gelsemium* influences a painful uterus." But further evidence, I said, has since come to light. I pointed out that in Stoerck's experiment which forms No. 18c of the provings in the 'Cyclopædia of drug Pathogenesy', we read of "short lancinating pains in the joints"; and that in No. 9 of the poisoning cases the action was still more marked. "All joints of fingers and toes, and also wrists and ankles, were very painful, and toes and fingers were painfully flexed at times. Pain in shoulder-joints succeeded, and, later, in hips and loins. It also increased in intensity, so that she said she thought she should go mad. Ultimately almost all the bones and joints were affected with pains, which were of a gnawing, digging character." In No. 8 also, I said, where seventeen persons drank from a bottle of *Vinum Colchici*, "severe pains were felt in the knee-joints by some, and in two cases were very marked in the left shoulder." I forgot, however, when then writing—though I had myself brought them before the British Homœopathic Society 1888,*—the later experiments of M. M. Mairet and Combemale. These were made with *Colchicine* upon eight men, three dogs, and a cat. In the human provers dull pain was felt in the joints; and in the cat, which was killed as soon as the effects of the poison began to manifest themselves, an autopsy showed congestion of some of the articular surfaces and of the "moelle osseuse" (? medullary canal). The reporters were constrained to recognise (as I have already mentioned) that "*Colchicum* produces its therapeutic effects by an irritant action," and that "in Gout it produces a substitutive irritation of the articular surfaces." Dr. Frederick Roberts gives, as the latest word of science, that "it is by no means settled how it acts."† I would present "substitution" to him as an hypothesis at least in accord with the facts; and if it leads him to Homœopathy, nothing could be more legitimate, or more to his advantage.

I conclude, then, that *Colchicum* is a similar to Gouty Arthritis;

---

* See M. H. R., xxxii., 473.
† Quain's Dictionary, 2nd Ed., Art. "Gout".

and that it is at least as reasonable to maintain that it acts Homœopathically in the treatment of the same, as to believe (with Dr. Searle) that the depressant influence of the drug on the circulation is localised in the affected joints, whose inflammation it thus removes Antipathically. It is indeed unnecessary and hurtful to give such large doses as will produce this depressant or drastic result. The bad effects so often traced to its employment, and which led Trousseau to dissuade from this altogether in the paroxysm, are entirely averted by reduction of the dose. We want to give just as much as is necessary to subdue the local pain and inflammation, and no more. I cannot affirm that any "dilution," however low, answers this purpose, and Dr. Yeldham's recommendation of five drops of the mother-tincture every four hours comes with all the weight of his experience —with which my own, as far as it goes, coinsides.

I have dealt thus fully with this point because it is a weak one in our Therapeutics, and (as I think) needlessly so; because we make it weak by shrinking from *Colchicum*, as in another place we are afraid of using *Quinine* (p. 254). But here, as there, we are not limited to the one "specific" upon which traditional medicine has chanced, but have several others as allies or substitutes. Thus there is no reason why the paroxysm should not be checked in its "forming" stage by the aid, in addition to elimination and (if you like) chemical neutralisation of the superabundant *Lithic acid*, of such medicines as **Nux vomica** or **Pulsatilla**, one or other of which usually corresponds exactly to the symptoms present. Later, when chills and restlessness announce the impending inflammation, **Aconite** comes in with unquestionable benefit, and is sometimes indicated in alternation with *Colchicum* throughout the attack. When Gout in the foot follows immediately upon mechanical injury (and you know how slight a cause of that kind will sometimes set it up), **Arnica** ought to be primarily of service. Dr. Drysdale has well-pointed out that these medicines have no necessary relation to the essential QUALITATIVE disorder we call "Gout"; that they meet the QUANTITATIVE disturbances locally induced by it, and would do so just as well if these were not Gouty at all. He thinks (but I know not on what ground) that *Colchicum* has true qualitative similarity. Symptomatically, *Belladonna* would seem indicated, not only by the intense redness of the affected joint, but by its hypersensitiveness to any jar.*

A word as to local applications. We of course agree thoroughly in the deprecation of any of a depleting or repressive character. But if *Colchicum* were likely to be useful when locally applied, we should certainly use it; and we are thus open to the recommendation of *Iodide of Potassium* so strongly

---

* See J. B. H. S., iii., 206, 323.

made by Dr. Belcher.* The solution he uses is of the strength of one or two drachms of the drug to six ounces of water.

When you have got your patient through his acute attack, you have to combat the morbid diathesis whose existence it reveals. I need add nothing to what men like Watson and Garrod have written on the diet and regimen necessary for patients thus affected. I can only add my testimony to the paramount importance of this part of the treatment, and refer you to the able writings of our own Ackworth † as enforcing with abundant argument and illustration the same truth. As regards medicines, it is possible that symptomatic resemblance (where there are any symptoms comparison) may lead you to a real Anti-gouty remedy; and so a moderate use of this method is justifiable. Dr. Ackworth states that he has seen much benefit from the administration of **Sulphur**, and the frequent determination of the poison of the skin in the form of Psoriasis or Eczema adds force to recommendation.

We have yet remaining for consideration the treatment of "Chronic Gout," and of the local manifestations of "Larvaceous" and "Anomalous" Gout. I follow Trousseau in this Nomenclature. By Chronic Gout he means that form in which prolonged and extensive attacks follow upon one another with only partial remission; so that there is structural change in the joints, and the deposit of tophus. Can we do anything for this? I should have said—nothing, save the treatment of the diathesis as specified above, with *Sulphur* and perhaps (as Jousset recommends) **Lycopodium**. But the very striking case recorded by Dr. Hirschel, in Volume XXVII of the BRITISH JOURNAL OF HOMOEOPATHY (p. 667), when combined the with the testimony of Dr. Belcher already cited, leads us to hope that **Kali iodatum** may do much for us here. Dr. Hirschel gave doses from 1/3 to 3/4 of a grain. Wherever practicable, its local application, as in the acute paroxysm, should be conjoined.

"Larvaceous Gout" is said to be present when the disease appears as a Neurosis or Phlogosis, or other affection unlike the frank arthritic paroxysm. Some of these will come under consideration among local diseases. I may say here that once certain of the Gouty nature of an inflammation, you can combat it (as a rule) more effectually with *Colchicum* than with any other medicine we have. The angina and Ophthalmia are figured pretty plainly in its pathogenesis; as is also Pleurodynia which is sometimes (though rarely) Gouty. The Gouty origin of a Neuralgia would lead us to **Coloynth** and **Sulphur** for its remedies in preference to such Anti-neuralgics as *Arsenic* and *Belladonna*.

The visceral diseases of "Anomalous Gout," as its Bronchitis and renal degeneration, will come under notice in thier respective places. I will only add a word here as to "Gout in the

---

* M. H. R., xiii., 152. † B. J. H., xv., 177; xvii., 83. ANNALS, iv., 481.

stomach," which I apprehend to be, in almost every case, a Neurosis of the solar plexus. Its danger would then be analogous to that of a blow on the epigastrium, or the rapid drinking of cold water when heated—viz., inhibition of the heart's action conveyed along the splanchnic nerves. **Nux moschata** has some reputation in our school in the treatment of this alarming complication. I should be disposed to give it in doses large enough to produce its stimulating effects.

I may add what I have mentioned in my 'Pharmacodynamics,' that Hering says of *Benzoic acid*, that the more it is used in Gout the more it will be prized. The swelling of the fingers noted by Nusser, one of its provers, points in this direction; and Dr. Ord reports* four cases, of various forms, in which the strong odour of the urine led him to prescribe it, and with the best results. He seems to have used the 1_x solution

I will also refer to Dr. Burnett's short Treatise on "Gout and its Cure," which appeared in 1895. Its main contribution to the Therapeutics of the disease is the recommendation of **Urtica urens** in five or ten-drop doses, of the tincture, as an eliminator of the Uric acid from the system. I have had no experience with it; but our late colleague evidently esteemed it very highly.

RHEUMATISM occupies a very different place from Gout both in our literature and in our practice. We have some capital medicines for it; and numerous Monographs on the subject are scattered throughout our Journals.†

---

* M. H. R., xxxix., 308.

† See Black in B. J. H., xi., 216; M. H. R., xiv., 731; Henriques in B. J. H., xii., 35; Mackechnie in IBID., xxviii., 764; Madden in IBID., xxix., 372; Vaughan-Hughes in IBID., xxvii., 177; xxviii., 103. To these may be added Dr. Russell's Clinical Lectures, which include five on this disease; and the statistical accounts of the cases of Rheumatic Fever treated at the Leopoldstadt Hospital, in Vols. xi, xix and xxxii, of the BRITISH JOURNAL, and Vol. iv., of the ANNALS. I have myself treated largely of "Rheumatism and the Antirheumatics in two of my Boston lectures ("The Knowledge of the **Physician,** Lectures VII and VIII., and shall draw to some extent upon those studies here.

The general impression you will derive from looking over the writings of our school is a very favourable one, as far as the treatment of Acute Rheumatism ("Rheumatic Fever") is concerned. There is an almost uniform testimony borne to the power of Homœopathic treatment over the disease, and a nearly universal agreement as to its main remedies. Moreover, our statistics compare very favourably with those of the old school. There, as you know. first the alkaline plan had been proved greatly superior to all others in Acute Rheumatism, and then the results of pure "expectancy" appeared to be equally good with those of alkalisation. The conclusion was inevitable that the latter was so much useless drugging; while the other methods were positively injurious. Our method, therefore, has to be compared with the expectant; and the result is that we shorten the average duration of the disease by from six to ten days.

And now as to the means by which this result is to be obtained.

You will, in the great majority of cases, commence your treatment by the administration of **Aconite**. I have pointed out that this medicine is Homœopathic, not only to the fever, but also to the local affections induced by the Rheumatic poison. It should be given, therefore, as Dr. Madden states, not as a mere anti-febrile, but as a specific antidote to the whole condition present. The brilliant results reported from its use by Lombard and Fleming have been especially confirmed among ourselves; and, as their example suggests, the lowest dilutions have been found most efficacious.

When *Aconite* seems to have exhausted its force, the medicine to follow it is nearly always **Bryonia**. I agree with Dr. Russell that those two medicines, and probably these only, positively neutralise the Rheumatic poison in the blood. *Bryonia* corresponds to the inflamed joints, intolerant of movement; and to the Pneumonia and serous inflammations which threaten to supervene. It is not less suitable, moreover, when the muscles are affected rather than the joints. It enjoys good repute with the advocates alike of the low and of the high dilutions.*

The only other medicines you are likely to have to consider

---

* See Bayes' "Applied Homœopathy," SUB VOCE: the cases appended to the Austrian raproving (ŒSTERR ZEITSCHR, iii.); and M.H. R., xxxv., 531. The last reference is to some cases by Dr. Lamb, of Dunedin, N.Z., in which the 30th dilution was used with much success Dr. Lamb's results were curiously balanced by later ones (Vol. xxxix., p. 397 of the same Journal), which shew still more rapid cures from 8-drop doses of the tincture every 3 hours. At both these extremes our colonial colleague reports himself better pleased than when he adopted what he calls the "Homœo-orthodox treatment of Rheumatic Fever", viz., the use of *Aconite* and *Bryonia* 1x, the preference of which dilution (of the latter) he ascribes to me. I do not know, however, where I have made such recommendation.

in acute **Rheumatism** are *Pulsatilla, Colchicum, Rhus, Mercurius, Lycopodium* and *Sulphur.*

Pulsatilla is suitable—and even sometimes excludes both *Aconite* and *Bryonia* from the commencement—in sub-acute cases, of synovial type; with little fever, and frequent shifting of the mischief from joint to joint; especially when the patient's constitution and temperament are those characteristic of this remedy. Its relation to the digestive organs, moreover, would point to it as specially applicable when faulty assimilation rather than chill had evoked the disease.

If **Colchicum** benefits Gout because in health it irritates the articular structures, two consequences should follow: it should act directly on the affected joints, and have no power over the diathesis; and it should have a corresponding effect in Acute Rheumatism. Well: the former is generally admitted to be the fact, and latter was so by the older physicians, though now the remedy has dropped out of mind. Watson says that "the preparations of *Colchicum* have sometimes an almost magical effect in subduing the disease"; and the tradation has been preserved in Homœopathic practice. Dr. Goodno has collected more than eighty cases treated by a solution of Merk's *Colchicine* in the proportion of a grain to the ounce. Of this 5-10 drops were given for a dose. "Relief of pain follows in most cases within 24 hours, and within 48 hours the patient is generally comfortable, the swelling, fever, sweats, etc., much diminished. By the third or fourth day it is evident the case is throughly in hand. By the fifth to the seventh day it is difficult to keep the patient in bed."* Dr. Colby has communicated† an equally favourable experience in sub-acute cases. It is of course, he says, especially useful in Gouty subjects; but even apart from this is well-indicated when the inflammation attacks chiefly the hands and feet;' shows central tenderness on palpation, moderate swelling, and a pink blush; causes constant pain, increased during the prevalence of damp East winds, and especially before a storm; and gives the affected members a sense of Paralytic weakness. He prefers the *"Vinum"* of the British Pharmacopœia, and thinks that nothing is gained by attenuating it.

Mercurius takes the place of *Bryonia* when the inflammation is obstinate in any one joint, and when the pains are much worse at night. It is said to be indicated when profuse sour perspiration is present, which nevertheless affords no relief; but this is always so more or less in Acute Rheumatism.

Rhus is indicated in those rare cases where the fever tends to an adynamic type, with great restlessness, the patients (unlike

---

* See M. H. R., xxxvi., 56.
† N. ENGL., MED. GAZETTE., March, 1895.

those who call for *Bryonia*) constantly shifting their position, finding their pains increased by lying still for any time.

Lycopodium was introduced as strikingly beneficial in Acute Rheumatism by the late Dr. Allan Campbell, of Adelaide.* His experience has been verified by Mr. Wilkinson. Both gave it in the 3_x trituration.†

Sulphur is invaluable to prevent the lingering convalescence, or the passing of the disease into a Chronic form.

I must add two other remedies as truly applicable to Acute Articular Rheumatism, but only (so far as we know) when particular localities are affected. These are **Viola odorata** and **Caulophylum**. For the value of the former in Rheumatism affecting the wrists (especially the right one) we have the unimpeachable testimony of Tessier and Kitchen ;‡ and Dr. Ludlam has shown the latter to be as curative as Dr. Burt has shown it to be pathogenetic of Inflammatory Rheumatism of the hands and fingers.§

As regards the complications of Acute Rheumatism those of the heart must be separately discussed in their place. We need no longer inquire whether, by refusing the aid of alkalies, we are losing a comparative immunity from cardiac complications which otherwise we might obtain for our patients. The result of expectancy have dissipated this idea, which I confess that at one time I myself held. || The occurrence of other inflammations in the course of the fever need not lead us to change our *Aconite* and *Bryonia*. To Pleurisy, Pneumonia, and Peritonitis these grand medicines are as suitable as they are to the general Rheumatic condition itself. Nor if we give the first of them full play, need we (I think) fear to encounter the hyperpyrexia ever and anon occuring in ordinary practice, which seems to require the heroic remedy of cold bathing to avert a fatal issue. "Cerebral Rheumatism" is sometimes a Meningitis ; sometimes according to Trousseau, a Neurosis only. In the former case the remarks made as to other intercurrent inflammations apply ; in latter I have suggested **Actæa racemosa** as a probable remedy.

While thus we are treating our patients at large, there is nothing that I know of to prevent any local medication of the affected joints which may relieve or improve their condition. Most of us employ water-dressing (or, which I think better, dry cotton wool covered in with gutta-percha tissue) in the acute stage ; but, when there is great pain, I have seen so much benefit from the warm Alkyline-opiate epithems recommended by Fuller and Watson, that I should be sorry to deprive a sufferer of them.

---

* M. H. R., xxxvii.
† J. B. H. S., iv., 160. See also M. H. R., xxxiii., 319.
‡ See. B. J. H., xxiv., 314, § See Hale's "New Remedies", Sub Voce.
|| See Annals., iv., 214, 385; M. H. R., ix., 748.

In CHRONIC Rheumatism a much larger number of medicines have to be brought into play. There is here little or no Toxæmia; and we have to combat the Rheumatic poison in the sphere of the tissues or organs it has affected. *Bryonia, Rhus, Pulsatilla, Mercurius* and *Sulphur* continue to find place; but to them we must add *Rhododendron, Ledum, Dulcamara Kali iodatum* and *bichromicum, Mezereum* and *Phytolacca*. **Bryonia** is indicated where the synovial membrane is affected rather than the peri-articular tissues; when heat, swelling and tenderness are present, and when the pains are increased by warmth and (especially) by movement. **Rhus** takes its place when stiffness is present rather than tenderness; when the tendons, fasciæ and ligaments are mainly affected; and when the pains, though increased by movements first, are by continued motion relieved. The causation, moreover, with *Rhus* is damp cold, with *Bryonia* dry cold. With **Rhododendron** the pains are like those of *Rhus*, in that they are worse at rest; but they are relieved at once by movement. It is the Electric rather than the hygrometric condition of the atmosphere to which they are sensitive, so that they are always worse before or during a storm, **Dulcamara** is suitable when the opposite relation to *Rhus* obtains, *i.e.*, when the pains are little affected for the worse by rest or motion, but decidedly so by cold and damp—to one or both of which they commonly owe their origin.* With **Pulsatilla** the knee, ankle and tarsal joints are the main seat of the trouble, and menstrual disturbance is often present. Its "conditions" here must specially be regarded; viz., that its pains are worse towards evening and at night, worse also at rest and in a warm room, and relieved by motion in the open air. The **Ledum** Rheumatism is generally in the lower extremities: the association of coldness is the only distinctive symptoms I know of it.† **Kali iodatum** and **bichromicum, Mezereum** and **Phytolacca**, are suitable to periosteal Rheumatism; **Mercurius** when its indications in the acute form are present; ‡ and **Sulphur** when the Rheumatic diathesis is very general and marked.

The six first-named remedies have gained most of their repute in Chronic Rheumatism in the higher dilutions, the rest in the lower.

---

* See J. B. H. S., viii., 253.

† See some good cases by Dr. F. B. Peroy in the N. ENGL., MED. GAZETTE of March 1895.

‡ See ANNALS. iii., and iv.

RHEUMATIC GOUT must, I think, still retain this name in preference to the "Rheumatoid Arthritis," the "Chronic Rheumatic Arthritis" or "Osteo-Arthritis" the "Arthritis Deformans" and the "Nodular Rheumatism," which have been suggested in substitution. The name is familiar to all; it well-expresses the phenomena and relationships of the disease: and we shall not be led astray by it as to its Pathology and treatment.

The cardinal facts about Rheumatic Gout, as bearing on the question of treatment, are first, the great predominance of women among its subjects; second, the frequent co-existence in them of menstrual perturbation or disorder;* third, the analogy between Rheumatic Gout and Gonorrhœal Rheumatism. The remedies suggested by this concatenation of uterine and Rheumatoid troubles are *Pulsatilla, Sabina* and *Actæa racemosa;* and with these in recent cases, or in such as begin with acute symptoms, we may do very much. **Pulsatilla** is best when the menses are scanty or suppressed, the digestion is disordered, and the mind melancholic. **Sabina** is preferable in the frankly inflammatory form, especially if there is Menorrhagia, **Actæa racemosa** has Dr. Ringer's high commendation; it is indicated when the pains are worse at night, and in wet or windy weather. It relieves these, he says, and the cramps which often accompany them, to a very considerable extent.

In cases of long-standing, knowing the disorganization of the joints which this implies, we can hardly hope to do much with internal medicines. I know of no expression of confidence or records of success on the part of writers of our school of medicine, save one case mentioned by Dr. Edward Blake, in which **Sulphur** was of decided benefit;† and the results of my own practice have been negative, save for one case, limited to the knee-joint, where **Colchicum** and **Guaiacum** achieved an unhoped-for success. You will do well, therefore, to fall back upon the measures recommended by Fuller, Garrod and Trousseau. The *Corrosive sublimate* and *Iodine* of the last-named and the *Fraxinus excelsior, Arsenic* and *Arnica* of the first chime well with our notions, and may find hereafter a defined place in our treatment. I have only here to tell you what Homœopathy can do, and how she does it.‡

---

* "In early life", writes Dr. Fuller, Rheumatic Gout is always hereditary or connected with disordered uterine function."

† See B. J. H., xxxv., 46.

‡ Dr. Cooper has had some good results with the *Arbutus andrachne,* given according to his ("arbori-vital") method (H. W., Nov., 1897); and a Dr. Zolatorin with *Lactic acid* (J. B. H. S., vii., 217).

Last, of

GONORRHOEAL RHEUMATISM.—Of the treatment of this disease I can say little. I have only had one case under my own care, and this seemed little influenced by any of the medicines I used. However, the patient made a good and complete recovery, which is more than occurs in many cases. Jahr speaks of having brilliant success in one case with **Pulsatilla** following *Aconite;* and others of the same (Hahnemannian) school have lauded **Sarsaparilla.** Dr. Nimier has recently spoken of a case in which the latter drug "acted marvellously." These medicines would of course be given in the higher potencies; Dr. Nimier used the 12th.

An old-school physician commends our *Thuja*—which he gives, however, in 4-6 drop doses of the mother-tincture.*

Before leaving the subject of Rheumatism, I must say a few words on its treatment by *Salicin* and its derivatives, which has been so fashionable of late. I cannot claim this for Homœopathy. It is only in large doses that anything noteworthy is effected by these drugs in Acute Rheumatism; and what they do is simply to reduce the fever and hush up the pain. That the essential malady is not touched appears from the fact that cardiac and other complications are at least as liable to occur, and that relapses are decidedly MORE frequent than when improvement has resulted from other measures. As compared with Alkaline treatment, for instance, heart mischief has been found nearly twice as frequent, and relapses occur three times as often.† Still, it might be said, giving due weight to these disadvantages, the benefit obtained is so great, and so unattainable by other means that the *Salicylic* treatment should not be withheld from our patients. But there is another demerit in it. The large dosage required is an evil which has not been sufficiently considered, either here or in the analogous instances of the *Bromide* treatment of Epilepsy and the *Iodide* of Syphilis. You cannot introduce these masses of foreign matter into the system without serious injury. That *Salicylic acid* and its *salts* are liable to such reproach is pretty well-known. As early as 1877, it had to be said that "in a considerable proportion of cases they give rise to disagreeable symptoms, such as Vertigo, Headache, Tinnitus Aurium and Deafness. Nausea and Vomitting after each dose, profuse sweating, great weakness, and occasionally a peculiar eruption on the skin. More rarely, the symptoms assume a dangerous complexion, violent delirium, Albuminuria, great prostration, with feeble pulse and pallid skin

---

* J. B. H. S., i, 283.
† See LANCET, Sept. 20, 1879.

ushering in fatal collapse."* Since then Necrosis (in a strumous child) of the bones of the legs and forearm, † hyperpyrexia and Hæmaturia are among the disastrous effects observed from this *acid*. *Salicin* is said to be exempt from such blame; but if, as Senator maintains, it is transformed into *Salicylic acid* in the system, the mischievous agent is still produced, and—though less manifestedly—does its injurious work.

I think, therefore, that on the whole we shall be doing most justice to our Acute Rheumatic subjects if we resist the temptation to hush up their pain and knock down their fever with *Salicin* and its derivatives. A man must make his choice; he cannot have every advantage and escape every drawback. Under Homœopathic treatment his disease will subside somewhat less rapidly, but no less surely; and he will run no risk of being poisoned during its course, or unduly weakened when he arrives at convalescence.

In so speaking, I am echoing the conclusions on the subject arrived at in our London Hospital. "Some years ago," writes Dr. Byres Moir, "I tried alternate cases, as they were admitted, with our ordinary treatment and the *Salicylates;* and while in certain cases the *Salicylates* seemed to have a specific action in relieving the joint troubles, and lowering the temperature in adults, in others the action was not so satisfactory. The tendency to relapse is much greater in the cases treated by *Salicylates;* and if continued too long they produce serious Anæmia. When there is Peri—or Endocarditis, the use of the *Salicylates* is, I think, often prejudicial." ‡

---

* Appendix to Vol. xvi. of Ziemssen's Cyclopædia.
† LANCET, Oct. 27, 1877.
‡ L. H. H. R., vii., 24.

LECTURE XXII.

GENERAL DISEASES

---o---

DIATHETIC VICES & BLOOD DISORDERS.

---o---

SCROFULA—CANCER,
SCURVY—PURPURA—PLETHORA—ANÆMIA—CHLOROSIS
—PERNICIOUS ANÆMIA—LEUCOCYTHÆMIA.

I have to speak to-day of certain DIATHETIC VICES—SCROFULA, TUBERCULOSIS and CANCER; and of the BLOOD DISORDERS—PURPURA, SCURVY, ANÆMIA (with CHLOROSIS and LEUCOCYTHÆMIA), and PLETHORA. And first of—

SCROFULA.—The doctrine of Scrofula and Tubercle has undergone many variations of late. In my student days, I was taught to think the latter an occasional manifestation of the former. Then we were led by Sir William Jenner to speak of "Scrofulosis" and "Tuberculosis" as distinct diatheses, differing from one another as essentially as either from Rachitis. Later, Niemeyer and his contemporaneous workers inaugurated another way of looking at the matter. Scrofula, with them is that vulnerability of the constitution which we call "delicacy," PLUS a tendency on the part of the lymphatic glands in the neighbourhood of any disordered part to take on hyperplasia and became enlarged. The other so-called strumous affections are in no way SPECIFICALLY distinct from the same diseases in non-strumous subjects. Tubercle, in the majority of cases is secondary to "cheesy" degeneration of simple inflammatory products of Scrofulous glands. It may even supervene upon vaccination, or result from an issue. But occasionally a primary Tuberculosis of the lungs and (possibly also of the cerebral meninges) is observed.

These views to a large extent harmonize the previous doctrines. Tubercle is often secondary to Scrofula, though mediatcly instead of directly; and Tuberculosis is occasionally met with as a distinct diathesis. The characteristic constitution with which the latter is associated, and the circumstances which constitute its predisposing and exciting causes, need further investigation. Pending this, I shall not speak of it here among General Diseases, but only when its local outbreaks (especially Phthisis) come to be considered. What I have to say at present concerns Scrofula only.

While Pathological theories vary, clinical observation remains unchanged ; and it has at all times recognised two leading types of Scrofulous constitution. Let me remind you of them in Professor Miller's graphic words:—*

"In the sanguine variety the complexion is fair, and frequently beautiful as well as the features. The form, though delicate, is often graceful. The skin is thin, of fine texture; and subcutaneous blue veins are numerous, shinning very distinctly through the otherwise pearly white integument. The pupils are unusually spacious; and the eyeballs are not only large but prominent, the sclerotic showing a lustrous whiteness. The eyelashes are long and graceful —unless Ophthalmia Tarsi exist, as not unfrequently is the case; then the eyelashes are wanting, and their place is occupied by the swollen, red, unseemly margin of the lid.

"In the phlegmatic form the complexion is dark, the features disagreeable, the countenance and aspect altogether forbidding, the joints large, the general frame stunted in growth, or otherwise deformed from its fair proportions. The skin is thick and sallow; the eyes are dull, though usually both large and prominent; the general expression is heavy and listless; but not unfrequently the intellectual powers are remarkably acute, as well as capable of much and sustained exertion. The upper lip is usually tumid, so are the columna and alæ of the nose, and the general character of the face is flabby; the belly inclines to protuberance; and the extremities of the fingers are flatly clubbed, instead of presenting the ordinary tapering form."

Now it seems reasonable that these differences of form in the Scrofulous constitution should be an important element in the data for choice of remedies for it. The hygiene and diet are much the same for both ; but the place which *Iodine* and *Ferrum* occupy in the treatment of the former variety is taken by *Sulphur* in the latter, while *Calcarea* embraces both. **Calcarea carbonica** is a medicine which, in our hands, inherits all the ancient reputation of *Lime-water* and the *Salts of Lime*. Its indications in Scrofula are a lymphatic temperament, a fair skin, plumpness rather than emaciation, and morbid tendencies of the glands, bones and joints. **Iodine** (whose relation to Scrofula I have fully discussed in my 'Pharmacodynamics) † suits the sanguine variety described above, especially when there is wasting ; and hence partly the value of Cod-liver Oil in the dietetic treatment of these subjects. **Ferrum** (in dynamic dosage) is the "tonic" of the same class of patients ; Dr. Cooper points to their clear skin and cruly hair as indications of their suitableness for it when weak. **Sulphur** is the great remedy for the second of our two forms, especially when the local manifestations tend towards skin and mucous rather than glands and bones. ‡

---

* Principles of Surgery," 3rd Ed., p. 21.

† An old-school physician, from an experience embracing some 200 cases cannot speak too highly of *Arsenicum iodatum* in the Eczemas, Ophthalmias, and Chronic Catarrhs of scrofulous children. He uses a 1 per cent. solution (L' ART MEDICAL, Dec., 1898).

‡ Dr. Jousset adds *Silicea* to the above remedies, speaking of it as "le grand medicament de la Scrofule." His account of the progressive evolution of the disease in its typical form, and his indication for *Dulcamarra, Viola tricolo* and *Conium* in its earlier stages, are very graphic and valuable.

You will, therefore, besides your all-important general treatment, prescribe one or other of these medicines in every instance of the Scrofulous diathesis which comes under your care. When I come to the various forms of strumous disease, we will consider how far diathetic remedies by themselves suffice for their treatment, and whether any of them act also on the affected parts. *

You may have questioned my stopping short with Niemeyer as regards the doctrine of Scrofula, and may feel still more dubious about my classing Cancer among General Diseases. While, however, I fully recognize the local origin of Cancerous growths, I cannot abandon the impression that there is an antecedent tendency, hereditary or acquired, which makes these growths occur in certain subjects, and not in others; which under similiar provocation of injury, of irritation, of heat, shews itself in such resentment, as we call malignant proliferation. You must indulge me in this, and now let me tell you what Homœopathy can do for—

CANCER—in its several forms. Let me say first that I do not think we can claim such results as to justify our urging patients to refrain from seeking the aid of Surgery in suitable cases. Were I a woman, and a Nodule appeared in my breast of undoubted or even suspected malignancy, I should undoubtedly seek its removal by operation. Drs. Marstone and McLimont, and Dr. Edward Madden, in our own ranks, † not to speak of more irregular practitioners elsewhere, have abundantly illustrated the value of enucleation by *Caustics* in Mammary Scirrhus, and removal by the knife is certainly growing rather than decreasing in favour among practical surgeons. But there are patients who will not endure such dealing with, and there are confessedly stages, varieties, and localisations of the disease which operative measures cannot reach; so that it will be of great importance if Homœopathy can prove itself efficacious in such cases.

The general impression one gains from reading the Homœopathic literature of the subject is that we have remedies which materially improve the general health of Cancerous patients, and

---

* Holding the above views of Scrofula and Tubercle, it may be imagined how gratified I felt at reading Sir Dyce Duckworth's Address to the Liverpool Medical Institution, published in the LANCET of November 9, 1901. That there is a "personal factor in Tuberculosis"; that that factor is the diathetic condition traditionally described as "Scrofula"; and that Scrofula is a morbid condition PER SE, having its own clinical history and manifestations, over and above the liability of its subjects to Tubercular deposit,—these are just the position which, for therapeutic purposes, I have taken up in the text.

† See B. J. H., xxi., 611; xxiii., 196.

which, by their elective affinity for the parts affected, tend in a greater or lesser degree to restore their healthy nutrition. I cannot say that I see evidence of any specific relationship between these medicines and the Carcinomatous diathesis, so that the one can fairly be expected to neutralise the other. Nevertheless, when you have done all you can by healthy living and generous diet, by *Iron* and by Cod-liver Oil to improve the general health of these subjects (and how much may be done in this way has been well-shown by Mr. Weeden Cooke,) you will find in our constitutional remedies the means of doing something more. The chief of these is **Arsenicum.** Under its use, in varying dilutions, you will seldom fail to observe an increase in strength, a better oxygenation of the blood, and a healthier performance of the functions in patients affected with Cancer. The lancinating pains, moreover, which annoy the affected part are frequently relieved by this medicine. Sometimes, where the general condition is characterized by great torpor, **Carbo** may be a better medicine even than *Arsenicum,* as in a case mentioned by Drs. Marston and McLimont (p. 633). The animal charcoal is generally used : but I sus-suspect that the vegatable product would act quite as well.

Approaching Cancer from another side, there are certain remedies to which we are led by the FORM of the disease present Thus, "Epithelial Cancer" has been histologically identified with such growths as Warts and Condylomata under the common title of "Epithelioma." Analogy would accordingly lead us to administer and apply **Thuja** in those cases, and to expect from it some at least of the power for good it manifests over the less malignant growths of the same order. Under this head it seems we are to group the Cancers of the lip, tongue, and scrotum, and the "Cauliflower Excrescence" of the os uteri. Perhaps Dr. Quin's case in the First Volume of the ANNALS (p. 177), though styled by him "Fungus Hæmatodes," was really Cauliflower Excresence ; and there *Thuja* was strikingly benificial. Epithelial Cancer of the lip, however, is so markedly under the control of *Arsenic,* that I should feel indisposed to resort to any other medicine. Its external use in the form of ointment (say gr. v. of the 3rd dec. trituration to 3j of Lard) is here advantageously conjoined with its internal administration. I should recommend the same treatment for "Cancer Scroti".

When Encephaloid Cancer assumes a fungous form, the power of *Thuja* over vascular as well as epithelial growths may be brought to bear with advantage. The celebrated case of Marshall Radetzky is possibly an illustration of its virtue. I say possibly, because the part taken by the medicine in the cure (the fungus grew from within the orbit) has been questioned. You will find the narrative of the case, with criticism and defence, in the First Volume of the BRITISH JOURNAL OF HOMŒOPATHY. But when the vascularity of the growth combines with its form to give it the name "Fungus Hæmatodes," the facts I have mentioned* under the head of **Phosphorus** must be borne in mind. You will notice how, in the case narrated there, **Thuja** rendered essential service towards the ultimate withering of the protrusion.

The third factor which guides us in our choice of remedies for Cancer is the PART AFFECTED. The elective affinities which we have ascertained to belong to our medicines are here brought into play with good effect. Thus *Conium, Hydrastis, Phytolacca* and *Carbo animalis* have more or less influence over Mammary Scirrhus. *Arsenic* and *Phosphorus* over Cancer of the stomach, and *Secale* over that of the womb : while *Aurum* and *Symphytum*, which are our chief osseous medicines, are said to have cured Cancer of the antrum. † But of these local remedies for the disease I shall speak under the head of the special organ attacked.

The only question which remains is, whether we have any general Anti-carcinomatous medicines, as we have Anti-syphilitics and Anti-sycotics. The few remedies which show any claim to the title are *Hydrastis, Cundurango, Calcarea,* and *Silicea*. I must refer you to what I have written upon each in my 'Pharmacodynamics.' That *Hydrastics* has seemed to arrest Cancer of the stomach suggests that its undoubted value in Mammary Scirrhus is more than the action of a glandular stimulant. **Cundurango** has gained still more frequent success in the former affection, even Fredreich and Nussbaum witnessing to its efficacy; and by Dr. Clotar Muller has been found very effective in malignant ulcerations of the surface, an experience Dr. H. Goullon corroborates. **Calcarea carbonica** and **Silicea** in substantial though small doses, seem capable of abating the pains of Cancer, and sometimes of causing its growths to wither. The *Gneiss,* introduced under the name of **Lapis albus** by Dr. von Grauvogl, ‡ appears to be a medicine of the same order, though it acts in more attenuated form.

With these internal remedies, and availing ourselves of what *Citric acid* and *Chlorate of Potash* can do as local applications, § we need not abandon any case of Cancer to despair. Even though life may ultimately be destroyed by the disease, much may be done towards prolongation of days and relief of sufferings ; while every now and then genuine cures may be effected.

---

* To these I may add the testimony of Jahr. "I have treated three cases of Fungus Hæmatodes," he writes, "the patients being children of 5-10. The fungi grew out of congenital claret-coloured spots. *Phosphorus* 30 removes the trouble perfectly in two or three weeks."

† B. J. H., xvii., 59; J. B. H. S., v., 200.

‡ See H. J. H., xxxii., 687; xxxiii., 571. (Also a case in J. B. H. S., iv., 345).

§ See IBID., xxiv., 518; xxv., 518.

So I wrote in 1877; and I have expressed myself similarly again to-day, because I think the mode of approaching the subject original and helpful. My last paragraph, too, has fairly represened the mind of Homœopathists on the subject as since expressed. I may refer you to the Paper in which Dr. Gutteridge put the possibilities of medicine in Cancer before out international Congress of 1881, and to the discussion which followed it. But the years have brought many fresh thought and facts to light, and I must make some further remarks on the treatment of Cancer before leaving the topic.

1. In Pathology, the most important point made has been the differentiaion between Carcinoma and Sarcoma. It may have more bearing on inferences from treatment than on the choice of remedies; but Dr. Helmuth, who contributed a valuable paper on the two forms of growth to the Congress of 1891, states that when Sarcoma can be definitely recognised, cure may often be looked for from *Thuja*—the tincture being given in drop doses internally and brushed freely over the growth. In the HAHNEMANNIAN MONTHLY for April, 1893, a similar experience appears in a case of Osteo-sarcoma of the thigh: and in the same Journal for February, 1895, a case of gaint-celled Sarcoma of the tibia, with hard and enlarged inguinal glands, is recorded, in which the persistent use of *Arsenic* removed the growth on a third recurrence after removal.

2. The relation of this great medicine to Cancer has of late years been notably accentuated, both on the pathogenetic and the therapeutic side. Mr. Jonathan Hutchinson, and also Uhlmann and others on the Continent,* have shewn that the continued use of the drug in medicinal doses may produce a form of Cancer which is of the epithelial variety, but presents certain peculiarities. Lassar, in the old school, has reported several cases of Cancerous growths and ulcerations disappearing under the influence of *Arsenic*. † Dr. J. S. Mitchell, of Chicago, some twelve years ago made a felicitous combination of the general and local influence of the drug on malignant ulceration by sprinkling 2x trituration on the sore while giving the 3x internally. In the NEW ENGLAND MEDICAL GAZETTE of July, 1895 (not long before his lamented death), he summed up his experience with the treatment, which had been very favourable. Dr. Helmuth had endorsed it in his paper of 1891; and in the number of the same Journal for february, 1901 Dr. van Deursen relates three cases of Epithelioma of the face in which the treament produced most satisfactory results.

3. The papillomatous form of Cancer corresponds to the growths over which *Thuja* has so much power. Dr. Ord relates ‡

---

* M. H. R., xxxii., 381; J. B. H. S., vi., 393; viii., 251.
† See BRIT. MED. JOURN., June 17, 1893.
‡ See M. H. R.. xxxix., 431.

a case of abdominal papilloma, ascertained to be such by abdominal incision. Singular improvement set in and was long maintained under the action of *Thuja* lx, though the patient ultimately relapsed and died.

4. The late Dr. William Owens had great confidence in **Acetic acid** as a remedy for Cancer. For eighteen years, he told us, at the Congress of 1891, he had treated all his cases with this *acid*, in a 4-10 per cent. solution internally and a 2 per cent. one topically. He could report a good number of cures of malignant ulceration of face, mamma and uterus under such medication. Dr. F. B. Percy has since corroborated his testomony. He reports a cure of the Epithelioma of the lips; a subsidence of all the gastric symptoms in a case of chronic diseases of the stomach, apparently malignant; and striking temporary improvement in one of Cancer of larynx. Here the local application was made by spray. *

I shall havte more to say about Cancer when I come to its local manifestation. For the present, what I have brought before you will show that our outlook in treating it is not altogether hopeless, and that medication on Homœopathic lines is capable of entering into fair competition here with '*Caustics* and the knife.'

I now come to what may be called, phenomenally at least, DISORDERS OF THE BLOOD.

SCURVY is a typical instance of a disease resulting from pure dieteic causes and requiring pure diatetic treatment. Sir James Simpson seemed to think that he had made a point against Homœopathy when he argued that Lemon-juice cures Scurvy, but is incapable of producing it. The argument is really altogether wide of the mark. Lemon-juice is only a convenient form of supplying certain necessary constituents of our food, the absence of which induces the condition we call scorbutic. It plays no essential part in the treatment of Scurvy It is generally sufficient to place the sufferers on the full diet of a hospital comprising as it does fresh meat and vegetables, with milk; and nothing more is required for the cure.

---

* N. ENG. MED. GAZETTE., Nov., 1896.

So I wrote in 1869. The editors of the MONTHLY HOMŒO-PATHIC REVIEW dissented * from my recommendation to treat Scurvy by dietetic means alone, and wrote:—"Raue, in his excellent 'Special Pathology and Therapeutics,' names fifteen remedies which are suitable for the various lesions consequent on Scurvy, and we should unquestionably give some of these, according to the individual specialities of the case, in addition to a proper regulation of the diet." I should like to know if Dr. Raue had ever treated Scurvy, and seen any of his fifteen remedies do what proper dieting was not doing, or not doing so fast. I can recall two (unsuspected) cases of (Land) Scurvy, in which the most careful medicinal treatment was effecting absolutely nothing, but which cleared up rapidly when the true cause of the symptoms was discovered and the deficiency of fresh vegetables supplied. It is not thus that diseases behave where medicines are of prime importance, and "regulation of the diet" is only a useful supplement. To the same effect is the experience lately had of Scurvy in young children resuting from the use of the artificial foods so much vogue. Nothing can be done with it till fresh meat-juice, milk and organes or lemons are added to the diet. † The only place for medication would be when hæmorrhagic effusion into the pleura or elsewhere had occurred Here we can readily follow Dr. F. F. Laird in esteeming *Phosphorus* as a valuable medicinal adjunct.

Again, Dr. Dyce Brown maintains § that Lemon-juice is Homœopathic to Scurvy. He refers to cases of poisoning by its too long-continued employment recorded in the 'Cyclopædia of Drug Pathogenesy,' where hæmorrhagic symptoms occured; and to the experience of Sir George Nares, that sailors to whom a double allowance had been given developed Scurvy very rapidly and often severely. I cannot check the latter allegation; but as regards the former would say that the condition produced seems to me one of Purpura rather than Scurvy. All the vegetable acids thin and liquefy the blood, and their over-use might well lead to its effusion; but Scurvy is much more than this.

PURPURA has been styled "Land Scurvy." I am convinced, however, that the resemblance is superficial only. In Purpura

---

* Vol. xiii., p. 236.   † J. B. H. S., ii., 27.
‡ IBID., ix., 179.   § IBID., ii., 39.

there is none of that excess of fibrin in the blood which analysis demonostrates to exist in Scurvy, and which shews itself in the plastic deposits which sheathe the muscles and mat the celluar tissue of scorbutic patients. Not is there in the majority of cases of Purpura any history of deficiency in the fulness or variety of diet. It seems to me a morbid condition SUI GENERIS,, developing itself under very various circumstances. I have gone somewhat into its Pathology and causation in a paper on the subject in the Twenty-Sixth Volume of the BRITISH JOURNAL OF HOMŒOPATHY. Referring you thither for details, I sum up here the conclusions arrived at as to its treatment.

Purpura appears under two forms, the Febrile and the simply Hæmorrhagic. The Febrile variety itself differs as it is sthenic or asthenic. Of Sthenic Purpura I have cited instances in my paper, and have noted the repute of venesection, purgatives and low diet in its treatment. With us the place of the first two would be taken by **Aconite**, which accordingly promises to be its most suitable remedy. Of Purpura with asthenic fever I have given two cases from the Homœopathic literature. Both were severe; and both recovered under *Sulphuric acid* and *Arnica*. I confess myself, however, quite unable to see the Homœopathicity of *Sulphuric acid* to the morbid condition here present. Its use seems a relic of old-school traditions rather than an induction from the Law of Similars; and it is difficult to conceive of the "astringent" action of the drug being exerted in the 1st and 2nd dilutions, which were those used in the cases cited. The claims of **Arnica**, indeed, deserve more respectful attention. The petechiæ of Purpura are unquestionably so many BRUISES (the term "Ecchymoses" is common to both) : only in this case the extravasation results from morbid change from within, and not from mcehanical violence from without. The influence of *Arnica* over Ecchymoses owing the latter cause is probably not merely local but dynamic and specific. It "determines" (in old-school language) "to the surface," ane so favours hæmorrhages; but there is nothing like Purpura, Simplex or Hæmorrhagica, in its Pathogenesis. A better remedy than either of these for Asthenic Febrile Purpura would seem to me to be found in **Mercurius**. This poison unquestionably causes Ecchymoses and hæmorrhages; and the second of the two cases cited reads so like an example of the Acute Hydrargyrosis that I wonder Mr. Willans did not treat with *Mercurius* throughout. **Arsenicum**, too, must not be forgotten; it is Homœopathic alike to the prosration and the petechiæ.*

Of the non-ferbile variety of Purpura, where the hæmorrhage

---

*An almost desperate case cured by this remedy is mentioned by Jahr. It was of the non-febrile form. Another is recorded by Dr. Hansen (J. B. H. S., iv., 237). There was no fever, but the patient was much troubled by tearing and burning pains in the legs. *Arsenicum* 2, given on this indication, cured, when *Phosphorus* had produced only temporary amendment.

is all in all, there is a good case in thee Fifth Volume of the
AMERICAN HOMŒOPATHIC REVIEW (p. 566). The symptoms rapidly subsided when, after six day's increase, on the seventh a high
dilution of **Phosphorus** was administered. The choice of the
medicine was determined by the hæmorrhagic symptoms ascribed
to it in Hahnemann's Pathogenesis. There is no doubt that
the abundant Ecchymoses observed in the subjects of poisoning
by *Phosphorus* closely resemble the symptoms of Purpura. The
weight of evidence hitherto has gone against these symptoms
being primary. They seem to occur only in connection with
the peculiar morbid changes induced by *Phosphorus* in the liver.
They point to the Purpuric symptoms which characterize Yellow
Fever and acute hepatic atrophy, rather than to the idiopathic
disorder. Still I do not hold the question as settled; and we do
well to keep the *Phosphorus* in reserve in the treatment of our
present malady,—in which Arnold, Clotar Muller, Jousset and
Goullon unite to esteem it the great remedy. Dr. Spiers
Alexander has contributed a paper to the Thirty-Seventh Volume
of the MONTHLY HOMŒOPATHIC REVIEW well-illustrating its
action.

Another candidate for the place of specific remedy for this form
of Purpura is **Hamamelis**. A case is recorded in Dr. Hale's "New
Remedies," in which the administration of this medicine rapidly
dissipated Purpuric symptoms supervening upon Varioloid.
I have myself, since writing the Paper referred to, cured very
speedily with it a case in which blood had been largely extravasa-
ted under the skin, and was passing in the urine. The anti-hæmorrhagic
virtues of *Hamamelis* are so considerable that I am dispossed
to credit it with much power over the morbid condition we are
considering.

Another position apparently Homœopathic to Purpura is *Serpent-
venom*. In my discussion of *Lachesis* and its congeners, I have
spoken of the "Purpuric or Hæmorrhagic form," which poisoning
by them often assumes. The Ecchymoses and hæmorrhages
which occur are shown to be dependent upon changes in
blood, which becomes diffluent and non-coagulabe. Whether
this is so in Purpura is hardly proved; but the phenomena
are so similar that one or other of the *Snake-poisons* used
in our practice should be fairly tried in its treatment. There
are two cases on record in which **Lachesis** was given
with rapid disappearance of the symptoms;* and Hasbrouck
notes the same of **Crotalus**.† Perhaps at the present day this
last remedy and *Phosphorus* are most in favour of all our means
of controlling Purpura.

---

* See B. J. H., xxii., 489; AM. JUUR. OF HOM. MAT. MED., iv., 66.
† J. B. H. S., vi., 300.

PLETHORA is a morbid condition which may be discussed in a very few words. I take it to be rarely met with now-a-days; and, when present, to result, from the transgression of obvious Physiological laws. Its treatment must accordingly be purely hygienic and dietetic, and no place for dynamic remedies can be with any plausibility assigned. If, however, a case should come before you in which the patient really does "make blood too fast;" if, in spite of spare diet and action exercise, the symptoms of Plethora still persist, medicines must be given. You would naturally propose to administer minute doses of some preparation of *Iron*. But if Dr. Drysdale be right in thinking that Lœffler's provings demonstrate a depressing action on sanguification as exerted by *Iron* from the first, we lose it as a Homœopathic remedy for Plethora; nor can I readily suggest another Dr. Hutchinson thinks that the pseudo-high health resulting in the Styrian peasants and Vienna horses from eating *Arsenic* is a Plethora of this kind, and infers the Homœopathicity thereto of the medicine. I should have thought, however, that it was rather from checking destructive metamorphosis than from increasing sanguification that *Arsenic* induced its Plethora. My MONTHLY HOMŒOPATHIC reviewer mentions that "in 1861 M. Lamare-Piquot announced the fact that small doses of *Arsenic* reduced the amount of red globules in the blood, and that he had found the remedy successful in cases where they were in excess, and the patients were suffering from cerebral congestion."

ANAEMIA present a wider field for inquiry. In one form indeed in which it occurs it is just the correlative of Plethora both as to cause and as to reatment. I mean when it results from deficiency of air, light and suitable food, and form other depressing causes. The only rational and permanently successful treatment of such cases must be removal of the injurious cause or the restoration of lacking SANANTIA. But even when these indications are satisfied, and still more when they can only partially be fulfilled, remedies acting Homœopathically upon the blood-making process are useful. That **Ferrum** is such a remedy I have already argued; and the experience of Dr. Bayes and others as to its value in Anæmia in the second and third decimal attenuation of the *Acetate* and *Iodide* confirms the inference drawn from its provings. Whether it should also be used as a dietetic agent is an open question; and we need comparative experiment to determine whether patients get on as fast without it. You, at least, would do well to begin by trying if they do. *Argentum* and *Zincum* are also truly Homœopathic

---

* See B. J. H., xxvii., 258.
† Applied Homœopathy, p. 91; B. J. H., xii., 376.

to Anæmia, and *Cuprum* and *Pulsatilla*, which have proved curative of it, * may be so.

There is another simple and intelligent form of the malady,— that resulting from excessive or long-continued losses of blood. I need hardly remind you of the value of **China** in these cases. † But this remedy goes no further than the exhaustion consquent upon hæmorrhage. Again we turn gladly io the well-tired *Iron* to help the generous diet we prescribed to make blood as speedily as possible. The direct feeding of the impoverished blood by the metal is here a plausible hypothesis enough.

But perhaps the most common form of Anæmia is that which comes before us in connection with disordered menstruation—

CHLOROSIS. A glance at a young woman who enters our consulting room gives us the whole group of symptoms. The Catamenia absent, or retarded, scanty and pale; frequent palpitation; breathlessness on slight exertion; debility, anorexia and low' spirits,—make up the patient's story; to which our examinaton adds the Anæmic murmur in the neck, the waxy, puffy skin, and the exsanguine mucous membrane. Now what is the relation between the Anæmia and the Catamenial disorder? It is common now to say that these patients do not menstruate because the ovaries find no blood upon which to draw. But very often the history of the case is this. A young woman in fair health gets a chill while menstruating, and the flow is checked. When the next period comes round, nothing is seen. Coincidently with this the general health fails, and the symptoms of Anæmia develope themselves. ‡ If now, under dynamic remedies (of which **Pulsatilla** is the chief), the Catamenia are restored, PARI PASSU the Anæmia departs.

I must not follow up the Pathological inquiries which such facts suggest. Their bearing upon treatment is party obvious.

---

* See J. B. H. S., vii., 84, 87. † See ANNALS, iii., 228.

‡ Compare the following case related by Trousseau :—"This young girl is seventeen years old; she has menstruated regularly until this last time, when, on her taking a cold bath on the last day of her menstrual period, the menses were immediately suppressed, and she shortly afterwards felt an acute pain in the region of the left ovary. Within a few days she had palpitation of the heart, got out of breath easily, and complained of disordered digestion and of vague pains; she had become Chlorotic." (CLINICAL LECTURES, transl. by Bazire, Vol. I., Lect. 17).

While you can hardly do anything but good by giving your chalybeate food as heretofore, Homœopathy enables you to strike at the root of the matter by her specific remedies for deficient menstruation. These will be considered in their proper place. For the present let me illustrate what seems to me the true plan of treatment for such cases by one of my own.

Emily G——,æt, 16, consulted me at the Dispensary on January 15th, 1866. In the previous February she had caught cold whilst menstruating, and the flow had prematurely ceased. She had seen nothing since; and had been growing weaker and weaker. She was very pale, and complained of breathlessness, palpitation, headache, &c.; in a word, she was thoroughly Anæmic. I ordered her to take two grains of the *Ferrum redactum* of the British Pharmacopœia once daily with a meal.

January 22nd.—No change. Continue *Ferrum*.

29th.—Feeling much better in health. Continue.

February 5th.—Much better and stronger, and colour returning, but no Catamenia.

Gave *Pulsatilla* 12, 6, and 3, in succession; each dilution for two days; a drop three times a day.

11th.—The Catamenia reappeared on the 8th (*i.e.*, while taking the 6th dilution), and were fair as to colour and quantity. She feels and looks quite well.

You may say, perhaps, that the Catamenia would have returned in time of their own accord when once the blood had regained its normal richness under the influence of the chalybeate. It may be so. But read the very similar case in Professor Hughes Bennett's Clinical Lectures (p. 890 of 3rd Ed.). It is said to have been dismissed "cured." But after two months' treatment by *Iron*, tonics, generous diet and rest, the Catamenia had not appeared.

This is Chlorosis proper, which I follow Immermann in defining as a change in the blood occurring in the early years of the woman's sexual maturity, and consisting in a diminution in the amount of hæmoglobin contained in the nutrient fluid. The red corpuscles may be numerous enough; but they are poor in quality. Chlorosis differs from ordinary Anæmia in the absence of any of the causal factors which belong to that condition, and in the limitation of the change to one constituent of the blood.

Now the treatment of this malady, as you know, is one of the things on which traditional medicine plumes itself. "There is scarcely any point in Therapeutics," says Immermann, "so fully established as the remarkable efficacy of *Iron* in removing all the symptoms of Chlorosis. . . . The blood and free use of *Iron* is of more importance than a meat diet, exercise, sleep, a coutry life, sea-bathing, mountain air, regulation of the emotional life. I do not hesitate to say that a couple of boxes of Steel Pills or any other active preparation of *Iron* will do a Chlorotic girl more good than the most complicated plan of treatment in which *Iron* occupies only a subordinate place." Is this Homœopathy? and, if not, can Homœopathy do better.

In my 'Pharmacodynamics,' I have gone at the length into the question, and have arrived at the following conclusions : —
 1. *Iron* probably hinders the formation of red blood in health and certainly promotes it in disease in the same manner in which other drugs affect the nutritive functions, as I have indicated in my Lecture VII. *
 2. It may thus be given for Chlorosis in small doses as a Homœopathic remedy, and should always be so administered in the first instance.
 3. *Iron* is also a food to the blood, and should be given as such unless improvement rapidly occurs under its use as a medicine.

Reviewing these statements in the light of subsequent information, I would say of the first that it is increasingly substantiated as times go on. Nothnagel and Rossbach (whose Article on the Metal I had not read when I wrote the above-named discussion) confirm Hahnemann's statement that "observations made upon those living in the neighbourhood of Iron springs, who use the Iron waters as a daily drink, have revealed a wonderful frequency of Anæmic conditions." † They shew, moreover, that this is only what might be expected. "We do not," they write, "believe in a so-called Plethora produced by long-continued use of Iron, at least not in the sense of an excess of red corpuscles. For an increase of these beyond the normal would necssitate a more rapid metamorphosis of material in the body, accompanied by a more rapid destruction of the corpuscles and increased excretion of Nitrogen and Iron ; they would thus be bringing about their own annihilation." One of our colleagues in Calcutta Dr. Younan, contributes an observation in the point. A patient asked him to look at a bird of hers which refused food and seemed so weak that it could hardly perch. Inspection shewed that it was suffering from Anæmia. Its back and legs, and the parts of the body stripped of feathers during the process of moulting, were pale and bloodless. On investigation, its water-cup was found to contain a dark-brown fluid and at the bottom lay a rusty nail. ‡

One the other hand, the thought of Iron as a food does not commend itself more to the mind as the facts grow upon us. Dr. Baruch reminds us § that "the Iron contained in the human system amounts only to 15-48 grains and in the worst cases of Anæmia the amount of Iron lost is only 3-4 grains,—which quantity can be furnished by a single pound of good beef." Dr. Bunge, of Bale, at the 1895 Congress of German Physicians, on the strength of similar facts urged the actual futility of

---

 * Page 90.
 † See also J. B. H. S., vi., 395.
 ‡ Calcutta Journ. of Medicine, May, 1895.
 § Med. Record, June 3, 1893.

Ferruginous medication in Chlorosis. And yet,—and yet,—it remains that within Iron there is no hæmatin, without hæmatin no red corpuscles, without red corpuscles no Oxygen-carrying, and without Oxygenation no bodily energy and activity of functions. It remains that by supplying this first link in the chain all the others start into being; so that in a Chlorotic girl taking 0.05 grm. of *Iron* daily for twenty-five days the red corpuscles increased gradually from three millions to four millions and a half per c. m. m., and she could be discharged cured.* It remains that up to a certain point increase of dose favours chalybeate action, and in severe cases may be carried almost to indefinite lengths, as Dr. Charles Taylor has shewn us. He took an extreme case of Anæmia, in a girl of 19, who had been getting gradually worse for two years. She was hardly able to move without Dyspnœa, and looked utterly bloodless. He gave a solution of the tincture of the *percloride,* of strength gradually increasing from 5 to 25 minims to the ounce, and told her to sip at it as she could day and night. She took it at the rate of two to three pints a day, improved most rapidly, and before she left the hospital, which she did in four weeks, was able to busy herself in the ward the whole day without fatigue. She took in 27 days 30 ounces of the tincture,—while, if she had taken the usual 20 minims three times a day, she wolud only have consumed 27 drachms. †

This looks feeding rather than medication—especially Homœopathic medication; and a similar inference may be drawn from Dr. Marc Jousset's remarks on the subject in L'ART MEDICAL ‡ *Ferrum* is indicated in Chlorosis, he tells us, when the menses are diminished or suppressed; in the menorrhagic form it is apt to increase the loss and so augment the malady. But this is just the reverse of what should happen, if the drug was acting as a similar remedy. Mennorrhagia, Hahnemann justly says, § is the primary action of *Iron;* and indeed for this trouble,, occurring in young subjects, there is no more useful Homœopathic remedy—of course in small doses. If it were behaving as such in Chlorosis, it should act upon the flux in like manner. In the same direction points the fact that it is only in Anæmia that *Iron* has to be given in any apprach to substantial doses. In the congestions, hæmorrhages, and vesical irritations to which its Pathogenesy leads us, it acts well in the attenuations from the 1st to the 3rd centesimal, or even higher; in Anæmia it is otherwise.

The conclusion must be, I think, doctrinally, that *Iron* acts here as it does when we water sickly plants with a solution of

---

* Nothnagel and Rossbach, SUB VOCE, *Ferrum.*
† BRIT. MED. JOURN., March 21, 1829.
‡ See note to § 141 of his pathogenesis of *Ferrum* in the 'Materia Medica Pura',

it, or when we secure its presence in the soil in which we plant them—knowing that only thus will Chlorophyll be developed in them, and their hues shine out and their fruit be borne. The Nonconformist minister did not use false image when he said to a Church Congress, "The thoughts of your great preachers and teachers have entered like Iron into our blood, and have coloured and inspired our whole ministry." And, practically, I, have long been forced to the conviction that my former advice to begin with fractional doses, as for Homœopathic action was hardly well-founded. The improvement taking place under the second and even the first decimal trituration of *Ferrum redactum* has been too tardy to satisfy my conscience; and I now, in Chlorosis, give (as I did in 1866) from the first a two-grain powder of the pure substance once daily. The results of this practice have been all I could desire in the cases I have seen, which have not been few; but I should be quite ready to increase the dose or the frequency of administration if need required. By so thinking and acting I seem to be doing most justice to my patients; while having the comfort of feeling that the value of *Iron* in Anæmia constitutes no exception to the Homœopathic law, it being mainly a matter of dietetics, with which SIMILIA SIMILIBUS has no concern.

You may fairly ask me whether in so reasoning and acting I have the concurrence of my colleagues. Practically, I may say I have. Bahr writes of *Ferrum*—"this medicine is a real specific for simple, uncomplicated Chlorosis : every simple case of this disease yields to the curative action of Iron." He recommends the first or second decimal trituration of the *Ferrum redactum* as the most suitable form. Jousset, in his "Elements," says that *Iron* is the medicine which oftenest corresponds to the ENSEMBLE of the symptoms, and of which we should make most frequent employment : he prefers the *acetate* or *protoxalate,* and gives about three grains of the first decimal trituration twice a day. Later, he has come to prefer the *Ferrum redactum,* giving about half a grain daily.* Dr. Galley Blackley, who has done so much good work in the field of hæmatic disease, uses the *Ferrous oxalate,* one or two grains three times a day. This preparation has, he says, the advantage that it does not constipate, but rather loosens confined bowels.

I must admit that when these writers face the question as to whether *Iron* acts here as a food or as a medicine, they all prefer the latter alternative. It matters little, as they agree in practice with what seems to me the more excellent way : only they have not the comfort of being able to account for their crude dosage as I do.† Hahnemann, at least the Hahnemann of 1811, would have countenanced them. In his "Defence of

---

* L'ART MEDICAL, Sept. 1900.
† J. B. H. S., vi., 282; L. H. H. R., vi., 6.

the Organon," which Dr. Dudgeon has lately given us in our language, he writes (p. 100),:—"What *Iron* contributes as a CHEMICAL remedy in such cases to the increase of the necessary quantity of Iron in the blood, is an altogether different question, which has nothing to do with the subject of Homœopathic cure by similarly-acting medicines." It 'is interesting to observe that Jhar says that "small doses" of *Ferrum* have not had the least effect in his hands. Since he probably means his usual globules of the 30th, the statement is not suprising, He tells us indeed that "in very many cases" *Pulsatilla, Sulphur* and *Calcarea*—given successively in this form—"are sufficient to bring about a blooming state of health"; but he does not mention how long the "cure lasts."

Bahr and Jousset agree that there are cases of Chlorosis in which Iron is not so effective as other medicines, and chief of these they count **Arsenicum**. To the latter, the co-existence of Menorrhagia is the great indication for it; the former recommends it where Iron has been abused and where there is "a high degree of debility, with excessive irritability, œdematous paleness, cardiac disturbances even during rest and complete Gastro-ataxia". It would also be suitable in the rare "Febrile Chlorosis" with its Dropsy and petechial effusion.

PERNICIOUS ANÆMIA, in which, since the initiative of Dr. Byrom Bramwell, it is generally recognised that *Iron* is of no avail, **Arsenic** taking its place. WHY it should do so on any ground but that of the Homœopathic method I cannot see,—the necrosis of the red corpuscles, the febrile symptoms and the Anasarca of Pernicious Anæmia, all belonging to the **Arsenical** Pathogenesis. The late Dr. Blackley, senior, communicated to the British Homœopathic Society in 1879 * four cases in which a cure was effected by the drug in doses much smaller than those generally employed; and his successor in practice at Manchester has appropriately followed these up by one of his own, in which the characteristic Poikilocytosis was well marked. Still more appropriately, his son, Dr. Galley Blackley, now Senior Physician to our London Hospital, has contributed another case, embodying it in an instructive post-graduate lecture on the disease. *Phosphorus* played some part in Dr. Blackley's results, and should not be forgotten as a possible alternative to the better-indicated metal; but its Homœopathicity is more dubious.

---

* See ANNALS, ix., 171.

Of—
LEUCOCYTHÆMIA I shall speak more fully when I come to the affections of the spleen, as it is on diseases of this organ that it seems to depend. If you should meet with it, however, as some have thought it does occur, without organic change, I will note that Erb finds **Picric acid** to produce a condition in dogs which he himself calls "an artificial Leucocythæmia"; and that a case of its infantile form, verified by blood examination, recovered under *Ferrum picricum*, five grains of the 1x trituration PER DIEM. * *Myrrh,* also, has been found to cause Lecucocytosis. †

---

* NEW ENGLAND MED. GAZETTE, Nov., 1900. Dr. Samuel Jones, who has done so much good work on *Picric acid* thinks the increased number of white corpuscles observed in picratisation comparative only, and due to the extensive obstruction of red corpuscles caused by the poison (HOM. RECORDER, Jan., 1912).

† IBID., April, 1898.

LECTURE XXIII.

GENERAL DISEASES.

THE VENEREAL MALADIES.

SYPHILIS—GONORRHOEA—SOFT CHANCRE—SYCOSIS.

In my present lecture I should speak of those Venereal Diseases which are of general character. But among these the last edition of our Nomenclature teaches us to include Gonorrhœa; and in this case Soft Chancre can hardly be shut out. We shall therefore discuss to-day VENEREAL DISEASE as a whole. And first of—

SYPHILIS properly so called. Comments upon its treatment occupy a large space in the field of Homœopathic literature. I refer you for them in the first place to our Journals generally; and in the second to two Monographs—Dr. Yeldham's excellant "Homœopathy in Venereal Diseases," and Jahr's "Veneral Diseases" translated with additions by Dr. Hempel, which, with some qualifications, also merits the commendatory title given to the other.* Bahr's Article on the disease will also well repay a reference.

In discussing the value of Homœopathy in Syphilis we shall always have to speak comparatively. I mean, first, that the Therapeutics of the old school are not here, as in the case of so many of the maladies we have had to consider, of a Nihilistic character : they are definite and specific, and claim unwonted success. "Anti-syphilitic treatment," as practised at the present day with *Mercury* and *Iodide of Potassium,* is affirmed to be capable of clearing away with remarkable rapidity most of the Secondary and Tertiary phenomena of Syphilis ; and such authorities as Ricord and Hutchnison have affirmed that the judicious treatment of the primary induration with the first-named drug may prevent the outbreak of constitutional symptoms altogether, and cure the disease in its primary stage.

Again, we have to take into account the results of the expectant treatment of Syphilis. It is allowed that both Primary and Secondary manifestations of the disease continue longer in existence under this method than when Anti-syphilitics are used.

---

* See Review in B. J. H., xxxii., 666.

But it is maintained that they are milder in kind and character; and that ultimately the infection disappears, and never goes on to the formation of Gummata and other Teritary phenomena.

The question before us, then, is this—Does the Homœopathic treatment of Syphilis give better results than expectancy? and does it render unnecessary the induction of the Physiological action of *Mercury* (which, however slight its degree, is always involved in the old-school use of the drug), and the administration of large doses of *Iodide of Potassium* -

Let us first inquire what Hahnemann thought on this point. Dr. Dudgeon's collection of his Lesser Writings' contains a very interesting Treatise on Venereal Diseases published by him in 1789—before, therefore, any conception of Homœopathy had entered into his head. In this work he maintains the entire sufficiency of *Mercury* for the cure of every manifestation of Syphilis; but states that to effect this it must be so administered as to set up a "Mercurial Fever" in the system. From eight to twelve grains of *"Mercurius solubilis"* were generally required for the purpose, given in divided but increasing doses. Evacuations—including salivation—were to be avoided; but a "drowsy" administration of the drug, insufficient to excite the specific fever, did no good, but rather harm. By setting up this fever both the primary Chancre 'and the general lues, however inveterate, might be cured in a few days; and if the treatment were adopted in the former stage, no general infection followed. He, of course, makes no distinction between Hard and Soft Chancres.

Writing forty-six years later, in the First Volume of the Second Edition of his 'Chronic Diseases' (1835), he is no less satisfied of the value of Mercurial treatment, though now he gives infinitesimal doses, and sets up no fever. 'In that stage of the Syphilitic disease where the Chancre or the Bubo is yet existing, one single minute dose of the best *Mercuriul* preparation is sufficient to effect a permanent cure of the internal diseaese' togethed which the Chancre, in the space of a fortnight." This "best preparation" he afterwards states to be the *Mercurius vivus;* and as the minute dose he says, "I was formerly in the habit of using successfully one, two or three globules of the billionth degree," i.e., the 6th centesimal dilution, for the cure of Syphilis. The higher degrees, however, even the decillionth —i.e., the 30th—"act more thoroughly, more speedily, and more mildly. If more than one should be required, which is seldom the case, the lower degrees may be then employed." He also says,—"In my practice of fifty years' duration I have never seen Syphilis breaking out in the system when the Chancre was cured by internal remedies, without having been mismanaged by external treatment." He thus recognises the continuity of his former and his later use of *Mercury*, different as it seems in dosage and effect.

Turning now to the general experience of the Homoeopathic school, we find that **Mercurius** in some form or other continues to enjoy universal confidence. Bahr may be taken as a fair exponent of the view of all. He regards "Simple Syphilis" as embracing the primary Chancre and Bubo, and the secondary erythema and superficial ulceration of skin and mucous membrane, with Condyloma and Iritis. All beyond this he considers Mercurio-syphilitic, or purely Mercurial. For this "Simple Syphilis," he says that the only remedy is *Mercurius;* nothing else is required for its complete cure.

But then the question arises,—Is this "cure" anything more than the "recovery" of expectancy? Hahnemann, as we have seen, claims much more for it, viz., the absolute prevention when the Chancre is treated, of secondary symptoms. Two of his followers—Jahr and Schneider*—concur in the same statement each basing it on an experience of thirty years, and the latter referring to more than a thousand cases. It is true that they, as he does, include Soft Chancre as well as Hard in the same category; but it is inconceivable that none of the latter should have occurred to them. Indeed, Dr. Schneider expressly states that the Chancres he treated "often exhibited the indurated condition," while "at most 2 per cent. went into the second period of infection." On the other hand, Bahr says that the indurated sore, in his hands, is generally succeeded by secondary symptoms; and Yeldham that, in his experience, "the appearance or non-appearance of secondary symptoms is a matter beyond the control, in most cases, of the very best treatment that can be adopted."

Whence is the difference in these results? If Hahnemann and Schneider only represented one side, and Yeldham the other, it might fairly have been argued that quantity determined the variation. The former gave their *Mercury* in rare and infinitesimal doses (6th to 30th with Hahnemann, 2nd to 3rd with Schneider); while the latter's smallest allowance to his patients was two grains of the first trituration three times a day. It is maintained by some that, *Mercury* in quantities sufficient to exite Physiological action, favours the occurrence of secondaries: it might have been supposed that Yeldham had been promoting these SEQUELAE, and not merely failing to avert them. But this explanation will not account for the results obtained by the remaining members, of the two groups. Jahr and Bahr treat Chancre almost indentically, the former giving half a grain of the first centesimal trituration morning and evening, the latter one grain of the second or third decimal trituration every other day. And yet Jahr sees his Chancres disappear in from fifteen to twenty days, without secondary symptoms supervening; while Bahr gives six to ten weeks even for the Soft Chancre,

---

* See B. I. H. xxii., 616 and xxxiv., 438.

and nine to fifteen for the indurated.—secondary symptoms commonly breaking out while the latter is still existing. When to these we add Schneider, with his morning and evening globules of the 4th to the 6th decimal potency of *Mercurius solubilis* (which, by the way, ought not to be prepared in globules under the 10th decimal), who allows six to eight weeks for the healing of the sore and the disappearance of the induration, but sees no secondaries,—the confusion is worse confounded, and there seems no rule for the variations.

Now I have argued at some length in my 'Pharmacodynamics' that *Mercury* has no essential similarity to the Syphilitic poison.* If it resolves the local infiltration and the indolent and indurated lymphatic glands of the true Syphilis, it is, I take it by its liquefacient (*i.e., Physiological*) action. Hence its obvious influence (but questionable advantage) in the hands of our old-school brethern; and hence, PERHAPS, Yeldham's satisfaction with it. But I must think that in such doses as those given by Hahnemann (in his later period) and Schneider, its action in the genuine disease in its primary stage is simply NIL, and that their absence of secondaries is either to be accounted for by imperfect after-observation, or is an unusually fortunate occurrence of expectancy.

Jahr's results would have more in their favour were they not neutralised by those of Bahr. Even as it is, I think his practice may well be followed by us, as it is uninjurious. We may heal the Chancre thereby: but I shall be surprised if we hasten the dispersion of the induration, or always or even usually escape secondary symptoms.

These are my own convictions as to the treatment of Chancre, and they are in accordance with what little I have seen of it. But it is fair that I should give you the recommendations of authors, representing as they do the common practice followed in our school, whatever may be their COMPARATIVE value. Here they are, in brief.—

1. For recent and hitherto untreated Chancre, Hahnemann would have given us one dose of *Mercurius vivus* 30; Schneider a dose morning and evening of *Mercurius solubilis* 4x to 6x; Jahr half a grain of the first trituration of the same with like frequency; Bahr a grain of the same preparation or of the *red precipitate* of equal strength every other day; Yeldham from two grains of the 2x trituration of *Mercurius solubilis* to three grains of the 1x three times a day.

2. For neglected (but not Mercurialised) Chanere, Jahr

---

* I am glad to be able to cite in support of this opinion the testimony of Hahnemann. In the Treatise of 1789, to which I have referred, he writes, "*Mercury* does not cure Syphilis by causing evacuations, but rather by the gradual or sudden ANTIPATHIC" (the capitals are my own) "irritation of the fibres of a specific nature" which it sets up (p. 195 of Dudgeon's Translation).

advised the *red precipitate* or *Cinnabar,* half a grain of the first trituration morning and evening.

3. For Chancre of some week's standing, that has been treated in old-school fashion with *Mercury,* **Nitric acid,** is recommended by all,—in the first decimal dilution by Yeldham, the first centesimal by Jhar, the third centesimal by Schneider. Bahr does not specify its dose. But all agree that it often needs supplementing by *Mercurial* preparations after a while ; and Jahr and Yeldham are disposed sometimes to begin these at once.

4. For Phagedænic Chancre, *Mercurius corrosivus* is warmly commended by Jahr, Hartmann and Gerson. Bahr thinks it and the *red precipitate* the best *Mercurial* preparations, but raher prefers *Nitric acid.* Jousset mentions *Nitric acid, Silicea,* and *Arsenicum* in high dilution ; but joins with them either cauterisation or the application of an ointment containing one part in a thousand of *Arsenic.* Yeldham gives a case in which Phagedæna set in while the patient was taking two grains of *Mercurius solubilis* 2x three times daily, and was arrested by *Nitric acid.* But he says of *Mercury* in general that "even in the Phagedænic Chancres, where its use is generally thought to be counter indicated, I have konwn it to arrest the ulceration when other remedies, ordinarily recommended for that condition had failed." I shall have to speak further of this trouble under the head of Soft Chancre.

5. Gangrenous Chancre is mentioned by Bahr, who says that *Arsenicum* is the sole medicine capable of arresting the destructive process ; and by Jahr, who says that the same remedy has never failed him.

When now from Primary we advance to SECONDARY Syphilis both theory and experience are in favour of the value of *Mercury;* and the general rule may be laid down that if this drug has not been hitherto abused in the treatment of the patient, it is the first to be employed in one form or other against these Secondary symptoms.

These must, I apprehend, be considered as elements of a specific febrile state, having its Rash and Sore Throat, with Iritis as its most frequent SEQUELA. The constitutional condition is one of Chloro-anæmia, with Rheumatoid pain (aggravated by rest and the warmth of bed) in the head and face, behind the sternum, and around the joints. To all this *Mercury is* strikingly Homœopathic, and should be employed persistently for its cure.

Then comes the exanthem,—Erythematous, Papular or Squamous. Yeldham prefers the *Iodides of Mercury* here,— two grains of the 2x or 3x trituration twice daily. Jahr gives either *Mercurius solubilis* or the *red precipitate,* more rerely *Cinnabar,* half a grain of the second or third centisimal trituration every other day. Bahr prefers the more intensely-acting

Mercurials here, among which he classes with especial praise *Mercurious vivus;* he gives the 3x trituration, Jousset prefers *Corrosive sublimate* in somewhat substantial doses; but, if he has to follow up with *Nitric acid,* he gives it in the 30th dilution. Schneider is content with *Mercurius solubilis* 3, alternated with *Nitric acid* 3. Where *Mercury* has already been fully given, Yeldham perfers *Kali iodatum* (two grains three times a day) to *Nitric acid;* and Jahr recomends *Phosphorus, Nitric acid, Sarsaparilla,* and *Lycopodium;* in the 18th to the 30th attenuations.

The more severe forms of Syphilitic cutaneous disease I agree with Bahr in thinking largely due to abuse of *Mercurial* treatment. Hence they nearly always require full doses of *Nitric acid* or *Iodide of Potassium* by way of antidotes. When the *Mercurial* element has been, as it were, dissected out by these means, we may proceed to treat the Syphilide occording to its character; as by *Arsenic* or *Borax* if it is Squamous, *Tartar emetic* or *Kali bichromicum* if it is Pustular, *Aurum* or *Hydrocotyle* if it is Tubercular. But now a few intermediate doses of the more potent *Mercurials* will greatly hasten the cure.

We have next the Secondary Syphilitic affections of the mucous membranes. Bahr believes these to be purely Syphilitic only when superficial, and treats them with *Mercurius vivus.* When they are Phagedænic, deeply penetrating, and threatening to affect the bones, he substitutes,—for the mouth, *Kali iodatum* and *bichromicum;* for the nose, *Kali iodatum* and *Aurum muriaticum;* and for the larynx, *Heper sulphuris* and perhaps, *Iodine* and *Kali bichromicum.* Jahr describes the ulcers of the throat as Chancres, and treats them with *Mercurius solubilis* if Simple, *Mercurius corrosivus* if Phagedænic,—half a grain of the 2nd trituration morning and evening. He recommends *Aurum* 3 where the nose is affected, and the *red precipitate* or *Nitric acid* for ulcers on the tongue. But he says nothing of what is to be done when *Mercury* has been fully given already; save that he prescribes *Lachesis, Lycopodium, Nitric acid, Thuja, Cinnabar, or Sulphur* in superficial erosions of the mucous surfaces thus occurring. Schneider is content with his alternate *Mercurius solubilis* and *Nitric acid.* Yeldham recommends that the throat be treated in the first instance for simple inflammation, as with *Belladonna* or *Apis,* and then with the *Iodides of Mercury* or *Nitric acid.* He also touches the throat with *Nitrate of Silver,* and attaches much importance to the administration of Cod-liver Oil.

My own experience in the treatment of these affections is in favour of *Kali bichromicum* [*] in indolent ulceration of the tonsils; of *Kali iodatum* when this is destructive as in the perforating ulcer of the soft palate; and of *Nitric acid* for ulceration of the

---

[*] See testimonies in its favour from Watzke and Russell in the "Hahnemann Materia Medica," Part I., and from Drysdale in the B. J. H., xv., 675.

mouth, and cracks about the commissures of the lips. For these last *Cundurango* promises to be useful.* There is a good case by Dr. Meyhoffer in Volume XXIV of the BRITISH JOURNAL OF HOMŒOPATHY (p. 363), illustrating the value of *Nitric acid* in the symptoms of mouth, throat, and larynx (while *Biniodide of Mercury* removed the exanthem, with headache and falling of the hair) of Secondary Syphilis.

Of this falling of the hair I have further to note that Bahr recommends *Hepar sulphuris* for it.

We have now to speak of TERTIARY Syphilis. Bahr again represents the general opinion of our school when he writes, "We are most assuredly of the opinion that Tertiary symptoms only set in consequence of the improper use of *Mercury;* our reason being that we are not acquainted with a single case of Syphilis where Tertiary symptoms showed themselves under Homœopathic management." We have seen that expectant treatment gives the same results. Bahr accordingly confines his remedies to two Mercurial antidotes. "The Tertiary phenomena require throughout a cautious but continued use of the **Iodide of Potassium.** It is only for single forms that other remedies are required—**Aurum,** for instance, for Syphilitic Lupus, for Caries of the facial bones, for suppurating tophi, and finally for Sarcocele." He also commends the Iodine-springs of Hall.

Bahr does not mention whether he gives the *Iodide of Potassium* in the full doses of the old school. Jahr is more explicit. He says, probably theoretically, that whenever this agent is capable of effecting a cure, it need never be given in doses larger than the one-hundredth of a grain; but of Tertiary bone and periosteal disease be writes : "I have likewise used *Kali iodatum,* even in large doses, as recommended by Allopathic physicians, and I have seen excellent effects from its use in such quantities; but they were never as lasting as the good effects obtained by means of small doses of other remedies. Usually the symptoms yielded to *Kali iodatum* in a very short time, but returned again in six or twelve months, which never occurred in cases that had been cured with the eighteenth or thirtieth attenuation of other drugs. This has induced me to adhere to the latter, without ever giving *Kali iodatum.*" The "other drugs" alluded to are those in general use in diseases of the osseous system, as *Mezereum, Phosphorus* and *Phosphoric acid, Staphisagria, Silicea, Fluoric* and *Nitric acids, Guaiacum* and *Sulphur.* But superior to all Jahr places *Aurum,* of which he gives half a grain of the third trituration every four days. Gummata he has only seen twice ; they were cured in the first instance by *Silicea,* in the second by *Arsenicum.* For the melancholy and prostration of the Syphilitico-mercurial cachexia he has given *Aurum* "with distinguished success."

* J. B. H., xxxxiii., 407.

Yeldham considers that "it is not enough, in the inveterate and deep-acting Tertiary affections to attempt to grapple with all their phases by *Iodide of Potassium,* as is originally done. That is a most useful remedy in many cases, but it is by no means of universal application." This author simply enumerates the various medicines suitable for Tertiary Syphilis according to the part affected; and in two of the cases he gives, *Silicea* (3x) which seems to have removed a Node (though very slowly), and *Graphites* 12 and *Lycopodium* 12, with Cod-liver Oil, to have dispersed Sarcocele.

I have given these citations at some length, because it cannot fail to be a serious question with you whether Homœopathy has anything better to offer in the treatment of Tertiary Syphilis than the full doses of *Iodide Potassium* which you have learnt to employ. When rapidity of action is required, as in painful Nodes, or when Gummata are exciting Neuralgia, Epilepsy, or Paralysis, I think that the common practice can hardly be excelled, and is imperative upon us for our patients' sake. If you would come at its rationale, I refer you to a very interesting Paper on the *Iodide* by Mr. Madden in the Twenty-Sixth Volume of the BRITISH JOURNAL OF HOMOEOPATHY. He points out that the Syphilitic and Rheumatic-gouty affections, and also the chronic indurations of glands, in which it is found so beneficial, are of the nature of organised new growths, which are therefore QUASI-parasitical to the organism, and require parasiticides to destroy them. That *Iodide of Potassium* is such an agent there is much reason to believe; and this accordingly seems to be the rationale of its action. It must hence be given for such purposes in full doses, and the indications for its use must not be expected to be found in its Pathogenesy.

Perhaps also some of the benefits of the *Iodide* here result from its power as a chemical antidote to *Mercury;* and this action also requires material doses.

But when time is not of such moment you may fairly act upon Jahr's statement of the more lasting effects of Homœopathically-acting medicines, and prescribe accordingly. The *Iodide* itself may be indicated in Tertiary disease of the tongue, which Mr. Langston Parker * has known it three times to simulate, and Dr. Yeldham has seen it (in ordinary doses) repeatedly to aggravate. In the same condition *Fluoric acid* may be, according to Dr. Laurie's and my own experience, of striking service. †
Aurum is a dynamic antidote to *Mercury* and acts powerfully upon the testicle and on osseous tissue: it is also a well-known anti-melancholic. It thus covers nearly the whole field of Tertiary Syphilis with its Cachexia; and Dr. Chapman and myself have put each a case on record illustrative of its

---

* See B. J. H., xi., 681.
† Pharmacodynamics, SUB VOCE.

virtues.* The other Anti-syphilitics, and also A-syphilitics (to use Hahnemann's Nomenclature), may come in when indicated, as the following case, taken from the NORTH AMERICAN JOURNAL OF HOMOEOPATHY, will show,—demonstrating at the same time how much may be done in confirmed Syphilis by pure Homœopathic medication : —

"A Portuguese, about thirty years of age, had been in the hospital at Lahaina for eighteen months; during this time he passed through all stages of the Syphilitic virus. When he arrived at Honolulu, the first day of July, he exhibited the most loathsome and disgusting appearance. The right side of his face was covered with a most fœtid ulcer of the Tertiary form of Syphilis: it developed itself over the right eye, down the outer angle and under the eyes to the nose, extending to the mouth over the whole cheek leaving the malar bone entirely bare and dry. There was carious affection of the frontal bone, extending over the right eye around to the temporal bone; the malar and nasal bones were more or less destroyed by the disease. The right eye was entirely closed. These ulcers were discharging a very fœtid and offensive watery fluid, and had a dark red appearance. In addition to all this he had Ascites, and was greatly bloated; from this he had suffered for last six months. The ulcers were very painful ; darting and gnawing pain, burning through the whole of the ulcerated surface, as he expressed it, as if, there were red-hot needles sticking in the ulcers.

"For these symptoms I selected *Ars. alb.* third, three doses a day for three days which greatly relieved the burning and mitigated the pain: but he was not relieved from the pain wholly until he took *Belladonna*, third, three or four doses. After these two remedies ceased to improve, I give *Acid. nit.* morning and evening; improvement followed; after the first week I gave but one dose per day, for two weeks. Under the action of these remedies, the ulcers put on a more healthy appearance, until the end of three weeks, when I could not discover any improvement. I then gave *Aurum muriat.* second, one dose per day. This seemed to stop all progress of caries, and the whole case looked favourable. I continued this remedy three weeks, with occasionally a dose of *Sulphur*, sixth. The healing of the ulcers was steady and permanent. His general health improved, appetite good. The digestive organs were completely restored. The urinary secretion became normal, he gained strength and flesh. A few doses of *Hepar sulph.* and *Ars. alb.*, were then given at intervals of three or four days. These last remedies removed all symptoms of Dropsy and Venereal disease about him. A more grateful person I never saw."

---

* IBID., SUB VOCE.

Besides all this, I do not think that we have yet sounded the depths of the value of simple **Iodine** itself, in minute dosage, in the treatment of Syphilis. From the old school we have the testimony of Dr. Guillemin, who finds the simple tincture do all, both in Secondary and Tertiary affections, that can be done by the *Alkaline iodide*. His doses, as Lancereaux says, "are very small compared with the usual doses of the compounds of *Iodine;*" he mixes five parts of the tincture with a thousand of water and gives two or three desert-spoonfuls twice a day on an empty stomach.* Zeissl, again, "calls attention to the fact that *Iodine*, in doses of two minims of the compound tincture, properly diluted, twice daily, brings about a more rapid disappearance of the affections of the mucous membrane than *Mercury* does. Moreover, according to him, *Iodine* in this stage exerts a weakening action on Syphilis, so that after its administration a few *Mercurial* inunctions suffice to bring about a permanent disappearance of the cutaneous rash."† Then, from our own ranks, we have the testimony of Dr. Jousset. After acknowledging the frequently marvellous results of large doses of *Iodide of Potassium* at the end of the second and throughout the third stage of Syphilis, he adds.—"On the other hand, in studying comparatively the various doses. I have obtained very rapid results with *Iodine* in the 30th, and even in the 500th dilution." At the World's Convention in Philadelphia moreover,, when the high potency men were challenged to say what they could do in Syphilis, their only champion, Dr. Macfarlane, stated his results as obtained with the **Iodide of Mercury** and added that the *Biniodide* acted better still. I suggested that this showed that the *Iodine* was in his mode of treatment more potent than the *Mercury*.

Considering, now, the power of *Iodine* to affect the mucous membranes and skin much as Syphilis—in its Secondary period —does, causing even pustular eruptions and Acne; and the statement of Trousseau, that "in some circumstances certain cachexiæ, and the Syphilitic among them, take a form identical with that ascribed by M. Rilliet to Iodism." § think we may expect it to play a more important part in the Homœopathic

---

* See Lancereaux's Treatise on Syphilis (N. Syd. Soc.), ii., 313.

† Ziemssen's Cyclopædia iii., 280. Dr. Larrien has lately come forward to announce a similar experience : JOURN. BELGE D' HOMŒOPATHIE, July—Aug., 1899.

‡ Such a cure of a Syphilitic adeuopathy as that reported by Dr. Bonino in the HAHNEMANNIAN MONTHLY of February, 1899, shows *Iodine* in other combinations working brilliantly as an Anti-syphilitic.

§ Colombini and Gerulli have shown its power of diminishing the red corpuscles and the hæmoglobin in the blood of healthy subjects, while it increases both in Syphilitics (M. H. R., xli., 575).

Therapeutics of Syphilis than it has hitherto done, and to make those Therapeutics still more effective than they are.

To the foregoing effect I delivered myself in 1877. You will naturally ask what changes or additions the years have brought since then.

1. I have no modification to make in my views as to the place of *Mercury* in the Homœopathic treatment of Syphilis. As regards *Iodide of Potassium*. I am bound to cite Meyhotter's statements, which bear out those of Jahr just adduced: "It has become the fashion," he writes in his "Chronic Diseases of the Organs of Respiration" (I. 190), "even among the disciples of Hahnemann, to exhibit the *Iodide of Potassium* in increasing doses; but we are convinced that this course is as useless as it is often injurious. From the moment the drug produces pathogenetic symptoms, it exaggerates the functions of the tissues, exhausts the already diminished vitality, and thence, instead of stimulating the organic cell in the direction of life, impairs or abolishes its power of contraction (qy. ? counteraction). We use, as a rule, the 1st dilution, from 6 to 20 drops a day; if after a week no decided progress is visible, one drop of the tincture of *Iodine* is added to each 100 of this 1st dilution." In this way he says, "the mucous tubercles, gummy deposits and ulcerations resulting therefrom in the larynx undergo a favourable termination." (It is of Laryngeal Syphilis that he is speaking). I have also to mention the Paper read by Mr. Knox-Shaw at the British Congress of 1891.* in which he defends the thesis that *Iodide of Potassium* is really Homœopathic to the lesions of Tertiary Syphilis having the power of causing similar phenomena. It seems to me (as I said at the time) that while Mr. Shaw well proved his points as far as the cutaneous lesions of the disease are concerned, there is as yet no evidence that it can cause anything like the gummatous deposits in the viscera and on the bones; while the dosage which is most effectual, and indeed ordinarily indispensable, is such as hardly consorts with the idea of a similarly-acting specific. Mr. Shaw promised to bring forward cases rendering nugatory the latter objection; but they have not yet made their appearance. His colleague at our London Hospital, however, Mr. Dudley Wright, could in 1893 express himself quite satisfied from his own experience that "the 1x dilution of *Iodide of Potassium* will, in the majority of instances of Syphilis, accomplish all that the drug undoubtedly does in larger doses." †

---

* See M. H. R., xxxv., 565.
† M. H. R., xxxvii., 346.

2. In his earliest study of the pathogenesis of *Kali bichromicum* Dr. Drysdale called attention to the similarity between its action and that of Syphilis, and thought we might fairly expect it to prove another remedy for that disease. His hopes have been often verified since in the treatment of lues affecting the nose, throat, eye, skin and periosteum; but their fulfilment has subsequently taken a wider range in the results obtained by Guntz, which our lamented colleague has epitomized in his latest presentation of the drug. I refer to his Article upon it, in the First and only Volume of the "Materia Medica, Physiological and Applied." You will find there that Guntz regards the *Chromic salt* a substitute for *Mercury* and *Iodine* in all stages of the disease. His cases seem to show that to abort the disease in its primary stage *Kali bichrcmicum* is more powerful than *Mercury*, and that it is at least equally curative in the constitutional symptoms, while it is, of course, much less harmful. He gives about half a grain daily.

3. If there be anything fresh of late years in our own Therapeutics of Syphilis, I should say it is in the larger use we make of *Nitric acid*. The cases by Dr. Kernler, summarised in the Third Volume of the JOURNAL OF THE BRITISH HOMŒOPATHIC SOCIETY (p. 216), well-illustrate its frequent usefulness, and that in purely dynamic dosage. I can cordially commend it to you in the ulcerations of the second stage, and in well-mercurialised subjects.

The other general disease of venereal origin, which our Nomenclature recognises is

GONORRHŒA. It can only, I suppose, become general by direct extension, or by local transmission : it does not infect the system by absorption, unless Gonorrhœal Rheumatism and Iritis are to be so accounted for. You have probably been taught to endeavour to abort this inflammation by injections. Let me caution you against doing so, save in its earliest incipience and its non-inflammatory forms; and then by mild astringents or antiseptics only. I will not urge you to try instead *Sepia* 30 night and morning, as recommended by Jahr; for I have not proved it. I can, however, confidently recommend the following treatment for the fully-established disease.

If your patient has it for the first time, and the inflammatory symptoms run high, put him on a low dilution of **Aconite** or **Gelsemium**, according to the amount and kind of constitutional disturbance, and trust to that alone. A case of Dr. Pope's in the Twenty-Fifth Volume of the BRITISH JOURNAL OF HOMŒOPATHY (p. 508) will show you what *Aconite* can do, and the virtues of *Gelsemium* find abundant evidence in Dr. Hale's 'New Remedies.' When the inflammatory symptoms have subsided, or if they have been moderate from the first, give **Cannabis sativa** steadily. It seems generally agreed that this medicine must not be much, if at all, attenuated. Even Jhar recommends the 3rd dilution; but most of our therapeutists use the mother-tincture, and are not particular about number of drops. The only other remedy likely to be required is **Cantharis,** which should be given (not too low) intercurrently with the other medicines when the urinary symptoms indicate that the inflammation is extending towards the bladder. It is also useful when painful erections occur.

The above has always been my treatment of Gonorrhœa, and it fairy represents that of our school. Bahr is the only marked exception. He would have us give *Mercurius solubilis* for the first ten or twelve days, and then (when the symptoms are less active) *Hepar sulphuris* till the close. He admits that four weeks are required for the duration of the disease under the medication, but asserts that Orchitis and Prostatitis hardly ever occur, and that in very few cases does a secondary discharge remain. He allows *Cannabis* to be preferable only in non-inflammatory cases. Jahr, giving the latter medicine alone, claims always to effect a cure in two or at the most three weeks. He recognises the value of occasiosal doses of *Mercurius* (*Vivus*, 2nd trit), if *Cannabis* hangs fire. Yeldham gives the same metal, in the form of *Corrosive sublimate* (five-drop doses of the 3rd decimal) in alternation with *Aconite* for the first week of inflammatory cases; and Jousset employs the *salt* in a weak injection to check lingering descharge. **Mercurius,** therefore, in some form or other, plays no unimportant part in the Homœopathic Therapeutics of Gonorrhœa as of Syphilis. **Copaiba,** which is quite Homœopathic to the morbid process—as I have shown in my Pharmacodynamics, is favourably spoken of both by Yeldham and by Jousset; but no distinctive place is assigned to it. The former also commends *Thuja*, which has produced a more outspoken Urethritis than has been obtained from any other drug; but which has been little used in Acute Gonorrhœa. Of the *Petroselinum* recommended by Hahnemann as an alternative to *Copaiba* we have no later experience; but may mention that Dr. Gilchrist prefers **Apis** to either, and thinks that, administered early in the inflammatory period, it will often abort the disease.

Chronic Gonorrhœa—"Gleet"—is not readily amenable to internal remedies. Those of which we have spoken in relation to the acute stage are sometimes of service, especially **Thuja** after which **Nitric acid** may come in usefully. We have also some testimony in favour of *Zincum muriaticum* 3 from Tessier, of *Kali iodatum* 3x from Franklin, of *Matico* 1x from Kafka, of *Sepia* 30 from Jahr, and of *Silicea* 6. More commonly, the best way of treating Gleet is to prescribe medicines suited to the state of the general health (which is nearly always depressed), such as *Sulphur, Nux vomica,* or *Ferrum* : and to medicate the urethra locally by injections. Those recommended by Dr. Yeldham are effectual and uninjurious, viz., : half a drachm of *Goulard's extract* to an ounce of Distilled Water, or an infusion of powered *Hydrastis* root in the proportion of an ounce to the pint.

Of the complications of Gonorrhœa I have spoken, or I shall speak, in other proper places.

SOFT CHANCRE, with its suppurating Bubo, is now generally recognised as a local, though specific and contagious venereal affection,—as standing, in fact, in the same category as Gonorrhœa. The very reason which have led me to maintain that **Mercurius** is Antipathic in relation to the Hard Chancre show that it is Homœopathic to the Soft; and you may rely upon it with the utmost confidence, and in quite moderate dosage. It cures, not because of the influence it exerts over the Syphilitic virus, but in virtue of its power of causing ulceration generally and at this particular spot. **Nitric acid** is here, as in ulcers of the mouth, an effectual ally to it; and the two medicines often come in usefully to reinforce one another's action when it is flagging.

Of the treatment of the accidents of Chancre I have discoursed when upon Syphilis. I have only now to speak of that of the Chancrous Bubo. Yeldham and Bahr concur in recommending that the *Mercurius* the patient is taking should be steadily continued when this complication appears, as its best remedy. **Hepar Sulphuris** may be substituted if suppuration appears inevitable. The former writer was in the habit at one time of opening the abscess early, but he has now so frequently seen it disperse without breaking that he gives it a last chance of doing so. Jahr and Caspari have had correspondingly good result from **Carbo animalis.** Of the treatment of Phagedænic Bubo I will speak in Dr. Yeldham's words. "It demands," he says, "the most careful management, both local and constitutional. The former consists, first, in the use of warm Linseed poultices; and, secondly, of *Calendula* lotion in the proportion of one part of the tincture to eight of water. Cotton-wool should be soaked in this, and laid in and over the wounds. The *Lotio nigra* may sometimes be advantageously substituted for it. The constitutional treatment consists in the administration of *Merc. sol.* or the *Biniodide of Mercury,* in from five to ten-gram doses of the 2nd decimal trituration, if *Mercury* have not already been given; or if it have, of *Acidum nitricum,* in ten-drop doses of the 1st or 2nd decimal dilution; or of *Kali hydriodicum,* in five-grain doses three times a day. The patient's powers should, at the sametime, be sustained by a generous diet, to which a table-spoonful of Cod-liver Oil every night is an excellent addition. He should also keep himself quiet, and as much as possible in the recumbent posture. Movement, from the peculiar situation of the disease, tends to retard the healing process." †

---

* Mr. Dudley Wright prefers the application of equal parts of *Glycerine* and the fluid extract with the help of the endoscope **(M. H. R.,** xliii., 129).

† Op. Cit., 3rd. Ed., p. 92.

Finally, I will follow Hahnemann in giving to SYCOSIS a separate place from Syphilis, and in reckoning it as general disease as Gonorrhœa may become. Of the nature and clinical history of the Condyloma which is its Chancre I have already, when speaking of *Thuja,* mentioned how diverse the opinions are. To the authorities cited then I may add Baumler, the Essayist on Syphilis in Ziemssen's Cyclopædia. He regards the Condylomata of the skin as identical with the mucous patches of the mouth, and both as modifications of the papule of Secondary Syphilis. But, he adds, "the so-called ACUMINATE CONDYLOMA (Mucous Papiloma), which has nothing at all to do with Syphilis, and is caused by irritation of the skin of mucous membrane with different secretions (particularly Gonorrhœal pus), and moreover is contagious, must not be confounded with the flat Condylomata."

However this may be, the following are the practical directions of Homœopathic therapeutists regarding the treatment of Sycosis phenomena :—

1. A true Chancre not uncommonly sprouts into Codylomatous vegetations before disappearing, or becomes transformed IN SITU into a mucous patch. If this is not the effect of large dose of *Mercury,* the continued use of that remedy in the manner already indicated for Chancre will lead to the disappearance of the phenomena; so say Bahr and Jahr. But if *Mercury* has been freely given, *Nitric acid* (1st dil.) or *Thuja* must (Jahr says) be administered.

2. For mucous Tubercles occurring elsewhere as concomitants or sequelæ of Chancre, the treatment of the same, with *Lycopodium* if they appear on the tonsils, or instead of being smooth, are jagged and rough. This last indication is from Espanet.

3. Excrescenes, "Fig-warts" (hence the name Sycosis), may also follow or accompany Chancre. In this case Jahr finds *Cinnabar* and *Nitric acid,** sometimes *Phosphoric acid* and *Staphisagria,* remedial. Bahr gives *Thuja* for them when they are accuminated and dry.

4. When Condylomata occur simply, or in connection with Gonorrhœa, all follow Hahnemann in treating them with **Thuja** internally or externally, or both. Jousset follows Petroz in believing such growths to be manifestations of a diathese epitheliale," and classing them with Warts and Polypi. But for all, the main remedy is *Thuja,* and generally in high (30th) dilution.

---

* A case by Dr. Henriques, in which the medicine (internally and locally) rapidly reduced them, may be read in B. J. H., xix., 64.

LECTURE XXIV.

DISEASES OF THE NERVOUS SYSTEM.

MALADIES AFFECTING THE BRAIN

CONGESTION—MENINGITIS—CEREBRITIS—SOFTENING
—CEREBRAL TUMOURS—APOPLEXY.

From the General Diseases—"Morbi Corporis Universi"—which have hitherto come before us, we pass to those of particular systems or organs—"Morbi Partium Singularum"; and take first, as of prerogative right, that organism within the organism whereby the animal differs in kind from the vegetable, and man differs in degree 'from other animals,—the NERVOUS SYSTEM. While in brain, cord and nerve we possess an apparatus of marvellous sensitiveness and flexibility for carrying on our higher physical and psychical life, it is one too liable to disorder and even disease, especially as civilization makes upon it its ever increasing demands. It is therefore very important to know what aid Homœopathy brings us in our dealing with the maladies of these organs so important to man in his place at the summit of creation.

A point I will make (before proceeding to special diseases), is that in its employment of *Belladonna* Homœopathy has made a contribution of the first importance to neurological medicine. If you look at the treatises on 'Materia Medica' of fifty years ago, such as those of Pereira and Neligan, you will find this plant classed as as a "narcotic," and recommended in disease—mainly locally—as anodyne and calmative. Already, however, its Physiological effect was so obvious as to lead Pereira to consider it (from his stand point) contra-indicated in ferbile and acute inflammatory cases; while from the other side Homœopathy saw in such conditions its indications. The Essays of Hartmann, "On the Principal Homœopathic Remedies," published during the decade 1830-1843 show that in the hands of Hahnemann and his followers it had even then become a polychrest of the utmost renown, and was esteemed in the treatment of most fevers, inflammations, and congestions as highly as in the neuroses to which its use had hitherto been restricted. I had myself, before being numbered with this band, taken much interest in the action of

Belladonna, and had written papers on it in the journals.*
I then, however, had been disposed to trace all its effects
to the stimulant influence it undoubtedly exerts on the vasomotor nerves, and the consequent contraction of the arterioles.
In 1862, after my conversion, I published in the BRITISH
JOURNAL OF HOMŒOPATHY a series of Cases of Poisoning
by *Belladonna*, with Commentaries"; and there maintained that
the nervous symptoms of the drug, with their accompanying
hyperæmia, were due to an inflammatory irritation set up
by it in the centres, analogous to that which, seen elsewhere, had led Christison to class it as a Narcotico-ACRID. In 1869.
Dr. John Harley issued, under the title of "The Old Vegetable
Neurotics," his Gulstonian Lectures of the previous year, in which
he comes to a similar conclusion. He calls the action "hyperoxidation of nerve tissue," but obviously means the same thing. The
only difficulty in the way of this hyphothesis was the Anæsthesia and
Paralysis 'occasionally present, especially in animals, from its
action; but this, with its dilated pupil and its tachycardia,
I showed in my 'Pharmacodynamics' of 1875 to be due to an influence
exerted on the function of the terminal extremities of the nerves,
and quite separate from that displayed in the centres. Pharmacology
has thus vindicated what symptomatology earlier led to:
and has given us in *Belladonna* a medicine curative. of,
because Homœopathic to, every form of nervous erethism and
hyperæmia, from a simple congestive headache to a fully-developed
Phrenitis or Myelitis.

You see at once what a potent weapon this gives us in our
combat with some of the most alarming disorders that affect
the human frame. A man falls down in an Apoplectic fit : he is
insensible, his face is flushed and warm. There may be no
circulatory tension or excitement such as would have led to
venesection in the past, and which we should relieve with *Aconite*
now. The condition is one for which the older physician would
have leeched or cupped, and against which now these measures
being hardly available, they are powerless. *Belladonna* will be
found to supersede the local as *Aconite* does the general bloodletting, and to reduce the cerebral circulation to a normal state.
It may come in again also later on, when reactive inflammation
is set up around the clot. I shall not readily forget my distress
at watching a brother of mine, who had been thus attacked
while walking along Piccadilly, and was carried into St. George's
Hospital. Every kindness was shown him, but the treatment
was absolutely Nihilistic: they noted the rise of temperature
most regularly and accurately, but they did nothing to subdue
it, as I knew *Belladonna* might have done. Again, a child is
seized with Convulsions,—it may be from Teething, it may be
during Whooping-cough. If hyperæmia accompany, as it

* LONDON MEDICAL REVIEW, 1860; BRIT. MEDICAL JOURNAL, Ibid,

generally does, *Belladonna* will nearly always prevent the recurrence of fits. Puerperal Convulsions are too generally uræmic to allow of similar medication being effectual; but if the urine is free from albumen, so that they seem to depend on abnormal reflex excitability, the indications for *Belladonna* may be followed with confidence. If you should ever see any variety of the "Brain-fever" so frequently spoken of in older literature—such as we should now call acute ' congestion, as from insolation, mental excitement, intemperance, or concussion; if you should have to treat Acoholism in the form of Mania-a-potu, or such acute Maniacal Delirium as Maudsley describes resulting from transfer of Erysipelas from the leg to the brain; if the Delirium of the Fevers or Exanthemata should be active and hyperæmic enough to require a special remedy—in all these circumstances *Belladonna* may be relied upon with the utmost confidence. Even in Tetanus and Hydrophobia—as we shall see—it may play a useful part. The co-existence of fever in such cases calls for no other medicine. *Belladonna* is one of the substances that can produce this state in health. De Meuriot, in his ETUDE of the drug, relates observations showing its power to raise the temperature in dogs from 1° to 4° degrees of the Centigrade Scale, and in man from $\frac{1}{2}$ to $1\frac{1}{10}$°. Higher ranges indeed than this have been noted in the human subject ; as in a recently reported case where a solution of *Sulphate of Atropine*, four grains to the ounce, dropped into the eye of a baby of a month old, twice caused fever—the temperature rising to 104·5° and 107·2° on the two occasions respectively.*

Nor is it only in these acute affections that the specific irritation set up in nervous tissue by *Belladonna* makes it a Homœopathic remedy. You know how many distinct forms of chronic nervous diseases have been brought into view, especially by the French Pathologists, during the last forty years: you may profitably read them—if you have not already done so—in the fascinating pages of Trousseau's "Clinical Lectures." Now there is one common feature of all these maladies—that they have, as their basis and inception, inflammation, followed by induration or atrophy, of particular tracts or elements of the cranio-spinal axis. Dr. Jousset has clearly exhibited them in this light, including in his survey Locomotor Ataxy, Multiple Cerebro-spinal Sclerosis (SCLEROSE EN PLAQUES). General Paralysis of the Insane, Spinal Paralysis of adults and infants, Labio-glosso-laryngeal Paralysis and Progressive Muscular Atrophy. To these may be added Pseudo-hypertrophic Spinal Paralysis and Lateral Sclerosis. When the stage of induration or atrophy has been reached, what little can be done for these maladies must be essayed with drugs of profounder action, like *Mercury*,

---

* See M. H. R., xxxix., 465.

Phosphorus and *Plumbum*. But their forming stage is the one hopeful time in which to take them; and here they have a SIMILE, and will often find a curative, in the great medicine we have been considering.

We continue to follow our official Nosology in giving preeminence in place among local maladies to the diseases of the brain. spinal cord, and the nervous system in general. When we come to details, however, it will be unwise any longer to tread closely in the foot-steps of our chosen guide. The Nomenclature of the College of Physicians was designed to facilitate statistical registration, to give greater exactness and uniformity to the reports made as to the occurrence and mortality of disease. Our object here is Therapeutics : we need to include and designate according as maladies meet us in practice, and call upon us for treatment. While therefore, I shall gladly use the catalogue of diseases given us by authority, so as to omit no disorder mentioned there, and also in choosing among the synonyms of the several maladies, I shall for the future to a great extent classify for myself.

I begin to-day the consideration of diseases affecting the BRAIN. I think I shall not omit anything of importance, if I treat, first, of its substantial disorders—CONGESTION, INFLAMATION, SOFTENING, and TUMOUR, with APOPLEXY, then of Mental Disorders (including DELIRIUM TREMENS). HEADACHE, VERTIGO, and the DERANGEMENTS OF SLEEP: lastly, of Injuries to the Head. From this list I shall exclude the many brain affections peculiar to childhood culminating in **Acute Hydrocephalus :** as these will be considered in the Section devoted to the subject of 'Children's Diseases.'

For my account of the Homœopathic treatment of these maladies I shall draw largely upon a series of treatises in which Dr. Peters. of New York, has embodied all the cases of cure collected by Ruckert with additions and comments.

I will first speak of

CEREBRAL CONGESTION,—The treatment of this condition will depend upon whether it is acute or chronic, active or passive, primary or secondary. I shall best handle these varieties by indicating the sphere of the leading remedies employed in their management.

Aconite is the remedy for acute active congestion resulting from cold or from violent emotion. There is tension of the circulation and coldness of the rest of the body.

Belladonna replaces *Aconite* where the concomitants mentioned do not exist,* or when hyperæmia remains after the action of

---

* Bahr gives "disposition to perspire", as a valuable indication for *Belladonna* in preference to *Aconite*.

the latter drug has exhausted. It has also a wide sphere of its own in simple active Congestion, with redness of face and tendency to Delirium; and in more chronic forms of the condition in delicate subjects. It is the primary remedy (as we shall see) for the Cerebral Congestions of childhood.

Glonoin supersedes *Belladonna* in more sudden and intense congestion, without fever. It is thus the great remedy in Sun-stroke, and in the cerebral effects of Menstrual Suppression.

Veratrum viride has lately been used* with much satisfaction in febrile conditions complicated with cerebral hyperæmia and excitement, where otherwise we should have to give *Aconite* and *Belladonna*.

Gelsemium is a valuable remedy for recent PASSIVE Congestion with Diplopia, Giddiness, etc. *Opium* replaces it when sopor is very marked.

Nux vomica stands midway between Acute and Chronic Congestion of the Brain. Not unserviceable in the former, as we shall see under Apoplexy and Headache, it is especially in hyperæmia of some-standing that it proves valuable, when occurring in strong frames and in persons of sedentary occupations, given to mental exertions, and in the habit of taking plenty of animal food and of *Alcohol*.

Arnica, Sulphur and **Iodium** are occasional remedies for Chronic Congestion, where *Nux* is not indicated. The former has much Vertigo: the two latter are suggested when the face breaks out into erythema or Acne. **Ferrum** is to be thought of where the hyperæmia relieves itself by Epistaxis.

Inflammation of the Brain comes before us in two different forms, according as the membranes or the substance of the organ are the seat—at any rate, the primary seat—of the morbid process.

I will begin with

MENINGITIS.—Theoretically, it would be correct to discuss under this heading inflammation affecting the dura mater, the arachnoid, and the pia mater respectively. But practically such a division is untenable. It is doubtful whether the arachnoid is ever primarily affected. Its upper layer is often involved in inflammation of the dura mater: its lower layer sympathizes with all that affects the pia mater. So that the practical division of the subject into Meningitis involving the dura mater and cranial arachnoid, and Meningitis involving the pia mater and cerebral arachnoid.

---

* See Pharmacodynamics, SUB VOCE.

1. The first form of Meningitis commonly comes before us as the result of external injury. It is that so graphically described by Watson :—

"A man receives a blow on the head; blow stuns him perhaps at the time, but he presently recovers himself, and remains for a certain period apparently in perfect health. But after some days he begins to complain; he has pain of the head, is 'restless, cannot sleep, has a frequent and hard pulse, a hot and dry skin, his countenance becomes flushed, his eyes are red and ferrety; rigors, nausea and vomiting supervene; and towards the end, delirium, convulsions or coma.

On opening the skull, the dura mater is found inflamed, and lymph or pus effused upon the superior surface of the arachnoid.

It is also occasionally caused by extension of disease from the internal ear. Of the latter the following case (from Peters) seems an example, and illustrates its treatment :—

"A youth æt. 18, had suffered from a discharge from the ear, which became suppressed by cold. He had violent piercing and insupportable pains darting from one ear to the other through the head, high fever, intolerance of light with very movable pupils, sleeplessness or starting up from slumber, violent cough with pain in the forehead, and constipation. He took *Bryonia* 2, one sixth of a drop every two hours. At the end of twenty four hours the discharge from the ear had returned, he had profuse prespiration, especially upon the head, the pain and fever were but slight, the skin only moderately warm, thirst not urgent, but he was restless, tossed about, thought he was going to die, slumbered a good deal, and had involuntary discharge of mucous from the bowels. *Hyoscyamus* 2nd dil. followed by the 1st, removed all danger in three days, and the patient was well in six."

It is to hospital experience that we should look for the proper treatment of Meningitis from injury; I cannot, however, find that any such is on record in Homœopathic literature. I can only suggest the use of **Arnica** from the commencement as a prophylactic, and administration of a low dilution of **Aconite** in frequently repeated doses as soon as inflammatory or febrile symptoms appear. If Delirium supervenes, you may alternate your *Aconite* with **Belladonna**, but do not omit it. Only if symptoms of effusion appear must it be abandoned in favour of the medicines of which I shall have to speak as suitable to the second stage of ordinary Meningitis.

2. Inflammation of the pia mater involving the arachnoid is the most common form of Meningitis. It is that which is set up by the Scarlatinal and Rheumatic poisons, and occasionally occurs in the course of Typhoid Fever and other acute diseases; it is sometimes the "Brain Fever," moreover, which is met with in the course of reaction from concussion without injury to the cranium, and as the result of excessive heat, mental excitement, intemperance, and such like causes.

Here, too **Aconite** is indispensable at the outset in primary inflammations while excitement is present. Give repeated doses until arterial tension relaxes and febrile heat departs in perspiration, and you will have won half the battle. All the good effects ascribed by Abercrombie and Watson to blood-letting in these cases will have been obtained, without spoliation of the vital fluid. Then, or in secondary Meningitis from the first, consider **Belladonna** and **Bryonia**. Jahr well indicates the differential diagnosis:—"I prefer *Bryonia* if the delirium is milder, and the pains are severe, shooting and tearing." That is, if the membranes are more affected than the brain itself. But it may often be difficult to decide between the two; and, in a complex condition like this, their alternation seems quite justifiable.

But it may be that, by the time you are called to your patient, the stage of excitement might be merging into that of depression and stupor, or this latter condition may be already developed. Remembering Trinks' canon as to the place of *Bryonia* in serious inflammations, viz., that it belongs to the period of effusion,* you will yet find it useful if the symptoms hitherto have been mainly meningeal. Should it fail to effect any change, your choice will lie between **Apis, Helleborus,** and **Sulphur.** The second would be preferable to the first when the cerebral depression was out of proportion to the amount of effusion, indicating that the brain-substance itself had been much affected; it would, in fact, follow *Belladonna* as *Apis* would *Bryonia*. But, should these directly Homœopathic remedies prove ineffectual, you would do well at once to fall back upon the inflexible and undoubted virtues of *Sulphur;* upon which, indeed, some of our therapeutists would have us rely exclusively as soon as the time for *Aconite, Belladonna,* and *Bryonia* has passed.

As long as the thermometer tells us that the heat of the blood is above the average standard (and it rarely falls throughout the course of this disease), I would not advise you to go beyond the truly Antiphlogistic remedy now mentioned. But, should inflammation really have ceased, and nothing but effusion or cerebral torpor remain, **Arnica** and **Zincum** may be thought of. The former would of course be specially indicated where Concussion had been the exciting cause; but, as promting the absorption of any serous effusion, it takes up the action where *Bryonia* and *Apis* leave it. *Zincum* occupies a corresponding third place in relation to *Belladonna* and *Helleborus;* even in advanced Paralysis from Encephalitis, with general coldness, it has been known to excite salutary reaction.

---

* See Pharmacodynamics, SUB VOCE.

Of the place and value of these medicines you will find abundant illustration in Dr. Peters' "Treatise on the Inflammatory and Organic Diseases of the Brain," and in Bahr and Jahr.* The inference both from the evidence adduced and from the agreement as to remedies, is much in favour of the power of Homœopathy over the diseases. On the other side we have Dr. Hammond's admission † that out of thirteen cases treated by him he lost ten, and that the good result in the three which recovered was not obtained with the orthodox medication he recommends—blood-letting, cold, purging, and Mercurialisation—but with large doses of *Bromide of Potassium.*

It is otherwise with Chronic Meningitis. We have here no definite Homœopathic experience or record; while, on the other hand, the therapeutists of the old school testify to results often surprisingly good with the large doses of *Iodide of Potassium* which they administer. In many cases the explanation of its beneficial effects is undoubtedly that the affection is Syphilitic, and the action of the drug is simply destructive to the new formation. But we may have Chronic Meningitis, especially at the convexity of the brain, from other causes, and still the *Iodide* is frequently beneficial, while smaller (though still substantial) doses are required. In the presence of this disease, therefore, I can say nothing about Homœopathic treatment, and should myself feel it a duty to give my patients the benefit of full and increasing doses of *Iodide of Potassium*. If, too, the *Bichloride of Mercury* helps its action in Syphilitic cases, and one of the *Bromides* in those otherwise caused, I know of no reason why they should not be employed.

So far of inflammation affecting the membranes of the brain. We come now to that which involves the BRAIN SUBSTANCE itself—

CEREBRITIS.—Inflammation of the brain, like that of the liver, may take place either in the essential elements of the organ—here the nerve cells and fibres—or in the connective tissue. In the former case it ends, if not checked, in Abscess; in the latter it leads to induration and atrophy.

1. Suppurative Cerebritis is always circumscribed, and presents itself in a sub-acute or chronic form, in the latter case

---

* A marked case of Cerebral Meningitis occurring in adult is recorded in CALCUTTA JOURNAL OF MEDICINE for July, 1805. The action of *Aconite Glonoin* and *Bryonia* was very decided.

† Treatise on Diseases of the Nervous System, 6th Ed.

constituting cerebral abscess. The symptoms of irritation and fever are never severe, and I do not think that *Aconite* and *Belladonna* find any place in its treatment. The most Homœopathic remedy for this condition seems to me to be **Mercurius**. I have mentioned, when speaking of this metal, that its influence on the cerebrum is very marked; and the symptoms it induces, which might belong to any degeneration of the organ, from its action elsewhere are best ascribed to inflammation. So when Sir Thomas Watson says, "I have known several obscure but threatening symptoms of brain disease clear entirely away when the gums were made sore by *Mercury* and kept slightly tender for some time,"* one is inclined to suppose that the power of the drug to cause cerebral disease had something to do with the cure, and that the Stomatitis was quite an unnecessary element in the treatment. I know, however of no intentional Homœopathic use of the drug for the purpose, or indeed of any recorded experience in the treatment of the disease. As regards our authors, Bahr suggests *Iodium* and *Plumbum,* giving a case of chronic poisoning by the latter metal in which the Autopsy disclosed Abscess of the Brain; and Jousset, reminding us of the harm which *Nux vomica* does in ordinary doses, justly infers that in minute quantities it might be beneficial.

2. Inflammation of the neuroglia of the brain causing induration thereof, and consequent atrophy of the brain substance, has only been recognized of late years. It may occur over one large tract, or in disseminated FOCI; hence we have "Diffuse" and "Multiple Cerebral Sclerosis.' The symptomatology of the affection, in these two forms is excellently given by Dr. Hammond; and its study may lead us to suitable remedies for the disease, among which *Baryta* deserves consideration, from the success which this writer claims from the administration of the *Chloride of Barium.* At present, I should suggest **Plumbum** as the drug best indicated by the nature of the lesion. Induration and atrophy are most frequently found POST MORTEM in the nervous centres of those subject to its influence; and the TREMBLOTTEMENT SATURNINE, as also the spasms and shooting or tearing pains it causes, have striking analogies in the phenomena of Cerebral Sclerosis. Dr. Halbert has had some good result from *Aurum.* †

SOFTENING OF THE BRAIN may be either Idiopathic, or secondary to obstruction of blood-vessels. In the former case the

---

* Mr. Jonathan Hutchinson, in Quain's Dictionary, speaks equally strongly as to the advantage of *Mercury* in cerebral inflammation.
† See the CLINIQUE, March, 1899.

morbid process is called an inflammation of the brain substance, though it has no tendency, as in true Cerebritis, to suppuration. If it be inflammatory at all, it seems analogous—again to use the liver in illustration—to Acute Hepatic Atrophy; and like that malady, it finds its correspondence in Pathogenesy among the effects of **Phosphorus.** I have shown, when speaking of this drug, that it is truly Homœopathic to Cerebral Softening; and the credit it is now receiving in its treatment in the hands of practitioners of the old school must be laid to its dynamic rather than to its nutrient operations on the nervous substance. Jahr speaks warmly of its power over the disease; and, from his description of the symptoms, it is evident that he has treated genuine cases. He always uses the 30th dilution.

The Softening dependant on dificient nutrition is Pathologically different from the primary form; but it may still find a useful medicine in *Phosphorus*. It is a Fatty Degeneration; and the powers of the drug to cause this morbid process in nearly every tissue of the body is now established. When, moreover, the obstruction to the supply of the blood arises from arterial Thrombosis, forming itself upon previous Atheroma, the drug would be as suitable to the cause as to the effect.* When the obstruction is from embolism, it would of course have no such influence; but there is nothing to prevent its aiding the starved part to avail itself of the collateral circulation as this becomes established.

Of
CEREBRAL TUMOURS, the prognosis given in the ordinary text-books is that they must necessarily kill unless they are Syphilitic, in which case they can nearly always be dispersed by full doses of *Iodide of Potassium*, with or without the *Bichioride of Mercury* to aid. I do not know that Homœopathy enables us to alter this statement in any particular. I can only add that **Apomorphia** has been found to check the vomiting and **Glonoin** to remove the occasional congestions incidential to the presence of these growths. Possibly, too, by remedies chosen from close symptomatic resemblance, and given in highest dilutions we may

---

* "In the case of a gentleman, aged sixty, with weakened brain and Bronchitis depending on adipose degeneration, I have seen, after five years of long and steady use of *Arsenic, Digitalis,* and *Phosphorus*, a very material gain in health and strength. A large arcus senilis diminished; a pulse, felt with extreme difficulty, now readily counted; and a weak-beating heart now manifesting in its clearer sounds a great gain in vigour" (Black).

palliate the atrocious pains they cause;* but, if not, we must resort to the ordinary *Anodynes,* among which Dr. Russell Reynold's *Indian Hemp* is the least objectionable.

The last disease of which I shall speak in this lecture is—

APOPLEXY.—Of the treatment of this very common disorder we have abundance of Homœopathic experience on record. I need not refer you to many books however; for you will find a very complete collection of all that had been published up to date on this subject in Dr. Petar's 'TREATISE ON APOPLEXY.'

There are three stages in the course of the malady in which we may have to consider the most appropriate treatment to adopt.

1. Our patient may be suffering under the well-known premonitory signs of this affection. Presenting constitutional evidence of tendency to Cerebral Congestion, or arterial degeneration or both, he complains of Headache, Vertigo, transient Deafness or Blindness, Double Vision, faltering speech, partial Paralyses or Anæthesiæ, failure of memory, drowsiness, dread, and so on. Here, besides the obvious hygienic and general measures, we have medicines of inestimable service. **Nux vomica, Belladonna,** or one of the others mentioned under Cerebral Congestion, will control the determination of the blood to the brain; and **Phosphorus** will do something to retard the advance of brittleness and obstruction of the arteries.

2. We may be summoned to a patient in an Apoplectic fit. If extravasation of blood or serum has already taken place, we cannot remedy that. But if either an excited state of the circulation or active Cerebral Congestion be present, they must be remedied, or further mischief will ensue. In the former case, withhold your lancet, and give **Aconite** at short intervals. You will be astonished at the rapidity with which the beneficial results formerly obtained by blood-letting will manifest themselves under the action of this potent drug. There are indeed few cases of Apoplexy—none certainly in vigorous or plethoric subjects—in which one or more doses of *Aconite* may not be given with advantage. If, however, the Cerebral Congestion be the most prominent feature in the case, another medicine will have to be selected. This must most frequently be **Belladonna.** Bahr and Jahr unite in giving it the highest praise; and the cases narrated by Peters show how often it has been efficacious. Its only rival is **Opium,** which is prefered when the congestion

---

* See B. J. H., xxvii., 467.

is less active, and the stupor more profound. To this also general consent is given. *Nux vomica* is more doubtfully spoken of, and is perhaps better suited for the previous stage.

Sometimes, especially in old people, neither arterial excitement nor Cerebral Congestion is present but the symptoms depend simply on the giving way of a long-diseased blood-vessel. They are then those of shock; and *Arnica* is the medicine to be administered.

3. When the primary Apopletic condition has passed away, medicine had best be suspended for a day or two, till you see whether Cerebritis is going to be set up. If it threatens, *Belladonna* is to be opposed to it. You will then endeavour to promote the resorption of the clot. *Arnica* is again helpful here; and, not less so, **Sulphur.** In aged persons the recovery of the brain from its shock seems aided by **Baryta carbonica.**

4. The Post-apoplectic Hemiplegia so often improves by the mere lapse of time, if the muscles be kept in exercise by passive movement and Galvanism, that it is not easy to say whether recovery under this or that medicine is a case of PROPTER or only one of POST. Bahr considers **Causticum** occupies the first place among its remedies; and after this ranges *Zincum, Cuprum,* and *Plumbum*. He recommends them in the higher potencies. Jahr also praises *Causticum;** and **Cocculus is another medicine** in repute here. Late contractions and rigidity of the paralyzed limbs were formerly supposed to be due to cicatrization of the lesion caused by the clot, and to be irremovable. There seems reason now, however, to ascribe them to secondary sclerotic processes in the motor tract of the cranio-spinal axis, which may be arrested. Dr. Hammond speaks very hopefully of the effect of Galvanizing the cord and Faradizing the muscles opposing those which are contracted; and the remedies I shall speak of under the head of Sclerosis of the Spinal Cord may do good service in aid.

---

* A good case, showing how rapidly this medicine may start a long delaying recovery in Hemiplegia, may be read in the REVUE HOMŒOPATHIQUE FRANCAISE for April, 1901.

LECTURE XXV.

DISEASES OF THE NERVOUS SYSTEM.

MALADIES AFFECTING THE BRAIN
(*Concluded*)

MANIA—MELANCHOLIA—DEMENTIA—GENERAL PARESIS, HYPOCHONDRIASIS—DELIRIUM TREMENS.
HEADACHE—VERTIGO—DERANGEMENTS OF SLEEP.
CONCUSSION OF THE BRAIN.

In my present Lecture I shall endeavour to give some idea of what Homœopathic treatment can do in MENTAL DISORDERS. When I last wrote upon Therapeutics, this field was so comparatively unworked that I could do little more than supply hints as to what might be done. All I had to draw upon, beyond the Pathogenesy of drugs, was the collection of cases of the successful treatment of such disorders made from our periodical literature by Ruckert, and arranged by Peters in one of his useful Volumes—"On Nervous Derangements and Mental Disorders":—this, and a Review of Jahr's Treatise. "Du traitment Homœopathique des Affections Nerveuses et des Maladies Mentales," in the Twelfth Volume of the BRITISH JOURNAL OF HOMŒOPATHY: where also are given the statistics of a private establishment for the insane in which the medicinal treatment was strictly Homœopathic, these being quite as good as could be expected.

Already, however, a brighter prospect was opening. The erection of the State Homœopathic Ashylum for the Insane at Middletown, New York, had began to afford an opportunity for Homœopathy to test its remedies on a large scale in Lunacy. I was able to quote from the Report of the first Medical Superintendent, Dr. Stiles, issued after the Institution had been open nineteen months for the reception of patients, and 168 had been admitted, the following encouraging statement :—

"Our medical treatment continues to be purely according to the Homœopathic law SIMILIA SIMILIBUS CURANTUR, and entirely without resort to any of the forms of *Anodynes,* sedative or palliative treatment so generally in use (even among physicians of our own school) in cases of mental disturbance. Not a grain of *Chloral, Morphine,* the *Bromides,* etc., has ever been allowed in our pharmacy or given in our prescriptions, nor do we feel the need of them even in our most violent cases of Acute Mania. A careful study of the mental and physical symptoms, together with a rigid adherence to the Hahnemannian principles of selection and administration of remedies, has enabled us to meet the requirement of each individual case with comfort and success".*

The principles and results here described have continued to characterize the Middletown Asylum throughout its subsequent career, extending now over nearly thirty years, during which it has been conducted mainly by Dr. Selden Talcott. He has frequently reported his practice there, to the American Institute and in the pages of our 'periodicals, and has now gathered up his long experience in a Volume entitled, "Mental Diseases and their Modern Treatment." The success of the Institution (which has now, I may mention, 1, 800 beds) appears from the Statistics of the ten years 1881-90 brought before our International Congress of 1891, their figures being compared with those of the three asylums under old school management in the same State. They show that the recovery rate at Middletown upon the numbers discharged each year during the decade was about 50 per cent: the death-rate, upon the whole number treated, about 4 per cent. In the other asylums calculations made on the same basis and for the same period show a recovery rate of less than 30 per cent, and a death-rate of over 6. The impression made by such results is best evidenced by the other institutions of the kind which different States of the Union have placed under Homœopathic management during the last twenty years—these being now six in number.

I shall draw largely on Dr. Talcott's Book in sketching the Homœopathic treatment of Mental Disorders. First, however, let us take into account certain General considerations.

1. It goes without saying that in our homes for mental disease, the improved general treatment of modern times is carried out in all its details—mental, moral, hygienic and dietetic. We should be unworthy of our Master were it not so; for Hahnemann, contemporarily though without concert, with Pinel, led the way in abandoning and condemning the harsh treatment of the insane prevalent in his time.* In this respect our asylums are fully abreast with those of the other school; but in another we go far beyond them. We do not poison with *Narcotics* the poor brains already so far gone from original righteousness. As at Middletown, so at Westborough—and I doubt not that the same is true at Fergus Falls, at Ionia, and at Fulton †—no medicinal hypnotic is ever administered. The physicians are under a self-denying ordinance in the respect, and the result has fully

---

* Dudgeon, "Lectures," p. xxxiii,   † See M. H. R., xiv., 254, for the last.

warranted the experiment. If only no harm had come from withholding this drugging, alienists ought to be grateful to us for providing that it is needless; but when we can show better figures than their own, surely not only our negative but our positive procedures should be imitated.

2. These consist, of course, in adding to the general management of insane patients the administration of small doses of medicines Homœopathic to their condition. In choosing a specific medicine for a case of Mental Disorder, it is more than ever necessary to take into account the "totality of the symptoms." I mean that the intellectual or moral disturbance is often intimately connected with a morbid state of the blood or of some organ of the body; and the remedy for the former must accordingly cover also the latter. I need hardly remind you of the Melancholia of hepatic disease and of Oxaluria, for instance Puerperal Mania and Melancholia, are examples of what I mean. And it is here that we gain so much by knowing the mental and moral characteristics of our medicines. There is no reason to suppose, for instance, that **Pulsatilla** has any direct relation to Physical disorders. But when we meet with its distinctive MORAL aggravated into Mental Disease, especially in uterine cases, we may prescribe it with the fairest hope of a cure. I shall refer to some instances of this when I come to speak of Female Disorders.

Your first step, then, will be to consider the morbid state of the whole organism, with a view to the choice of a specific remedy. In this way medicines like **Nux Vomica** and **Sulphur** may often be the best to administer. The former is invaluable in "Hypochondriasis"—i.e., Melancholia accompanying, but out of proportion to, Dyspepsia—when the gastro-intestinal symptoms are (as they generally are) those of this drug. *Sulphur* is a remedy often given with advantage when the cutaneous symptoms indicate an impure state of the blood.

Hahnemann has some valuable remarks on this point in his 'Organon' (ccx.—ccxxx.). He points out that the mental diseases do not constitute a class distinctly separated from all others, since in the so-called corporeal diseases "the condition of the mind and disposition is ALWAYS altered, and in all cases of diseases we are called on to cure the state of the patient's disposition is to be especially noted, along with the collective symptoms, if you would trace an accurate picture of the disease, in order to be able therefore to treat it Homœopathically with success." On the other hand, Mental Disorders are rarely anything more than corporeal diseases, in which the accompanying derangement of the mind is in excess, even to the extinguishment or at least suspension of the bodily ailment. The latter, however, though it may not be apparent at the time of our examination of the patient, must be diligently ascertained for the complete picture of the morbid state to be constructed. Drugs, in like manner have each a state of disposition characteristic of them, which they produce in the healthy and cure in the sick. Our choice of them in corporeal disease is often largely determined by the Psychical disturbance present, and in Mental Diseases we have but to attach additional weight to this element of the similarity. The remedies, he adds, for chronic or recurring Mental Disorders should be sought among the class of Antipsorics, *i.e.*, the medicines of deep and slow action; while, if Insanity suddenly breaks out as an acute disease, it should be managed in the first place with such remedies as *Aconite, Belladonna, Stramonium, Hyoscyamus, Mercury,* etc. What these can do, in the "minute, highly-potentized" doses which he recommends, he does not say, but of chronic forms of Mental Disorders he writes;—"Indeed, I can confidently assert, from great experience, that the vast superiority of the Homœopathic system over all other conceivable modes of treatment is nowhere displayed in a more triumphant light than in Mental Diseases of long-standing, which originally sprang from corporeal maladies or were developed simultaneously with them."

As regards the varieties of INSANITY, it is doubtless abstractly correct to classify them as PERCEPTIONAL, IDEATIONAL, EMOTIONAL, and VOLITIONAL. As a matter of fact, however, these elementary morbid states come before us for treatment in the concrete forms of MANIA, MELANCHOLIA, DEMENTIA and GENERAL PARESIS, under which headings I shall consider their medicinal treatment.

And, first, of
MANIA.—Excluding the Puerperal form of this disease (of which I shall speak in its proper place), your choice for its remedy will nearly always lie among the three *"Mydriatics"*— **Belladonna, Hyoscyamus** and **Stramonium.** * You will remember the differential characteristics of these medicines, as I have sketched them in my 'Pharmacodynamics'—the more furious rage of *Stramonium,* the marked hyperæmia of *Belladonna,* and the altogether less active and sthenic type of the delirium of *Hyoscyamus.* Dr. Talcott concurs in this preference and these indications. He adds, as regards *Belladonna,* "a fixed and savage look, with now and then sudden ebullitions of rage and fury", restlessness, destructiveness, and rapid alterations of mental state. When erethism is well-marked, he prefers the dilutions from 3rd to the 30th : when there is heaviness and dull rage, he gives the 1, and 2. For *Stramonium* he considers hallucinations, which cause the patient great terror, a main

---

* *Duboisia,* whose action is so similar to that of *Belladonna,* has found much favour in Mania of late (J. B. H. S., i. 376; ii., 219).

indication, and the dread and horror itself, even without the illusions, another; for *Hyoscyamus*, a tendency to expose the person. When this last symptom exists with marked immodesty and lasciviousness, **Phosphorus** is strongly recommended by Jhar—of course in high dilution; when it is more Physical than Psychical, Dr. Talcott relies upon **Cantharis**.

Veratrum album is the only other remedy I would mention. Its reputation among the ancients has been confirmed in our practice. Dr. Talcott has verified the indication I have given for it in extreme anguish of mind. This is often associated, he says, with the physical prostration and coldness of the drug—which he classes with the three *Mydratics* as the "Big Four" against mania.

Whichever of these medicines you choose, you must persevere with it,—not expecting any rapid results. Dr. Talcott gives three to six months as the probable duration of mania, even under the most favourable circumstances. In chronic cases, and in the recurrent form of the malady, you may gain time by making a strong impression on the brain by a single full dose sufficient to excite Physiological effects. The advantage of doing this with *Hyoscyamine* (of which Alkaloid he gives a grain for a dose) has been illustrated by Dr. Lawson. He says justly that the drug produces in man a subdued form of Mania, accompanied by almost complete Paralysis of the voluntary muscles, and finds that by inducing this state Chronic Mania is subsequently improved to a striking extent.*

MELANCHOLIA is sometimes simply a mental feature of Dyspepsia, hepatic disease, Oxaluria, or disordered ovario-uterine functions. It then yields, with the other symptoms of such statess, to the remedies suitable for these. *Nux vomica* and *Pulsatilla; Mercurius* and *Carduus marianus; Oxalic* or *Nitro-muriatic acid Actæa, Lilium tigrinum* or *Platina*—these medicines, in their respective spheres, have restored many a patient to cheerfulness. But there is a Melancholia which is out of all proportion to any bodily disorder on which it is engrafted; which is traceable, to inheritance or acquirement to Psychical causes; and which requires remedies of another group. I am glad to find that Dr. Talcott confirms my recommendation of **Ignatia** as the best medicine in recent cases. He emphasised the

---

* PRACTITIONER, Vol. xvii. See also B. J. H., xxxv., 162.

suspension of the power of weeping as calling for it, where also "the grief that cannot speak.
Wrispers the o'erfraught heart, and bids it break.*
Where the patient weeps overmuch, and the physical state is of the Anæmic, atrophic state characteristic of it, **Natrum muriaticum** may take the place of *Ignatia*. In more confirmed cases our choice generally lies between **Aurum** and **Arsenicum**. Dr. Talcott has been disappointed in the former metal; but this is probably because his hospital patients are in too low a physical condition to render it suitable. The testimony borne to it by Hahnemann himself and several of his followers is too strong to be neglected. It is, as you know, when suicidal tendencies manifest themselves in Malancholia that *Aurum* has so much repute among us; and I have suggested that its mental state, though urgently demanding treatment on its own merits, is one primarily engrafted on hepatic or testicular disease. But while vindicating the traditional claims of *Aurum*, I fully subscribe to all that Dr. Talcott has written in praise of *Arsenicum*. Patients calling for it, he says, are "much emaciated, and have wretched appetites. They present a dry, red, tremulous tongue; they exhibit a shrivelled skin, and a haggard and anxious countenance. They look as if they had suffered the tortures of the damned." That *Arsenicum* is imperatively called for here there can be no doubt. Its patients may not be so suicidal, but they are "apt to mutilate the body by chewing the fingers, pulling out the eyelids" (? eyelashes), "by scratching holes in the face and scalp, and by torturing the flesh generally." They are also very restless.*

These (with *Veratrum* when its bodily conditions are present) are the leading medicines for Acute Melancholia with anguish. There is a form of the malady, however, where stupor predominates,— "Melancholia Attonita" of auothers. Fever is often present here, possibly threatening life, and **Baptisia** is most frequently called for to subdue it. Following it, or from the first in apyretic forms, we have to think of **Helleborus,** of **Opium,** and (again) of **Veratrum.** The first two seem best indicated, but Dr. Morris Butler—who has worked with Dr. Talcott at Middletown—writes (in a valuable study of Melancholia Attonita) †:—
Veratrum album has proved, in our experience, the most valuable remedy in our Pharmacopœia for combating this formidable disease. Many of these patients, who for weeks had passed their days sitting with heads bent and hands resting on their knees, noticing nothing with their mental and physical vitality reduced to

---

* Some cases illustrating the sphere of *Arsenicum, Aurum* and *Pulsatilla* in the Melancholia, by Dr. Junge, may be read in J. B. H., S., iv., 137.
† NORTH AMER. JOURN. OF HOM.; Feb., 1837.

the lowest ebb, we have seen, under the influence of this drug, renewed and restored to their normal activity of mind and body." *Opium* is more renowned in the old school than with us.* Melancholy, however, is characteristic of *Opium*-eaters; and the Constipation so constantly present in the Idiopathic disease is an important element in the Homœopathicity of the drug.

I come now to
DEMENTIA. I need hardly say that in its senile form this malady is unsusceptible of cure, save so far as good diet and surroundings can conduce to it. But Dementia may be acute. I have said hitherto that when occurring in the young it is nearly always the result of masturbation. Dr. Talcott, however, has well-pointed out that it may be induced by "monotony of thought and feeling, or mental inanition." Factory life, prison life, stationary sailor life are in this way conducive to it, and such factors are specially operative on the youthful, as yet unstable, nervous system. In either case be agrees with me that **Phosphoric acid** is its great medicine—especially, he says, when the flow of urine is profuse. I have added **Anacardium**. Dr. Talcott only recommends this medicine when the patients are inclined to swear, which in Dementia they surely are rarely energetic enough to do. It is gaining in repute of late. Failure of memory is the great indication for it, and even in incurable cases may be benefitted by its administration. Delusions, also, will clear away if it be given as soon as a new one crops up. † When Melancholia co-exists in masturbatic patients, **Conium** is said to be useful.

These are primary Dementiæ; but another possibly curable form of the disease is that which sometimes follows upon an acute attack of Mania or Melancholia. For this *Helleborus*, or, in more confirmed cases, *Zincum*, would seem indicated.

GENERAL PARESIS, as Dr. Talcott gives good reason for calling it, appears to be in all cases connected with a diffuse inflammation of the cortical substance of the brain and the

---

* See Hammond, OP. CIT., p. 372.
† So Drs. Taylor and McCracken, from alienist experience, in the CLINIQUE for July, 1899.

—ghbouring membranes. This would indicate, in its early stage, the persevering administration of **Belladonna**. When the symptoms of mental exaltation so characteristic of it as it advances are present, I think we should try whether benefit might be obtained from **Cannabis Indica**. This medicine has been much used in mental derangement of recent years, but its Homœopathicity thereto seems quite ignored. Great exaggeration of perceptions, ideas and emotions is the mental disorder produced by it: and here, if anywhere, it finds opportunity for exerting a curative action on similar phenomena.

Dr. Talcott speaks very despairingly of the treatment of this disease. Dr. Elias Price has published a case seemingly of it, which recovered under *Plumbum and Zincum*, 24 and 30. It is worth-mentioning, moreover, that as a subject of *Iodoform-poisoning* (through the uterus) the cerebral symptoms became chronic, and ended in General Paresis, from which the patient died two years and a half later.

Hypochondriasis and Delirium Tremens must finally be discussed ere we leave the subject of Mental Disorder.

HYPOCHONDRIASIS has been already alluded to in its most common form, i.e., of Melancholia accompanying, but out of proportion to, Dyspepsia: and the value of **Nux vomica** in such a conditioned mentioned. But there is also what Jousset calls a HYPOCHONDRIE ESSENTIELLE, which is a real mental disease. It is defined by Drs. Gull and Anstie, in their Article upon it in Reynolds 'System of Medicine', as "mental depression, occurring without adequate cause: and taking the shape, either from the first or very soon, of a conviction in the patient's mind that he is the victim of serious bodily disease." Dr. Jousset says that England is the country of Hypochondriasis; but it seems to be Germany than by us at the present day. Hartmann goes very fully into its remedies; and Bahr has an excellent Article on the disease. Besides *Nux vomica* and *Sulphur* he commends **Staphisagria, Natrum muriaticum** and **Conium;** the first being specially indicated when the affection is caused by long-continued depressing emotions; the second when there is much Cachexia and Constipation; the third when forced sexual abstemiousness seems the origin of the trouble. He also transcribes Hartmann's strong recommendation of **Stannum** which I have cited when speaking of that drug, viz., that it is good when severe abdominal pains are present, relieved by movement, which, however, exhausts.

Besides these medicines, I must mention **Arsenicum** and **Ignatia**. The latter will control the occasional semi-delirious exacerbations of mental distress which afflict the victims of **Hypochondriasis**. The former is indicated by the burning pains so characteristic of the disease and the mental condition present corresponds closely with that induced by the poison. Dr. Black* speaks highly of its value in association with *Mercurius*.

DELIRIUM TREMENS is confessedly an instance in which more patients have died of the doctor than of the disease. Treated of old as an inflammation, the Antiphologistic measures and regimen adopted were (so Watson tells us) "positively injurious." But now the same imputation is cast upon the *Opiate* treatment which in his eyes seemed their rational substitute. "Great mischief" is ascribed in one of the latest treatises on Medicine to such belief and practice; and we are told that "the idea that patients in Delirium Tremens require to be narcotised into a state of repose may now be said to be abandoned by those best-qualified to speak upon the subject." The treatment of the present day seems to be one of almost pure expectancy,—"the successful treatment of Delirium Tremens, in nine cases out of ten, depending on the regular and continuous supply of suitable nutriment, whereby the functions of the nervous system are supported during the struggle towards recovery."

I have no Statistics to bring forward bearing on the question whether Homœopathy can add anything to the success of expectancy here. But I think it highly probable; and shall endeavour to give you the indications for certain medicines to be used in its treatment.

You will generally require two,—one to control the cerebral disorder, the other to meet the gastric and general nervous symptoms of the Alcoholised patient. The former you will find in **Hyoscyamus, Belladonna, or Stramonium,**—far most commonly the first. It is rare that the Delirium is inflammatory enough for *Belladonna*, or sufficiently Maniacal for *Stramonium*. The medicines of the latter class which will do you good service are **Tartar emetic** and **Arsenicum**. The former answers best where there is much MUCOUS gastric derangement, as when Beer has been the intoxicating agent: the profuse cool sweats also indicates it. The tendency to supervention of Pneumonia in cases of Delirium Tremens is another proof of the Homœopathicity of *Tartar emetic*. *Arsenic* comes in when the condition of the stomach is one of Gastritis, and when the nervous disorder is considerable, as shown by the prostration and the muscular tremors, which last it remarkably controls.

---

* Hahnemann Mat. Medica, Part i., p. 25.

By giving one of the latter medicines by day, and one of the former by night, you will, I think get very satisfactory effects in Delirium Tremens. For some illustrative cases I refer you to a paper on the disease by Dr. John Moore of Liverpool, in the Eighth Volume of the BRITISH JOURNAL OF HOMŒOPATHY. I agree with him in thinking that *Hyoscyamus* requires to be given here not higher than the first decimal dilution, I would also commend to your notice a paper on the disease by Dr. A. P. Williamson in the HAHNEMANNIAN MONTHLY of October, 1896. He thinks **Cannabis Indica** more often called for than the other deliriafacients. Dr. Olive, of Barcelona, has recorded a good case in which it exhibited marked curative power.*

Delirium Tremens is now described as "Acute Alcoholism," and is viewed in connection with a series of changes in the nervous functions occurring in drunkards, to which the term "Chronic Alcoholism" is given. Muscular tremors and morning vomiting are the most common of these; grave degenerations of the nerve-centres, as indicated by Paralysis and mental alienation, stand at the other extremity of the scale. I need hardly say that, if such patients are to be treated successfully, their vicious habit must be broken off. But, besides this, you may obtain great benefit by the administration of **Nux vomica** in these cases when the mischief has not gone too far. In more advanced forms of the disease I suppose we could hardly do better than what Dr. Anstie recommends viz., endeavour to improve the nutrition of the nervous centres by **Phosphorus** and fatty foods. We ought, moreover, to utilise Dr. Marcet's favourable experience with the preparations of **Zinc** in such cases, as the remedy is throughly Homœopathic to the morbid condition.

Having now concluded the substantive diseases of the brain, I must, before passing to the spinal cord, speak of certain phenomena, proximately cerebrale, but of very various origin, which frequently come before us for treatment. These are Headache, Vertigo, and the Deragements to which Sleep is liable.

First, of
HEADACHE. It is one of the glories of Homœopathy, that it has brought within the range of curative treatment a multitude of minor ills hitherto thought unworthy of the practitioner's attention. Who ever contributes to the LANCET and its fellows a case of chronic or recurrent Headache successfully treated? It is one of the most prevalent of complaints, especially in women; but it has come to be regarded as a necessary evil, and neither physicians nor patients think of it as curable. It is just the

---

HAHN, MONTHLY, March, 1896, p. 201.

reverse with Homœopathy. Our literature abounds with cases of the cure of Headache—Dr. Peters had collected 169 in his treatise on the subject; and the relation of many of our medicines to this form of pain is accurately fixed. For full details I refer you to the "Treatise on headaches" by Dr. Peters, which I have mentioned; to the admirable papers "on Headaches" by Dr. Black in the Fifth Volume of the BRITISH JOURNAL OF HOMŒOPATHY; and to a semi-popular but really excellent sketch of the subject by Dr. Shuldham, entitled "Headaches; their Causes and Treatment." I will myself endeavour to sketch for you the treatment of the leading forms of the malady.

Of TOXÆMIC (Syphilitic, Gouty, Rheumatic) and SYMPATHETIC Headaches I need not speak particularly. Their treatment must be that appropriate to the blood-poison or the disordered organ on which they depend. Nor will I deal here with Migraine. Recent study of this affection has given it a place among the neuroses, with which we shall consider it. The three great types which come under our present notice are the NERVOUS, the CONGESTIVE, and the "SICK" Headaches.

I. By the "NERVOUS HEADACHE" I understand a hyperæ-thesia of the brain itself or of some of its issuing nerves, depending on a morbidly excitable condition of the cerebral substance. We have two leading remedies for this trouble—**Belladonna and Nux vomica.** The former is, as a rule, most applicable to women and children; at any rate, to young slender subjects of nervo-sanguineous temperament and otherwise fairly healthy. *Nux vomica* is preferable for men; when the well-known constitution, temperament, habits and conditions characteristic of this medicine are present; and when errors in diet readily excite the attacks. Hyperæsthesia and hyperæmia are features common to both. When the pain takes the form of "Clavus" in nervous and excitable subjects and when depressing emotions will at any time bring on the attacks, *Ignatia* will replace either. With it the face is pale during the paroxysm (unlike that of *Belladonna* and *Nux vomica*); chronic spasms are frequent concomitants; and diuresis often constitutes the crisis. One or other of these medicines will both relieve at the time, and by their continued use will greatly lessen the morbid susceptibility upon which the suffering depends.

There are three varieties of NERVOUS HEADACHE which must be specified here, as they require their own medicines.

1. The first is a Chronic, persistent ache, somewhat resembling the Syphilitic, but with no such anamnesis; generally occipital in seat and thence coming forward: relieved by warmth, increased by mental and physical exertion. Here *Silicea*, in medium dilution, will often work wonders.*

---

* See J. B. H. S., vii., 438; viii., 160.

2. The second is the Headache traceable to INJURY, whether physical or mental. It may be from over-work, from exposure to too much light or noise, or from Concussion, that the damage has been wrought; but damage has been done, the brain is a bruised one, and aches. **Hypericum** is the *Arnica* of such injuries as you may see in Dr. Lambert's interesting study of the drug in the Eighth Volume of the JOURNAL OF THE BRITISH HOMŒOPATHIC SOCIETY.

3. The third is the Headache of EYE-STRAIN. For this the excellent therapeutist I have just mentioned has given us one remedy in **Natrum muriaticum;*** and American experience has furnished two from among their indigenous plants, both named from Virginia —the **Epiphegus** and the **Onosmodium.** I have frequently verified the recommendation of *Epiphegus*—the provings of which show a clear Homœopathicity, and a power of inducing Headache which SIMILIA SIMILIBUS ought to utilise yet further. † To the testimony in favour of *Onosmodium*, Dr. A. B. Norton has lately given his weighty accession. Even where the proper correction of refraction cannot be made, he says that great amelioration will follow the use of the drug. A tired feeling, locally and generally, he describes as a sure indication for it. ‡

II. I come now to CONGESTIVE HEADACHES. Here, as is only to be expected, the remedies for Cerebral Congestion itself find place again; and I need to repeat what I have said as to the distinctive indications for *Aconite, Belladona, Ferrum, Glonoin, Gelsemium, Nux vomica* and *Opium.* I would add to the list however, *Bryonia, Chininum,* and *Melilotous.* **Bryonia,** like *Nux* suits the Congestive Headaches connected with Dyspepsia and Constipation. The pain is in the forehead, and accompanied by giddiness; both being much increased by movement, and also by stooping, which causes a sensation as if the brain would fall out. The *Nux* headache is rather occipital, and is specially aggravated by mental exertion. The headache of **Quinine** is general and continuous, with a tendency to Deafness and noises in the ears: in this I have often found the first three triturations of much benefit. Dr. Bowen has lately come forward again to testify his confidence in **Melilotus.** There is frequently Epistaxis with its Headaches to show their congestive basis. ‡

---

* L. H. H. R., vii 144.

† Dr. J. C. Andrews affirm that it is as effective in Headaches from excitement of any kind as it is in those of eye-strain. He gives the 3x dil. (J. B. H. S., v., 191).

‡ NEW ENGL. MED. GAZETTE, March, 1901.

$ See J. B. H. S., ii., 360; vii., 223.

§ The following case is not given in Dr. Peter's Treatise. It is related by Dr. Chapman in the Seventh Volume of the BRITISH JOURNAL OF HOMŒOPATHY (p. 505) :—

Dr. Claude has good reason to believe that the Headache of over-work is associated with congestion—not of the arteries but of the veins of the head. He is sustained in this connection by Dr. Parenteau, who finds in the cases Dr. Claude has sent to him, marked enlargement of the veins of the fundus oculi, with corresponding shrinking of the arteries. Dr. Claude has long-treated such Headaches mainly with *Pulsatilla*, and has found the mother-tincture aggravate, while the dilutions from the third upward have shown most beneficial effects.*

III. I have yet to discuss "SICK HEADACHE." I do not mean mere Dyspeptic Headache,—the remedies for which are the Antidyspeptics indicated. I mean a periodically recurring attack, of which pain in the head is one symptom, and vomiting another; but whose clinical history points to a gastro-hepatic rather than a cerebral origin. The following case will illustrate what I mean, and exhibit the action of one of the remedies:—

Agnes F—, æt. about thirty, had suffered, on and off, from recurring "Sick Headaches" for the last eight years, I had treated her at times in the past, but with little result. On May 6th 1870, she again applied to me to see if I could help her in this respect. When I come to inquire into her condition, I found that the symptoms had acquired so typical a form that I was able to promise her almost certain relief.

"A lady arrived at Liverpool from South America in a great state of suffering. From the time she went on board the ship until she landed she had been constantly Sea-sick; was never free from Nausea and vomited frequently. During the last fortnight of her voyage there had been Hæmatemesis several times. The bowels had not been relieved for upwards of a fortnight, though she had taken pills frequently, which only increased her Nausea and the distress of her stomach.

"Her face was very red; she was very giddy; she could not stand, and could scarcely sit. She had considerable Headache; a sensation of great fulness in the bowels. The slightest movement increased her sufferings, which were partially relieved on lying down and keeping quite still. The colon was distended, and to the touch seemed loaded with fæces. Notwithstanding her repugnance to it, had an ounce of Castor Oil with a few drops of *Laudanum* was given to her. She retained it, and discharged an enormous quantity of fæces.

"The next day, though the distension of the bowels was relieved and the long-accumulated fæces had been removed, all her symptoms of Sea sickness continued—the flushed face, the giddiness, the Headache and the Nausea: the distress increased on any movement. A drop of *Bryonia* of the 3rd dilution was given her: the next day she was quite well, and travelled to London."

* M. H. R., xiv., 489.

Every fortnight regularly this patient began to feel much pain in the right hypochondrium, which gradually increased in severity. As it grew worse the head began to ache, especially in the right forehead and temple. This also rose by degrees to its acme; and, as it did so, the nausea which had been present to some extent from the first resolved itself into vomiting, chiefly of bile. This continued for some hours, and then the symptoms as gradually declined, the whole attack lasting nearly three days. In the intervals there were occasional feelings of Headache, sickness, and pain in the side, but in a slight degree. The secretions and the uterine functions were normal.

The medicine I had fixed upon in my mind as I heard her story and from which I was able to promise such certain benefit, was *Chelidonium.* I gave her these drops of the 3rd dilution night and morning.

May 30th.—The attack came on at the usual time, but was less severe. Continue medicine.

June 15th—It is now three weeks since the last proxysm, and no further one has occurred. She feels altogether better, Continue medicine, 3rd decimal dilution.

June 25th.—An attack came on the day after I saw her, but was quite a slight one. She feels little of the nausea and pain in the side. Continue medicine.

This was the last of the Headaches for a long time. Patient discontinued the medicine at the end of July. I have seen her occasionally since, but once only for an attack of this kind, which is now a rare occurrence.

It is seldom that the hepatic origin of the attack is so obvious as in this case. When the symptoms are more obscure I would direct your attention to **Iris.** It will often cut short the proxysms; and its continued use, with proper attention to diet and Hygiene, will be much to obviate their recurrence. It is said to be especially useful when the attack commences with a blur before the eyes, as in true Migraine—of its place in which I have yet to speak.

For other Headaches not falling within these three classes, and not mentioned under the head of Catamenial or Climacteric sufferings. I must refer you to the Clinical Index to my 'Pharmacodynamies,' and references to its text there given.

The list of symptons of nearly every medicine given in the schematic Pathogenesis begins with

VERTIGO. In the presence of this EMBARRAS DE RICHESSES you will be glad to have the results of experience in the treatment of the symptom in question.

Symptom it is, and nothing more, in organic disease within the cranium, in Apoplexy, and in gastro-hepatic disturbance. Persistent in the first case, temporary in the two latter, in either it affords no point for special treatment. But Vertigo not uncommonly comes before us unconnected with either of these causes, and sufficiently prominent to require special attention and medication. It may depend on disorder of the intra-cranial circulation, and this in the way either of excess or of defect. When Congestion is present, and accompanied by Headache, the medicines already recommended for the latter consequence will remove the Vertigo also. But cases often occur, especially in old people, in which Chronic Cerebral Congestion causes much giddiness, but little or no aching. In this affection I have derived singular benefit from **Iodine** in about the 3x dilution. *Sulphur*, also, must not be forgotten. Still more frequently, however, Vertigo testifies to deficient supply of the brain from an enfeebled heart. This is the "Essential Vertigo" of Dr. Ramskill.* In such cases we shall have some palpitation and breathlessness, a slow and feeble pulse, and a tendency to Syncope. Here **Digitalis** is our grand remedy, given in small doses (say the 1st dilution), as a direct tonic to the muscular fibre of the heart. The disappearance of the Vertigo is generally the earliest sign of its taking effect. Another Anæmic Virtigo is that to which Epileptics are subject. It is from a contraction of the cerebral arteries, not strait enough to amount to the "Petit mal"; and it finds an effective medicine in **Hydrocyanic acid**.

Much light has been thrown on Vertigo in recent years by the researches made as to the functions of the cerebellum. They are well brought together by Dr. Ferrier, in the Fourth and Sixth Chapters of his "Functions of the Brain." The cerebellum appears to be the centre of equilibration, the seat of association of those combined impressions and movements which result in the preservation of balance under all circumstances. The impressions which convey the sense of need of adjustment come through three channels—the eye and optic tracts, the semicircular canals of the internal ear with their afferent nerves, and the paths of tactile sensibility—these last being the posterior columns of the cord, which transmit the sensations caused in the soles of the feet by walking and standing. The cerebellum being connected with all these central paths, and receiving their impressions, transmits them peripherally through the motor paths, with which it is equally connected by means of its middle peduncles; and here they are transformed into such movements as are requisite to preserve or restore the balance.

Now, through its superior peduncles the cerebellum is connected with the cerebrum, the seat of consciousness; and here loss of balance finds its subjective complement in Vertigo— the sense of giddiness. Let the posterior columns be affected with Sclerosis, as in Locomotor Ataxy; and if the optical aid to equilibrium is removed by closing the eyes the patient immediately feels as if he would fall, and has to grasp at some support. Conversely, let a full dose of *Hemlock*, which paralyses the ocular muscles, be taken; and here the ingester will be unable to walk steadily as long as his eyes are open, while on closing them the giddiness immediately passes away. The part played in equilibration by the semi-circular canals, was ascertained experimentally by Flourens, and has been confirmed Pathologically by the phenomena of Meniere's Disease. Vertigo, then, may evidently be set up through disorders occuring in any of these paths; and will require medicinal remedies accordingly. *Quinine, Salicylic acid* and *Chenopodium* will be indicated when Tinnitus and perhaps Deafness indicate the ear as at fault; *Conium* and *Gelsemium* when the trouble lies in the optical apparatus, as shown by exacerbation on changing the focus or direction of vision.* There may be also a real "Essential Vertigo," *i.e.*, one where the cerebellum itself is primarily at fault; and certainly giddiness does not uncommonly come before us where no exciting cause or Pathological explanation can be found for it. In such cases I am in the habit of prescribing **Cocculus,** and with fair success; though Jousset considers **Tabacum** preferable (in the 6th dilution).

If these indications prove insufficient, you must consult the 'Materia Medica'; or you may save yourself a long hunt by referring to Dr. Kafka's exhaustive treatise on the subject, which is translated in the Thirty-First Volume of the BRITISH JOURNAL OF HOMŒOPATHY. As for our other authorities Bahr, simply considers the Vertigo of old people, and treats it according as the brain seems hyperæmic or Anæmic,—in the former case with *Belladonna, Arnica, Nux vomica* and *Lachesis;* in the latter, with *Siliiea, Baryta carbonica, Graphites, Lycopodium, Ambra,* or

---

* In Russell Reynolds' System of Medicine, Vol. ii. Art. "Vertigo".

Flouric acid. Jahr gives a good many symptomatic indications and says that *Phosphorus* "displays great curative powers in every imaginable case of Vertigo, more specially in the Vertigo described as NERVOUS." Dr. Guernsey speaks of a giddiness on the least mental or physical exertion as under the control of *Argentum nitricum.*

It is probable that Primary Vertigo may be classified as Headache into Nervous, Congestive, and "Sick"—the last-named being understood to be cerebral and not of gastro-hepatic origin. Then we shall have as our main remedies,—for the first form, *Phosphorus, Ambra, Argentum nitricum;* for the second, *Iodium, Arnica, Nux vomica, Sulphur;* for the third *Tabacum* and *Cocculus.*

Here are two more excerpts bearing on this subject.

1. In a case of poisoning by a grain of *Morphia,* recorded in the HOMŒOPATHIC PHYSICIAN for December, 1945, a marked symptom was Vertigo from the least motion of the head. In the March number, Dr. Skinner relates a case in which this symptom, tending even to "Petit-mal," after resisting *Nux* and *Lycopodium,* yielded rapidly to a high potency of *Morphia muriatica.*

2. Dr. Colby calls attention to the marked Vertigo experienced by those who have taken Pomegranate root for the expulsion of tæniæ, and says that he has come to regard *Granatum* as quite the leading remedy for Vertigo when occuring as a substantive symptom of a case. This is from the NEW ENGLAND MEDICAL GAZETTE of November, 1900.

I come finally to the

DERANGEMENTS OF SLEEP.—Sleep is too important a part of the life of the brain not to be subject to disorder, and not to require remedial means when that disorder is considerable or persistent. The most common form in which its disturbance comes before us is SLEEPLESSNESS. When this is part of a general systematic derangement, the treatment — medicinal and hygienic—suitable thereto will nearly always favour sleep; and, indeed, improvement in this respect is one of the best signs, alike in acute and in chronic disease, that the remedies chosen are agreeing with the patient. But it not uncommonly happens that Sleeplessness comes before us as the main element in a condition of nervous erethism, and demands primary consideration in our choice of medicines. You will generally find its remedies among the group consisting of **Aconite, Actæa racemosa, Chamomilla, China, Coffea** and **Iodine.** Of these *Coffea* has been, in my experience, by far the most frequently useful; it is indicated when the patient cannot get to sleep for simple cerebral activity, thoughts crowding upon him and clinging to him in spite of all his efforts at detachment. I have found the 6th and 12th better than the lower dilutions.* The habitual use of Coffee as a beverage, if not taken in excess, is no counter-indication to its exhibition as a remedy. In cases, however, where the Sleeplessness is traceable to its immoderate use—especially when it is drunk by students to keep themselves awake—it must be discontinued, and *Nux vomica* or *Chamomilla* given as an antidote. *China* is good when the erethism is rather emotional, and when its subject is weak from some drain on the system. It is also the remedy when excessive Tea-drinking has been the exciting cause. The Sleeplessness of *Iodine* is connected with palpitation, that of *Aconite* with vascular excitement generally, that of *Actæa* and *Chamomilla* with bodily restlessness (motor erethism). You will also remember *Nux vomica* when the patient wakes at two or three A. M., lies awake for some hours, and then sleeps heavily when he ought to be getting up; and *Pulsatilla* when he cannot get to sleep during the early part of the night.

Again, the sleep may not be absent, but morbid; it may be disturbed by dreams, made hideous by nightmare, or entirely altered into the Pathological condition known as SOMNAMBULISM. Dreams when unusual in frequency, vividness, or persistence of character, are no unimportant indication of the state of the brain, or the body generally, and deserve more attention than they ordinarily receive, Hahnemann enjoined the taking account of them in examination of patients, and frequently in his Pathogenesis records their production by drugs, with the peculiarities they assume. For information as to them in parti-

---

* Sometimes, however, the *Berry* in its ordinary form is efficacious; and thus we have an old-school writer saying, "Although the effect of Coffee is generally such as to induce Sleeplessness, there are cases in which its action is directly the reverse" (Hammond 'SLEEP AND ITS DERANGEMENTS', 1869).

cular cases you will of course consult your Repertories. I would just say that **Hyoscyamus** and **Cannabis Indica** are very useful when dreaming is simply too frequent and vivid. For Nightmare and Somnambulism the *Bromide of Potassium* is in much use in the old school, and, as I have shown from Laborde's experience how entirely Homœopathic it is, we can hardly do better than employ it. **Pænio**, also, is good for Nightmare.

Finally, sleep may be excessive; and such soporose conditions may occur independently of other symptoms of cerebral or general disorder. You will naturally think of **Opium** here, and it will often wake your patient up. But another good medicine for it is **Nux moschata.** The face is inclined to redness with the former drug, to paleness with the latter.

I need hardly say that the general management of patients with disturbed sleep is of the utmost—often of primary—importance. For many useful suggestions on the subject I may refer you to Dr. Hammond's Treatise on "Sleep and its Derangements," and to a Paper by Dr. Ker in the Eighteenth Volume of the MONTHLY HOMŒOPATHIC REVIEW.

On the subject of INJURIES of the HEAD I have only to speak of.

CONCLUSSIONS OF THE BRAIN.—You had best give **Arnica** here while the symptoms are those of Shock;* but as soon as reaction sets in, your chief aim will be to moderate this with repeated doses of **Aconite.** If it should be already established when you see your patient, and inflammation should be threatening, you will combat it with **Belladonna.**

---

* "The medicine that is most essentially serviceable in the treatment of Concussion is *Arnica;* and its early administration, if the injury be not extremely severe,, will not only prevent many of the evil consequences that may result, but by its influence upon the vessels may limit the extravasation of blood within the cavity of the cranium" (Helmuth, SYSTEM OF SURGERY, 4th Ed., p. 620).

Other remedies, however, may conceivably be required. If, for instance, Spinal Congestion should be met with as a recent affection resulting from cold, or from suppression of a menstrual or hæmorrhoidal discharge, the timely administration of *Aconite* might restore the disturbed balance of the circulation without further aid. Where excessive muscular exertion was the cause, and a strong man the subject, I should be disposed to employ the indubitably Homœopathic action of *Nux vomica* or its Alkaloid. Dr. Aitken mentions that the difficulty in walking after recumbency characteristic of Spinal Congestion "may be temporarily induced by *Strychnia or Nux vomica*"; and it is equally significant that Dr. Radcliffe should speak of "*Nux vomica* now and then in small doses" as part of the successful treatment of the illustrative case he relates, and that Dr. Hammond—who is addicted to large doses—should enjoin "that *Strychnia* should never be administered in Congestion of the Cord".

SPINAL IRRITATION receives from Dr. Radcliffe a descrip tion which separates it distinctively from Hysteria on the one hand and from Myalgia on the other. Dr. Hammond draws a very similar picture of it, and thinks that its Pathological basis is Anæmia of the posterior columns of the cord. However this may be, the pain, tenderness to pressure at certain points, and the eccentric symptoms of Irritation of the spinal nerves, make a group of symptoms familiar to most of us, and having an undoubted clinical history of their own. What can we do for them? Bahr is the only one of our authors who characterizes the malady distinctly; but for its treatment he sends us to our 'Repertories', save in the form resulting from Onanism in which he recommends *Nux vomica* and *Sulphur*. **Ignatia**, **Actæa racemosa** and **Agaricus** are the remedies which have commended themselves to me. In a case reported by Dr. Chepmell in his "Hints for the Practical Study of the Homœopathic Method" the first-named medicine did much good in conjunction with *Platina*, the latter being given on account of the uterine symptoms present. *Actæa* is suitable when the latter troubles are the exciting cause of the disease. The reproving of *Agaricus* under Professor Zlatarowitch displayed a striking action of the drug upon the cord; and the symptoms are those of Spinal Irritation rather than of Congestion. Dr. Clifton writes. "In Spinal Irritation, in weakly women of low and feeble habit of body, with weak pulse, tenderness over the spinous processes of the cervical and dorsal vertebræ, attended with headache, constriction across the chest, and flatulent eructations, I have frequently found it useful".*

---

* M. H. R., xii., 402.

LECTURE XXVI

DISEASES OF THE NERVOUS SYSTEM

—o—

MALADIES AFFECTING THE BRAIN

—o—

SPINAL CONGESTION—SPINAL IRRITATION—SPINAL MENINGITIS—MYELITIS—SPINAL PARALYSIS—LABIO-GLOSSO-LARYNGEAL PARALYSIS—MULTIPLE SPINAL SCLEROSIS—LATERAL SPINAL SCLEROSIS—LOCOMOTOR ATAXY—PROGRESSIVE MUSCULAR ATROPHY—SOFTENING—HYDROPHOBIA—TETANUS.

From the Diseases of the Brain I pass on to those of the SPINAL CORD. I shall first speak of its non-organic disorders—CONGESTION and IRRITATION; and then of its INFLAMMATION, including under this heading the various forms of SPINAL PARALYSIS. In this novel and somewhat obscure region I shall assume as my basis for Pathology and diagnosis two recent contributions on the subject,—Dr. Radcliffe's Article on "Diseases of the Spinal Cord" in the Second Volume of Reynolds' 'System of Medicine', and the section treating of these maladies in the Sixth Edition of Dr. Hammond's "Diseases of the Nervous System".

In Discussing the treatment of these maladies I regret that I can do little more than give hints and suggest probabilities. There is an almost utter absence of well-diagnosed spinal disease in Homœopathic literature. I can only hope that by noting this deficiency I may stir up some of our practitioners, and especially those attached to hospitals, whose large experience must have included cases of this kind, to tell us what they can do for them, and with what remedies. An excellent beginning in this direction has been made by Dr. Goldsborough in connection with our own London Hospital, and we cannot have too much of such work as his.

SPINAL CONGESTION is excellently characterized by our two authorities, and is no very uncommon affection. I have myself seen several cases of it, and have found **Gelsemium** in the first or second dilution most effective in its removal. In one instance there was Paresis of both arms and legs and of the sphincter vesicæ, with numbness and tingling in the extremities; in another (in addition to the usual symptoms) some difficulty in speaking and writing, with loss of the memory of words, *i.e.*, incipient Aphasia. In all the dull, burning aching in the spine and the aggravation after recumbency were present. I have not required the aid of heat or cold, or of Electricity, in this malady.

In my 'Pharmacodynamics,' noting the tenderness of some of the vertebræ felt by Dr. Caroll Dunhum during his proving of **Tellurium,** I said it should cause the metal to be remembered in Spinal Irritation. Dr. Shelton has reported three cases in which great pain and sensitiveness of the spine were prominent symptoms, and which recovered under this medicine in the 5th dilution.*

I must acknowledge that I have found Spinal Irritation a very intractable disorder. I have only succeeded in CURING two cases of it—one with *Ignatia* the other with *Actæa* and *Agaricus,* all in the first decimal dilution. Whether I should have done better with higher potencies, I cannot say. But I feel ashamed of my own Homœopathy, at least, when I find Dr. Hammond stating that, of the hundred and fifty-six cases occurring in his private practice during six years, a hundred and thirty-three were thoroughly cured, and that, as his examples show, in no long space of time. Of the constituent elements of his treatment, based upon his Anæmic theory of the disease, I cannot adopt the Blisters, or the large doses of *Strychnia, Phosphorus, Phosphoric acid,* and *Opium*; but the hot-water bag to the spine, and the passage through it of the continuous Galvanic current, are auxiliaries as unobjectionable as they are rational. The *Secale* moreover, which in large doses is his favourite remedy for Congestion of the Cord, might in small doses be beneficial to its Anæmia. In the Cramps of Spinal Irritation Dr. Hirsch has found the medicine very beautiful. Dr. Brown-Sequard's Article on the disease in Quain's Dictionary contains some practical suggestions for its management.

SPINAL MENINGITIS—I am now on untrodden ground, for I know of no recorded experience with this disease,† and I have not myself met with it. In its acute form, however, the analogy of Cerebral Meningitis would leave little doubt of the usefullness of **Aconite** and **Bryonia.** The pain on movement characteristic of the latter medicine is nowhere so marked as in Spinal Meningitis : and its Pathological appropriateness, as also that of *Aconite,* is obvious. In the chronic form of the malady Dr. Hammond concurs with other observers in placing much reliance upon *Iodide of Patassium,* of course in full doses, conjoined, when there is a Syphilitic history, with the *Bichloride of Mercury.* Here, as in Cerebral Meningitis, Homœopathy has no counter-experience to show ; and you will have to consider

---

* M. H. R., xxxvi. 548.
† Since writing the above, I have met with a well-characterized case from Dr. H. Goullon (J. B. H. S., iii, 214). Here the action of *Bryonia* 3 was very satisfactory.

whether your duty to your patients requires you to use accredited measures, which are nevertheless out of the range of your ordinary practice.

MYELITIS is also conspicuous by its absence in Homœopathic Therapeutic records. Bahr, who notes the fact, accounts for it by the rarity of its cure; for it is not so uncommon a disease. He himself relates an acute case which recovered under **Mercurius** (3x trituration), and to this medicine, preceded or accompanied by **Belladonna**, I think we may safely trust in recent instances of the disease. In more chronic cases the two medicines I should suggest for consideration are **Oxalic acid** and **Arsenicum**. In describing, in my lectures, the phenomena of poisoning by the former drug, I have said that I think there can be no doubt of their pointing to inflammation of the membranes and substance of the cord. A Myelitis involving the meninges to some extent would best correspond to them. I have also described, from Dr. Imbert-Gourbeyre's materials, the *Arsenical-Paralysis* and shown that its seat is in the cord. Congestion only had been found POST MORTEM up to the time of writing; but, Velpeau now announces that he has succeeded in developing an acute Myelitis by it in a dog, and three undoubted cases of the disease in the human subject have been traced to its influence. The absence of Meningitic symptoms distinguishes the *Arsenical-Myelitis* from that of *Oxalic acid*. Dr. Ravel, from whose remarks in L'ART MÉDICAL (XLIII. 48) I have taken these later facts about *Arsenic*, mentions a *"Plumbic* and *Phosphoric-Myelitis"* also; but I think that they belong to other diseases of the cord than the simple inflammation of which I have now been speaking. More pertinent is Dr. Simpson's case of Diffuse Myelitis in the MONTHLY HOMŒOPATHIC REVIEW of 1894 (p. 639). Here *Lathyrus* proved curative.

By "Myelitis" I have meant (as explained) SIMPLE INFLAMMATION of the whole thickness of the cord. But recent investigations—especially those of the French school—have (as I have already said—see Lecture XXIV.) led to the recognition of Inflammation, followed by induration or atrophy of particular tracts or elements of the cranio-spinal axis, as being the Pathological basis of a number of hitherto diseases. You cannot find the results of these discoveries better summed up than in an Essay by Dr. Jousset "On Chronic Inflammation of the Spinal Marrow and of the Brain", which is translated in the Thirty-Third Volume of the BRITISH JOURNAL OF HOMŒOPATHY. The maladies he groups here around this common lesion at its various seats are Locomotor Ataxy, Multiple Cerebro-spinal Sclerosis (SCLEROSE EN PLAQUES), Gentral Paralysis of the Insane, Spinal Paralysis of adults and infants, Labio-glosso-laryngeal Paralysis, and Progressive Muscular Atrophy. To these Dr. Hammond, in his Chapter on "The Inflammations of the Spinal Cord", adds Tetanus, Pseudo-hypertrophic Spinal Paralysis, and Lateral Sclerosis. Of these affections I have spoken of General Paralysis of the Insane among Mental Disorders; and shall reserve Infantile Paralysis for the Diseases of Children. Tetanus I must class with Hydrophobia as a spinal malady PER SE. I shall therefore, here discuss the SPINAL PARALYSIS of adults (Jousset's Essential or True Paraplegia), LABIO-GLOSSO-LARYNGEAL PARALYSIS, LATERAL SCLEROSIS, MULTIPLE SPINAL SCLEROSIS, LOCO-MOTOR ATAXY, and PROGRESSIVE MUSCULAR ATROPHY.

SPINAL PARALYSIS (Poliomyelitis Anterior Acute) appears to be an inflammation of the anterior grey cornua of the cord. Beginning with pains in the back, which radiate to the limbs, it rapidly shows itself in Paralysis, which is followed by atrophy. The sensory disorder of Myelitis is absent; there are no cramps or bed-sores; and the sphincters nearly always escape. We know nothing of its Therapeutics, and should consider whether the large doses of *Secale* with which Dr. Hammond starves the inflammation by occluding the spinal arteries merit employment. Of our own remedies. **Belladonna** would be indicated by the Pathological condition in the early stage,* and either **Phosphorus** or **Plumbum** when atrophy was threatening. The latter medicine would even seem earlier indicated. Dr. Jousset has communicated to L'ART MEDICAL (XLIII., 269) a striking case of acute Paralysis of the muscles of the neck and those of deglutition, with abolition of electric contractility, rapidly cured by *Plumbum* 30. There can be no doubt, he thinks, of the presence here of the specific lesion which lies at the bottom of so many of the Spinal Paralyses, *i.e.*, inflammation of the grey substance— in this case of the anterior horns. He considers the acute Myelitis which Vulpian has found *Plumbum* to cause an affection of this nature. *Phosphorus* is undoubtedly most appropriate to non-inflammatory Softening of the Cord; but the case of *Phosphoric-Paralysis* I have cited in my lecture on the drug presents some features of the commencing atrophic stage of the present malady.

Probably, however, the use of localised Electricity is of more

---

* Trousseau and Pidoux speak of Bretonneau as having obtained in several cases of Paraplegia a cure as unexpected as inexplicable by the use of *Belladonna*.

importance in confirmed Spinal Paralysis than any medicinal treatment; and it seems to give excellent results.

LABIO-GLOSSO-LARYNGEAL PARALYSIS* is probably the more precise modern name for the "PARALYSIS OF THE TONGUE" of which we sometimes read in the older Homœopathic books. *Anacardium* is said to have cured it; and *Oleander* is recommended for it on the strength of some symptoms in its Pathogenesis, which, however, I think is misinterpreted. But as the lesion here is identical in form with that which obtains in general Spinal Paralysis, and differs only in seat, I think our most promising remedies must be the *Belladonna* and *Plumbum*—especially the latter—there recommended.

The disease hitherto mentioned (with Infantile Paralysis) appear to be inflammations of the grey substance of the cord going on to degeneration and atrophy of its cells. In the three now to be discussed the latter process seems secondary to an inflammation of the neuroglia—the connective tissue of the cord; and the thickening of this substance leads to such induration, partial or general, that the affections resulting from it are named "Scleroses." The process may be disseminated here and there in the cord, or may attack its lateral or its posterior columns exclusively. The Paralysis caused is always more or less of the "spastic" kind.

MULTIPLE SPINAL SCLEROSIS is the same affection as the disseminated inflammation of the neuroglia of the brain which we have already considered : it is one form of the SCLEROSE EN PLAQUES of the French. The *Aurum, Barium* and *Plumbum* already suggested there would be applicable here ; but the rigidity and contracture which characterise its Paralysis strongly suggest the phenomena of *Lathyrism,* and point to **Lathyrus** as a promising remedy. The promise has received fulfilment in at least one case—that contributed by Dr. Dewey to the MEDICAL CENTURY of January, 1900, where the 3x and 6x dilutions were employed. If the spinal mischief be of traumatic rather than spontaneous origin, **Hypericum** would be casually indicated, and Dr. Speirs Alexander has communicated two excellent cases in which complete cure resulted from its use.†

LATERAL SPINAL SCLEROSIS is similarly characterized, but the Paralysis is more general. There is one form of it which strikingly reminds one of the effects of *Cuprum*; that, namely, where the affected muscles are atrophied (the "Amyotrophic"

---

* Now more commonly known as "Progressive Bulbar Paralysis".
† J. B. H. S., v., 41.

form). If the description I have given in my 'Pharmacodynamics' of the palsied arm of a Copper-worker be compared with the plate at p. 576 of Dr. Hammond's work, illustrating this disease, the correspondence will be found exact. There is no recorded experience with this Metal in the disease; but Dr. Halbert has given us a well-diagnosed case in which immense improvement has taken place under the persistent use for nearly a twelve-month of **Argentum nitricum**, first in the 3x and finally in the 30x dilution.

Sclerosis of the posterior columns—more strictly, of the posterior root-zones with their intra-cranial continuations—constitutes the interesting disease known formerly (as in Romberg's time) as "TABES DORSALIS," but now called—

LOCOMOTOR ATAXY. †—There was very little to be found in Homœopathic literature, when I wrote my 'Therapeutics,' regarding the treatment of this disease; and I confined myself to suggesting *Belladonna*, in the incipient stage, and mentioning some results obtained from *Agrentum*, *Aluminium* and *Zincum* in more advanced cases. We have more material of the kind now; and the "much may be done by drugs" which is stated by Sir William Gowers in his Article on the disease in Quain's Dictionary is confirmed by the experience of our school.

1. The Syphilitic anamnesis so frequently obtaining in this disease has not, as is generally the case, aided in its treatment. Gowers speaks of the "the almost invariable inefficacy of Anti-syphilitic remedies". The "almost" is borne out by a case of Dr. Delamater's in the MEDICAL ERA of October, 1897, where a course of **Mercurius corrosivus** 3x, with one fortnight of *Secale* 1x, effected a complete cure in six months.

2. The probable commencement of the disease is an inflammatory process, and the analogy between its symptoms and those of the drug, have led me in time past to urge the employment of **Belladonna**, at any rate in the incipient stage, when the "douleurs fulgurantes" and other erethistic symptoms are present. I think I have checked a commensing case with it. My reasonings have lately been supported by Dr. Jousset ‡ He prefers the drug in the form of *Atropine* which he gives in the 3rd trituration during alternate fortnights with *Strychnine* of the same strength. From that medication, he says, he has in the first stage of the disease obtained gratifying results.

3. *Argentum*, in the form of the *Nitrate*, and of course in substantial doses, has in the hands of Wunderlich and others played a considerable part in the old-school medication of Locomotor Ataxy. I am unable to claim for Homœopathy any

---

* CLINIQUE, July, 1896.

† Quite recently, there seems a tendency to reversion to the old name; but I cannot think it—appropriate.

‡ See BULL. DE LA SOC. MED. HOM. DE FRANCE., xxxi., 43.

virtues it may have, and I observe that Gowers places it below *Arsenic* and even **Aluminium**. Both of those are ours,—the former by the similarity of its pains to those of the disease, the latter by the experience of Bœnninghausen to which I have already referred. * It has been verified of late among ourselves. Dr. Simpson, of Liverpool, contributes a case having all the features of the disease, in which *Aluminium* 6 relieved the muscular weakness, the formication, the numbness of the feet and the tottering gait. *Phosphorus* 6 was then given for some time, at the end of which "the patient expressed himself free from pain and discomfort, and strong to labour and endure," † Dr. Clarence Bartlett says that he has used it in a couple of instances with good effect : ‡ and in the four cases contributed by Dr. Goldsborough in the MONTHLY HOMŒOPATHIC REVIEW of June, 1901. *Aluminium* played an active part in the improvement effected. Bœnninghausen states that he was led to this remedy by the Pathogenesy of *Alumina;* and though it is difficult to follow him here, the dosage employed by himself and his followers forbids any but a Homœopathic explanation of its efficacy.

4. The suggestion of the phenomena of Lathyrism in the direction of spastic Paralysis has been paralleled by that of *Ergotism* an regards Locomotor Ataxy. If you will read some of the descriptions of the results of living on spurred Rye collected in the Cyclopædia of 'Drug Pathogenesy' you will at once see the resemblance of the two series of symptoms, and will ask whether **secale** should not find an important place among our anti-tabetic medicines. It has already begun to do so. Besides Dr. Delamater's case already mentioned, I can refer you to one of Dr. Ord's, where arrest of the disease and an endurable life seems to have been secured by the use of the 1x dilution —*Stramonium*—1x helping head symptoms and *Carbo vegetabilis* 3x gastric crises. §

5. Even in incurable cases, something may be done to relieve symptoms, especially those calling most loudly for help—the lightning pains. These being to what may be called the fluctuating, functional, dynamic, and therefore modifiable element in the disease; and, besides the *Belladonna* or *Atropine*, already specified, have proved amenable to several of our remedies. **Agaricus** developed in the heroic Austrian provings a marked action on the spinal cord; and among the phenomena were fugitive neuralgic pains along the spinal nerves. Dr. Dyce Brown, in a valuable study of the Pathogenesis which appeared in the Twentieth Volume of the MONTHLY HOMŒOPATHIC REVIEW suggested its appropriateness to the pains of Ataxy. I said that I could not quite follow him here as the inflammatory induration which lay at the basis of these was

---

* See p. 54. † M. H. R., xxxix, 442
‡ J. B. H. S., iv., 127. § M. H. R., xl., 465.

beyond the range of action of the drug. They answered rather, I suggested, to those of Spinal Irritation. So far I was right, but the DOULEURS FULGURANTES may be just an expression of such irritation, which intervenes—as it were — between them and the Sclerosis. Dr. Brown's recommendation was well-founded; and Dr. Sauer has since spoken of having obtained at least temporary benefit from the remedy. You will remember that the neuralgic pains of *Agaricus* are compared to sharp ice touching the spots, or cold needles running through the nerves, —in this contrasted with those of *Arsenicum*, where the imaginary needles are red-hot. Coming now to the drug last-named, I would say that while the "Myelitis" which has been observed from it is hardly that of Locomotor Ataxy, so that it has no fundamental relation to the disease, the *Arsenical-Paralysis* is always accompanied by neuralgic pains and usually with loss of sensibility, and least to everything but cold. A similar exemption of the sense of temperature is often seen in the anæsthesia of Ataxy, which, too, not uncommonly sets in with BURNING pains in the soles of the feet. A case is recorded by Dr. Mackechine in which the lightning pains were almost entirely removed by the 3x trituration of the *Iodide,* the patient reporting himself also as wonderfully better in every repect.* We also have high commendation of *Ammonium muriaticum* from Drs. George Martin and Dewey,† and cases showing great benefit from *Plumbum iodatum* (3rd dil.) from Dr. Allen and of *Guaiacum* from an Indian practitioner (this last case occurred in a highly Syphilitic subject). ‡

Another troublesome symptom is the Enuresis, Dr. Tessier has seen this disappear under *Ferrum phosphoricum* 3x and *Equisetum* 1x given alternately. § The painful sexual excitement which is sometimes present in the earlier stages of the malady may be relieved by *Picric acid* ; and the Perforating Ulcers of the Soles have been seen to heal under *Silicea.*

PROGRESSIVE MUSCULAR ATROPHY is the last malady of this group. It was for some time uncertain whether it was a disease in the first instance of the muscles themselves or of the cord. The question is settled in favour of the latter—the anterior cornua being the seat of the degeneration; and hereby is made complete by the resemblance of the phenomena to those of chronic poisoning by Lead. When lecturing on **Plumbum** I have shown

---

* M. H. R., xli., 32.
† J. B. H. S., iv., 349; v., 294.
‡ IBID., 396; vii., 419.
§ IBID., v., 293.

how close is the analogy here, and have only to repeat the recommendation made, that the medicine be given a full trial in the first case which comes before any of us, and the result reported. I am bound to add, however, that Sir William Gowers speaks of hypodermic injections of *Strychnine* as "certainly capable of arresting the disease" when occurring in subjects not too advanced in life. The hundredth-grain doses he gives somewhat commend this medication to us, but we cannot claim it for Homœopathy.

"There is", I wrote in 1877, "another form of this disease, in which the muscles, though impaired as to function, are increased instead of lessened in bulk. It is the Pseudo-hypertrophic Paralysis of Duchenne. Fatty degeneration and deposit appear to be the essence of the muscular change, while the central lesion is identical with that which obtains in ordinary Spinal Paralysis". This last statement seems to require modification now, as in the great majority of cases the spinal cord exhibits no morbid changes. It does not, however, impair the recommendation I made of **Phosphorus** for it, some thirty years ago : and which has since been carried out with success by several of our practitioners. You will find the whole evidence well brought together by Dr. Goldsborough in a Paper appearing in the Fifth Volume of the LONDON HOMŒOPATHIC HOSPITAL REPORTS. From the 3x to the 6 dilutions have been employed.

So far of the inflammations of the spinal cord. A few words now upon its

SOFTENING, which may be primary and non-inflammatory. I think that this is the malady which as frequently as Locomotor Ataxy, is designated in the old books as "Tabes Dorsalis" ; for the condition thus styled is said to be a common consequence of sexual excess, and the form of disorder set up by this cause is Softening. We have two excellent medicines for it in **Phosphorus** and **Picric acid** both of which have caused the lesion in the brute and the symptoms of it in the human subject, and both of which are in relation with the usual exciting cause. They may not indeed, be able to effect regeneration of substance already softened, but they ought to be able to check any advance of the morbid process. *Picric acid* has shown its power of so doing in a case described by Dr. Lilienthal.* He cites it as an instance of Locomotor Ataxy ; but I cannot so read it, nor do I see any symptoms of this condition in the Pathogenesis of the drug. The animals poisoned by it died paralysed, and their spinal cords were found white, soft, and diffluent, while the weakness

---

* NORTH AMER. JOURN. OF HOM., xxiv., 63.

and heaviness of limbs experienced by the provers seem to be of the same kind to bear the same significance.

It remains that I speak of Injuries affecting the Cord. These may be either intrinsic or extrinsic. Of the former class is Spinal Hæmorrhage, where, if any good is to be done, it will probably be (as Dr. Jousset recommends) by **Aconite** and **Arnica**; and Concussion of the Spine, for whose effects we seem to have a very promising remedy in **Hypericum**. I mean, of course, when these effects have not gone on to congestion or inflammation, in which case the medicines appropriate to these conditions would come in. As Injuries of the Cord of extrinsic origin I class the two important maladies known as HYDROPHOBIA and TETANUS. And, first, of—

HYDROPHOBIA, which is the name of the nervous disorder induced when the TRAUMA is the bite of a rabid animal. Homœopathy has of course nothing to say against the attempt at removal of the exciting cause. Indeed, the excision of the bitten part is as much the duty of the Homœopathic practitioner as of his brother of the old school; and nothing we can offer in the way of prohylaxis or cure supersedes its paramount necessity. But having done this, we can advance to further treatment with larger resources and fairer propects of success.

In my Fifteenth Lecture I referred, in passing, to the "Mithridatism" now coming into vogue, as not content—like the ancient king of Pontus—with seeking generally from poisons to be made proof against poison, but requiring the defensive to act similarly to the offensive agent. I illustrated this by the use of *Tansy* as preventive of Hydrophobia and *Strychnia* of Tetanus. Now that we are upon the class of maladies to which these two belong, we may look further into the subject, with a view to the Therapeutics of the formidable diseases so named.

In a Paper by M. Peyraud, presented by the late Dr. Brown-Sequard in 1887* the former tells us that, since 1872, he had been led to think that substances which were isomeric atomically were also isomeric Biologically, and VICE VERSA. Experimenting on animals with the *Tanacetum vulgare*, our common *"Tansy"*, he found it produce convulsions of the Hydrophobic rather than the Epileptic type—as with its congener *Absinthe*. "All the phenomena of RAGE are seen: hallucinations, convulsions without loss of consciousness, opisthotonos, spasms of the muscles of the pharynx, larynx, and the entire thorax, abundant salivation, asphyxic phenomena, sensorial excitability, tendency to bite, characteristic hoarse cry, diminished sensory and motor activity, momentary Parylysis, foamy and bloody mucus in trachea and bronchi, sub-pleural hæmorrhages, sanguineous

---

* See BULL. DE LA SOC. MED. HOM. DE FRANCE., xxxix., 570,

infarctions in the liver". You may read these experiments in detail, with some corroborative poisoning cases, in the 'Cyclopædia of drug Pathogenesy'. They led M. Peyraud to believe that the virus—whether primarily animal or a chemical product of bacilli—which produces Hydrophobia. must be isomeric with *Tansy*, as the two act so similarly; and therefore that it might take the place, in the "Vaccination" of persons presumably bitten by rabid animals, of the extract of poisoned cords used by Pasteur. He tested his idea upon five rabbits with brilliant results: two drops of an essence of *Tansy* seemed sufficient to neutralise the effects of an injection of rabic virus which had previously killed two of their comrades.

Nothing further seems to have come of these researches; but they are surely conclusive as far as they go. A plant acting similarly to the Hydrophobic virus—a "simili-rage" as M. Peyraud calls it—is found to inhibit the development of the latter's action. Whatever value these ingenious theories about Isomerism may have, phenomenally at least (and that is all we care for) the practice is one of Homœopathic prophylaxis. Nor is it the first time that this thing has been done. I recalled, in my 'Therapeutics', the results obtained by the pastor Munch and his sons with *Belladonna*—a drug, if you will consider some especially of its older poisonings, as truly Homœopathic to the disease as *Tancy*, in the human subject perhaps more so. They treated with it 176 persons who had been recently bitten by mad dogs, and not one of these was attacked by the disease. According to the most recent and moderate estimate, one-third of these persons should have become Hydrophobic. I think that these results may compare favourably, to say the least, with Pasteur's; and that the method of such prophylaxis is obviously preferable to his. The wholesale destruction of animal life and happiness required for the latter, the loss of time and money and the positive risks of "Rabies Paralytica" and other accidents incurred by the subjects of his injections,—these might be tolerated if the results were commensurate, and if they could not otherwise be obtained. But when an equal immunity promises from the simple administration of non-lethal herbs, should not their influence be sought rather than the Pasteurian "vaccinations"?

I went on to show that here, as elsewhere, Homœopathic preventive is also a curative. "Bayle relates six cases treated by *Belladonna*, and of these four recovered. Hempel has collected five other cases of supposed cure with it; and three are recorded by practitioners of our own school in which it was the leading remedy" *Tancy* has not yet been tried: it should be, I think, first tested in the canine rabies it so vividly simulates.

---

* B. J. H. vii., 146; viii., 81; xi., 140.—Another has since been added; see J. B. H. S., ix., 182.

Till this is done, the best ally of *Belladonna* would be its sister plant *Stramonium*. This is reputed a specific for the disease in China; and might, as I have said, be chosen in preference when the general nervous irritability and delirium—such as it causes—were extreme.

The Homœopathic treatment of—

TETANUS was not, at one time, brilliantly successful. In our Austrian hospitals there were received, during the years 1832-1848, ten cases of this disease, of which only four recovered—one of these being non-traumatic. This is hardly worse than in the opposite camp, where 24 deaths out of 44 cases seems to be regarded as an average mortality; but we ought to do better. So, it seems, we do now; for in the Cook County Hospital at Chicago, recent statistics show in the Homœopathic wards two deaths out of twelve cases admitted; while during the same period, the same number treated on the other side gave a mortality of ten. One would like to know whether this advance is due to a more thorough reliance on the great SIMILLIMUM of the disease—*Nux vomica* and its Alkaloid. Of the curative action of the former two cases have been lately published,* in which it was given in quite high dilution—one of them being an example of the dreaded Tetanus Neonatorum. On *Strychnia* as remedial here we have really heard more from old-school writers than from our own. Sir Thomas Wason justifies its recommendation in a most naively Homœopathic way. "We know," he says, "that *Strychnia* acts upon the spinal cord, affecting apparently those parts and those functions of the cord which are affected in Tetanus; and in so fatal a malady, it would be justifiable, I conceive, to give the *Strychnia* in the hope that it might occasion a morbid action which would supersede the morbid action of the disease and yet be less perilous and more manageable than it. This, were it successful, would be a cure according to the Hahnemannic doctrine SIMILIA SIMILIBUS CURANTUR." Stille cites eight cases of the traumatic form in which its use was followed by cure, gr. $\frac{1}{8}$ to 1/16 being given for dose. He is more puzzled than Watson was at such results being obtained, but like him suggests that the *Strychnine* acted "substitutively," which we know to be equivalent to saying that the process is Homœopathic. We should probably adopt less perturbative dosage than he used, and should especially choose the medicine—in preference to its alternatives, *Aconite* and

---

* IODIAN HOM. REGIEW, March, 1895; PACIFIC COAST JOUR. OF HOM., June, 1895.

Hydrocyanic acid—when reflex excitability was very marked; but it should certainly be our leading Anti-tetanic.

And here too it appears that besides cure Homœopathy affords prophylaxis. Starting from the recognised facts as to the TOLERANCE of poisons which may be induced by their continued use Rummo "sought, by establishing a tolerance for *Strychnia*, a substance producing Physiological effects much resembling those of Tetanus, to protect animals against that disease. With considerable difficulty he was able to produce a fair amount of tolerance to *Strychnia* in a small series of guinea-pigs, so that they resisted a dose of $3\frac{1}{2}$ milligrammes when introduced into the stomach. All these, as well as several controls, were then inoculated with a culture of Tetanus. The controls all died in from six to ten days; some of the less saturated guinea-pigs developed slight symptoms of Tetanus, from which, however they recovered; those in which a maximum degree of tolerance had been set up did not develope any sign of the disease." * Here by another hypothesis—the establishment of tolerance for the same or similar poisons, the Homœopathic preventive has been reached; but that it is Homœopathic and might readily have been reached by applying SIMILIA SIMILIBUS to prophylaxis as well as cure, cannot be questioned. We must claim for Homœopathy, though not for Homœopathists, the credit of the piece of practice in question; and I trust that we shall hear of its adoption in our hospitals.

The adoption at the present day of a bacillary origin for Tetanus seems to have paralysed its ordinary treatment proceeding on the lines of a starting-point in injured nerves. We still, however, act in accordance therewith,—not so much by stretching or dividing the nerve trunk leading from the wound as by medicating this internally with **Hypericum**. Dr. Henser has cured two cases with the 1x dilution. Dr. Majumdar relates a case occurring in a young lady, where the lesion was a jammed finger. *Hypericum* 3 relieved the pain in a couple of hours and soon dispelled the spasms. Dr. Charles W. Smith reports a case of no slight severity, resulting from a lacerated wound where *Hypericum* was first given alone, then in alternation with *Nux vomica* 1x and subsequently the latter with *Hyoscyamus* till the termination of the case in complete recovery. Another case, recovering under this drug constitutionally and topically used, has been reported later. †

The Homœopathicity of *Strychnine* to Tetanus has needed no demonstrations. It is one of those facts that go to prove the fundamental character of the Law of Similars, since we see Nature herself making provision for its application. That

---

* BRIT. MED. JOURN., 1894, i., p. 35 of 'Epitome of Current Literature'.
† See, for the above, J. B. H. S., v., 109; viii., 185; M. H. R., xiiv., 740,

Aconite can cause Tetanus is less generally known, but the reference to cases of poisoning which I will give in a note will set the fact beyond a doubt.* Here, too, we have some old-school experience, showing it to be Tetanifuge as well as Tetanigenic. In a second note you will find references to records of nine cases treated by it (eight being traumatic), of which eight recovered. † It was stated that at one time it was the one remedy given in every case of the disease at the Middlesex Hospital. It is hardly surprising that such practice should bring the remedy into contempt. *Aconite* would be most applicable when exposure to cold and wet formed some part at least of the exciting cause of the disease. It would thus find its chief place in the idiopathic form, and would be least appropriate when the symptoms arose purely from eccentric irritation. Its spasms are more continuous than those of *Strychnia* and depend less upon reflex excitement.

The Homœopathicity of **Hydrocyanic acid** to Tetanus was pointed out by Dr. Madden and myself in an Article on the poison which he published in the Twentieth Volume of the BRITISH JOURNAL of HOMŒOPATHY. It does not seem to have been known as a remedy for the disease either in the old school or in our own. But in the Twenty-Fourth Volume of the same Journal Dr. George Moore reported a traumatic case successfully treated by drop doses of Scheele's preparation of this *acid*. It will not do to lay too much stress on this one case, for the patient might have recovered spontaneously. Still, during the first forty-eight hours of the treatment which was commenced with *Aconite* and *Belladonna*, the spasms were more numerous and violent; and the patient much more prostrate. Improvement commenced on the night after the *Acid* was begun. A similar account may be given of a case by Dr. Stopford, published in the MONTHLY HOMŒOPATHIC REVIEW of 1886 (p. 472). I cannot suggest any differential indications for this medicine.

I would add that the source of most of the experience cited above seem to render it necessary that, if we would emulate its success, we should give tolerably full doses of whichever of these medicines we select, Jahr, however, states that in the Insurrection in Paris in June, 1832, he treated a case with *Angustura* 30, which soon controlled the convulsions. I presume he means the *Angustura spuria;* and this, as is well-known, is only *Nux vomica* in another form.

---

* BRIT. MED. JOURN., Dec. 1, 1860; LANCET, Oct. 6, 1860 (two cases); "Hahnemman Mat. Med.," Part 1., Art. *Aconite,* sympt. 664; Fleming on *Aconite* (two cases).

† Braithwaite's Retrospect. 1846, i., 484, 494; BRIT. MED. JOURN., Jan. 28, 1860; Oct. 26, 1861; LANCET, Aug., 1860; Stille, ii., 316.

LECTURE XXVII

DISEASES OF THE NERVOUS SYSTEM
―o―
THE NEUROSES.
―o―
EPILEPSY—CHOREA—TREMOR—HYSTERIA
CATALEPSY—NEURASTHENIA

In this Lecture I propose to discuss the Therapeutics of a group of maladies which, though obviously belonging to the Nervous System, are not definitely referable to either of its divisions, and possibly involve both. They are EPILEPSY, CHOREA, TREMOR, HYSTERIA and CATALEPSY. They form, together with certain other disorders (as Neuralgia, Migraine, etc.) elsewhere treated of, the group of NEUROSES.

And first, of—
EPILEPSY.—Under this name I speak solely of the Idiopathic disease. All symptomatic and toxæmic convulsions, however Epileptiform in appearance, must here be excluded, if we wish to avoid confusion. In this I follow all writers—Trousseau, van der Kolk, Brown-Sequard, Russell Reynolds, Sieveking, and Radcliffe—who have of late years written upon the disease. To supplement these works on the therapeutical side Homœopathy has many recorded cases of relief and cure, most of which up to that date are contained in a collection by Dr. Baertl, which you will find translated in the Twenty-Second Volume of BRITISH JOURNAL OF HOMŒOPATHY. You should also read the two lectures on Epilepsy in Dr. Russell's 'CLINICAL LECTURES'; and the account of Dr. Bojanus' experience with it given in the Thirty-Ninth Volume of the Journal last-named.

You may possibly enquire, however, whether it is worth while going any further until we know whether Homœopathy can do better than in old-school practice, which is done by the new universally used *Bromides*. I have fully considered this question when speaking of the *Bromide of Potassium* in my 'Pharmacodynamics,' and I came to the conclusion that the large and continued doses of the drug which were necessary to suspend the fits were themselves so prejudical, that the *Bromic*-treatment of Epilepsy was not to be adopted save when the frequency of the convulsions was threatening life or reason, and then only as a temporary palliative. My mind is not altered by anything I have read or seen since. Dr. Hammond, who has himself had three cases of death from *Bromism*, and admits the Cachexia induced by the large doses necessarily given, considers nevertheless, that the induction of such a condition is favourable to the eradication of the Epileptic tendency, and therefore endeavours to produce it as soon as possible. Strangely enough, however, he goes on to say that one of the *Bromine* compounds—that which it forms with *Zinc*—has in several cases proved exceedingly efficacious in arresting the paroxysms where other *Bromides* had failed, but that Bromism is not an attendant upon its administration. He nevertheless considers that the *Bromine* of the compound exercises considerable curative influence. When, moreover, he speaks of prognosis, he says that "recent cases can often be cured, but those which have lasted for several years are rarely brought to a favourable termination." Dr. Brown-Squard, who wrote the Article on Epilepsy in Quain's Dictionary, did not hold out much better hopes. He treated all his patients with a stock mixture of *Iodide of Potassium, Bromide of Potassium* and *Ammonium,* and *Carbonate of Potash,* giving also *Strychnine* or *Arsenic* as a "Tonic." This, he says, may be, continued for years "without any marked bad effect"; but he admits that like medical treatment generally, it only issues in cure or improvement in 7 per cent. of the cases. Dr. Bojanus, in a series of 54 cases, can report 22 as cured, and 11 as considerably benefited. The comparative results of the *Bromic*-treatment thus hardly outweigh its disadvantages; and as Homœopathy does not need to poison its patients in the process of curing them,* I think you may with a clear conscience keep your hands off the *Bromides* when you have Epileptics to treat, and be content to do your best for them according to the method of Hahnemann. Should, indeed, this method itself lead you to them, as where (in a case of Dr. Carpenter's†) much mental hebetude existed, or where minute doses as Dr. Love's 25 centigrammes daily of the 1x trituration†) suffice to produce the effect desired, you will do well to avail yourselves of any specific action there *Bromine* has upon Eclamptic conditions. I only advise not to keep your patients in a chronic state of *Bromic-poisoning* because they occasionally have Epileptic fits.

Let us consider what the condition is which in patients afflicted with this disease we have to treat. It is a chronically morbid state of a certain portion of the nerve-centres (generally perhaps, the medulla oblongata), which leads to an irregular production of its force, and occasional explosive discharge of the same. This morbid patch may be an inherited infirmity, or it may be acquired under the influence of depressing emotional

---

* See Dr. Weir Mitchell's enumeration of the evil effects of Bromic intoxication in J. B. H. S., v. 88. He may well "strongly inveigh against deluging patients with *Bromides,* especially in Epilepsy". To the same effect Dr. Goodhart has spoken in his Address in Medicine at the Meeting of the British Medical Association in 1901. "The *Bromide* treatment of Epilepsy," he affirms, "often does a great deal of harm, and I am by no means certain that it does any equivalent good." (BRIT. MED. JOURN., Aug. 3rd, 1901).

† J. B. H. S., viii., 257.   ‡ IBID., p. 157.

or other causes, or from continued eccentric irritation. In any case itself is the proximate cause to which our medication must be directed : the paroxysms are only tht indication of its presence.

Our available remedies for this condition are of several kinds. There are, first, certain *vegetable poisons* from whose acute operation Epileptic convulsions are apt to occur. These are *Hydrocyanic acid;* the three Umbelliferæ. *Œnanthe crocata Cicuta virosa,* and *Æthusa cynapium,* and *Belladonna.* Next we have some mineral substances, and a vegetable one whose long continued operation sometimes gives rise to similar phenomena : I speak of *Copper, Lead* and *Arsenic,* and of *Absinthe.* Lastly, there are drugs which, though never causing Epileptiform paroxysms, have an ascertained relation either to over-excitability of the nervous centres or to their imperfect nutrition. In the first class are *Strychnia* and its ores (as they may be called) *Nux vomica* and *Ignatia;* in the second, we have *Calcarea* and *Silicea.* These drugs constitute our Anti-epileptic armoury ; it is rarely that you have to go beyond them. Let me sketch to you the adaptation of them to Epilepsy in its several stages and forms of occurrence.

First, as to the FIT itself,—can you do anything to ward it off, when the occurrence of premonitory symptoms gives us time and opportunity ? If we can, I think it must be employing the Antipathic rather than the Homœopathic method,—though one of the drugs with which we carry it out is (or once was) peculiar to the school of Hahnemann. I am speaking of **Glonoin**. In lecturing upon that substance, I assigned reasons for believing that it acts immediately upon the medulla oblongata, and thence upon the vaso-motor nerves of the head and face, causing its well-known throbbing and flushing. It thus occupies the same ground and traverses the same path as the Epileptic NISUS, while its influence is precisely contrary thereto ; and it acts with almost equal rapidity. It thus answers in all respects to the requirements of an effective Antipathic palliative, and ought to be very useful in such a capacity. I suggested its employment here many years ago;* but have had no sufficient opportunity of testing its efficacy. In the meantime, however, another agent of the same kind, but acting more quickly still, has been introduced into the ordinary practice,—**Amyl nitrite.** Drs. Weir, Mitchell and Crichton Browne at once perceived its applicability to check the Epileptic paroxysm, and have reported very favourably of its employment. Dr. Hammond also praises it, but jtstly simits its use to those cases in which the face ordinarily becomes pale in the very inception of the attack. He has found it, as might be expected, of no curative power whatever when given systematically. The *Amyl nitrite* should be inhaled ; with *Glonoin* the first decimal dilution may be touched with the tongue.

---

* See 'Manual of Pharmacodynamics', 1st Ed. (1867), p. 289.

The treatient we adopt in the interval of the paroxysms, with the view of averting their recurrence, will be somewhat modified according as the disease is recent or of long-standing. For Epilepsy of recent origin we have two very valuable remedies, which are of little power in confirmed cases. These are *Ignatia* and *Hydrocyanic acid*.

Ignatia is of much value on account of the frequent origin of Epilepsy in emotional disturbance. I have mentioned that it was in use for the disease when thus caused before Hahnemann's time, and that he confirms its usefulness from his experience with small doses.—limiting its sphere, however to recent cases, or to those in which the fits never occur save from disturbance of this kind. Dr. Baertl relates several instances in which it was curative, and two are given by Dr. Bojanus. It is especially suitable for Epilepsy occuring in children, without being inherited by them.

The Homœopathicity of **Hydrocyanic acid** to Epilepsy was first argued out by Dr. Madden and myself in a Paper of this subject contributed to the Twentieth Volume of the BRITISH JOURNAL OF HOMŒOPATHY. I have several times since returned to the subject, and maintained our position, defending it against the only assailant it has had—our late colleague Dr. Russel ; and in a communication to the proceedings of the World's Convention of 1876, which is published in its Transactions, I have finally stated the whole matter. You will find there the complete argument of the conclusion that *"Hydrocyanic acid is exquisitely Homœopathic to the Epileptic paroxysm ; that its effects as closely and truly resemble that disorder as those of Strychnia resembling Tetanus."* Of this I think there can be no doubt ; but the inference as to its curative power over the disease cannot be made without considerable reservation. In Tetanus it is 'the paroxysm that we have to treat, in Epilepsy it is the morbid condition of the nervous centres from which at times paroxysms start. It is not so certain that we can modify this with the drug, which has moreover (as Dr. Russell justly pointed out), a very evanescent action. Nevertheless, as it will sometimes cure, in a most rapid and striking manner, such recurrent spasmodic attacks as Gastrodynia and Pertussis, there is no reason why it should not be occasionally remedial in Epilepsy. I have cited, in the Paper last referred to, several recorded instances of cure by it, even in cases of long-standing. I have myself many times obtained great benefit from it here, and when the disorder was of recent origin, actual cure. In one very interesting case the patient was the subject of Angina Pectoris also and both affections yielded to the *Acid*. I have had better results since I gave stronger, more frequent, and more continued doses It is my present practice to administer from five drops of the 3rd decimal attenuation to three drops of the 1st centesimal four times a day.

In Epilepsy of some standing the leading remedies among Homœopathists are *Belladonna, Calcarea* and *Cuprum*.

Belladonna still holds in our affections that high place which it once occupied in the old school until dethroned by the *Bromides*. I have mentioned in my 'Pharmacodynamics' Trousseau's favourable estimate of its powers ; and from Dr. Stille's Article upon the drug, it appears that its systematic use was intitiated by Debreyne, and consisted in giving daily doses increasing in quantity up to the maximum of toleration, and continuing this course with occasional relaxations and intermissions for three or four years. From the cases collected by Dr. Baertl and those reported by Dr. Russel it appears that it can sometimes cure in much smaller and less frequent doses, to complete the recovery. Bahr justly remarks that "the Epileptic *Belladonna-Convulsions* are the consequence of an intense intoxication of the organism; while running their course they may recur several times, but never in the form of a chronic affection, as is the case with *Cuprum* and *Plumbum*. Hence the *Belladonna-Convulsions*, as we indeed know from experience correspond rather to Eclampsia, which has been very properly designated as Acute Epilepsy." We shall see, when Puerperal and Infantile Convulsions come before us, how important a place *Belladonna* holds in their treatment. It is indicated in Epilepsy the younger the patient is, and the more sanguine his nervous temperament. It acts (we may suppose) by modifying the irritability and hyperæmia of the discharging centre. We can quite follow *Echeverria*, therefore, in expecting good from it in "Vertiginous Epilepsy;—the PETIT-MAL of the French writers. It may be tried in the form of *Atropia* also before abandonment.

That **Calcarea** has proved not less frequently and more permanently useful is evident from the cases in Dr. Baertl's Paper. It is of course especially indicated when the constitutional condition is one for which this great nutrition-modifier is suitable. But it seems often to have acted well when no symptoms of this kind were present. and to be peculiarly suitable for re-inforcing and perpetuating the action of *Belladonna*.

Cuprum, which once had some reputation in the old school as an Anti-epileptic, has a big one in ours. Bahr, Jousset and Bayes concur to give it the first place among our remedies for the disease; and Dr. Baertl cities a number of cures of chronic cases. Dr. Bayes thinks it indicated in proportion to the violence of the Convulsions.—The last two medicines have done most in the higher dilutions and rarely repeated doses; and Bahr thinks this practice to be best in the treatment of Epilepsy generally.

A few words may be said upon certain other medicines which may in exceptional cases become serviceable.

Argentum nitricum has well-known traditional reputation. Dr. Gray of New York says that it is often curative—without the need of including Cyanosis in the process—in cases arising from moral causes, as impassioned lay preaching. Dr. Brown-Sequard relates two cases in which $\frac{1}{8}$ gr. doses effected a cure. *Arsenic* has undoubtedly caused Epilepsy, but we know nothing of its power to cure it; it would perhaps be indicated if the paroxysms recurred periodically, *Cicuta* is credited with some cures, and so also is *Cocculus*, as I have related in my '*Pharmacodynamics.*' *Opium* is said to have cured cases where the fits occurred only in sleep. *Plumbum* is highly commended to us by Bahr, but rather upon the ground of its Homœopathicity than from any experience with it. *Silicea* is recommended in Epilepsy when the constitutional condition and concomitant symptoms of the patient are such as to suggest this remedy: it also (like *Opium*) is indicated by the occurrence of the Convulsions during sleep. The latter feature is Dr. Hammond's indication for *Strychina*, of whose successful use in Dr. Tyrrell's hands I have spoken when lecturing on that drug, *zizia aurea** appears to act as a poison much like *Œnanthe* and *Cicuta*. It has cured in Dr. Marcy's hands two genuine cases of Epilepsy of some standing. He gave the third decimal dilution.

I need hardly say that in Epilepsy, as everywhere, whenever the maxim TOLLE CAUSAM is practicable, it ought to be implicitly obeyed. Whether the CAUSA be an intestinal parasite, a depression of the cranium, or a Syphilitic growth, it must be removed by the measures appropriate for the purpose.

In these Therapeutic suggestions I have mainly reproduced what I wrote in 1877. The lapse of years since then has brought some further experience to light.

1. The use of **Œnanthe crocata,** which of the three Umbelliferæ most closely simulates Epilepsy, has been growing of late, Dr. Dewey has summarised the published evidence of its remedial power in the HOMŒOPATHIC RECORDER for December, 1899, and there is really a good body of it. Among others, Dr. Talcott praises it as improving the Epileptics among his patients in the Middletown Asylum. He gives it in the mother-tincture. †

2. Dr. Colby, of Boston, who is a nervous specialist, writes: "I have now been trying **Indigo** in nearly all my cases of Epilepsy for the past twelve years, and the percentage of actual cures has been so much greater than from the *Bromides* that I still continue to employ it, with 10 per cent. of apparent cures, *i.e.*, patients who do not have an attack of GRAND or PETIT MAL for over two years." ‡

---

* See Hale's New Remedies, 2nd Ed. SUB VOCE.
† J. B. H. S., i., 280.
‡ NORTH AMER. JOURN. OF HOM., NOV., 1899.

3. In the Supplementary Lecture of my 'Pharmacodynamics' I have mentioned the repute of the **Artemisia vulgaris** in Epilepsy both in the hands of the common people and in those of Nothnagel; and have called attention to the power in the *Artemisia absinthium*, when habitually taken as "*Absinthe*," to set up an Epileptic condition. My inference that we should get better results from this species of the genus has hardly been verified; on the other hand Dr. Sprague, from his experience at the Nebraska Institution for the feeble-minded, is inclined to place the *"vulgaris"* species at the head of our Anti-Epileptics, and seems to have used it in the dilutions.*

4. I have also, in the same place, quoted testimony to the virtues in the sphere of the poison of the toad, which we call **Bufo.** I omitted to mention that to this remedy, in the medium dilutions, Dr. Bojanus owed the majority of the cures and improvements he has reported.

5. Dr. W. M. Butler, whose experience, like that of several of the foregoing, has been gained in a public institution, has had his best results from *Cuprum* and *Hydrocyanic acid*. Of the former, he says that he has not been able to define its exact indications; but that several cases, apparently hopeless, which had been for years under old-school medication, he has promptly and permanently cured with it. Nor has it been inefficacious in recent cases, though for these he generally prefers *Hydrocyanic acid*. "We have found," he writes, "exceedingly satisfactory, and have permanently cured several cases through its agency. In some instances, where we have ultimately had complete success, we have found that it did not at first check the Convulsions, but rendered them much milder and shortened their length, the patient retaining partial consciousness during the seizures." The lower dilutions are recommended. †

The next Neurosis of which I have to speak is the well-known "St. Vitus's Dance"—

CHOREA. For Therapeutical purpose I think we may speak of three varieties of Chorea. The first is that induced by a

---

* North Aer. Journ. of Hom., Sept. 1894
† Ibid., May, 1901.

definite exciting cause, whether mental or material, as fright or the presence of worms. There is doubtless some fundamental instability of the nervous centres here; but when the cause can be removed or neutralised, the disturbances ceases. In the second the Chorea seems to be an expression on the part of the nervous system of a general diathesis or constitutional condition, as Chlorosis, Rheumatism, or Tubercle. The third form, in our ignorance, we must class as Idiopathic.

1. There seems no doubt that Chorea, like Epilepsy, may arise from a sudden and profound emotional impression, such as fright. Trousseau records two well-marked instances of the kind. In these cases we should expect the same benefit, from **Ignatia** as in recent Epilepsy thus caused: and the Pathogenesis fully favours the expectation. Jahr recommends *Causticum* where *Ignatia* is indicated, but proves insufficient. Like Epilepsy again, Chorea may be a symptom of the presence of worms in the intestinal canal. I have referred, when lecturing on **Cina,** to a very pretty case in which severe Chorea subsided on the expulsion of Ascarides consequent upon the administration. It will generally be the appropriate medicine where worms are suspected to lie at the bottom of the symptoms. Another which may fairly be named here is **Spigelia**, whose relation to Rheumatism strengthens the indications for its use in Chorea.

2. *Iron* is deservedly a favourite remedy in the old-school for Chorea; and the frequent co-existence of Chlorosis and Anæmia with this disorder explains its efficacy. In such cases Homœopathy has nothing better to suggest, and you had better give **Ferrum redactum** as you had a simple case of Anæmia before you. On the other hand, Trousseau's statement that Chorea is not uncommonly an expression of the Tubercular diathesis leads me to call attention to the place of **Iodine** in its treatment. Something very like the twitchings of Chorea appears among the phenomena of *Iodism;* and from my observation of the action of this precious medicine on the Nervous System in general, I should look for good results from it in cases of this kind. Jousset recommends it in the graver forms of disease, and there is old-school experience in its favour.

But by far the most important diathetic relationship of Chorea is that which it bears to Rheumatism. I do not mean through the medium of cardiac vegetations, causing embolism; but immediately. Wherever you can trace this relationship, I advise you to depend upon *Actæa racemosa* in its treatment. The cases recorded in the Second Edition of Dr. Hale's 'New Remedies' and those communicated by Dr. Gibbs Blake to the Sixteenth Volume of the MONTHLY HOMŒOPATHIC REVIEW, will encourage you in this course; and will also, I think, lead you not to go much above the mother tincture for the most suitable dose.

3. In the treatment of Idiopathic Chorea we are in much the

same plight as our brethren of the other school. We have so many remedies that we question whether any of them really cure or whether the disease does not get well of itself. The **Arsenic** and **Zinc** so much relied on by them we also use, adding **Cuprum.** We have also the group of vegetable neurotics, **Belladonna, Hyoscyamus** and **Stramonium;** and **Agaricus.** The last-named has perhaps been credited with most cures in our school; and its Austrian proving shows its perfect Homœopathicity to the disorder. The characteristic of the Convulsive movements of this drug mentioned by Dr. Clifton,* that they cease during sleep, is an almost invariable feature of Chorea. While with this medicine and *Cuprum* we may combat the ordinary cases of the disorder, *Belladonna, Hyoscyamus* and *Stramonium* will be more suitable in nervous and delicate children, *Zincum* where the nervous centres and the general nutrition are much depressed; and *Arsenicum* in those graver forms of the disease where even life is threatened. As the Pathology of such cases seems to be a condition of active hyperæmia at the base of the brain, the **Veratrum viride,** so much commended by Dr. Cooper,† might be a useful adjunct.

Another class of remedies of some repute in Chorea are the venomous spiders. The alleged connexion of the convulsive epidemics of the Middle Ages with the bite of the **Tarentula** has yet to be demonstrated; and Dr. Nunez's proving has not added much to our real knowledge of the subject. His preparation of the spider, however, has gained a good deal of repute among the Spanish and French Homœopathists in the treatment of Chorea, Dr. Jousset stating that it has given him more successes than any other remedy. While I am referring of authors, I may say that Bahr and Jahr concur in placing *Cuprum* and *Stramonium* at the head of Anti-choreic remedies. The former employs *Stramonium* in severe cases till the violence of the paroxysms is reduced, and then—or in "Chorea minor" from the first—gives *Cuprum.*

Here also, as in Epilepsy, the years which have passed since I wrote thus have brought their changes, though rather in the way of addition than of modification.

1. Dr. Goldsborough has given us two valuable studies of the Therapeutics of Chorea, in Sixth Volume of the LONDON HOMŒOPATHIC HOSPITAL REPORTS and the Eighth of the JOURNAL OF THE BRITISH HOMŒOPATHIC SOCIETY respectively. They are based upon the experience gained in our hospital, and I am glad to say that they confirm the suggestions I had so long ago made. *Ignatia* where simple nervous instability seems present, or mental emotion has been the exciting cause; *Actœa*—in fullish dosage—where a Rheumatic element is present; *Arsenic*

---

* M. H. R., xii., 400.
† B. J. H., xxix., 163; xxxiv., 279.

in severe cases, especially when there is Endocarditis; *Agaricus* or *Stramonium* when spinal cord or brain seems involved; *Cuprum* for sharp spasm and *Zincum* in depressed nervous systems with bad surroundings—these are his remedies as they have been mine and my former colleagues'. Brilliant and rapid results are not to be expected, but satisfactory recoveries can nearly always be depended upon.

2. Dr. Halbert has several times given, in the CLIOINUE so ably edited by him, illustrative cases of the treatment of Chorea. In Non-rheumatic cases he depends mainly on *Agaricus,* giving it in the form of its Alkaloid—*Agaricine.*

3. Here again, as in Epilepsy, *Argentum nitricum* receives commendation. Dr. Gross, of Regensburg, finds in it—in the 2nd to the 4th trituration, probably decimal—more effective than any of our ordinary remedies, and relates four cases illustrative of its power.*

Under the head of—

TREMOR several distinct affections might be included. Trembling is a marked feature of the SCLEROSE EN PLAQUES of the French Pathologists, whether occurring in the brain alone, or in the brain and cord conjointly. There are attacks of Convulsive Tremor which are connected with Epilepsy, differing from it mainly in that there is no loss of consciousness. But over and above these there is an essential tremor which is apt to invade the body,—either beginning in the head and gradually spreading from thence, or primarily involving the hands and associated with Paralysis. In the former variety (often called Senile Tremor, though by no means peculiar to old) I think **Agaricus** very useful. I once rapidly cured a case of long-standing in an old man with deep doses of the mother tincture of this drug; it had the peculiar feature of the twitchings of the arms ceasing when he used them in his work of shoe-making. The other kind of essential Tremor is "Paralysis Agitans," though its English equivalent "Shaking Palsy" probably applies to both. For this disorder **Mercurius** ought to be useful as it is strikingly Homœopathic; but Dr. Jousset says he has used it and other medicines without benefit. From the other school we have reports in favour of **Hyoscyamus** from Dr. Oulmont, and this is Homœopathic enough. Dr. Hammond speaks of obtaining excellent results from Galvanism and the *Bromide of Zinc.*

Good effects in Paralysis Agitans have been noted more

---

* ALLG. HOM. ZEIT., vol. lxiv., No. 24.

recently, by Dr. Goldsborough from *Mercurius solubilis* 12 **and** 30 and by Dr. Halbert from *Zincum picricum* 3x.* *Hyoscyamus* is also receiving enhanced favour in the Termor both of this complaint and in that of disseminated Sclerosis. In the latter Dr. Delamater uses the 4x trituration of Merck's preparation of the *Hydrobromate of Hyoscyamine* with much satisfaction. †

HYSTERIA is the next in order of our Neuroses. Here, besides the all-important mental and moral treatment, we can do a good deal by medicines,—thus advancing a step beyond the old school, which, according to one of its latest expositors, knows "not one single drug which exerts any specific action on the disease."‡ We have such a drug in our **Ignatia**. Besides removing many of the pains and spasmodic phenomena occasionally present, its continued use in varying dilutions will almost certainly modify favourably that morbid impressionability—emotional, sensory and reflex—in which so much of Hysteria consists. With **Moschus**, moreover, we can sometimes arrest and always shorten the Hysteric paroxysm. It should be given in the lower dilutions of the tincture, as its odour has much to do with its rapid action.

These are the medicines on which experience has taught me to rely. Jousset, however, considers **Tarentula** of at least equal value with *Ignatia*, especially when Hysteria assumes the Convulsive form. When this amounts to "Hystero-Epilepsy," the old-school recommendation of Duboisine may be considered.§ Bahr has a very full and detailed Article upon the disease, mainly taken from Hartmann, and gives indications for a number of remedies, as *Nux moschata, Valerian, Secale, Aurum, Pulsatilla, Conium, Cocculus, Asafœtida, Sepia*, &c. One would have been glad of some practical recommendations for special Hysterical affections. One of these is vomiting, which is often very obstinate; but it will sometimes give way to *Kreasote*. Hysterical pains in the joints will often yield to *Ignatia* or *Chamomilla*, or—if of longer-standing—to *Argentum*. For Aphonia, Paralysis and Anæsthesia occurring in connection with Hysteria, we have generally to call in the aid of Electricity. When Hysteria takes the form of sopor, *Opium* will prove curative;** when of Catalepsy, *Cannabis Indica*.***

---

* J. B. H. S. iii., 141; vii. 329.
† IBID., vi., 101.
‡ Dr. Russell Reynolds, in his 'System of Medicine', ii., 327.
§ See J. B. H. S., i., 121.
¶ See J. B. H. S., v. 296.
*** See IBID viii., 156, I have myself had a similar experience.

CATALEPSY itself is so rare a disease that there is little likelihood of the question of its best Homœopathic treatment being brought before you. Nevertheless, it is well to remind you of the perfect picture of its phenomena occasionally presented by susceptible persons under the influence of the **Cannabis Indica** I have spoken of in connection with the Hysterical simulation of the condition.

I can find no better place than this for the affection so much noted of late, and described under the name of—

NEURASTHENIA—It is our old "Nervous Debility" scientifically recognised and elevated to the rank of a distinctive malady. Where it occurs in women, without any ascertainable exhausting cause, and when emaciation co-exists, I have no doubt that the plan of treatment devised by Dr. Weir Mitchell of Philadelphia, and carried out here by Dr. Playfair, is the best that can be adopted. When, however, Neurasthenia is distinctly traceable to over-strain or other nerve-depressing causes, much may be done for it by ordinary Hygiene and Homœopathic medication. Of our old remedies, **Phosphoric acid** and **Silicea** stand out pre-eminent,—the first where grief or chagrin has lowered the system or sexual excess had drained it, where there is diuresis and too ready perspiration, and where the memory shows notable failure; the second where there is more erethism present and more tendency to Headache and other pains. I have signalised these medicines in my 'Pharmacodynamics', and have generally been content with them; but I am glad to note the aid brought to *Silicea* by **Picric acid and to** *Phosphoric acid* by Schussler's **Kali phosphoricum.** Dr. Halbert finds no remedy for Neurasthenia equal to or surpassing *Picric acid*; and Dr. W. E. Taylor finds it curative even when the nervous depression threatens Insanity.* Dr. Gorton, of Brooklyn, assures us that we shall be helped by drop doses of the tincture *of Scutellaria lateriflora* when the brain symptoms are marked.†

---

* J. B. H. S., viii., 75 ix., 101.
† M. H. R., xxxvii., 109.

LECTURE XXVIII

DISEASES OF THE NERVOUS SYSTEM
---o---
LOCAL NERVOUS AFFECTIONS
---o---
NEURITIS—NEURALGIA—MEGRIM—LOCAL SPASMS—FACIAL PALSY

Having now completed the consideration of the general disorders of the nervous system, I shall devote this lecture to those which are of a more localised character. I shall speak of NEURITIS and NEURALGIA, of MIGRAINE, of LOCAL PARALYSIS, and of LOCAL SPASMS.

NEURITIS has only recently been recognised, but it embraces several affections to which we have hitherto given other names, as "Rheumatic" Neuralgiæ and Paralyses. I shall still speak of the treatment of those under their former headings; and will only say here that **Aconite** (preferably in the tinctures of the root) is the great remedy for them. The most interesting form of Neuritis is that called "Multiple Peripheral." Its special interest to us arises from its frequent causation by mineral poisons, as *Lead, Arsenic,* and (in India-rubber workers) the *Bisulphide of Carbon* : for in these substances we get remedies for it when occurring as an effect of Alcohol or a sequela of Influenza or Diphtheria. In the Fifth Volume of the LONDON HOMŒOPATHIC HOSPITAL REPORTS, Dr. Galley Blackley relates five cases of its having the latter origins, in four of which the **Carbon bisulphide** certainly contributed to the cure. Dr. George Black has related a cure of a case of long-standing, having its seats in the right sciatic, by the 3x dilution of this drug; and Dr. Hawkes has reported an Alcoholic case successfully treated by **Plumbum**.

In Neuritis of traumatic origin, you will of course think of **Hypericum**. A case where it was consecutive to Neuroma was practically cured by it in Dr. Colby's hands.†

---

* M. H. R., xxxvii., 594; xxxix., 121.
† J. B. H. S., 1., 280.

And now of—

NEURALGIA.—Of the Homœopathic treatment of this painful malady I am able to give you a most favourable account. Without the blistering and hypodermic Morphia, or even the Electricity, which seem at present the main resources of the old school, you need seldom fail to effect a rapid cure of the ordinary varieties of the disease, and even the intractable "Tic Douloureux" will sometimes yield to our remedies. If you need further encouragement than my assertion affords, let me ask you to read the cases of the diseases recorded by Dr. Quin in the Fourth, by Dr. Morgan in the Thirteenth, and by myself in the Twenty Second Volume of the BRITISH JOURNAL OF HOMŒOPATHY. I can also refer you to Dr. Burnett's little volume on the disease.*

In my Lectures on the 'Materia Medica' I have endeavoured to characterize the sphere and kind of action of our most noted Anti-neuralgics. I would ask you to read what I have written there about *Aconite, Arsenic, Belladonna, Colocynth, Phosphorus, Spigelia* and *Sulphur* in this relation; and will here, without repeating myself, take up the subject from the side of the disease, and endeavour to apportion our remedies to its several forms and varieties.

The primary classification to be made of them relates to the history of the malady,—whether it is recent or of long-standing inherited or acquired, and whether its subject is young and impressionable, or sufficiently advanced in life to be undergoing degenerative changes. A Neuralgia of recent origin in any one yet on the sunny side of the grand climacteric requires such remedies as *Aconite, Belladonna, Colocynth* and *Spigelia* : it is pretty sure to be more or less Rheumatic or inflammatory (if not reflex) in origin. But when a patient inherits a morbid nervous system; when Neuralgia sets in with him to all appearance spontaneously, and settles in time into a chronic and obstinate misery; or when it begins late in life,—you will have to resort to deeper-acting remedies, like *Arsenic, Phosphorus* and *Sulphur*. You have degeneration to deal with, and must select your remedies accordingly.

Let us now pass in review the local varieties of Neuralgia, with the object of seeing what has been or may be done for their treatment.

1. Neuralgia of the trigeminal nerve (PROSOPALGIA) are among the most frequent we are called to treat. Many of these affect its supra-orbital branch alone. The sympathetic Neuralgia of gastric disorder generally attacks this nerve (some persons cannot swallow an ice without being attacked by it); it then finds it remedy in **Kali bichromicum.** The 'Hahnemann Materia Medica' contains two cases cured by it in the 6th and 12th dilutions. "Brow-ague," again is a supra-orbital Neuralgia, and when truly Malarious, finds its best remedy in **Quinine** which may also prove serviceable in the disorder otherwise occurring, Dr. Anstie agreeing with Valleix as to the doubtful value of this remedy in

---

* "Neuralgia" its causes and its remedies 2nd Ed., 1894.

Non-malarious Neuralgia, except "the Ophthalmic form." In this Buzzard also commends it. And the following case shows that infinitesimal doses of the drug may suffice for the cure, which could hardly be unless it were Homœopathic to the condition,—as indeed the provings of Dr. Schulz have proved it to be.*

Mrs. Des V—, æt. about 50, consulted me on December 12th, 1867. About a week previously, she had had a chill, the immediate effect of which was a cold in the head. With this her appetite had gone off; and in a day or two a pain had set in above the left eye, which, after wavering about for a little, had become a periodical supra-orbital Neuralgia. For the last three days the pain had come on daily at noon, and continued till between four and five p.m. It shot from the supra-orbital foramen up the scalp on the same side, and one spot over the parietal bone was especially painful, and tender to the touch. The eye did not become bloodshot during the attack, nor did it water, but the eyelids quivered much. The distribution of the supra-orbital nerve readily accounts for all these phenomena.

I found the appetite quite absent, a clammy taste in the mouth, and the tongue rather thickly coated with a greyish fur. The urine was loaded with Lithates, but the bowels were normal. No other symptoms worthy of note were ascertainable. I prescribed *Kali bichromicum* 6, a drop three times a day.

Dec. 14th. The tongue was cleaner and the appetite better, but the attacks of pain had recurred without diminution or variation. Continue *Kali bichrom.*

Dec. 16th. The gastric symptoms are now quite removed, but there is no real change in the Neuralgia. The periodicity of the paroxysms and the Lithate-loaded urine were the only symptoms upon which I could found my choice of a remedy. They led me to *Quinine*, which I prescribed in the 3rd centesimal dilution, a drop four times a day.

Dec. 18th. Since beginning the *Quinine* there has been hardly any pain worth-mentioning, but during the usual hours of attack there has been an occasional slight stab in the brow and quivering of the eyelids. Continue.

Dec. 21st. No supra-orbital nerve symptoms has appeared these three days. The urine is much clearer.†

In RIGHT supra-orbital Neuralgia, especially in connection with hepatic disorder, you may do well to bethink yourself of **Chelidonium,** which indeed its prover, Dr. Buchmann extols as sovereign remedy for most superficial affections of this nature.‡ **Nux vomica** also is appropriate here, and is commended by Jousset even when Malaria is the exciting cause.

Neuralgia of the Superior and inferior maxillary branches of the fifth (often including the Ophthalmic) is met with under two forms, the one recent and readily curable, the other chronic

---

* 'See Cyclopædia of Drug Pathogenesy', ii., 738.

† Abridged from report in B. J. H., xxvi., 131.

‡ See Vol. xxv. of the same Journal p. 30 : and vol. xx., p. 47.

and very intractable. A good number of remedies have gained repute in the former; and possibly some of them may be applicable to the latter. I will therefore give the indications for in each in order.

Aconite I have formerly described as "invaluable in quite recent cases, where the phenomena are Congestive or Rheumatic in character," referring to Dr. Morgan's first case as illustrating such adaptation. Since, however, I became acquainted with Schroff's provings, showing its power of setting up a true Trigeminal Neuralgia, I have much extended the range of its usefulness, saying that "in recent Prosopalgia, especially when caused by exposure to dry cold, it will prove curative, even when the terms 'Congestive,' and 'Rheumatic' are out of place." This is Dr. Dudgeon's experience as well as our own.* Dr. Gubler's results, cited in my 'Pharmacodynamics', would lead us to trust to it in more chronic and deeply-rooted cases; but here, I think, it should be given in the form of the tincture of the root or of *Aconitine*.

Belladonna is the remedy in sub-acute cases, even of some standing; in comparatively young and florid subjects; where in each attack of pain the face flushes up (especially, sometimes only, on the side affected), the cheek being hot and the eyes suffused. Its Neuralgia differs from that of *Aconite*, which otherwise—in the congestive form—it so closely resembles, in having hyperæsthesia present, so that any jar aggravates the pains. These, moreover, are apt to come and go suddenly.

Colocynth is recommended where the disorder has arisen from exposure to damp cold, or occurs in Rheumatico-gouty subjects. The pain is tearing; aggravated by touch or movement of the facial muscles; relieved by warmth and rest.

Spigelia in Bahr's opinion, "deserves the first place in the list of remedies for Prosopalgia." The indications are those of *Colocynth* (*i.e.* the "Rheumatic" character), with anxiety at the heart and great restlessness. The pain, too, is as much jerking or pulsating as tearing. Jahr adds periodical recurrence as a characteristic; others aggravation by stooping.

I confess that I have had no successful experience with the last two remedies in Rheumatic Prosopalgia. I have always got on, if *Aconite* has not been sufficient, with **Rhododendron** and **Pulsatilla**. The first has answered well in recent cases, where the whole half of the face seems to ache; in one such case where it failed, *Kalmia* succeeded, as recommended by Dr. Bayes. *Pulsatilla* comes in where the disorder is of longer-standing, and the pains are of the character so graphically described by Hahnemann—"as if a nerve were put upon the stretch and then let loose again suddenly causing a painful

---

* See "Materia Medica, Physiological and Applied," i., 134.

jerk." The other characteristic of the drug are also usually present.

Verbaseum, Mezereum, Platina and **China** find also an occasional place in the treatment of Prosopalgia. The pain of the two former is seated in the infra-orbital foramen, and is a stupefying pressure. Dr. Cretin thinks highly of *Verbascum* (in the mother tincture): its pains, he says, are readily excited, the face is red, and there are acid eructations.* Syphilitic or Mercurial influence would especially suggest *Mezereum*. *Platina* and *China* are (like *Aconite* and *Belladonna*) exactly antithetic in one important particular, viz., that the pain of the former is accompanied by numbness, while with the latter the face is so sensitive that the least touch aggravates. *Cedron* and *Plantago* also should be considered. †

Last, though not least, but greatest comes **Arsenicum.** In purely Nervous Prosopalgia (as from Influenza, Malaria, or Simple Debility) this remedy stands FACILE PRINCEPS. I have fully given the indications for it in my 'Pharmacodynamics,' I may add here Bahr's testimony to its efficacy. *"Arsenicum"*, he writes, "quiets nervous pains better than any other medicine. Its effect is rapid, and sometimes rivals a powerful dose of *Opium*. It is characteristic of *Arsenic* to exert this soothing influence only" (I should rather say "especially") "in the case of pains that become worse at the approach of night, reach their climax about midnight, and are accompanied by an extraordinary degree of nervous restlessness." I quite agree with this author in preferring the higher dilutions of *Arsenic* (and, indeed, of most other Anti-neuralgics, save *Aconite* and *Belladonna*) to the lower.

It is mainly by such use of *Arsenic* that the true TIC DOULOUREUX—the "Epileptiform Neuralgia" of Trousseau—can be (when it ever can) removed out of the category of incurable disorders. Several of the cases recorded by Dr. Quin were unmistakenably of this nature—in the first the Neuralgia had actually superseded Epilepsy; and all were of some standing. *Arsenicum*, in high dilutions (30-39), was his chief remedy, though it was sometimes powerfully reinforced by *Belladonna*. The cases are too long to cite, but their attentive perusal will well repay you. The other medicines deserving of consideration in this frightful malady are **Sulphur, Phosphorus,** and **Thuja.** Although none of Dr. Copper's recorded cases of cure by the first-named drug ‡ can be referred to this category, yet some of them were severe and obstinate enough to suggest its further trial; and in a case I have myself treated it has so far effected a cure that the

---

* A case resembling Tic Douloureaux, in which this drug in the 3x dilution was of great service, may be found in the J. B. H. S., Vol. vii., p. 420.

† See Ibid., p. 87, and Vol. i., p. 374.

‡ "Sulphur as a remedy for Neuralgia and Intermittent Fever," by Robert T. Copper M. D., 1869.

patient suffers very little as long as she continues to take it. The mother-tincture (tinctura fortissima of the Pharmacopæia) is the form in which its victories have been achieved. Very similar remarks may be made about *Phosphorus.* None of the cases continued in Mr. Ashburton Thompson's Book, or of those cited from the medical literature of both schools in the Article upon the Subject which commences the Thirty-Second Volume of the BRITISH JOURNAL OF HOMŒOPATHY, were of true TIC DOU-LOUREUX, but many were of very violent and chronic character. The relation of *Phosphorus* to nerve degeneration would make it specially applicable to this form of Neuralgia. It has hitherto done most in tolerably substantial doses; but Dr. Jousset speaks of having had success with it in a case of the kind in the medium attenuations. This writer mentions cures effected by him with two curious medicines—*Thuja* and *Coccinella** in alternation, giving the third dilution of each. This was an old medication of his master Tessier's—how arrived at I know not. Some trials by Dr. Escallier and himself have indicated the *Thuja* as the really potent agent in this combination. Dr. Cooper was the only English physician, who seems to have employed it—and this rather in "Face-ache" (Alveolar Periostitis) than Prosopalgia. His experience was gained, though not published, in 1868-9. In 1881, Dr. Burnett was led, as I have related, to his views about "Vaccinosis," and to the practice of treating such blood-infection with *Thuja*. In 1882, a case of this kind (as he considers) came before him with, as its chief symptom, a severe Post-orbital Neuralgia (so diagnosed by all the oculists consulted); and it was cured by *Thuja* 30. Other cases (see pp. 64 and 88 of his book on "Vaccinosis") were similarly characterized and cured. In his Book on Neuralgia he reproduces these three cases, and adds two more,—the pain in all instances being seated mainly in or about the eyes. Whatever we may think of Dr. Burnett's theory, the action of his remedy seems indubitable; and, with Tessier and Jousset also warranting it, we may give it in suitable cases with much hope of success.

2. Sub-occipital Neuralgia has no special Therapeutics of its own; Intercostal Neuralgia will be discussed under the head of Pleurodynia; and the various Visceral Neuralgiæ will come before us in connection with the organs they affect. I have, therefore, here only to speak of the malady as it is seen in the limbs.

Neuralgia affecting the arms—"Brachialgia," as it may be called—is not, I think a very common affection. You will bear in mind Mr. James Salter's observations, cited by Anstie, † of its frequent dependence on carious teeth; and will not neglect TOLLERE CAUSAM in such cases. Where it cannot be traced to

---

* Not *"Coccus cacti"* (See B. J. H., xxxvi., 184).

† "On Neuralgia and its Counterfeits," 1871—See a good illustration of such causation in M. H. R., xxxviii., 610.

such origin you will find some indications in Jousset (who seems to have seen the affection often) for *Bryonia, Rhus, Mercurius, Nux vomica, Pulsatilla,* and *Sulphur.* All he says from direct experience, however, is that he has cured a patient, who suffered cruelly at night and when at rest, with the third dilution of *Veratrum album.* My own successes here have been gained with *Aconite*-root and *Kalmia.*

Neuralgia of the lower extremities may attack the crural nerve, but this is a rare occurrence. Pain along the course of this nerve is generally, I think, sympathetic of ovarian irritation and finds its remedy in *Xanthoxylum* or *Colocynth.* The seat of pain in Neuralgia affecting the leg is nearly always the great sciatic :

We have to deal with

SCIATICA.—There are two principal forms under which this malady is encountered—the purely Nervous, seated in the nerve itself or its origin; and the Thecal, where the sheath is the part affected.

(*a*) Pure Sciatica, like Prosopalgia, differs in character according to the age of the patient, as Anstie has well-shown. In young persons of nervous temperament, **Chamomilla** will often suffice for the cure. The pain is worse at night, and the sufferer complains of it as intolerable: it is of a drawing or tearing character, and accompanied by a paralytic or numb sensation. Sometimes **Ignatia** is preferable, as in a case recorded by Dr. H. Nankivell in the Fifteenth Volume of the MONTHLY HOMŒOPATHIC REVIEW (p. 30). Great restlessness, so that the patient must walk about to relieve the pain, is the chief indication for it. In persons more advanced in life and subjected to fatigue, exposure, or constant sedentariness (whence pressure on the nerve), we have a more severe form of the malady (though it must be said that Dr. Nankivell's patient was fifty years old, and of sedentary habits). Here, in recent cases, **Colocynth** has always justified in my hands the high repute it has in Sciatica. Dr. Jousset says it is especially useful when the pain is cramplike, and there is a sense of constriction round the haunch.* But when the affection is of longer-standing I have been disappointed with this medicine, and have fallen back with success on **Arsenicum,** which Bahr and Jousset concur with me in commending. Case xxviii. in my series is a capital instance of its virtue. Here Sciatica of eleven months standing yielded, after the failure of *Colocynth,* to one day's administration of *Arsenicum* 30. I may mention that this man died two years later of cardiac disease, but had no return of the Neuralgia. In

---

* A typical case of the Sciatica calling for this drug is reported by Dr. Hobart in the MEDICAL ERA of January, 1893. The pain had commenced in the stomach and left ovary, then shifting to the left leg, where it had continued at intervals for a year. It was drawing, crampy and throbbing. *Colocynth* 3x cured in four days.

chronic and obstinate cases you may think of *Lycopodium,* as recommended by Bahr, or of *Plumbum,* with which, writes Dr. Jousset, "I have succeeded in an utterly rebellious case. I employed the 12th and 30th dilutions." *Sulphur** and *Phosphorus,* also as mentioned under Prosopalgia, must not be lost slight of.

(*b*) THECAL SCIATICA (shown to be such by the tenderness to pressure which is present) is sometimes Syphilitic, and then yields to the usual treatment for the diathesis. A case cured by *Mercurius corrosivus*, 2, is reported by Dr. Crawford. † Far more frequently, however, it is Rheumatic. When the affection is recent it yields readily to **Aconite**, which I have always given here in the 1st decimal dilution, or, better still, the 1st centesimal of the tincture of the root. In more chronic cases **Rhus** will rarely fail to relieve, as my thirtieth case shows: of this remedy I prefer the medium and higher dilutions. Sometimes, as in Rheumatism occurring elsewhere, **Bryonia** may replace it. Dr. Jousset speaks of having obtained "very fine results from it in the second and first triturations, even in chronic cases, and where atrophy of the limb was present." He does not say if the characteristic increase of pain by movement was observed. An acute case of the kind, where this symptom was present, is reported by Dr. Fisher in the MEDICAL CENTURY of January 1894. Here a single dose of the 3, relieved so completely that no more had to be taken.

Besides the above-mentioned remedies for for Sciatica, I would say a few words upon *Arnica, Gnaphalium* and *Iris.*

A patient suffering from this malady swallowed a wineglassful of tincture of **Arnica.** His pains increased considerably, and he had a bruised sensation in the joints; but after six hours this subsided, and with it went all trace of the Sciatica. This case led Dr. Lambreghts to try the drug in obstinate cases of the disease. He mentions five as having yielded to it, after resisting *Rhus, Colocynth,* &c. Four to six drops of the tincture were given daily for several days. It was especially useful when compression of the nerve seemed to be the exciting cause; and to cases having such origin or aggravation I should confine its use. ‡

The power of **Gnaphalium** both to cause and to cure sciatic pain has been noted in my "Pharmacodynamics" and its repute has been growing since, especially in the hands of those who have not feared to give substantial doses. §

Iris so far differs from *Gnaphalium* that it is only in diluted form that it has proved pathogenetic here, and that no application

---

* See J. B. H. S., iii., 456.
† IBID. ii., 228.
‡ JOURNAL BELGE D' HOMŒOPATHIE, May—June, 1893. p. 217.
§ See M. H. R, xxxxii., 491,

has been made of the fact in practice. It must not be forgotten, however, as a possible Anti-sciatic medicine.

For further suggestion in troublesome cases of Sciatica, I would refer you to an excellent Paper upon it by Mr. Wilkinson in Vol. xxxviii. of the MONTHLY HOMŒOPATHIC REVIEW.

From Neuralgia I pass on to another local nervous affection which I will follow most recent writers in calling, not by its Greek name HEMICRANIA, nor by the French derivative MIGRAINE, but by the old-fashioned English corruption of the latter—

MEGRIM,—It is under this name that Dr. Robert Liveing and Dr. P. W. Latham have described it—the latter in Quain's Dictionary, the former in a Monograph taking high rank in medical literature. † Megrim is known as "Sick-headache,' from two of its most constant and distressing features. Some persons, for similar reason, describe it as "Blind Headache." It may occur, however, without either sickness, headache, or disturbance of vision. Dr. Liveing, studying the malady MORE HANNEMANNIANO, has been able to construct a complete picture of its phenomena, seen in full only in the most typical cases, but so occurring by one, two, or three as to leave no doubt of their coherence one with another and with the essential disease. "The forms of Megrim," he sums up, "range from the simplest, Hemi-cranial pain, transient half-vision, or sick-giddiness, to cases which present a complex assemblage of phenomena and wide range of sensorial disturbance." In a well-developed example, the attack is ushered in by a peculiar disturbance of vision, and culminates in Headache and vomiting; but during the culminating process there may occur numbness and tingling on one on other side of the body, and disorder of speech or thought; and at any time throughout the attack there may be Vertigo, hyperæsthesia and hallucinations of the other special senses, and emotional disturbance, especially "a vague and unaccountable sense of fear." The face in generally pale and sunken; the heart is slow and the pulse contracted. Dr. Liveing regards Megrim as a true and independent Neurosis, like Epilepsy, Asthma and Angina Pectoris; shows that like these it is hereditary, paroxysmal, approximately periodical, violent in direct proportion to the length of the interval since the last attack, and

---

* "On Megrim, Sick-headache, and some allied Disorders," 1873.

interchangeable with other forms of nervous disorder. The whole paroxysm is a nerve-storm.

I have given these details (others may be found in Dr. Latham's Article, and in the literature of the subject summarised in the First Volume of the LONDON MEDICAL RECORD) that we may look for medicines truly similar to its essential features. Before doing so, however, let us see what our older writers have to say on the subject. Clotar Muller and Trinks have discussed* at some length on the disease (whose distinctive Pathological character they fully recognise) and its remedies : and Bahr's Article may be consulted with advantage.

HEMICRANIA (these all say) is a disease which requires to be closely individualised. When you have selected what seems the SIMILLIMUM, administer it in frequent doses during the paroxysm, in rare ones through the interval, and give it a thorough trial before you change it. In chronic cases three months should be the shortest time of testing. Do not give one medicine in the intervals, and another during the paroxysms; and especially, as long as you have any hope of curing your patient, do not resort to palliatives like, Coffee, Guarana, and Chloral. It is significant that the old-school treatment of the malady resolves itself into the use of these; on the CURATIVE measures to be adopted between the attacks, its writers are vague and brief.

The medicines between which your choice will commonly lie are (they say) these :—*Belladonna, Calcarea, Ignatia, Nux vomica, Sepia* and *Stannum.*

Belladonna is generally the best medicine we can prescribe if the Headache is of recent origin, and occurs in young, slender subjects of nervo-sanguine temperament and otherwise fairly healthy. Vaso-motor complications confirm its choice; and the tendency of Migraine to pass over into genuine Neuralgia (as shown by Dr. Anstie) still further substantiates it. I agree with Dr. Muller that the medium dilution (3-6) are preferable to the lowest for this purpose.

Calcarea vies with *Sepia* as the radical remedy for chronic and obstinate cases. In lymphatic subjects especially of Scrofulous diathesis, and where (in males) there is an unhealthy state of the reproductive organs it is indicated. The symptoms of the paroxysm which call for it are coldness of the head, and much acid in the eructations and vomiting. The *acetate* seems the best form of administration.

Ignatia is commended here also, as in ordinary nervous Headache, when the pain has the form of "Clavus." It is indicated (as there) in nervous, Hysterical patients, and when depressing mental emotions will at any time bring on the attacks. The face is pale during the paroxysm (unlike that of **Belladonna** and **Nux vomica**):

---

* B. J. H., xxi., I, 276.

clonic spasms are frequent concomitants, and diuresis often constitutes the crisis.*

Nux vomica cannot fail to do something for Migraine when the well-known constitution, temperament and conditions characteristic of this medicine are present, and when errors in diet readily excite the attacks. But neither it nor *Ignatia* is allowed place in the first rank of its remedies by our writers.

Sepia has the largest and most unanimous testimony in its favour as a radical remedy for this disease. Its finds its sphere in chronic cases, occurring chiefly in women of disordered sexual function with much Leucorrhœa, and subject to hepatic disturbance and abdominal congestion. A florid countenance, inclined to be yellow, indicate it; also the so-called "Sudor Hystericus" in the soles or axillæ.

Silicea is only mentioned by Bahr, but his indications are precise. They are—"rush of blood to the head, great sensitiveness of the scalp, falling off of the hair, much perspiration on the hairy scalp." To these I would add—pain ascending from the nape into the head.

Stannum is unnoticed by any of the three writers I am quoting, but it is a favourite medicine of mine. The CRESCENDO DECRESCENDO character of its pains first directed my attention to it in Migraine, where this feature is often very marked. Its action is not so profound as that of *Calcarea* and *Sepia;* but after these I am inclined to claim the highest place for it.

Returning now to the picture of Megrim as drawn for us by Dr. Lieving, let us take the disturbance of vision as our starting-point in the search for remedies. The affection is a blind spot, most frequently central, but sometimes assuming the form of Hemiopia, and then almost always lateral, very rarely superior or inferior. The blur is dark against a bright ground like the sky, but luminous on closing the eyes; and is generally surrounded with zigzag coruscations, often compared (in shape) to the bastion-work of a fortress. It spreads peripherally or laterally, according as it is central or hemiopic; and the vision clears at the primary spot as the obscuration widens. Its course is a brief one, and then comes the Headache. It seems to be bilateral in all cases (though beginning, Dr. Latham says, on the side opposite to that on which the pain subsequently developes) : and is unconnected with any change (appreciable by the Ophthalmoscope) in the retina.

In hunting for remedies on the scent, we are first of all led to *Ignatia* and *Nux vomica* again. Hahnemann observed sixteen hours after taking a dose of the former, circle of brilliant

---

* See a good paper on "The Ignatia Headache" by Dr. Shuldham, in the Fifteenth Volume of the MONTHLY HOMŒOPATHIC REVIEW. His sketch of the subject in his treatise on Headaches is less detailed.

white glittering zigzags beyond the visual point when looking at anything whereby the letters on which the sight is directed become invisible, but those at the side are more distinct"; and again he notes, after thirty hours, "a zigzag and serpentine white glittering at the side of the visual point, soon after dinner." In a note, he directs attention to these symptoms as "very much resembling Herz's so called Spurious Vertigo". I cannot trace the allusion, but should think it most probable that Herz was describing the visual phenomena of Migraine, of which giddiness is often a potent element. Looking then to the other features of drug and disease, we find that the Headaches caused by *Ignatia* were frequent and severe, though only once associated with inclination to vomit; that difficulty of thinking and speaking was noted by two of Jog's provers of it; and that hyperæsthesia of the special senses and emotional disturbance are very characteristic of it. *Ignatia*, therefore, would be well-indicated for Migraine beginning with central blur and coruscations, and going on to severe pain with such concomitants as those mentioned.

Nux vomica also has produced the visual phenomena which Hahnemann compares to the Vertigo Spuria of Herz;* so that it would seem as if the *Strychnine* common to the two were their real exciting cause. In the Pathogenesis of the Alkaloid, however, though herocially enough obtained, this symptom has not appeared; and our wisdom will be, for the present at least, to use the matrix drugs. We thus, moreover, get two remedies instead of one, for *Nux* and *Ignatia*, as you know, have many points of distinction. The patient whom the former suits is one of different temperament and habits (often also of sex) from those which call for the latter; and (remembering how it is indicated for brain-workers) it is note-worthy how many men of high intellectual power — Woolaston, Herschel, Airy, Lebert, Du Bois Reymond—have furnished narratives of their personal experience with Megrim to Dr. Lieving's Book. The *Nux vomica* Migraine would, from its Pathogenesis, have more Vertigo in it than that of *Ignatia*, as much hyperæsthesia, but less strictly emotional excitement,—if anything of this sort were disturbed, it would be what we call the "temper". Errors in dier might well be its exciting cause; but I do not think that any stress must be laid on vomiting in the course of it, as only once has the Headache of *Nux* had this concomitant, and then it came on after dinner, and was sour,—very different from the way it occurs in Migraine.

When first the visual symptoms of Megrim were definitely described in our day, they recalled to several results obtained by Purkinje with **Digitalis**. Experimenting on himself on two occasions with the extract and infusion, he both times noticed

---

* 'Materia Medica Pura', Transl. by Dudgeon, § 145

much flickering before the eyes, and makes this comment on some of his experiences:—"The figures formed by the flickerings have been described as FLIMMEROSEN, because the outline of the rose is their type. In place of the round spots in the middle of the field of vision observed in the first experiment there now occurred a space bounded by four deep oval circular lines, forming four large round identations, and the waves of light and shade surrounding it show the same indented form but less pronounced. These figures, which first appeared on the second day, were formed when they reached their height on the third by curved (but flater) lines having five indentations, and were surrounded by waves of light and shade exhibiting a similarly five-fold but not deep indentation". Now one may agree with Dr. Lieving that the resemblance between these "roses" and the "fortification pattern" of Megrim is not striking; yet it is near enough to call attention to the drug, and on looking further we find in its visual and other symptoms a close parallel with the disease. In a patient of Baker's taking it, muscæ volitantes were seen before the eyes on looking at distant objects, which, when the eyes were covered, became luminous. Brunton, when proving *Digitaline*, saw a large bright spot advancing before him; and Bahr, under the same circumstances, had the upper half of his field of vision covered with a dark cloud. In him, moreover, a parietal Headache set in the morning, became worse in the afternoon, and "increased in the evening to a violent Migraine". This was indeed not an unprecedented occurrence with him, but it was different from his ordinary attack, in that then it was always at its worst in the morning on rising. Headache, moreover, often sever, is a frequent effect of both *Digitalis* and its Alkaloid. Vertigo is not less marked from it, and its vomiting is of cerebral origin, slow of coming on, but when excited, violent and long-lasting. Remember also the slow pulse of Migraine, and the pale face and contracted arteries—the last being often so prominent a feature as to lead Du Bois Reymond and Latham to suppose the disorder a Vaso-motor Neurosis; and you have in forms of it frequently appearing a complete picture of the effects of *Digitalis*. Dr. Marc Jousset has made a beginning of the suggestion herein conveyed:* I hope that other experience may confirm his good results.

Again, of the Austrian provers of **Cyclamen** seven had more or less obscuration of sight, and four had flickering before the eyes. One of these, whose eyes were weak and required glasses had this symptom after two doses of the drug for six days in the right eye, for three weeks—though less severely in the left. It began, too, with violent Headache, which lasted unchanged for two days, diminished on the third and disappeared on

* L. Art MEDICAL, lx., 126.

the fourth. At one time he speaks of seeing a "luminous ball" before the eyes; at another, "with the eyes opened or closed, he seemed to see at a distance of about two feet a disk as large as a two-groschen piece, which seemed frequently to be pierced by brilliant lightnings". Vertigo and mental confusion appeared in the provers, and have been verified by a good cure. In this case they occurred in a women at the Climacteric; and Dr. Eidherr had long before given us several cases in which the head and eye symptoms of the drug had co-existed with Catamenial derangement such as it causes, and which had yielded to it. *Cyclamen,* therefore, should be useful in Migraine occurring in such subjects and under such circumstances; especially where its character was such as to lead to its being called "Blind Headache"

Of **Iris**, I have nothing to add to what I have written on it in my 'Pharmacodynamics'; but as it was the "blur before the eyes" preceding a Sick Headache which first led to its employment in true Migraine, it could not be omitted here.

I will also refer you to what I have written in the work just mentioned regarding **Sanguinaria,** * **Theridion** and **Zincum sulphuricum;** and will end with two quotations from the JOURNAL OF THE BRITISH HOMŒOPATHIC SOCIETY :—

1. "Translating a Paper of Dr. Jousset's on the treatment of Migraine, Dr. Pritchard adds some bits of experience from Dr. Puhlmann and himself. The former, for the radical cure, has most reliance on *Sepia* and *Calcarea carbonica* in alternate weeks. Dr. Pritchard has had personal experience of the Ophthalmic variety, where 'fortifiration-patterns' and zigzag flashes are seen before the affected eye. It was brought on in his case by the over-use of Tobacco and want of rest. After trying several remedies unsuccessfully he took *Nux vomica* 1, which relieved him in two minutes".

2. "Dr. H. Moser has a Paper on the treatment of this malady in the HOMŒOPATHISCHE MONATSBLATTER. No. 2 of 1893. His experience is that one can never hope to cure a case without getting the patient to give up Coffee entirely; that *Sanguinaria* and *Iris* are the leading remedies; and that **Niccolum,** when indicated 'will surprise'. Its pain is most severe in the forenoon, from 10 to 11, and may be so intense then that the patient cries out in anguish. It appears first on the left side, then possibly jumps over to the right. In the evening it disappears".

To sum up :—Megrim is a Neurosis like Epilepsy, having its periods of incubation and its paroxysms. The latter should be treated with drugs corresponding to their features,—of which we have studied *Belladonna, Ignatia, Nux vomica,*

---

* See also M. H. R., xl., 750.

Digitatlis, Cyclamen, Niccolum, Iris and *Sanguinaria.* Sometimes one or other of these will control the morbid tendency; but more frequently we have to deal with by means of deeper-acting medicines such as *Calcarea, Sepia, Silicea, Stannum,* and *Zincum*— medicines which deal with the general disorder of which the paroxysms are but an expression. By the use of both these classes of remedies in their respective place we are best likely to control the disease now under consideration.

Under the head of—
LOCAL SPASMS I propose to speak of several forms of involuntary muscular contractions. Tonic or Clonic, which, although localised, will not come under notice among the disorders of particular organs.

1. The more common of these are well-known CRAMPS OF THE CALVES. Seen at their highest intensity in Cholera they are symptomatic of the forms of instestinal irritation, or may result merely from fatigue. In the latter case *Arnica* will check them, in the former *Nux vomica;* but a more potent remedy than either is *Cuprum* which is so valuable for the Choleraic Cramps. Jousset says that he always succeeds in such cases with the 12th dilution; but suggests the wearing of plates of the metal on the legs when the affecttion is obstinate. Dr. Hirsch makes a similar recommendation of *Ferrum,* binding an Iron key to the soles or introducing it beneath the bed-covers.

2. A more general and continued form of CRAMP of the EXTREMITIES has been described by Trousseau and others under the name of "TETANY." The kind of contractions here present and the numbness, tingling and formication with which they begin, forcibly remind us of the pathogenetic effects of two medicines, **Aconite** and **Secale.** The facts which lead Trousseau to 'consider the affection of a Rheumatic nature, the occasional presence of febrile symptoms, and the benefit observed from blood-letting, all point to *Aconite* as the most important remedy. That Tetany occurs so frequently among nursing or pregnant women confirms the indication for *Secale,* and would lead us to choose it for such patients when no decided *Aconite* symptoms were present. The similarity of the symptoms of Tetany and of

Ergotism has been pointed out by Dr. Maxon; and Bauer actually applies the name to the phenomena induced by eating the spurred rye.* It is quite in accordance with these facts that Dr. Jousset recommended **Solanum nigrum** for the present malady.; for it has been chosen, on the ground of the similarity of its effects, as the best remedy for Ergotism; and has proved of much benefit in its treatment.

3. In the facial muscles we meet with Clonic Spasms in the complaint known as "TIC NON-DOULOUREUX," or "HISTRIONIC SPASM OF THE FACE." In young persons it is a kind of local Chorea, and **Hyoscyamus** is useful in its treatment. In adults it is a very intractable disorder, being probably deeper-seated : "its treatment," writes Erb, "is one of the most thankless problems of medical practice." I have only seen one case of it, in a woman close upon sixty : the affection had been increasing upon her for four years. There was a history of much painful emotional depression, and of violent Headache on the right side of the head, the facial spasm being on the left. She had a tendency to stagger on walking. Some of the concomitant symptoms led me to give **Argentum nitricum;** and under this medicine in the third and third decimal dilutions, the spasms had entirely left her after about five months' treatment, and she was much stronger and firmer on the legs.

4. "TRISMUS" is the Tonic Spasm of the masticatory muscles. Excluding its appearance as a part of Tetanus, it arises either from Rheumatic cause when **Aconite** will help; or as a sympton of Hysteria, when the indications for **Ignatia** will be plain. In two cases of traumatic origin reported by Dr. Owens, *Physostigma* sufficed for the cure. † Its action would seem of Antipathic nature. "Trismus Neonatorum" will come before us among the Diseases of Children; as also will Carpo-pedal Spasms.

5 "TORTICOLLIS," in its Clonic form, is as yet unknown to our Therapeutics. I suspect that it is nearly always of central origin, and should be disposed to try the continued use of such medicine as *Strychma, Belladonna* and *Agaricus.* Perhaps *Magnesia phosphorica* might come in usefully here. Dr. McNish relates a case of a man of 60 who nineteen years before coming under his care strained his back while digging. The effects soon passed off, and he believed himself well, when he was suddenly seized with a Cramp in the lower dorsal and upper lumber region, which twisted him round until he "faced to the rear." The Spasm, which was very painful, was repeated several times. After an interval of some weeks he had another attack, and from that time forward they had increased in frequency, until he had one or more daily. *Magnesia phosphorica* 6x was given four

---

* See Ziemssen's CYCLOPŒDIA, xi., 368.
† MEDICAL ERA, Jan. 1893, p. 8.

times daily for a month, and for eighteen months thereafter, when the report was made, they had not recurred.* The Tonic form of Torticollis may be of "Rheumatic" origin, being indeed only a more acute form of "STIFF-NECK"; it will then like that yield readily to **Aconite**.

6. "WRITTER'S CRAMP" is the last of these Local Spasms I shall specify here. It is included by Dr. Russell Reynolds with the disorders Pathologically similar to it in the following definition— "A chronic disease, characterized by the occurrence of Spasm when the attempt is made to execute a special and complicated movement; the result of previous education; such Spasm not following muscular actions of the affected part when the special movement is not required.' It may, however, be more Paralytic than Spasmodic in character, as its old name of "Scrivener's Palsy" would suggest. Certainly, the medicines which have helped it most have been Paralysers rather than Spasm-exciters. Dr. Halbert records a severe case in which, with static Electricity, **Picric acid** 4x was administered. (Electricity in all forms had been vainly tried before) Complete recovery, with great improvement in general health, occurred in three months though the patient did not relinquish the type-writing which was her occupation.† Again, an old-school physician published a case in which the affection—occurring in a pianoforte player —yielded to moderate doses of the tincture of *Gelsemium*; and this experience has been varified with yet gentler doses in our own ranks (among others by myself). It would be in cases of apparently local origin, not presenting the constitutional Asthenia of *Picric acid*, that *Gelsemium* would seem preferable. As an alternative, that close analogue of *Gelsemium*, **Conium,** may be named. Dr. Wingfield relates a case of a female clerk in an insurance office who for six months had suffered from loss of power of the right fore and middle fingers, with Stiffness, numbness, and excruciating pain. After the failure of *Gelsemium* to give more than temporary relief, *Conium* 1x 2 drops every 3 hours, was ordered. In two days the symptoms had disappeared, and three weeks later had shown no sign of return.‡ when the symptoms are traceable to over-exertion (which is by no means always the case) **Arnica** might be a useful auxiliary to the obvious prescription of rest.

---

* AMER. HOMŒOPATHIST. Oct. 15, 1897.
† HAHNEMANNIAN MONTHLY, Jan. 1899, p. 15.
‡ M. H. R., xxxix., 579.

After Local Spasms would naturally come Local Paralyses; but I find that nearly all affections of this kind will be more naturally treated of in connexion with the organs—as the eye, bladder, and rectum—which are their seat. The only exception is—

FACIAL PALSY, of whose Therapeutics a few words must be said in this place. I am speaking of course of the Peripheral form of the malady. It is so frequently of "Rheumatic" origin, and owning inflammatory swelling of the nerve-sheath as its Pathological basis, that **Aconite** should always be given in recent cases. When of longer-standing, there is a general consensus as to the value of **Causticum;*** and its administration need not exclude the Faradisation of the paralysed muscles.

---

*Dr. Cowperthwaite, contributing to the MEDICAL ERA of August, 1898, an interesting study of *Causticum* (which he regards as *Potash* preparation, says, "Some years ago I published the reports of a large number of cases of Facial Paralysis.... brought on by exposure to cold winds... cured in a very few hours with the aid of *Causticum* 30."—One would like to have the reference to this publication.

LECTURE XXIX

DISEASES OF THE EYE.

OCULAR APPENDAGES—CONJUNCTIVA.

BLEPHARITIS—HORDEOLUM—BLEPHAROSPASM—PTOSIS—
CHALAZZION—DACRYO.CYSTITIS—FISTULA LACHRYMALIS—
LACHRYMATION—CNNJUNCTIVITIS SIMPLE—PURULENT
CONJUNCTIVITIS—GONORRHOEAL OPHTHALMIA—STRUMOUS
OPHTHALMIA—PHLYCTENULAR CONJUNCTIVITIS—
CONJUNCTIVITIS MEMBRANOSA—CONJUNCTIVITIS
TRACHOMAEOSA—PTERYGIUM:

It is perhaps rather presumtuous in me, who am neither oculist nor aurist, who am not even of the surgical side of the profession from which such specialists are usually drawn, to say anything EX CATHEDRA (that is, here, from a lecturer's—not seat, but stand) on the treatment of Diseases of the Eye and Ear. I do so only because I have to speak of HOMŒOPATHY in such diseases; because by means of this method, Drug-therapeutics has penetrated so much further than it could reach before, that the work of oculist and aurist among us has become very largely Medical rather than Surgical, and the physician can feel at home in their department. As long as *Mercury* was the only medicine known, which, taken internally, could influence ocular inflammations, and then only by inducing its Physiological effects, such affections were, naturally, left to the surgeon. Now we have a score of drugs which exert such power, and after the Homœopathic manner—the whole Physiological being absorbed in their Therapeutic action. They cannot hurt, and they do heal; and while we value the aid of our experts for diagnosis and mechanical work upon the eye, we treat it mainly as we do other parts of the body when inflamed, and its maladies of this kind become the subject of the art of the ordinary practitioner of medicine.

What Homœopathy ean do in EYE-DISEASES received a severe test some twenty years ago, when the New York Ophthalmic Hospital was by its manager placed under practioners of the system. These brave men, having no special experience in Ophthalmology, but confident in the fruitfulness of the method of Hahnemann, undertook to supply the needs of the patients of the charity—hitherto cared for by the best oculist of the old school. Instead of falling off, its CLIENTELE steadily increased, and it has become a most flourishing institution, and one from whose wards skilled students have gone forth to carry Homœopathic Oculistry into all the cities of the States, The experience gained by its work, moreover, has been embodied in a Treatise on "Ophthalmic Therapeutics". The First Edition was written by Drs. T. F. Allen and George B. Norton, the original physicians to the Hospital ; the second by the latter alone ; and the third, since his lamented death, by Dr. A. B. Norton, who has embodied all that his brother had collected for the purpose of such a re-issue. Before we had this work, our literary sources of information of the subject had been very limited. We had only the series of papers on the various forms of Ophthalmia by Dr. Dudgeon, in the Sixth and Seventh Volumes of the BRITISH JOURNAL OF HOMOEOPATHY ; and the Treatise on Disease of the Eye, by Dr. Peters, founded on Ruckert's collection of cases. This last includes the non-inflammatory affections of the eye— Cataract, &c., and also the morbid states of the ocular appendages ; but its Pathology is necessarily of an imperfect character owing to the time at which most of the cases gathered by Ruckert were treated. I shall use it, and Dr. Dudgeon's materials, as freely as I can, and shall also draw upon the Volume "On Diseases of the Eye" by Dr. Angell, of Boston ; but my main source of information will continue to be the Treatise of the Nortons.

Even in the Old World, though it is hard to spare them from general medicine, we have oculists in the Homœopathic ranks ; among whom I may name our own Knox Shaw, the late Dr. Dekeersmaecker of Brussels, and Dr. Parenteau of Paris. The last-named has lately, at one of a series of Conferences Eubliques sur l' Homœopathie", treated of "Homœopathy and the diseases of the Eyes,* and has spoken in the most appreciative manner of the resources the method lends us in this sphere. He had been for twelve years attached to the Hospital Saint-Jacques, and for seven years to the Dispensaire Alix Love—a children's charity, at which during the space of time mentioned, more than 140,000 consultations are registered as having been given. Speaking from the large experience thus gained, he says —"It is my deep-seated and reasoned conviction that wsth our globules, at which people laugh, and our few grains of powder, I have obtained cures much more numerous, more rapid, and above all more durable than with the Allopathic treatment employed by me previously during the five years I served as clinical assistant under my excellent master and friend Dr. Abadie".

With this encouragement, let us proceed to consider in detail the Homœopathic treatment of Ophthalmic Disorder, beginning with the Diseases of the APPENDAGES OF THE EYE,

---

*L' ART MEDICAL, Aug,, 1893.

DISEASES OF THE EYE

First, of the LIDS.

BLEPHARITIS, when acute, requires different medicines according to its precise seat. Thus, if it affects the skin and cellular tissue outside the lid, it is of an Erysipelatous character, and demands the remedies for that disorder viz. *Belladonna, Rhus,* or *Apis,* according to the indications I hsve given when treating of Erysipelas itself. When it invades the lining mucous membrane (Conjunctivitis Palpebrarum), it yields to the remedies for Catarrhal Ophthalmia. Its distinctive form however, is that assumed when it is seated at the edges of the lids, in which case it is kdown as Tinea (better, Ophthalmia) Tarsi. I have generally found **Hepar sulphuris** very effective here, but Dr. Angell relies upon **Mercurius**. They are both truly Homœopathic.

A peculiar form of inflammation of the LIDs is

HORDEOLUM, "Stye", I must agree with Hartmann that its progress may generally be arrested by a few doses of **Pulsatilla**. Should there be a disposition to frequent recurrence of these little troubles, it seems agreed that **Staphisagria** is commonly the best remedy to obviate it. Other authors, however, speak of *Sulphur, Thuja, Grapihtes* and *Phosphorus* as useful for this purpose ; and Allen and Norton used to think nothing so good for it as *Pulsatilla* itself.

Inflammation of the Lids most frequently comes before us as a chronic process, forming, if at the edges, "Lippitudo", if inside, Granular Lids and "Pannus" or Vascular Cornea. The former I think still best treated in many instances with *Hepar sulphuris*. I have had a case in an infant of six months, in which this condition had lasted nearly since birth. It disappeared in three days under *Hepar 6*. If M*ercurius* is required, the *Red oxide* seems the most suitable form. Other remedies to be considered are *Alumina, Calcarea, Graphites, Petrolium** and *Sulphnr,* for which minute indications were given by Allen and Norton. They say that the ramedy which comes nearest to being a specific in the disease is **Graphites,** and recommended its local as well as internal administration. Dr. A. B. Norton maintains their commendation of this drug.+ Chronic Conjunctivitis Palpebrarum is generally, if not always, a sequel of an Acute "Granular Ophthalmia", or "Trachomatous Conjunctivitis" ; and I shall speak of it under this heading.

---

* See a striking case illustrating the virtue of this drug in J.B.H.S. i., 93, Lashes absent for 17 years grew again under its use. See case in X, A. J. H., Feb., 1893, P. 116,

DACRYO-CYSTITIS

Spasmodic and Paralytic affections of the eyelids, causing the phenomena known as Ectropium, Entropium and Lagophthalmos must be carefully traced to their causes if we desire to treat them successfully. They will then come under other headings of this part of our subject. I will only speak here of BLEPHRROSPASM and PTOSIS.

BLEPHAROSPASM may be Tonic or Clonic. In the former case it is secondary to some irritation of the ocular surface, as in Strumous Ophthalmia : in the latter it may be (apparently at least) primary, and comes before us as "Nictitation". There is general agreement as to the value of **Agaricus** here , and Dr. A. B. Norton srys that it should be given in four drop doses of the tincture before being abandoned. *Codeia* has caused such twitchings, and should do something towards curing them : the same may be said of *Physostigma*. Jahr recommends *Hyoscyamus* and *Ratanhia* has proved remedial * When the Clonic Spasm only amounts to a Quivering, such as people describes as 'live-blood," it will generally yield to *Pulsatilla*, or, in very nervous subjects, to *Ignatia*.

PTOSIS, when distinctly traceble to cold, will yield to *Causticum* if this was dry, to *Rhus* or *Dulcamara* if it was damp. In the absence of such exciting cause, *Gelsemium* or *Conium* should be curative.

Of TUMOURS OF THE LIDS I have only to speak of—

CHALAZION, MEIBOMIAN CYST. This has disappeared more than once under *Calcarea carbonica*.† In Tarsal Tumours projecting like a Condyloma, *Thuja* is much commended.

I will now say a word or two about the diseases of the LACHRYMAL APPARATUS. Some of these of course require mechanical treatment : I shall only speak of what may be done by internal remedies.

DACRYO-CYSTITIS, inflmmation of lachrymal sac, was once rapidily cured, in Dr. Dodgeon's hands by **Silicea 6**, after getting worse under other remedies.†† I have myself had a very

---

* J.B.H.S., v., 102. † See ANNALS, i., 272. †† B.J. H., xiii., 135.

similar case. Dr. Norton would assign this medicine to phlegmonous case, or when suppuration threatens to supervene in the catarrhal form : in simple cases of latter kind he depends upon **Pulsatilla.**

So far I have been speaking of Acute Dacryo-Cystitis. In its chronic form or stage it comes before us as Epiphora, with distension of the lachrymal sac or at least hyperæmia of the passages. Dr. Tessier has related a series of such cases in which cure resulted from the use of *Graphites*, *Calcarea* and *Silicea*; or, where the os unguis or the periosteum seemed involved, *Mercurius* and *Hepar*. The 12th dilution was mainly used.* Dr. Kafka has put on record a case of incessant lachrymation of the right eye, caused by exposure to a strong North wind. *Natrum muriatium* 6 cured in four weeks ; and was equally efficacious when, on later occasions, the trouble returned.†

FISTULA LACHRYMALIS is reported to have been cured by *Natrum muriaticum* and *Stlicea* ;†† in other cases by *Calcarea, Fluoric acid,* and *Causticum.* Some of the cases so named were simply such obstruction of the nasal duct, with Stillicidium Lachrymarum, as I have just mentioned. However, the rationale of treatment is one and the same. Restore the mucous membrane of the duct to its norm by medicines, and the tears will flow through their natural channel, and the Fistulous opening (if any) will close. Dr. Junge has reported** two good cases, in which this was evidently accomplished by *Petroleum 3,* and Dr. Roche relates another cured by *Mercurius corrosivus* and *Sulphnr* ; ‖ while of the latter remedy Jahr writes,—"I have not yet treated a single case where *Sulphur* did not render cure." One would hardly have supposed, however, that "many cases" of this affection would have came under the care of a general practitioner, even during "forty years' practice."

LACHRYMATION, when not due to such obstructions as I have mentioned, or to displacements of the puncta, may often (Drs. Cladue and Parenteau write ††) be remedied by **Guarœa.**

With these few hints upon the treatment of the Diseases of the Ocular Appendages, I pass to the consideration of the affections of the CONJUNCTIVA—the OPHTHALMIAE proper.

---

* REV, HOM. FRANCAISE., Oct., 1895. † J.B.H.S. ii., 222.
†† B.J.H., xxvii., 567 ; AMER. HOM. REV., v., 390
** J.B.H.S., v., 204. ‖ M.H.R. xiv., 500. †† J.B.H.S., i., 177.

CONJUNCTIVITIS SIMPLEX

CONJUNCTIVITIS SIMPLEX, Catarrhal Ophthalmia the common "Cold in the Eye," yields readily (when Actue) to Homœopathic treatment, without the need of any local application. The following are Dr. Dudgeon's detailed instruction as to the choice of its remedies :—

"When the affection is recent, and symptoms are, dry itching or smarting sensation in the eyes and lids ; feeling as if something had got into the eye ; frequent winking, and occasional discharge of tears, the conjunctiva being partially or uniformly injected ; little or no mucus secreted ; the conjunctiva of the lids being comparatively redder than that of the ball ; a dose or two of *Sulphur,* in almost any dilution, usually suffices to effect a rapid cure. When, in the commencement of the disease, there is great dry burning feeling, with frontal Headache, and symptoms of Congestion of the Head, *Belladonna,* preceded or not by *Aconite,* will often be found of use. If the flow of tears is considerable, and even of an acrid character, with corresponding watery discharge from the nose, sneezing and other indications of Coryza, *Euphrasia* is the remedy indicated. Where, along with copious flow of tears there is much smarting and burning pain, the tears being particularly acrid and corrosive, or if there is Chemosis or œdematous condition of the lids, *Arsenicum* will be found useful. If at the outset of the disease there is considerable mucous discharge, *Chamomila* should be borne in mind. Where the mucous secretion is excessive, the injection considerable, and the caruncula particularly inflamed and enlarged, *Argentum nitricum* will, I imagine, prove specific. When the Meibomian glands seem much affected, and the edges of the lids red and swollen the secretion forming during sleep, yellow crusts on the ciliæ, *Mercurius solubilis* or *Hepar sulphuris* will be given with advantage. When the evening exacerbations, which are usually present, are very well-marked, *Pulsatilla* will be found useful."

I give these directions in case of need, and because the characteristics of the remedies in Ophthalmia generally are so clearly given. But I doubt much if Dr. Dudgeon has ever had occasion to use more than three or four of these medicines in Simple Conjunctivitis. For myself, I have always got on with **Euphrasia** or **Belladonna** ; though I think that. if the patient be of unhealthy constitution, a dose of *Sulphur* should initiate and may conclude the treatment. *Euphrasia* is preferable where there is much lachrymation, *Belladonna* where the ocular surface is dry.

I may add that Bahr thinks *Aconite,* if given early, capable of curing nearly every case single-handed. I would certainly begin with it if the inflammation was acute ; and the same may be said of similar conditions occuring in any of the coats of the eye. He gives indications, besides the remedies already mentioned, for *Euphorbium* and *Rhus*; and says, that "when locally applied, *Euphrasia* often has a very excellent effect, even after its internal administration had proved absolutely useless." Jahr appears to use *Arsenicum* and *Euphrasia* most frequently; but agrees in beginning the treatment of nearly every ocular inflammation with *Aconite*. Jousset thinks with me as to *Euphrasia* being the principal remedy for Catarrhal Ophthalmia; but his colleague Dr. Cartier would have us substitute *Duboisine*.* When there is much Chemosis, Dr. Claude commends **Guarœa**.

It is in the Chronic form that we are most frequently called upon to treat this affection. The common practice is to do so by applying local irritants, the *Nitrate of Silver* and the *Sulphates of Zinc* and *Copper*. This is true Homœopathy, though of the crudest sort. Dr. Liebold has well shown that these substances are no mere "astringents," but such as, when applied to a healthy conjunctiva, inflame it ;† and I am far from denying that their application may sometimes be the best plan to follow. But I would urge upon you to try internal remedies throughly, before you resort to this less desirable mode of proceeding. The *Argentum nitricum* itself is one of these. The specific irritant influence of this medicine on the conjunctiva was strikingly displayed in Dr. Muller's beautiful proving; and it is recommennded by Dr. Norton when the conjunctiva is scarlet red and the papilæ hypertrophied. *Mercurius corrosivus* and *Kali bichromicum*, also, are here as in most chronic mucous inflammations of curative power; but **Arsenicum**, in this instance surpasses either. In Simple Chronic Conjunctivitis, I would advise you to try no other treatment until you have given this great medicine a full opportunity of doing good.

I may also mention *Sulphur* as a valuable ally in unhealthy subjects, and cite what Bahr says of *Staphisagria*: with this remedy we have cured several cases of very obstinate Chronic Catarrah, with considerable Swelling of the Lids, after others had entirely failed.

Leaving now the Simple Conjunctivitis, we have come to its Purulent form, of which we have three varieties—OPHTHALMIA NEONATORUM, EGYPTIAN OPHTHALMIA or SIMPLE PURULENT CONJUNCTIVITIS and GONORRHOEAL OPHTHALMIA. Of the first I shall speak among the Diseases of Children; the two latter will come before us here.

---

* See REV. HOM. FRANCAISE, Jan. 1901, p. 8.
† See Transactions of Amer, Inst. of Hom, for 1867.

PURULENT CONJUNCTIVITIS.—Of these diseases I can speak only from the experience of others. Dr. Peters states. that he and a colleague "treated over forty cases of Purulent Ophthalmia in children, at the Home of the Friendless, without the loss of a single eye, although three or four cases proved exceedingly intractable." Mild local applications were employed; but I suppose that the unusual success must be ascribed to the internal medication, which consisted, in most cases, of **Hepar sulphuris** night and morning, and **Rhus** every two to eight hours, according to the severity of the symptoms, Both were given in the attenuations from the first to the the third. Drs. Allen and Norton, while allowing the occasional value of these medicines, described **Argentum nitricum** as "the remedy, PAR EXCELLENCE, for all forms of Purulent Ophthalmia. "We have witnessed", they say, "the most intense Chemosis with strangulated vessels, most profuse purulent discharge, and commencing hazines of the cornea with a tendency to slough, subside rapidly under this remedy, internelly administered. "We have yet," they add, "to see the first case go on to destruction of the cornea." They gave the thirtieth potency; and, while believing that there is no need of cauterisation, allowed that weak lotion of the drug, applied externally, aided in the cure. It is due to Dr. Dudgeon to say, that he was the first (in the papers I have mentioned) to point out the specific action of *Nitrate of Silver* upon the conjunctiva, and to recommend its internal administration where hitherto it had been known only as a *Caustic*. Dr. A. B. Norton vouches for his predecessors' experience, though he says nothing of their dosage; and Mr. E. Lucas Hughes, our oculist, at the Hahnemann Hospital, Liverpool, bears a later testimony to the drug in the 6th or 3rd potency.*

Should you need additional help, I may mention that Dr. Jousset treats all his cases of Purulent Ophthalmia by instilling into the eye, every two hours, a solution of twenty drops of the first attenuation of *Mercurius corrosivus* in a hundred grammes (about two ounces) of water. Dr. Dakeersmaecker states that he had adopted this mode of treatment in every case, and with very encouraging success.

GONORRHŒAL OPHTHALMIA.—I think it very important to distinguish between two forms of this disease. In the one it is a constitutional effect of the virus, analogous to Gonorrhœal Rheumatism, with which it is frequently associated: both eyes are here affected simultaneously. In the other, it is the result

---

* J. B. H. S., ix., 132.

of acidental contact with the diseharge ; and attacks, at least at the outset, one eye only.

The former variety will, there is good reason to believe, yield to internal treatment alone. "In all such cases," writes Jahr, "I first give *Aconite*, with a view of moderating the inflammation, after which, if the discharge still continues *Nitric aicd* completes the cure, or perhaps *Pulsatilla*, if the discharge had suddenly stopped". As the iris is the part chiefly affected here, I should prefer **Clematis**. But the other kind of Gonorrhœal Ophthalmia is so strictly local a disease, that if every topical treatment is to be relied upon, it is here. You may begin with what Bahr recommends, viz., **Mercurius corrosivus** internally and externally ; and, if all goes well, **Hepar sulphuris**, in the same manner, to complete the cure. But so rapidly does the mischief spread, that unless after twenty-four hours of treatment it is declining rather than advancing, I would advice you no longer to delay the local and pretty strong application of *Nitrate of Silver*, giving it internally at the same time. In so acting, you may comfort yourself with the admission of Watson, "Mr. Guthrie," he says, "considers this to be a local disease of a peculiar charaeter ; and, acting upon the aphorism of John Hunter (an aphorism, however, which requires some qualification), that two diseases or actions cannot go on in a part at the same time, he proposes to set up in the inflamed conjunctiva a new action which shall supersede the original disease, and create another that is more manageable. In this point of view MR. GUTHRIE'S ratio medendi AGREES WITH THAT OF HAHNEMANN, about which there has been so absurd a noise made of late years"* The strength of the *Solution* according to Dr. Angell, should be from one to fifteen grains to the ounce, according to the severity of the symptoms.

I need hardly say that in all forms of Purulent Conjunctivitis the removal of the matter which collects and the prevention of its re-accumulation by frequent ablution, is attended to by Homœopathic practioners as carefully as by others.

As it is the Conjunctiva which is chiefly affected in that curious form of Ophthalmia which so often arises spontaneously in Scrofulous subjects, I shall go on next to speak of this malady.

STRUMOUS OPHTHALMIA is one of the most annoying

---

* Dr. Dudgeon, indeed, considers that, even when thus locally applied, *Argentum nitricum* acts specifically ; and that no mere irritant, with affinity for the inffamed tissue, would have the same effect.

diseases we are called upon to treat, the frequent replaces causing repeated disappointment. Nevertheless, the treatment I shall sketch out for you is sure ultimately to succeed, though whether it contrasts favourably or not with that of the prevalent school I am unable to say. It is, at any rate, pleasanter. Dr. Angell, usually so partial to local applications, finds them nearly always unnecessary in this disease ; and this looks like a comparative verdict in favour of Homœpathic treatment.

You must first take into account the constitution of your patient, and give him accordingly, besides attending to his Hygiene, a course of **Sulphur** or **Calcarea**. This I regard as indispensable in all cases, *Sulphur* is most suitable when the Ophthalmia is the only sign of Scrofulous taint, or when the latter shows itself chiefly in unhealthiness of the skin. As subjective symptoms, Drs. Allen and Norton give a sharp and pricking character of the pains in the eye, and in intolerence of the parts of water. *Calcarea* is better when the diathesis is strongly marked, especially by enlargement of the lymphatic glands : our authors add that, when it is indicated, there is a general aggravation of the symptoms during damp weather, or from the least chill, to which the patient is very susceptible. A course of one or both of these drugs, with the occasional aid of the milder remedies for inflammation and Photophobia, will sometimes be sufficient to effect a cure.

To the same effect speaks Dr. Parenteau, who takes for his first example of the superiority of Homœopathic treatment in the affections of the eye called "Strumous". It is curious to watch the "organician" tendency of present-day Pathology, though one's interest is chequered by regret at the localising of treatment which follows with it. Scrofulous Ophthalmia was once a well-recognised ocular malady, as much so as the Catarrhal and purulent forms. Then, having regard to its Anatomical seat and features, it was called "Phlyctenular", and classed among affections of the conjunctiva or (as in Lawson's Book) the cornea ; its constitutional origin being barely allowed. In Mr. Brudenell Carter's Article on Diseases of the Eye in the last Edition of Quain's Dictionary it is altogether absent. And yet it throngs our dispensaries, presents a distinct clinical form and history, and without treatment is indefinite in duration and often damaging in after-effects. Dr. Parenteau depicts it in its several varieties of Blepharitis, Conjunctivitis, and Keratitis ; sketches the treatment, either, inert or violent, to which its subjects are liable in the ordinary way ; and then contrasts its management under Homœopathy. Instead of external revulsives and internal "tonics which are irritants, I nearly always limit myself", he says, "to the alternation of two constitutional remedies (*Calcarea carbonica* or *phosphorica, Iodine, Sulphur Arsenic, Graphites,* &c.) in the form of a little pinch of trituration, or of a few globules. That is all. Yet after a few days or weeks (according to the gravity or the nature of the case) the parents are astonished to see the local symptoms disappear and therewith the general state alter for the better,—avowing that never under the Allopathic treatment had they seen so prompt a cure."

In most cases, however, the employment (I of course mean internally) of the more intensely operating local remedies will be required. I speak especially of the irritant Salts of **Mercury**,— the *Bichloride*, the *Biniodide,* and the *Nitrate*. Drs. Bocker and Kidd have satisfactorily illustrated the value of *Corrosive sublimate* in Strumous Ophthalmia ; * Dr. Angell speaks highly of the *Biniodide* ; and Drs. Gray and Liebold concur, from large experience, in praising the *Nitrate*, which they use both internally and externally. † The lower potencies of all have been those employed. The only rival of *Mercurius* here is **Hepar sulphuris**. Numerous cases illustrating the action of this medicine will be found in Dr. Peters' Treatise. It is one in which I have great confidence when numerous repeated ulcers form.

There are two somewhat exceptional medicines now to be mentioned, which often play an important part in the treatment of Strumous Ophthalmia. There are forms occcasionally assumed by this disease which have led some pathologists to set it down as an eruptive disorder, and others to class it among the Neuroses. When the former seem right, when the Ophthalmia appears but as a part of a general Eczema of the face, then **Rhus** will generally prove the best medicine, though **Graphites**, as indicated by Allen and Norton, must also be considered. When, on the other hand, the inflammation seems too fugacious to be real, and nervous element in the case is predominant, **Arsenicum** will do what no other medicine can. You will find ample illustrations of these statements in the cases furnished by Dudgeon and Peters.

In whatever way you are treating Strumous Ophthalmia, you will find it usual to employ intercurrent remedies to check inflammatory exacerbations and to relieve Photophobia. For the former purpose **Belladonna** or **Euphrasia** will serve, the one where the mucous membrane is dry, the other when there is much acrid lachrymation and discharge. For PHOTOPHOBIA **Conium** is singulary efficacious when there is little visible inflammation, as in the *Arsenicum* cases ; and Dr. Angell speaks highly of **Tartar emectic**, which would work well with *Rhus*. But where (as often happens) the dread of light is connected with the intensity of the mischief in the cornea, I think that you will best relieve it by acting on that tissue of the eye with **Apis**. Dr. Jousset, who has much confidence in this remedy in Strumous Ophthalmia, lays stress on the importance of having it prepared directly from the bee-virus, having been disappointed when using a trituration of the entire insect. He premises *Ipecacu-*

---

* B.J.H., Vols. iii. and xxii. †Angell, p. 113, Allen and Norton p. 195

PHLYCTENULAR CONJUNCTIVITIS 421

anha* when much Conjunctivitis is present, and finds *Aurum muriaticum* very useful to complete the restoration of the cornea to its integrity. *Aurum*, indeed, in one form or other plays an active part when Strumous Ophthalmia is mainly a Keratitis, There are some good illustrative cases in the Eighth Volume of the old NORTH AMERICAU JOURNAL OF HOMOEOPATHY ; and Dr. Dahlke has lately recorded a severe one in which he was led to it by noticing that whenever the patient was worse there was determination of blood to the head.†

Bahr and Jahr, whose treatment is much the same as that which I have now sketched, concur in recommending **Nirtic acid** in protracted and obstinate cases ; and Dr. H. Goullon cites evidence to the same effect. I am referring to this physician's excellent Treatise on Scrofulous Affections, which we have in an English Version. It is significant that he writes : "There is hardly a disease which, in its appearence and course, is so well-fixed and conservative as Scrofulous Ophthalmia" ; and again "It is not practical, though ophthalmologists do so, to separate Scrofulous Conjunctivitis from Keratitis. They appear too often simultaneously, and too frequently run into each other." This is a true clinical classification, as opposed to one that is merely Anatomical.

The subject of Strumous Ophthalmia was brought before our Congress of 1896 by a Paper from Dr. Bushrod James, of Philadelphia. If you will read this, and the discussions which followed it, I think you will find what I have now said to be generally agreed to in the Homœopathic ranks.

Dr. A. B. Norton though fully assenting to the predominantly constitutional treatment of Strumous Ophthalmia treats of it under the title of "Conjunctivitis Phlyctenularis." I have preferred to give prominence to the diathetic relationship of the disease ; and moreover, I am disposed to think that the local lesion designated by this name may arise entirely apart from Scrofula. I will, therefore, speak of—

PHLYCTENULAR CONJUNCTIVITIS as an independent disease. It seems so generally agreed that the local application of *Colomel* is specific here, and it is so harmless a measure, that there may be little else to be done. Dr. Lawrence Newton says that he has more than once signally failed to disperse the vesicles without it. Dr. Angell too, strongly advises the treatment. I

---

* Dr. Wanstall concurs with him in esteeming this drug highly in what he calls "Pustular Conjunctivitis" (see Norton's Appendix, SUB VOCE)

* J. B. H. S., iii., 441,

am bound to say, on the other side, that I have several times seen this affection, chiefly in girls at boarding-school, yield nicely to the internal administration of **Rhus**.

CONJUNCTIVITIS MEMBRANOSA appears in two forms —the DIPHTHERITIC and the CROUPOUS, the former presenting an interstitial infiltration, the latter having a superfical pellicle. Here, too, local measures are obviously indicated, and least objectionable of these are the Lemon juice and the *Liquor chlori* mentioned by Dr. Norton. Internally, **Apis** and perhaps **Guaroea** should control Diphtheritic Conjunctivitis when forming, **Mercurius cyanatus** later ; for the Croupous form **Kali bichromicum** is without a rival.

CONJUNCTIVITIS TRACHOMATOSA "GRANULAR OPHTHALMIA," appears to be one of the forms of the "EGYPTIAN OPHTHALMIA" observed where (as in that country) there is much hot wind and dust ; it is apt to arise where many children are thronged together, and is undoubtedly contagious. In this Acute form it is often amenable to treatment, as with *Aconite* and *Belladonna*. In the Chronic stage *Alumina, Arsenicum Aurum, Natrum muriaticum* and *Thuja* are beneficial ; but Granulations of long-standing seem almost extra-vital, and are, I fear, amenable only to local and mechanical treatment. Dr. Norton uses pressure as his chief agent. Dr. Angell gives some cases illustrating the good effect of this proceeding and the occasional application of irritants—of which latter Dr. Liebold esteemed burnt *Alum* most highly.

If "PANNUS" should remain after the Granualations of the Lid which cause it have been removed, you may disperse it, as Dr. de Couman has done by the steady use of *Aurum muriaticum* and *Hepar sulphuris* ;* or by *Kali bichromicum*. †

PTERYGIUM is the last of the affections of the conjunctiva of which I have to speak. Generally supposed to be amenable to Surgical treatment alone, Homœopathy has found internal medicines capable of curing it. On the other side of the Atlantic they seem to depend upon **Zincum**,—especially, Dr. Norton says, when the Pterygium extends from the inner canthus. In this country the remedy which has most frequently succeeded has been **Ratanhia**, as I have shown when speaking of this medicine.

---

* J. B. H. S., v., 208   † Norton's appendix, p. 459

LECTURE XXX

DISEASES OF THE EYE (*continued*).

SCLERA, CORNEA, IRIS, CHOROID & RETINA

SCLERITIS—KERATITIS—CORNEAL-OPACITIES—IRITIS—CHOROIDAL CONGESTION—CHOROIDITIS—GLAUCOMA—RETINAL HYPERAEMIA—RETINAL HAEMORRHAGE—RETINITIS—DETACHMENT OF THE RETINA—RETINAL HYPERAESTHESIA.

We have now considered the morbid states of the conjunctival covering of the eye, with its prolongations. Our attention must next be directed to those of the constituent elements of the EYE-BALL itself.

We will first take the diseases affecting its fibrous investment, the SCLERA and the CORNEA.

SCLERITIS constitutes, I think, the most common form of "Rheumatic Ophthalmia." It is the inflammation which, in subjects without Rheumatic taint, follows exposure to cold winds; and shows itself by severe pain in and around the ball, with straight-lined and crimson injection of the surface,—thus both in sensation and appearance differentiated from Catarrhal Conjunctivitis.* In this affection we have two excellent remedies in **Aconite** and **Spigelia**. *Aconite* acts here so well not only because the constitution sympathises with the local mischief, but because the sclera is one of the few tissues which it has the Pathogenetic power of inflaming. I advise you to depend upon it at first alone, and my experience indicates the lowest dilutions as most serviceable. But if its action should seem exhausted, and further help be required, I think you will get it from *Spigelia*. The pains indicating this remedy are of a stitching character, whereas those of *Aconite* are more diffused.

In Patchy Episcleritis the two chief candidates for favour are **Thuja** and **Terebinthina**. The former is Dr. Norton's main remedy: the latter is chiefly indicated when its characteritic

---

* I believe that the affection would now be regarded as seated in the sub-conjunctival tissue, inflammation of the sclera itself being accounted very rare, and its hyperæmia occurring in patches. But the description I have given above will enable the disorder treated of to be plainly recognised.

dark and scanty urine is present.* Kalmia has sometimes proved useful.

Inflammation of the CORNEA,

KERATITIS, may be SIMPLE, SCROFULOUS, or SYPHILITIC; and, again, INDOLENT or SUPPURATIVE. The chief medicines which help us to modify favourably inflamed states of the cornea are *Apis, Arsenicum, Aurum, Cannabis sativa, Hepar sulphuris* and *Mercurius corrosivus*.

Apis is, I think, specific in simple Diffuse Keratitis. It is also of great value, as I have said, when the phlyctenulæ of Strumous Ophthalmia invade the tissue.

Arsenicum is strongly recommended by Dr. Angell when ulceration threatens, especially when—as is then generally the case—the patient is feeble and cachectic. More indolent ulcerations may often be met satisfactorily by *Sulphur, Calcarea* or *Silicea* + if the constitutional condition indicating these remedies is present.

Hepar sulphuris is the medicine to be depended upon in Suppurative Keratitis, and in Abscess of the Cornea (Onyx).

Cannabis sativa, Mercurius corrosivus and Aurum are the medicines for the interstital Keratitis of the subjects of Hereditary Syphilis. The first is praised by Dr. C. C. Boyle when the cornea is opaque and very vascular, without much pain or Photophobia. * *Mercurius corrosivus* is suited to more active cases, where the Syphilitic diathesis is marked. But *Aurum*, whether *metallicum* or *muriaticum*, holds the highest place in the treatment of this severe affection, and has wrought brilliant cures. $ It, and indeed all the corneal remedies, seem to require the lowest attenuations in which to exert their power.

Ipecacuanha, ‖ *Kali bichromicum* and *Zincum* $ have at some hands, received high commendation for their power over corneal inflammations and ulcerations.

---

* See case in J. B. H. S., iv., 341   + J. B H. S., i., 90
✝†IBID., iii, 442 ; see also Norton's Appendix, SUB VOCE.
$ IBID, i, 375 : iv.' 128 ; M. H. R., xxi., 58,
‖ J. B. H. S., iii., 100.   ** IBID,, ii , 100,

CORNEAL OPACITIES may arise from interstitial deposit of lymph (nebula, albugo), or from the cicatrization of an ulcer (Leucoma). The latter is probably incurable. The former will often disappear under the continued use of the medicine which cured the original inflammation, especially when this has been *Corrosive sublimate*. Some cases from the pen of the late Dr. Ozanne, illustrating its virtues here, may be read in the Third Volume of the ANNALS; and Druitt states that "Gooch used to cure Opacities of the Cornea even of long-standing, with full doses of the drug." But we shall sometimes do better with such medicines as **Calcarea carbonica** and **fluorata, Cannabis sativa** and **Causticum**. Cases showing the power of these remedies are related in Peter's Treatise.* The second is most in repute, and there is some reason to believe that it has caused the affection.

I come now to the disease of the UVEAL TRACT, the vascular coat of the eye. This includes the IRIS, the CILIARY BODY, and the CHOROID. which may be affected separately or together, so that we may have IRITIS, CYCLITIS and CHOROIDITIS, and also IRIDO-CYCLITIS and IRIDO-CHOROIDITIS. A new class of remedies will now come into action, distinct from those on which we have drawn for affections of the mucous and fibrous tissues or the eye. But it must be remembered that, besides pigmentary and muscular elements, we have in the IRIS a serous membrane with which to deal, in the form of the capsule of the aqueous humour, the membrane of Descemet, I apprehend that not only in the so-called "Keratitis Punctata," where its corneal portion is attacked but also in Syphilitic and Rheumatic Iritis, this membrane is the primary seat of the inflammation, and that from it the lymph is exuded. Hence Iritis having such causation may be a different thing from the same affection when traumatically induced, or when occurring as an extension of Choroiditis.

With this preface, let us proceed to speak of—
IRITIS, in its SIMPLE RHEUMATIC, and SYPHILITIC forms.

SIMPLE IRITIS, hardly going beyond hyperæmia, may occur from over-use of the eye, when it is often continuous with a similar condition in the choroid, and is aided by the *Santonine* I shall recommend for that. Of the traumatic form, I have seen two well-marked cases, and both yielded very rapidly and completely to **Belladonna**, of which two drops of the first dilution were given every two hours. The Traumatic Iritis which is apt to supervene after the extraction of Cataract is said to yield nicely to *Aconite* and *Arnica*. A "Serous Iritis" is also described, in which the pupil instead of being contracted is dilated; in

---

* Also, for *Calcarea flourata* see J. B. H. S., iii, 206, and iv. 236 for *Kali bichromieum*.

which the tension of the globe is increased, and hypopyon may be present. Here **Gelsemium** is described as almost specific.

RHEUMATIC IRITIS is the severer form of "RHEUMATIC OPTHALMIA," and its painful, damaging, recurring character is well known. **Mercurius**, in some form (most frequently the *Corrosive sublimate*), is commonly relied upon by Homœopathists in the treatment of this affection : 'its various combinations," Drs. Allen and Norton said, "are our sheet-anchor in the treatment of all forms of Iritis" ; and Dr. A. B. Norton repeats the statement. I must confess, however, that my own observations have disappointed me as to its possessing any great power over the disease. Should it not have this, you will say, seeing how readily it sets up Iritis ? I am by no means certain of this Homœopathicity on its part. I examined the question in a paper which you will find in the Tenth Volume of the ANNALS OF THE BRITISH HOMOEOPATHIC SOCIETY. I there showed that the two authorities usually cited in favour of the production of Iritis by *Mercury*, Graves and Travers, both recognise in their cases the presence of two other factors of much greater importance—Syphilis, and cold with damp ; while it has never been observed among the workers in the metal. A single exception made by Travers to his statement that all his patients were Syphilitics, and an observation of Basedow's in which an "Iritis Mercurialis" appeared in a patient being treated with the drug for Hepatitis, were the sole evidence I could find of the possibility of the disease being induced by it. In taking up the question again in 1884, in my Boston Lectures, I had before me Huber's exhaustive collection of effects of *Mercury* and its preparations, then in course of appearing as a supplement to the NORTH AMERICAN JOURNAL OF HOMOEOPATHY. In all this long list I could only find three observations which with reasonable probability bore out such Pathogenetic power of the metal. While, therefore, I do not deny that *Mercury* CAN cause Iritis, I do dispute its readiness and frequency in so doing ; and am not surprised at its comparative inertness even in the Rheumatic form of the Idiopathic disease.

Still more unable am I to recognise its Homœopathicity to SYPHILITIC IRITIS. This is essentially a plastic inflammation, and *Mercury* is as essentially an antiplastic, a liquefacient drug. I think it has yet to be proved ihat it exerts any influence in the resolution of the Gummata, save at the cost of inducing its Physiological effects on the system. That in some cases the gain may be worth the cost I do not deny ; but there is no doubt that Syphilitic Iritis may often get well without Mercurialisation and I think that in most cases we may safely treat with other remedies. I am myself well-satisfied with **Clematis** here, as with **Euphrasia** and **Kali bichromicnm** in the Rheumatic form. *

---

* See for these, B. H. J., xli., 21, 114, 118,—*Kali bich*. is commended by Dr. Norton in Descemetitis.

Others of our collegues have had good effects in the former variety from *Aurum* and *Cinnabar* (which is not a true Mercurial) ; and in the latter from *Rhus*.* Conversely, the Therapeutic evidence adduced by Huber goes against the Homœopathicity of *Mercury* in Syphilitic Iritis, as his two clinicians of most weight—Kafka and Payr—find it necessary to resort to inunction of the drug, as did Dr. Dudgeon in a case referred to in my Paper.†

But whatever medicine we are giving internally, there is no doubt that we must apply *Atropine* locally to dilate the pupil. It is mainly a mechanical proceeding. We want to hold the iris away from the capsule of the lens, lest it should adhere there ; and to prevent the contraction of the pupil, which might become permanent. To effect this by a mydriatic is surely open to no objection. But since in all probability, *Atropia* dilates the pupil by stimulation of the sympathetic nerves of the part, it must also contract the blood-vessels, and in this way help to subdue the inflammation. It keeps, moreover, the iridal muscle at rest, and perhaps abates the ciliary pain. This last indication may also be carried out by the intercurrent use (in highish dilution) of medicines suggested by the subjective sensation complained of, as *Spigelia, Calocynth, Cedron, Prunus* and *Chamomilla*.**

Les you should ever meet with Tuberculosis of the Iris, I will note that in a case of Dr. Schepen's *Arsenicum, Sulphur* and *Kali bichromicum* were without effect, while *Tuberculinum* (Kochii) 6 given twice a day caused immediate arrest of growth and speedy clearing away of the deposit.††

I have nothing to say about MYDRIASIS, as it is nearly always a symptom of some deep or distant mischief.

I pass on, therefore, to affections of the CHOROID.

CHOROIDAL CONGESTION is, I think, the condition of the eyes in sufferers from over-work of the organs, when it is not one simply of Asthenopia from muscular fatigue. *Ruta* and *Rhododendron* have been recommended for it in past times ; but we have, I think, a much more potent remedy for it in **Santonine.**

---

* See J B.H.S., i., 375 ; 443, 453 ; iv., 407.

† I have been glad to see that Dr. Allen supports me in this agreement.

** See B.J.H., xxvii., 467. †† JOURN. HOM. BELGE. Jan.—Feb., 1898.

CHOROIDITIS may be SIMPLE (serous), DISSEMINATED or SUPPURATIVE.

SIMPLE CHOROIDITIS has been caused and cured by *Ipecacuanha* ;* and *Arsenicum* has once at least proved capable of removing it † But *Belladonna* and *Gelsemium*, in recent cases, with *Phosphorus* in those of longer-standing, were Drs. Allen and Norton's recommendations; and they scem borne out by the known action of the drugs. Photopsia and Chromopsia are congestive Headaches in those calling for the first. The *Gelsemium* condition is less active. *Prunus spinosa*—a little known remedy—is recommended by these authors when pain is severe, of a crushing or pressing-asunder kind.

DISSEMINATED CHROIDITIS seems generally connected with Syphilis. It is natural, therefore, to treat with **Mercurius** and **Kali iodatum**. Both, however, have proved useful in the Non-syphilitic form; and the latter is regarded by Dr. Angell as having quite a specific action on choroid. Allen and Norton give a good case of Non-syphilitic. Disseminated Choroiditis cured by it in the first centesimal dilution.

SUPPURATIVE CHOROIDITIS, often called "Panophthalmitis," is a very serious dlsease. If there is any remedy on which dependence can be placed in it, it is **Rhus**. I know of a case in the malady supervened upon Pyæmic infection from dissecting wound; but by the use (mainly) of this medicine both eyes have beeen saved, and very tolerable sight rcgained. Mr. Knox Shaw says he has satisfied himself that *Rhus* and ice-compresses will sometimes abort a threatened Panophthalmitis after Cataract extraction. **

Besides these experiences, I may mention one of Chronic Headaches traceable to Choroiditis, recovering under Dr. Cooper's treatment by single doses of *Viola odorata* ;✛ and two of the Disseminated form, apparently Non-syphilitic. In one *Belladonna* proved curative ;∥ in the other pain and Photopsia were markedly relieved by *Tabacum*.✛✛

It is in this place that I must consider the treatment of the obscure but very interesting malady known as—

GLAUCOMA.—The benefit or iridectomy (or sclerotomy) in

---

* B.J.H., xli., 118.   † IBID., xxii., 568.
** L.H.H.R., vi., 31.   ✛ IBID., 318.
∥ J.B.H.S., ii., 363; iii., 105.   ✛✛ IBID., iii., 83.

very acute Glaucoma is so undoubted, and the danger of prolonged tension of the globe so great, that I cannot think ony one justified in neglecting it in favour of medicinal measures. But when a premonitory stage exists, and we can catch the patient in it; or when Glaucoma is chronic in character, and the occasional inflammatory exacerbations leave intervals of complete remission, I think we can do a good deal by remedies. Dr. Parenteau is hardy precise enough here : but this at least he tells us, that the well known action of *Atropine* in augmenting intraocular tension and aggravating the Glaucomatous phenomena may be utilised Homœopthically by the adoption, in similar Idiopathic states, of the internal administration of the drug in sufficiently attenuated doses. Of course, so far as the obstruction of the filtration-apparatus (on which the increased pressure in the eye seems to depened) is mechanical, as from rigidity of the sclera or enlargement of the lens, drug-treatment cannot help, and iridectomy or sclerotomy is the most-rational as the most effective measure. But that simple congestion (or is it inflammation ?) will cause it, appears from the observations of the occurrence of Glaucoma as one of the vaso-motor or trophic disorders incident to Trigenimal Neuralgia. Anstie in his Treatise on Neuralgia, devotes several pages to this subject (pp. 102-04, 150), referring to six recorded instances of the kind. One of them he relates at length, and it shows the typical symptoms of Glaucoma coinciding with each occurrence of pain, but subsiding in the intervals, until at last the Neuralgia departed, and therewith all impairment of vision, Mydriasis, tension and other morbid phenomena in the eyes.

Mr. Brudenell Carter, whom Ansite quotes as inclining to the nervous origin of some forms of Glaucoma, in the Article in Quain's Dictionary describes it as of purely mechanical origin, and susceptible only of mechanical relief, the inflammatory and Neuralgic symptoms being secondary only. The evidence of Therapeuties, however, goes against him. From our own school we have, besides Dr. Parenteau's statement, the testimony of Dr. Dekeersmaecker to the value of *Aconite* in Glaucoma, when the ocular affection is associated with Anæsthesia or Neuralgic pain in the parts supplied by the trigeminus, suggesting (as he says) its own dependence on some disorder at the origin of that nerve.* The power of *Aconite* to set up such disorder, exhibiting itself in such forms has been definitely ascertained by Schroff. Again there are several cases on record in which *Phosphorus*, given on account of the pain present, seems to have restored soundness and vision to undoubtedly Glaucomatous

---

*L'HOMEOPATHIE MILITANTE, 271. "I have seen proof, positive of this action," he writes "and hope to publish it one day. That I had to do with veritable Glaucomas there can be no doubt : the diagnosis was strict and confusion impossible." It is greatly to be regretted that the writer's too early death prevented him from following up this subject.

eyes.* The power of this drug over Neuralgia, always recognised in our school, has been substantiated very fully by Mr. Ashburton Thompson ; and to such power, I think, we must trace its Antiglaucomatous properties.

Besides **Atropine**, therefore, we have in **Aconite** and **Phosphorus** medicines promising on every ground to be of value in this serious ocular disease. When tension and Chromatopsia are more marked than Neuralgic pain, I think we have another candidate for honours here in the shape of **Digitalis**. It was noted by several of the English physicians—Lettsom, Withering, Mossmann and others—who in the Eighteenth Century used the *foxglove* so largely in Phthisis and Dropsy, that it had peculiar effect upon vision. Those under its influence complained that their sight was dim and indistinct ; or that the colouring of objects was altered, so that they seemed blue, yellow or green ; or all things appeared as if covered with snow, and faces assumed a corpse-like whiteness. At another time motes floated before the sight, which on covering and pressing the eyes appeared as sparks ; then flashes and balls of fire were seen, and objects appeared brilliant with a fiery halo around them. If the use of the drug was pushed, blindness might occur, which in one case lasted for a month after omitting it ; the sense of pressure in the eyeballs which accompanied the initial symptoms being exchanged for throbbing pain and sense of fulness and enlargement. All this will be found in Hahremann's "Materia Medica Pura" ; but the 'Cyclopædia of Drug Pathogenesy adds some further features of the kind from later experimentation. These I have sketched to you in Lecture XVIII., when speaking of Migraine. The suggestion in all this of early Glaunoma must be admitted to be very strong, and I think it ought to lead to practical results.

Oculists must decide in any given case of the disease whether it is safe to try medical action, or whether operative interferences must be at once resorted to if the eye is to be saved. Of course if Mr. Carter's later view be the true one, the question can never arise : but I rather sympathize with Anstie. "I think", he writes, 'that there is now sufficient evidence to show that Glaucoma is sometimes entirely, and very often in considerable part Neuralgic in its origin········· I am necessarily without the means of personally observing Glaucoma on a large scale, but I have now seen two cases in which, if I possess any faculty of clinical observation whatever, the whole genesis of the disease was a Neuralgic disorder of the trigeminus ; and it was to me a melancholy reflection that nothing better than iridectomy in one case, and excision of the eyeball in the other, could be done in the present state of ophthalmic science." Perhaps in

---

*See B.J.H., xxxii., I. I can speak from personal observation of its power of abolishing pain in Glaucomatous eyes.

our *Belladonna* and *Digitalis*, our *Aconite* and *Phosphorus*, he might have found—had he lived to try them—the better thing for which he longed. *

In writing on this subject in former years. I have said that a good deal of information as to what drugs can do in Glaucoma may be obtained from the German experience of the Homœopathic treatment of "Arthritic Ophthalmia," many recorded instances of which are unquestionable examples of the former disease. The cases cited by Peters show that *Arsenicum, Colocynth* and *Spigelia,* given according to symptomatic indication, have often proved of great benefit in the atrocious Neuralgic pains of the malady; while *Cocculus* and *Sulphur* seem to have met it successfully in even advanced stages. An analysis of these cases, by a competent oculist, so as to determine the exact operation of the medicines employed, would be very useful. I have also reminded my readers of what I have said about the "excessive tension" and horizontal Hemiopia noted by the provers of *Aurum.* ✛ Drs. Allen and Norton have shown that when the latter symptom (the upper half of bodies being invisible) is present in chronic affections of the eye, the drug is always more or less beneficial ; and I do not see why Glaucoma should not be among them, though a Chronic Choroido-Retinitis would be a more common cause, I have little now to add. Dr. A. B. Norton contends himself with giving the symptomatic indications for remedies bequeathed by his brother, avowing that to him the results from the use of them are somewhat problematical. He evidently would depend on the local use of *Eserine* in non-operative cases in preference to internal medication. Dr. Fellows, Professor of Ophthalmology in the Hahnemann Medical College of Chicago, communicates some favourable experience with *Gelsemium* 1x and *Spigelia* 3x. Dr. Parenteau has added to his former contributions to the subject an experience in which *Cocaine,* instilled into the eyes for Scleritis, developed a Glaucumatous condition therein when used too freely. It speedily passed on omitting the application. He has taken the hint, and has used the drug internally, in dilutions from the third to the twelfth, in Glaucoma itself, finding it specially useful when this process supervenes upon Iridal, Ciliary of Choroidal affections.

---

* Curiously enough he reports later in his book an experience very like Dr. Parenteau's. "I believe that in these cases I have succeeded, by prompt injection of *Sulphate of Atropine* ($\frac{1}{80}$ to $\frac{1}{40}$ grain), in saving a Neuralgic eye from damage, possibly from destruction, from impending Glaucoma (p. 189).

✛ I have examined these more in detail in a Paper contributed to the NEW ENGLAND MEDICAL GAZETTE for December, 1893 (p. 545).

I have now to speak of the diseases of the nervous elements of the eyeball—the RETINA and the OPTIC NERVE.

RETINAL HYPERAEMIA "frequently depends," as Allen and Norton write, "upon some anomally in the Accomodation or Refraction of the eye which should be corrected by suitable glasses, after which the retina resumes its normal condition." If this cause is absent, we may generally find another in over-use of the eyes, when *Santomine* or *Ruta* will be of service; in cardiac disorder, where Dr. Angell finds *Cactus* of great benefit; or in menstrual suppression, in which case it will often yield to *Pulsatilla*. In cases owning no such origin, but presenting marked hyperæmia, *Duboisine* should be thought of.

RETINAL HAEMORRHAGE, when occuring as a separate affection must be treated like sanguineous effusions elsewhere. *Lachesis* is the remedy which seems to have done most in favouring re-absorption. When it is part of a general hyperæmia of the fundus (Retinitis Apoplectica), *Mercurius* in some form is recommended.

RETINITIS may be SIMPLE ALBUMINURIC or SYPHILITIC.

1. For SIMPLE Inflammation of the Retina, when recent, we used to rely upon **Belladonna**; and there is good evidence of its power over the disease, even where the nerve-entrance is involved (Optic Neuritis). 7 A red conjunctival streak along the line of fissure of the lids is said to indicate it in hyperæmic states of the retina. The excellent proving of **Duboisine**, however, by Dr. A. B. Norton, has shown a yet more striking hyperæmia of the fundus, with the symptoms usually associated therewith; and Dr. Deady has made a beginning of its Therapeutic use in such states, as you may read in the other's book. In Chronic cases **Mercurius** should be thought of, and perhaps *Plumbum*. With the former there is special sensitiveness of the eyes to the glare of a fire.

2. Still stronger is the evidence for the two last medicines in Albuminuric Retinitis. **Mercurius corrosivus** is the standing remedy for it, and may cure it even though the accompanying renal malady shows its virulence by killing the patient. as in a

---

* See ease in J. B. H. S., vii, 220.
7 See Art. Belladonna in Part II. of Dr. Norton's Book.

case recorded by Dr. Speirs Alexander in the Forty-Second Volume of the MONTHLY HOMOEOPATHIC REVIEW. * In longstanding cases *Plumbum* promises most, † but I would call attention to the retinal changes induced in dogs by *Picric acid* as presenting a curious resemblance to those of our present malady.

3. In the Syphilitic from **Kali iodatum** will probably be the best remedy, it having to us the recommendation of having caused (as has *Iodine* itself) a corresponding affection.

DETACHMENT OF THE RETINA is an affection in which I happen to have personal interest, but which on its own merits I may fairly commend to study from a Therapeutic stand-point. We used to consider the fluid which effects this separation an effusion from the choroidal veins; but the tendency here also is to mechanical views, and we are taught to look for the causation of the DETACHMENT to a shirnking of the vitreous (from senile change or post-inflammatory contraction), dragging on the retina, and so rupturing it that the humor in front flows in and lodges behind it. If this be true, the "great sphere of usefulness for" *Gelsemium* in this affection, inferred by Allen and Norton from its power over Serous Choroiditis, becomes indefinitely narrowed; and yet some good results are reported from its use. In one case "DETACHMENT had been present for three weeks, and was dependent upon an injury. It was accompanied with diffuse haziness of the vitreous and serous inflamation of the choroid and retina. In a month, under-*Gelsemium* 30 the vision improved from mere perception of light to $\frac{90}{70}$, and the retina became completely re-attached." Dr. George Norton, who cites this case, adds—"Since then similar results have been obtained from its use in detachment from Myopia." *Aurum*, too, which has caused Horizontal Hemiopia such as would result from DETACHMENT of the lower half of the retina, seems occasionally to be of service here, ⊕ especially when there was a history of Syphilis and prolonged dosing with Anti-syphilitics. These results do not amount to

---

* See also Norton, Art. Mercurius corrosivus.
† See J.B.H.S., vi., 313. ⊕ See p. 400 of Dr. A.B. Norton's Book.

much; but if drugs, in infinitesimal doses are of any use whatever in a such a condition, it cannot be wholly dependent on traction and rupture and influx of fluid, as now believed, but must have a vital and dynamic origin. It should therefore be amenable to drug action ; and for the sake of many condemned to hopeless blindness from its presence, I urge a further effort towards its medical treatment.

In essaying this, besides the drug I have mentioned above, I would direct attention to that crystalline product of Tar known as *Naphthalin*. We had already used it for sometime (I know not how we came to do so) in spasmodic affections of the respiratory organs, like Whooping-Cough and Asthma, when in 1889 Panas, experimenting with it on rabbits, found very curious changes developed in the eyes. Serous effusion into all spaces—between the hyaloid membrane of the vitreous and the retina, between this and the choroid, between the lens and its capsule, and between the fibres of the lens itself—seems to be the essence of its action. Panas' experiments—which have been confirmed by Magnus, Dor and others * —were brought before the Homœopathic Congress held in Paris in 1889 by the late Dr. Ozanam, ✝ and their bearing on Homœopathic treatment indicated. Infiltration of the optic papilla (choked disc), Soft Cataract and Detachment of the Retina are named by him as ocular affections to which it corresponds ; but I have looked in vain through the published volumes of our JOURNAL OF OPHTHALMOLOGY AND OTOLOGY to find any application of it to practice. I asked Mr. Knox Shaw whether he had had any experience with the drug. He kindly replied as follows ; "When studing *Naphthalin* with regard to its action on cataract, I had noted its possible use in Detachment of the Retina. Panas' experiments show that the drug might be useful in such Detachment in highly myopic eyes with Choroiditis, but we do not seem at the Hospital to have had any appreciable results with it so far clinically. I cannot say that I have seen any real benefit from any drug in this affection. I have tried *Aurum, Apis, Cantharis, Kali iod*, and others. In most cases of Detachment there are not the same coarse changes seen, that were found to exist in the vitreous, retina, lens and choroid of the animals experimented on "

I think that Mr. Knox Shaw does some injustice here to his own practice. Dr. Lambert and Mr. Spencer Cox, who have both worked with him at the London Hospital, speak more cheerfully of their results. The latter says that though he never saw a complete cure, there was a good deal of improvement obtained ; and the former reports one complete recovery —under *Apis 6*. ✝✝ It is thus also in America. Dr. A. B. Norton

---

* See Cycl. of Drug Pathogenesy, iv., 653.
✝ See its Transactions, p. 169.   ✝✝ J. B. H. S., 74, 78.

speaks very sceptically about any gain resulting from medicinal treatment; but a Meeting of the Homœopathic Medical Society of New York County in 1900, Dr. Ruth Worrall cited cases treated successfully with pressure and *Gelsemium*; Dr. Boyle stated that he had cured one case with this drug, and had found the retina perfect nine years after when he operated for Cataract; and Dr; Deady related an instance of Alcoholic origin twice recovering from an attack so brought on under the influence of *Kali Iodatum* 1_x.*

RETINAL HYPERÆSTHESIA, if accompanied by hyperæmia, will yield to the remedies for that condition, especially **Belladonna.**† If occuring without ophthalmoscopic evidence of change in the fundus, *Nux vomica* ✝✝ (or *Strychnia*) may be required, and perhaps *Conium*; I agree with Dr. Angel in thinking its best remedy to be *Macrotin*—the "concentrated preparation" of *Actæa racemosa*.

I might speak next of RETINAL ANÆSTHESIA, meaning by that name FAILURE of VISION occuring without any obvious cause, But as this trouble may arise from other conditions of the retina than simple anæsthesia—as Anæmia from embolism of the arteria centralis—I prefer to speak of it among the other derangements of vision, which I will take up at our next meeting.

---

* IBID., viii.' 359.   † See Norton p. 404

✝✝ An observation of Allen and Norton's recalls a case of my own in which *Nux* acted finely. "Hyperæsthesia to this Retina," they say, "with frequent pains to the top of the head, sleepless nights, and awakening cross in the morning, was promtly relieved by *Nux vomica*." The "pains to the top of the head", reminded one of Dr. Ferrier's localisation of the ultimate visual centres at that point. My patient had, on first looking at daylight in the morning, a dazzling blinding distress extending just two spots on each side of the sagittal suture; and use of the eyes at any time caused pain there, The case was one of Brain-fag.

LECTURE XXXI

DISEASES OF THE EYE. (*Concluded*).

VISION, LENS, OCULAR MUSCLES, REFRACTION & ORBIT.

AMBLYOPIA—HEMIOPIA—NYCTALOPIA—CATARACT
—ASTHENOPIA—OCULO-MOTOR PARESIS—MYOPIA—STRABISMUS
NYSTAGMUS—ASTIGMATISM—ORBITAL CELLULITIS—
ORBITAL PERIOSTITIS

Besides the derangements of visions connected with inflamation and other lesions of the retina or optic nerve there are some which are not traceable to any definite alternation herein, and which for all practical purposes must be treated as substantive affections. I will begin with AMAUROSIS, or (as the loss of VISION is sometimes incomplete)—

AMBLYOPIA.—LOSS OF SIGHT may be sudden. If from exposure to cold, it will often yield to **Aconite**, and shown by two cases related by Dr. Hirish in the Thirty-Third Volume of the BRITISH JOURNAL OF HOMŒOPATHY (p. 172). It sometimes occurs in connexion with the Albuminuria of pregnancy and the prognosis is bad ; but two cases are on record where recovery ensued on the use of *Kali phosphoricum* 6_x.* More frequently it supervenes, gradually and is traceable to debilitating causes. When there have been loss of blood or other exhausting discharges, it will sometimes yield to the **China** which, with suitable diet and Hygiene, recruits the general strength. If in spite of all this it persists, it must be treated on its own merits, and then **Phosphorus** will generally be found the most helpful medicine, unless the symptoms (central scotoma, &c.) should resemble those of smokers' Amaurosis when (as in a case of my own) **Tabacum** may be prescribed with the utmost advantage. Tobacco-blindness itself is now, with that of Alcohol, ascribed to a Retro-bulbar Neuritis. The obvious treatment is the reduction or cutting-off of the noxious indulgence ; but in both forms help may be obtained from **Nux vomica**. "The results following its use are often," Drs. Allen and Norton say, "marvellous." The first dilution has generally been required.

---

* J. B. H. S., vii., 417.

CATARACT

HEMIOPIA, if not dependent on serious ocular or intra-cranial changes, may yield to the medicines which have been known to produce it. These are *Aurum* and *Digitaline*, when the upper half of objects is invisible; and *Ammonium bromatum*, *Arnica*, *Ferrum phosphoricum*, *Lithium*, *Morphia* and *Titanium** when the Hemiopia is vertical (generally on the right side).

NYCTALOPIA appears, from the researches of Mr. Tweedy, to be the traditonal and correct name for Night-Blindness, which I with others have hitherto called HEMERALOPIA. It is sometimes merely a symptom of Pigmentary Retinitis, † and sometimes one of the features of Scurvy or inanition. In such conditions medicines would probably play little part; but in the not unfrequent cases where Night-Blindness occurs in consequence of exposure to too much light and heat, remedies are quite available. **Belladonna** and **Nux vomica** ✝✝ have frequently proved successful, and seem suitable enough to the alteration present. The same can hardly be said of *Lycopodium*, but Dr. A. B. Norton repeats the strong recommendation of it in 'Hemera lopia" contained in the old "Ophthalmic Therapeutics" and I cannot but note it.

Other derangements of Vision, PHOTOPSIA, CHROMATOPSIA, &c., must be treated by pure symptomatic resemblance. The materials for so doing are specially abundant in the Repertory to the 'Cyclopædia of Drug Pathogenesy.'

I have now gone through the coats of the eye-ball, and have only to speak of the diseases of its media and of its muscles.

Of the media, the crystalline LENS is subject to the important lesion known as—

CATARACT.—Dr. Parenteau gives this as his second example of Homœopathy in Oculistry, which may seem surprising; but let us hear what he says about it. "Certainly, I do not pretend to cure all Cataracts, any more than my colleagues profess to cure all the Pulmonary Catarrhs and the Pleurisies which are given them to treat. But what I can affirm here, without fear of disproof, is that in a very considerable number of cases where this affection is taken in time, before the lens has undergone degeneration and indelible alternation, I have succeeded in

---

*See a case where this derangement of vision coincided with Vertigo and both yielded to *Titanium*, in J. B. H. S., x., 109

† As I have not mentioned this rare disease among the varieties of Retinitis I may here say that Dr. Copelend reports some favourable experience with *Phosphorus* in it (MED. CENTURY, Dec. 15th 1855.)

✝✝ J. B. H. S., iv., 939

checking the Cataract and sometimes even in causing it to take on retrograde action"

A statement like this, coming from a competent observer should lead us to look further. Dr. Burnett is again among the number of those who have so looked. Moved by the success of internal treatment in a case he tentatively undertook he made research into both the Homœopathic and the general literature of the subject, and was suprised to find the amount of testimony and evidence extant as to the "Curability of Cataract with Medicines." Under this title, he published (in 1880) one of his little volumes containing all he had found about it, with some experience of his own. Dr. Burnett does not profess to be an oculist ; and those who do, when they read his pages, must not expect to find the scientific precision in which they (justly) delight. They must not be prejudiced thereby into resisting the impression which his book must otherwiee make on the mind, that in a fair proportion of cases, vision impaired by commencing Cataract may be materially improved and so maintained ; and that in a still larger percentage the progress of Blindness may be checked, so that its subject conserves what slight he has, and is spared the risks and other inconveniences of an operation. This is what patients want : the exact determination of opacity and visual range is immaterial to them, as long as they can see and be immune from the knife. If Homœopathy can supply their need in this way they will bless it.

A similar conclusion, viz., : that the prognosis in Cataract is not so hopeless as is ordinarily supposed, has been come to by two leading oculists of our school—Mr. Knox Shaw of London, and Dr. A. B. Norton of New York ; but on rather different grounds. Dr. Norton published in the NORTH AMERICAN JOURNAL OF HOMŒOPATHY for December, 1891, a tabulated statement of 100 cases of incipient Cataract treated by Homœopathic remedies. The value of these to check its progress he considered brone out by the fact that one-half of all the cases under observation for two years or over showed no failure in vision and no increase of the opacity, and that in about one-third more there had been but a vesy slight loss of vision. Mr. Shaw also (his paper appears in the "Reports" of our London Hospital for 1893) bases himself on a series of cases, 125 in number, of the diseases in its incipient stage and simple (*i. e.* primary) form. His results are nearly if not quite as good, but drug-treatment does not seem to have played a prominent part in his hands. The point he makes is the frequent co-existence of Refractive error and Accommodative difficulty, and the corresponding commencement of the the opacity rather in the equatortial region of the lens than in its central nucleus. His measures therefore are directed to correct those errors ; and to deal, medicinally and hygienically, with the eyes as a whole. Simple Cataract, he holds, is not PER SE a senile change ; the prime factor in its development is eye-strain; its rate of advance is slow, and in many cases it may never reach maturity; and the means specified above will delay its progress, and in some cases cause (at any rate for a time) actual improvement in the condition of the lens.

I think, therefore, that Dr. Parenteau's claims, large as they may seem, are borne out by experience; and may be acted on. To encourage us further, Dr. Burnett has reminded us that Embryology shows the lens to be a dermoido-epithelial structure, like skin and mucous membrane, arguing therefrom that it should like these be sensible to medical treatment; and I long ago pointed out * that the development of opacity in it has followed on retrocedent Gout, menstrual suppression, and the drying up from without of cutaneous eruptions and of habitual perspiration of the feet. Other affections so arsing are amenable to specific remedies; why should this not be so?

These last considerations bring Cataract into the category of Hahnemann's "Psoric" disease, and suggest his "Antipsorics" as affording its most appropriate remedies. Experience has proved them so, at least in respect of the great triad – *Sulphur*, *Calcarea* and *Silicea*; perhaps also as regards *Magnesia carbonica*, with which a Frence physician, Dr. Pirel, has obtained some fairly satisfactory results. * *Causticum*, though ranked by Hahnemann as such a medicine, and stated by Dr. Norton to have undoubtedly proved of most value in his hands, I agree with Mr. Shaw in thinking of it as acting rather upon the Accommodative apparatus – to which, as he justly says, the symptoms for which it is prescribed mostly belong. The same may be said of *Phosphorus*. Of other drugs which have proved useful I may mention *Colchicum* and *Sontonine* as having been found capable (in animals) of inducing opacity of the lens, and *Chelidonium*, *Conium* and *Pulsatilla* as possessing some empirical reputation against this change. *Narum muriaticum*, *Naphthalin* and *Secale* are other substances which have caused the lesion. With the first, however, the phenomena is probably a physical one, such as occurs in Diabetes; in the two latter it is—Mr. Shaw thinks—Secondary to grave alteration wrought in the retina and ciliary region. We have already examined the question as regards *Naphthalin*; but excluding it and its fellows, enough choice of remedies remains to give us a good chance of fitting an effective agent to most cases of Cataract which come before us in the forming stage.

A Paper by Dr. Malan in the Fifth Volume of the BRITISH JOURNAL OF HOMOEOPATHY, and the section in Peters' Treatise, contain all the cases of Homœopathic cure or improvement of Cataract with which we were acquainted of old times. Some of these are of dubious value; but even when they are eliminated, the power *Sulphur*, *Silica*, *Cannabis*, *Pulsatilla*

---

* 'Manual of Therapeutics,' 1st Ed. (1869), p. 195
† BULL DE LA SOC, MED. HOM. DE FRANCE, Vols. v. and vi.

and *Calcarea* must remain unquestioned. **Silicea** has been most frequently successful ; it should be especially thought of when suppressed perspiration of the feet seems to have been the exciting cause. **Sulphur** ranks next : its value is obiously best marked when the trouble dates from repercussion of a cutaneous eruption. **Cannabis** would be suitable when the Cataract was capsular—the result of inflammatory action. Should we catch such a Cataract in the act of formation— i. e., in the inflammatory stage - it seems probable, from one of Peters' cases, that **Belladonna** might be relied upon to disperse it. **Pulsatilla** was a reputed remedy for cataract in the hands of Storck. It acted very satisfactorily in one of of Peters' cases where a Chronic Catarrhal Ophthalmia calling for it was present ; and would be specially indicated where suppression of the menses was the exciting cause. **Calcarea*** would natuarally be thought of in Strumous subjects, as in the following case :—

"A farmer æt. 51, of small stature, and with light-brown hair, had suffered for the last few weeks with impaired sight ; the patient had formerly been troubled with Scrofula.

"The patient sees with the right eye only those objects which are above him, and with the left only those which are at his side ; but in al other directions everything appears as dark as n:ght to him. Partial opacities of the crystalline lenses were clearly obscrvable ; the one in the right occupied the larger, and that in the left the smaller half of the pupil.

"*Cannabis* 2, three drops daily in water for three weeks, was without benefit. *Calcarea 3*, six doses ; at first one dose a day for two days. afterwards one dose every week. Before the last dose had bzen taken, the patient had entirely recovered his sight" (Peters, 221).

There is a form of Cataract known as "Traumatic" and it is said to have been occasionally cured by **Conium**. A case of this kind is mentioned by Dr. Bayes. It is true that the Pathology of the affection shows that spontaneous recovery is at least a probable issue. The aqueous humour, rushing in through the ruptured capsule, at first renders the lens opaque ; but, unless the rent closes, will ultimately dissolve it and so clear the vision. In Dr. Bayes' case, however, Blindness had continued for eighteen years. Dr. Talbot esteemed *Conium* highly in Cataracts otherwise arising ; and in the MEDICAL CENTURY for January, 1893, † published two well-marked cases practically cured by it.

I add a note furnished me by Dr. Henry Madden, who had unusual experience in the treatment of this disease. "In the early stage, when vision is but clouded, and streaks only of

---

* Mackenzie states that Cataract is a common disease in all countries where Wine is so cheep as to be the habitual beverage of the lower orders. Has this anything to do with the lime and flint so commonly found in natural Wines ? ✝ See also M. H. R., xxxvii., 107

opacity are seen by the ophthalmoscope, a check to further deposit may often be expected. If there is nothing more than smokiness of the lens' it may clear away entirely. The medicines I have found of most service are *Mercurius, Calcarea* and *Phosphorus*, all in the higher dilutions."

I must not leave Cataract without telling, you what has been done for it by local treatment- The distinguished Wiesbaden oculist, Pagenstecher, has praised *Iodide of Potassium* in the incipient stage. He uses an ointment of it abont the eye, and has no doubt that it can bring the Cataractous process to a standstill, and in some cases increase the vision. In our own school the instillation of the *Cineraria maritima* has gained some credit. In a case treated thus by Dr. E. D. Perking great and progressing improvement occurred and instead of a dull lustreless eye, with muddy congested conjunctiva, the patient showed a bright, clear, healthful-looking organ.*

Of the other media of the eye I have nothing to say save that *Senega* has been found effective in clearing away opacities of the vitreous humor.

Affections of the OCULAR MUSCLES.
ASTHENOPIA is defined (in Quain's Dictionary) as "any condition in which the eyes cannot be used for long without fatigue, pain, or other symptoms." It may be "ACCOMODATIVE," when the ciliary muscle is at fault, and there is no confused or donble vision ;† or "MUSCULAR," in which the extrinsic muscles of the eye are the seat of debility. You will remember that all these are, like the ciliary, supplied by the third nerve, save the inferior oblique and the external ractus, to which (for the independent action they subserve) the fourth and sixth nerves respectively are devoted.

It is, I think, ACCOMODATIVE ASTHENOPIA that **Ruta** has gained its repute in ophthalmic affections. Hahnemann (as I have said in my 'Pharmacodynamics') mentions that *Rue* was commended by Rosenstein, Swedjaur and Chomel for dimness

---

* J. B. H. S., vi., 394.

† Accomodative Asthenopia, too, may itself be of two kinds, as Dr. Norton suggests ; it may be Paralytic, when the medicines come in of which I have spoken above, or Irritable, where the Myotics — *Physostigma, Muscarine* and *Pilocarpine* —would be indicated. Dr. Norton uses *Jaborandi* 3 in such cases with marked effect.

of vision caused by over-exertion of the eyes, and points to S.44 and 45 of his Pathogenesis of the plant as showing that it causes what it cures. These symptoms* are, "His eyes feel as if he had strained his sight too much by reading." "weak pressive like pain in the right eye. with dimness of surrounding objects, as if from having looked too long at an object and fatigued the eyes." A Hungarian physician, of the name of Elgajaki, has drawn attention to the same double series of facts. Allen and Norton gave us an alternative, but mainly for MUSCULAR ASTHENOPIA, in **Natrum muriaticum.** With this there is aching on moving the eyes in any direction, and the muscles feel stiff and tense. They also commended *Ammonium Corbonicum*, where the origin is strain. **Argentum nitricum** suits the Asthenopia of Neurasthenia, which Nettleship ranks as quite a distinct variety.* Dr. Angell finds *Macrotin* very effective in relieving the evil effects of the use of Asthenopia eyes, such as hyperæmia and Photophobia— an experience I have frequently verified. If pain alone occurs at every attempt to use the eyes, you may bethink yourself of the benefit obtained in such an affection by Dr. Kafka from *Kali carbonicum* 6. ☥

In bad cases of Asthenopia the remedies for—
OCULO-MOTOR PARESIS must come into play. These are *Causticum* and *Rhus* ; *Gelsemium* and *Senega* ; and *Phosphorus*. **Causticum** ☥☥ and **Rhus** are most suitable when the Paresis is of "Rheumatic" origin ; the former (Allen and Norton think) being preferable when the patient has been exposed to dry cold. the latter when the cold has been conjoined with damp. **Gelsemium** and **Conium** correspond to simple Paresis of the ocular muscles, without any definite cause ; the first aught to be specially useful when the external, and *Sen'ga* when the superior, rectus is at fault. *Phosphorus* has proved curative in more pronounced forms of the malady, as from Spermatorrhœa or sexual excess.

For Paralysis of the Accomodation, *Atropine* would be exquisitely Homœopathic ; but when occurring after Diphtheria I find *Gelsemium* very effective

Spasm of the ocular muscles is rarely seen in the lids, where I have already spoken of it. But the fact that spasm of the ciliary muscle is a leading element in acquired —

---

* See B. J. H., xxxii., 739 ; UNITED STATES MED, INVESTIGATOR, vi., 539 ; M. H. R., xxii, 152. ☥ J. B. H. S., ii , 220

☥☥ Dr. Van Royers, of Utrecht, relates in a very scientific manneer a case of Paralysis of the oculo-motorius occuring in his own person, in which, after *Spigelia*, *Argentum nitricum* and *Natrnm muriaticum* had sailed, *Causticum* in the 8th dilution, effected a cure (J.B.H.S., ii, 208).

MYOPIA led the late Dr. Woodyatt, of Chicago to a very pretty piece of Homœopathic therapeutics. You will remember that **Physostigma** (the Calabar bean) temporarily causes short sight by stimulating the accomodating apparatus, just as *Atropia* sets up Presbyopia for a time by paralysing it. He has accordingly given this medicine, in the second and third decimal dilutions, in a number of cases of Acquired Myopia, and with most satisfactory results. *

STRABISMUS, when Paralytic, must be treated accordingly ; when dependent on Ametropia, must be corrected by suitable glasses. But it not uncommonely comes before us in children as a sympathetic disturbance, as a relic of Convulsions or a symptom of Helminthiasis. In the former case *Belladonna, Hyoscyamus* and *Cicuta* ; in the latter *Spigelia, China* and *Cyclanen* have gained successes.

NYSTAGMUS, an involuntary and morbid oscillation of the eyeballs, finds—lika Nictitation in the lids—its most frequent remedy in **Agaricus**.

I have a few words to say about—
ASTIGMATISM. —A prover of *Lilium tigrinum*, a married lady, who took two doses of the third dilution daily for six days after suffering much inconvenience in the eyes, found that an Astigmatism, under which she had laboured for a twelve-month past, had disappeared. Dr. Woodyatt's attention was drawn to the medicine, and he found that it acted like *Physostigma,* and corresponded to spasmodic conditions of the ciliary muscle. Astigmatism was his special indication for it ; and he has published several cases in which this condition, when dependent on muscular irregularity, has been removed by iis use. Dr. L, Hooper has had a corresponding result with *Physostigma* itself.✝

Lastly, of affections of the ORBIT.
ORBITAL CELLULITIS presents itself in two forms, the Œdematous and the Phlegmonous. The former yields readily to **Apis**. The latter, in children, has found a remedy in **Phytolacca** : in adults it is a more serious malady, but is generally under the control of **Rhus**.

ORBITAL PERIOSTITIS is generally of Syphilitic origin and whether so or not seems always to demand **Kali iodatum**, in not too attenuate dosage.

---

* See United States Med. Investigator ii., 375 ; v., 390 ; and vi., 44.
✝ J. B. H. S., vi., 222.

LECTURE XXXII

DISEASES OF THE EAR
——o——

AURICLE, MEATUS, TYMPANIC CAVITY & AUDITION.
——o——

ERYSIPELAS AURIUM—ECZEMA AURIUM—OTITIS EXTERNA—
OTORRHOEA—EXOSTOSES—THROAT-DEAFNESS—TYMPANITIS
—DEAFNESS—TINNITUS AURIUM—MENIERE'S DISEASE

I enter to-day upon the consideration of the maladies affecting the organ of hearing. When I wrote upon the subject in my 'Therapeutics', the Homœopathic literature pertaining to it was but scanty. It is far more copious now. Dr· Houghton, the surgeon to the aural department of the New York Ophthalmic Hospital, has gathered up his occasional papers in our journals, and his whole otiatric experience, in a handsome volume of "Lectures on Clinical Otology." Dr. Cooper, who acted in the same capacity in our London Hospital, has published his Lectures on 'Inflammation and other Diseases of the Ear' delivered at the London School of Homoeopathy in 1877-78 ; and has otherwise contributed to our knowledge of these maladies, as we shall see in proceeding. The German otological literature has been well collected in a series of papers by Dr. H. Goullon in the INTERNATIONALE HOMOEOPATHISCHE PRESSE for 1676, which have been translated in the BRITISH JOURNAL for the year ; and there are some English contributions to the subject by Dr. Dudgeon, * Mr. Cutmore † and Mr. Dudley Wright.

In spite, however, of the illumination thus bestowed upon Aural Therapeutics, we have much to learn regarding them. I was led to think that further light might be thrown on their comparative obscurity by considering the homologies of the eyu and ear. The morbid states of the former organ, and the medicine which influence its component parts are so (comparative) well-known, that they become stepping-stones of no littlle trustworthiness on our road through the darker regions of the latter. I made a study, therefore, of these homologies, and published it in the MONTHLY HOMOEOPATHIC REVIEW of 1868 : whence I transferred it to the Ear Sectton of 'Therapeutics' of 1878. Curiously enough, the same thought occurred in 1894 to Dr. Ord. (wirhout, he tells me, any recollection of my treatment of it), and he brought it before the British Homoeopathic Society in the October of that year. ** In reproducing my own

---

* B.J.H., Vol. xxi.   † ANNALS, Vol. iii.   ** See J.B.H.S., Vol. iii.

DISEASES OF THE EAR

paper here, I shall embody any sidelights it may gain from his, and shall discuss any points at which our respective views diverge.

Let us compare the organs of the two senses of sight and hearing as to their healthy structure and function.

We find at the base of the brain two sets of ganglia, themselves independent centres, but intimately connected by branching fibres with the gray matter of the cerebral hemispheres. They are the CORPORA QUADRIGEMINA and the AUDITORY GANGLIA respectively – the former being connected with the sense of sight, and the latter with that of sound, either as their ultimate recipients or (as now seems more probable) as their immediate transmitters to localised centres in the cortex cerebri. To obtain the impressions which they thus perceive or convey, they send to the outer world feelers- the OPTIC and the AUDITORY NERVES. Each, on passing beyond the cranium, expands into a receiving surface: the optic nerve becomes the RETINA, and the auditory nerve spreads itself out upon the walls of the LABYRINTH.

So far the correspondence is obvious; but let us preceed from behind forwards. Immediately in front of the auditory expansion lies the serous-like MEMBRANE OF THE LABYRINTH, enclosing the LIQUOR COTUNNII. The importance of this fluid in transmitting the sonorous vibrations needs no comment. What has the eye answering to this? Why immediately in front of the retina lies the VITROUS HUMOR, contained in the meshes of the HYALOID MMBRANE. The different consistence of the two media precisely corresponds to the difference between the two kinds of undulations they are designed to transmit.

Next, we observe that the waves of sound which set the labyrinthine fluid vibrating, are communicated to it through a chain of OSSICLEs. The last of these (stapes) is separated from the vestibule of the labyrinth only by the membrane of the fenestra ovalis, on which it rests. In like manner, also, the light which has reached the vitreous humor has come to it last through the Lens, which parted only by its proper capsule,* impinges upon the hyaloid membrane. I am anticipating somewhat; but I cannot resist pointing out the morbid homologies of these two structures. Whatever ancillary office they occupy in relation to the nervous expansions beyond, it is certain that these are able, in cases of necessity, to dispense with their services. Let the ossicles be disconnected, or even

---

* The posterior capsule of the lens, therefore, corresponds with the membranous septum of the fenestra ovalis. It is interesting accordingly to notice how a branch from the central artery of the retina penetrates the vitrous humor to supply the neighbouring surface of the capsule as though recognising the fellowship of the two **membranes.**

destroyed by disease ; let the lens be extracted by the surgeon, and hearing and sight will still be preserved, It is otherwise, however, when these media, retaining their place, become incapable of transmitting their messages. If the lens be rendered opaque by Cataract, or the stapes be anchylosed to the margin of the fenestra, there is little left that the ear can hear or the eye can see.

Let us go forward. The outer extremity of the chain of ossicles is connected with the MEMBRANA TYMPANI. This membrane is stretched across the passage along which sound makes its way, the transmission of which it regulates by the antagonistic ac.ion of its two muscles the tensor and laxator tympani. It thus performs for the ear the office which, in the eye, is discharged by the IRIS. The latter is, indeed, itself muscular, and its two sets of fibres dilate or contract, as is required, its central aperture through which the light-rays pass. I hardly know whether to lay any stress on the presence, in each of these membranes, of a circular and a radiating layer of fibres. In the membrana tympani both sets are attached to the malleus, but at different parts. The tendons of the two muscles, are also inserted into distinct points of this bone. A study of the action of the muscles might possibly show that each acted upon one of the layers of fibre. But a more important question relates to the nervous supply of the two structures. The ciliary nerves, which control the movements of the iris, all proceed from the ophthalmic ganglion ; but experiment has proved that the filaments which supply the circular fibres (contractor pupillæ) come from the third nerve, while those which go to the radiating fibres are from the sympathetic system. In the ear, the chorda tympani supplies the laxator tympani, while the tensor tympani receives a branch from the optic ganglion. It is quite possible that here also it would be found that sympathetic filaments from the ganglion supply the latter muscle, while the former is under the influence of the cerebro spinal fibres, probably from the facial, which the chorda tympani unquestionably contains.

So far the parallel has been indubitable. But now we encounter a difficulty. This is not raised, however, by the cornea. The cornea really belongs to the iris, although it projects forwards, that it may gather together the luminous rays. It is the pane of glass, so to speak, which fills the window of the pupil. If the selerotic, instead of curving forward, were to dip down vertically into the curtain of the iris, having the transparent cornea for its centre, the correspondence with the membrana tympani, with the central fibrous layer, would be complete. The trouble arises at the next step we take, In the eye we come upon mucous membrane, the conjunctiva. In the ear our next tissue is the skin of the external meatus. It may be said, skin and mucous membrane are essentially indentical, differing only according to situation, whether external or internal; they are even capable of transformation of the one into the other. But the awkward fact is that the ear does possess a true mucous membrane, prolonged from that of the pharynx through the Eustachian tube, lining the tympanic cavity and enveloping its ossicles, and finally terminating in the mastoid cells. Does this answer to the ocular conjunctiva? I think not. To do so, the latter ought to lie, not where it does, but between the cornea and the vitreous humor, lining the walls of the chamber, reflected off at the margin of the lens to cover this in, and finally prolonged into the ethmoid cells, whose neighbourhood to the eye reminds so much of that of the mastoid cells to the ear. The closed "capsule of the aqueous humor," if such an entity be anything more than hypothetical, fills this place; but neither in structure, functions, nor connexions is it a mucous membrane.

I conclude, therefore, that the eye has nothing truly answering to the mucous membrane of the tympanum; and that the conjunctiva finds its homologue in the dermic layer of the membrana tympani. Its communication by the lachrymal and nasal ducts with the mucous membrane of the nose is merely a provison for carrying off the TEARS of which the CERUMEN of the auditory passage is the representative. Nor is the MEATUS without its homologous structure. We have only to imagine the ORBIT deepened and narrowed and rather bent, and the eyeball pressed back as far as it will go, and we should have to use a speculum to ascertain the state of the conjunctiva and cornea, as now we use it to explore the membrana tympani.

(I must have forgotton this argument of mine when I listened to Dr. Ord's paper, for in the discussion which followed I seem to have maintained the contrary position to that taken up here about the relation between the conjunctiva and the tympanic mucous membrane. On grounds of homology he is (as I was) right about them, and he makes a fresh point in the same direction when he argues that the prolongation which constitutes them is from the respiratory tract with the former, from the alimentary with the latter. Nevertheless, I must agree with Mr. Dudly Wright that as regards morbid processes and the actions of drugs the two have much in common, and that we may—tentatively at least—argue from one to the other.)

Lastly, the EYELIDS and the AURICLE are undoubted homologues. Each consists of cartilage, covered with skin and cellular tissue. Each belogs to the meatus of the organ, though the one stands at the outer, the other at the inner, extremity of the way. To each it belongs to guard the passage which they cover, for which purpose they are moved by their appropriate muscles,— in their movements subserving also the purposes of expression. Both orbicular and auricular muscles are accordingly supplied by the facial—the nerve of emotional expression. In the lower animals, as is well-known, the auricular muscles have sufficient power to direct the ears towards the point from which the sound proceeds. In the eye this duty is performed by the recti and oblique muscles of the globe.

I now proceed to consider the various diseases which affect the EAR. In doing so, I shall mainly follow the classification of Toynbee, though availing myself freely of the additional researches of von Troltsch.

The AURICLE, like the eyelid, when attacked with inflammation usually has it in the Erpsipelatous form. I shall therefore speak of—

ERYSIPELAS AURIUM.—Here, also, as in its homologous part, the choice lies between **Belladonna, Rhus** and **Apis**; but it is rare to see the pale-red and œdematous condition which indicates the last remedy.

Sometimes, however, the DERMATITIS has such a character as to lead us to call it—

ECZEMA AURIUM.—This affection, when recent, will often subside pretty rapidly under the general remedies for Eczema, as *Rhus*, *Croton* and *Mezereum*. But it more frequently comes under treatment as a chronic affection, when, as you know, it is liable to extend into the meatus, and to eause Deafness by blocking up the passage with exfoliated epidermis. Mr. Cutmore has contributed two good cases of this affection to the Twenty-Second Volume of the BRITISH JOURNAL OF HOMŒOPATHY. The curative effect of *Arsenicum* and *Clematis* in the first case was very marked. When Eczema affects the back of the auricle and the adjacent mastoid surface, it is a most obstinate affection. *Muriatic acid, Graphites* or *Oleander* may do something for it; but it rarely gets well without some local application, such as *Glycerine* or *Tanin*. Dr. Houghton speaks well of *Petroleum*, locally and internally; or of a trituration of *Graphites* suspended in concentrated *Petroleum*, and topically used.

I have now to speak of the numerous diseases which attack the EXTERNAL MEATUS, I do not include among these mechanical obstruction, whether from foreign bodies, or from accumulated cerumen; since with us, as with all the remedy here is the syringe. I cannot say that we have any medicine which checks the over-activity of the ceruminous glands, on which the accumulation referred to may possibly depend; if we have, it seems to be *Conium*. Mr. Cutmore thinks we have in *Spongia* an excellent remedy for the opposite condition, viz., where there is a total deficiency of wax.

OTITIS EXTERNA, when acute, has in my experience assumed two different forms requiring different remedies. The former is the "inflammation of the connective tissue" of Kramer, * confined to the outer half of the meatus, whose orifice becomes an almost imperceptible slit. Here **Belladonna** is generally indicated (though Dr. Jousset prefers *Pulsatilla* and *Mercurius*); and with the aid of a moist heat continuously applied, will effect resolution as speedily as possible. In the other form the mischief is in the dermis itself, and chiefly in the deeper part of the meatus, where there is no connective tissue. The exreme sensibility of the dermis in this place makes the inflammation a horribly painful one ; and when (as often happens) it spreads to the mambrana tympani, distressing head-symptoms occur. Of this latter complication more anon. It is to this form of inflammation of the meatus, I think, that Dr. Bayes' experience belongs, with which my own entirely coincides : "in Otitis, of which I have seen many severe cases, **Aconite** 1st decimal, has proved rapidly curative, in 2 to 5-drop does every hour or two hours until the pain is relieved. I have never seen the higher dilutions of *Aconite* or *Pulsatilla* or *Chamomilla*, of any marked service in the maddening pain of Acute Otitis, while *Aconite*, *1*st decimal, has acted admirably," †

Chronic cases of this disease consist sometimes in the repeated recurrence of the acute attacks. Dr. Dudgeon mentions one such case, in which the tendency was checked by the presistent use of *Nitric acid* 3. Not uncommonly the recurring trouble comes in the shape of Boils. I think you will find the usual treatment of Boils sufficient here, viz., repeated doses of **Belladonna** *1* at the time, and **Sulphur** to check the recurrence ; though Dr. Houghton speaks of having obtained better results from *Picric acid* for the latter purpose. His experience has been verified by that of many other observers, among whom I may specify Dr. Gurnee Fellowes. † Chronic inflammation of the meatus, when continuous, may be with or without discharge. The latter is too much of a local affection for internal medicines to do much and although you may administer *Arsenicum, Graphites,* or *Mercurius corrasivus* with possible advantage, I think you will do best by the local application of *Nitrate of Silver*, say gr. j to the ounce. So Mr. Cutmore also advises.

---

* B J. H., cxi., 243.
† "Applied Homœopathy," p. 45. † J. B. H. S., ix., 97

The more common form, accompanied with discharge, constitutes in most cases what we call—

OTORRHOEA.—I think it is practical still to treat of this symptom as a disease, though it doubtless depends upon more than one Pathological condirion. The important point is that when chronic, it is nearly always connected with impaired general health on the part of the patient, and requires constitutional treatment accordingly. The two leading forms of Otorrhœa are, first, that dependent on primary ehronic inflammatiou of the dermis of the external meatus and membrana tympani ; second, that symptomatic of catarrh of the tympanic mucous membrane. In the former of these, the dermis becomes a kind of mucous membrane, suffers a "catarrhal" inflammation, and pours out a milky discharge. Besides daily syringing (which, however, should be gentle), or cleansing with cotton, you will often get very good results in these cases from medieines like *Mercurius, Hepar sulphuris* and *Nitric acid* ; but if these fail you, you will do well to fall back upon *Sulphur, Calcarea*, or *Silicea*, according to your patient's constitutional symptoms.

The second form of Otorrhœa, belongs to the affections of the middle ear (though it may occur without the perforation of the membrana tympani), in which category I shall consider it.

POLYPUS AURIUM is a frequent accompaniment of Otorrhœa, with the removal of which these growths will often spontaneously disappear. A case in point, in which *Mercurius* was the curative medicine, is given by Dr. Dudgeon : the Polypus appears to have been of the "raspberry celluar" form of Toynbee. Where a Polypus, being of such a mucous kind, requires a remedy of its own, this many sometimes be found in the curious power of *Thuja* over such growths. I have myself recorded one such case ; * and Drs. Speirs Alexander and George Black have each contributed two more, †—the medicine in all being in the 30th dilution. When the fibrous predominets ouer the cellular element in such a growth, I should have less expectation of cure from internal treatment, and should follow Dr. Houghton in applying locally a saturated solution of *Bichromate of Potash.*

---

* See M. H. R., xiii., 536. † J. B. H. S., i.,299

THROAT-DEAFNESS 451

EXOSTOSES of the external meatus are described by Toynbee as of no infrequent occurrence. He connects them with the Rheumatic and Gouty diatheses, and reports much benefit from the topical use of *Iodine* and the Internal of *Iodine of Potassium*. I know nothing about their Homœopathic treatment ; but results obtained elsewhere would suggest the trial of *Hecla lava* or *Calcarea fluorata*.

Of the Affections of the MEMBRANA TYMPANI it is needless to say much. The outer dermic layer belongs to the external meatus, in whose diseases and their treatment it shares. Its inner mucous membrane is part of the tympanic cavity. Relaxation of the membrane appears always connected with a morbid state of the middle ear and is curable by the remedies which influence the mucous membrane. The only part peculiar to this membrane is its fibrous layer ; and when the symptoms point to this as the seat of inflammation, I would suggest **Bryonia** and perhaps **Aconite** as their most likely remedies. The evening exacerbations of this malady remind one forcibly of Rheumatic Ophthalmia, of which it is obviousiy the homologue.

The EUSTACHIAN TUBE contributes its quota to aural disease by frequently suffering CLOSURE OF ITS FAUCIAL ORIFICE. This is the familiar—

THROAT--DEAFNESS.—I assume your acquaintance with all that is now known respecting the Physiology of the Eustachian tube, and with the various mechanical expedients (inflation by Politzer's method, or through the catheter) adopted to obviate its closure. When you have ascertained its want of potency, and the dependence of this upon an unhealthy state of the faucial mucous membrane, you will naturally turn to the remedies we have for modifying the latter condition, Mr. Toynbee has some good remarks upon the merely palliative action of mechanical measures and topical application here- "There arises a THIRD suggestion," he writes, "to ascertain the signification of this thickened mucous membrane, to make out what Nature may be endeavouring to effect by thickening it. And if the patient be a child, perchance it may be that Nature, through this thickened membrane, is endeavouring to rid Herself of the Scrofula taint ; or, if the patient be a middle-aged man it may be that Nature through this thickened membrane is endeavouring to rid Herself of the Gout poison. And if we address ourselves to the assistance of Nature, we shall, so to speak, ward off the necessity of her thickening the membrane ; this will then return to its natural state, the Eustachian tube will be opened by its muscles, and the Deafness disappear, in this case permanently."

This is the principle of our treatment of such cases. When the affection is recent—the relic of a catarrh—**Pulsatilla** will generally do all that is required to make the relief given by inflation permanent. In more chronic cases I have generally obtained such excellent result from *Iodine* (which I have given in the third decimal dilution) that I have felt it unnecessary to resort to any other remedy; but I would mention *Petroleum, Graphites* and *Manganum* as medicines which have been found useful and which are quite suited to the disorder. Jousset says he has had the best results from *Sepia*. In the Gouty cases of which Toynbee speaks, *Sulphur,* and perhaps *Hamamelis,* ought to be useful.

The following case will illustrate what *Iodine* can do in this affection, even without mechanical aid or local applications.

Miss L. æt. twenty-one, has always been somewhat deaf with the left ear. Her throat has been unhealthy for years past, the tonsils being large, and secreting much cheesy matter. In March, 1890, she had an attack of Acute Tonsillits which was subdued without proceding to suppuration by *Baryta carbonica*. A hoarse cough succeeded this attack, for which, on May 21st, I was asked to prescribe. She then told me that since the Quinsy, her right ear had been gradually becoming deaf like the left. She got *Hepar sulphuris* for the cough, and I did not see her again until June 7th, when an attendance began upon her sister, which lasted some weeks; and during this time I was able to treat Miss L. steadily for the Deafness, which had now become so great as entirely to exclude her from the conversation of the room. An examination with the ear-speculum showed there was nothing wrong with the tympanum or external meatus; and the whole history of the case pointed to the Eustachian mucous membrane as the seat of the obstructive mischief. A week of *Pulsatilla 2* having produced no effect, I put her upon *Iodine,* third decimal, two drops three times a day. In a few days a snap was felt in the ear, and the hearing for some hours became acute, but then the Deafness returned, though not to its former degree. Another similar report was followed by like results; and in the course of three or four weeks the hearing of the right ear became perfect. Nor was this all, but the left ear with which she had been deaf as long as she could remember, became much more sensitive to sound.

Toynbee draws a distinction between the "thickened" and the "relaxed" mucous membrane of the throat in this cases : and future observation may determine the relation between such varieties and the medicines I have mentioned.

Obstruction of the Eustachian tube at the tympanic orifice really belongs to the affections of the MIDDLE ear, to which I now return. The Pathological importance of this portion of the organ of hearing arises from its being lined by that offset of the pharyngeal mucous membrane which passing through the Eustachian tube, ends finally in the mastoid cells. The readiness of this membrane to take on inflammation under the influence of cold or of the Exanthemata—especially when, as in Scarlatina the throat itself is affected—makes its morbid states of frequent occurrence and prime importance,

Congestion, or sub-acute inflammation, of the tympanic mucous membrane appears to be, in most cases, the substratum of—

OTALGIA.—There is, doubtless, a truly Neuralgic Ear-ache, at any rate as sympathetic of Carious teeth, when **Chamomilla** (or **Plantago***) will at least give temporary relief. But this is rare as compared with the sub-inflammatory form. It is here that **Pulsatilla** plays another of its great parts in affections of the middle ear. Remembering that you are using it against a real lesion, and not a mere morbid sensation, you will not leave it off too soon when the pain is relieved. The membrane is apt to get permanently thickened by repeated attacks whose consequences are only partially removed.

Fully-developed inflammation of the tympanic mucous membrane I will speak of as—

TYMPANITIS.—This is the "OTITIS INTERNA" of the older authors ; and Hartmann is very strong upon the usefulness of **Pulsatilla** in checking its progress. He makes an exception only on behalf of *Belladonna* when consensual cerebral symptoms show the tendency of the inflammation to be inwards rather than outwards ; and Dr. Rafael Molin, of Vienna, endorses the choice of this latter medicine Dr. Copper follows Hartmann in thinking *Pulsatilla* the main remedy ; and Dr. Houghton agrees in commending it, even when the inflammation is suppurative from its origin, though he admits that it is still more effective in the catarrhal form, it being then rare that any other medicine is required. Should it need reinforcement here, it may find this form Schussler's **Ferrum phosphoricum**. Pulsating character of the pain is said to be a special indication for it. †

In the SUPPURATIVE form OTITIS MEDIA (as this inflammation might well be called) I agree with Molin that **Belladonna** should be the primary Antipyretic and Antiphlogistic. It may sometimes need the aid of **Aconite** in very acute cases, or where the general symptoms are those characteristic of this medicine and where the inflammation involves the mastoid cells, it has generally to give place to **Capsicum**, The symptom of Hahnemann's Pathogenesis, "On the patrous bone, behind the ear, a swelling painful to the touch", had attention called to it by Dr. Allen ; and Dr. Houghton as early as 1873 published cases showing its value in acute Mastoiditis. ✢ His later experience is fully corroborative, and I can join him in praising the remedy. It

---

* See M.H.R , xxxvii., 44 , xxxviii, 669.   † J.B.H.S. viii, 78
✢ See N. Y. JOURN, OF HOM., i., 61

has more than once enabled me to dispense with the free incision down to the bone recommended by most aurists—to which, however, you must always be prepared to resort if head-symptoms of grave character supervence. The same thing may be said of incision of the membrana tympani in case of Abscess forming within the cavity it bounds. **Hepar sulphuris** supercedes all other medicines in such a condition, and may sometimes avert the use of the bistoury; but do not let your patient suffer needlessly for want of it.

It is in the treatment of ACUTE inflammation of the middle ear that Homœopathy, by means of its specially-acting medicines, is at so great of advantage. When this condition comes before us in the chronic stage, it has yet to be proved that we can do as well by our attenuated internal remedies as the aurists of the old school with their local astringents and *Causties*. Dr. Searle, summing up in 1877 our position as regards Ophthalmology and Otology,* thought that we could rarely dispense with such aids; and the cases given by Dr. Houghton show that such has been his experience also. More especially is this so in Chronic Aural CATARRAH. There is generally inspissated mucus here in the tympanic cavity; and nothing seems better calculated to dissolve and dislodge it than the warm Alkaline applications ordinarily employed. In chronic suppuration of the middle ear, with perforation of the membrana tympani, injections for cleansing purposes as in Purulent Ophthalmia, are obviously necessary; but I think that they need not always be of an astringent character. There is sufficient evidence of the value of such medicines as *Colcarea*, *Hepar Sulphuris* (especially where the mischief is Post scarlatinæ), *Mercurius*, *Nitric acid* and *Silicee* † here to lead to their thorough trial when indicated; and there is nothing to prevent their being locally applied also ⚜ as in the eye. This would be more satisfactory practise than drying up the mucous membrane with *Zinc* or *Lead*. Besides these well-known remedies, attention should be given to two unusual ones—*Elaps coralinus* and *Tellurium*. The former is suitable when much naso-pharyngeal catarrh co-exists: the latter when the discharge is thin, acrid, and of disagreeable odour. When the still more offensive smell charrcteristic of necrosed bone is present, or when there is Caries of the Mastoid Process, besides *Mercurius* and *Nitric acid*, **Aurum** is indicated.

The cases of Otorrhœa which Dr. Copper has appended to the Second Edition of this book bear out these recommendations; and they add to the drugs I have mentioned. *Hydrastis* and

---

* See B.J.H., xxxv., 211.

† Or its congener "*Lapis albus.*" See J.B.H.S., ii., 224; viii., 79.

⚜ From Dr. Clifton's experience it seems that with *Calcarea* at least this may sometimes be done by snuffing up a trituration. See M.H.R., xxxiv., 200,

Natrum chloratum—the former acting best when the discharge is thick, the latter when it is thinner. The same thing. as regards ordinary remedies, may be said of the reports collected by Goullon from Homœopathic literature in the Journals referred to, and also in his Treatise on "Scrofulous Affections." Drs. Copper and Alexander* have each reported a case cured by *Thuja* : and the former, one where *Viola adorata* was effective. † There is thus no lack of successful experience on record, or of remedies to choose from. I cannot at psesent give you, established differential indications for these : their general action must be our main guide in their selection.

The remaining affections of the TYMPANUM come before us in connexion with deafness rather than as substantive affections : and under that heading, therefore, I will consider them.

In speaking of—

DEAFNESS, I am brought into the region of the INTERNAL EAR But I propose to take here a comprehensive view of this affection, as regards its treatment by medicines.

It is obvious that HARDNESS OF HEARING may be a concomitant of many of the aural disorders already mentioned ; and in this case it may be expected to subside with their cure. But on the other hand, it often comes before us without association with inflammation, discharge, pain, or obstruction of either the meatus externus or the Eustachian tube. We must here enquire into the exciting cause, which have come from without or from within.

1. Of the external exciting causes of Deafness the two most obvious are Concussion and Cold. When the former has operated, the most hopeful remedy is **Quinine**. The Deafness confessedly caused by large doses of this medicine appears to me to be brought about by an action on the auditory nerve very much resembling that of Concussion ; and it is probably to such an affection that Dr. Brown-Sequard refers when he naively remarks that it is curious that some forms of Deafness should be curable by *Quinine*, which so often causes it. Mr. Dalby thinks that in some of these cases (especially when the Concussion arises from a blow) there may be some effusion of blood within the labyrinth ; in which case you will think of **Arnica** †

J. B. H. S., i., 303. *IBID ii., 101

† See some cures with it, in substantial dosses, in Goullon's Essay (B. J. H., xxxi., 550.)

When exposure to Cold has been the exciting cause, we have a congestion present ; and **Aconite** in quite recent cases, **Belladonna** in those of longer-standing, may be expected to prove of good service Dr. Goullon cites some cases illustrating the power of the latter remedy.

2. When no such origin can be ascertained. the next inquiry to be made in whether the Deafness has followed upon any illness (such as the Continued Fever of which it is a well-known concomitant), or can be traced to mental or bodily exhaustion. In these eircumstances, and when the absence of substantive change leads you to set down the Deafness as "nervous", * you will often get excellent results from **Phosphoric acid**, to which *Anacardium* and *Ambra* may be useful adjuncts. Dr. Jousset speaks well of the Serpent-venoms—*Lachesis*, *Naja* and *Elaps*. When the deficiency is one of hearkening rather than of hearing, when noise is audible enough but the patient cannot distinguish the sounds of speech, a Paralytic state of the muscular apparatus of audition may be diagnosed, and **Causticum** given with advantage.

In the absence of sncn indications as these, we must fall back upon the patient's diathesis. If he is Scrofulous, it may be that he has the hypertrophy of the mucous membrane of the tympanum described by Toynbee, causing the drum of the ear to resist the passage of the sonnd-waves. Here *Caclearea* may be given with every hope of benefit. It would appear that this condition may also be set up by the suppression of an eruption on the scalp, as in a case recorded by Carroll Dunham, ✛ in which a complete cure was effected bp *Mezereum*, as being the remedy most Homœopathic to the eruption itself. If the patient is Rheumatic or Gouty, or the subject of Rheumatoid Arthritis, a graver prognosis must be given. There may be here, Mr. Toynbee says, either rigidity of the tympanic membrane, or Ankylosis of the ossicles, especially of the base of the stapes to the fenestra ovalis.* The former he considers THE cause of Deafness in advancing years '; If any good can be done under such circvmstances, it might be by *Sulphur* or *Kali iodatum*. Lastly, there is a Syphilitic Deafness, which may cither appear in the course of the secondary stage of the acquired disease, or in the subjects of its inherited influence. In the one case it will subside with the symptoms it accompanies ; in the other it is rebellious to the most potent Anti-syphilitics of the ordinary practicc, and we have no experience of our own to offer.

A good deal of fresh informativn has since I wrote what I

---

* The Deafuess apt to follow Cerebro-spinal Meningitis is said to be due to suppuration within the labyrinth. Dr. Searle has succeeded in checking an incipient ease ; *Silicea* was his chief remedy.

✛ See "Homœopathy the Science of Therapeutic," p. 462.

have just enunciated, been brought to bear on Deafness and it' treatment.—mainly from the fertile brain and industrious pen of Dr. Copper. He divides it into obstructive (whether from the meatus or the Eustachian tube). Nervous, and Vascular—including under the last term all those cases hitherto called "Sclerotic" or "Proliferous," and set down to stiffness of the conducting media. He has published a special treatise on this form of the trouble,* which is well-worth reading. The most useful medicine for it he considers to be the *Ferrum picricum*, which he seems to give in about the 3, dilution ; but it requires long-continued treatment. Pure Nervous Deafness he finds more amenable to *Gelsemium* and *Magnesia carbonica*—the former low, the latter high—than any other remedies. In a Paper presented to the International Congress of 1896, he described a fourth form of Deafness which may be called Nutritional,—occurring in growing children and often congenital ; in this he gets striking results from *Calcarea carbonica*, in high attenuation.

In the discussion which followed Dr. Copper's Paper, Mr. Dudley Wright, while recognising the value of *Calcarea* in the subjects indicated, would also mention *Mercurius biniodatus* when an inherited Syphilitic taint was present. The Transactions which contain these meterials have also a study and repertory of the drugs which have caused Deafness by Dr. Hayward, senr., from which oftentimes a remedy may be drawn.

I have lastly to speak, among affections of the external ear. of TINNITUS AURIUM.—I know of course that in many cases noises in the ears are due to affections of the tympanum or its cavity, even to those of meatus and the Eustachian tube, and will subside on their removal. But even here they are probably due to pressure, through the membrane of the senestra ovalis, upon the fluid contained in the labyrinth ; and there are many instances in which no such external cause can be found, and we must think of the seat of mischief as being that sequestered and sinuous cavern in which the auditory nerve lies dispread till the waves of sound break upon it. Some congestion, some irritation, some spontaneous undulation of the water-cushion on which its fibres rest, makes it thrill continuously or intermittingly ; and we have the roaring, humming, buzzing, ringing of

---
* "Baeic Aural Dyscrasia and Vascular Deafness." London : Balliere Tindal and Cox, 1886.

which our patients so often complain, and of which our drug-pathogeneses are so full.

There is, I say, plenty of caused Tinnitus in the Materia Medica, but there is not a corresponding fulness in the record of cured Tinnitus in Homœopathic literatnre. It is time that we set ourselves to fill up this gap. The way has been smoothed for us from the clinical and Pathological side. Hitherto the treatment of the subject in aural treatises has been of the scantiest and vaguest character ; but Dr. Woakes' original little book on "Deafness, Giddiness and Noises in the Head" is full of information and suggestion. We want a corresponding study from the pathogenetic side, whica our own school alone is capable of adequately furnishing ; and then, reaching by medicinal affinities the parts so shut off from topical treatment, we might be able to still the noises so many unfortunates carry over with them, and steep their sense in blessed silence. The drugs which most notably cause this symptom when over-acting, *Quinine* and the *Salicylica*, have hardly, 1 fancy, proved so effective in its treatment as might have been expected : they have certainly on the whole disappointed me. We perhaps need to know their action more minutely ; but we must also investigate that of the *Bisulphide of-Carbon*, *of Chenopodium*, *of Coca* ' and of a number of other substances ere we have full material for coping with Tinnitus.

In such stndies we shall, certainly in the case of the two first-named drugs, probably in that of others, come upon associated symptoms which remind us of

MENIERE'S DISEASE, or, as it is now more appropriately called, LARYRINTHINE VERTIGO. There may be no history of sudden giddy falling and immediate setting-in of Deafness and Tinnitus, such as the French observer had described as resulting from hæmorrhagic exudation into the labyrinth ; and yet it is plain that the contribution made by the auditory nerves to the equilibrating function of the cerebellum is in some way hindered—supended altogether or transmitted fallaciously. When it is so—when with impaired hearing and subjective sounds we have more or less giddiness, the essential condition is there however incipient and unorganized, which Meniere wrote of as it is in its full development. It is just here, as with nervous disease generally, that we can catch it with the best hope of effecting improvement. It is encouraging to us, but curious in itself, that the only substantial benefit reported in the old school therapeutics of this disease has been obtained with the very drugs I have mentioned as causing most of its symptoms. Charcot found good results from *Quinine*, and Sir William Gowers has had reason to commend in print the *Salicylate of Soda*. That our own men should do this, that McClatchey and and Dyce Brewn * should have published cases of the kind treated successfully with the *Salicylate*, is not surprising ; but why Sir William should have chosen the drug for the disease, while ignoring the Law of Similars, does not seem obvious. Perhaps it was an instance of the same unconscious cerebration as that which we heard of sometime ago,—when, wanting an alternative metal to *Arsenie* for the pains of Locomotor Ataxy, he stumbled quite by accident upon such an unusual one as *Aluminium*.

At the same Congress I have just mentioned, Dr. Dudley Wright contributed a Paper on this affection, which he called "Aural Vertigo."✝ *Bryonia* and *Aurum* were the medicines most commended by him. In the subsequent discussion, Drs. Dudgeon, Clifton and McClelland expressed themselves entirely satisfied with *Quinine* and *Salicylic acid*, in medium dilutions ; and successes with *Conium*, *Silicea* and *Tabacum* were mentioned.

Dr. Cooper was not one of the speakers on this occasion, but in his Essay on Deafness he has mentioned some interesting experience with *Kali iodatum*, which he generally gives as high as the 30th. It is simple Tinnitus, with little or no Deafness, that he finds it most useful ; and this brings us back from Meniere's symptoms to noises in the ears themselves. Isolated cures have been reported from *Carbon Sulphuratum* ✝ and *Graphites* ; $ but the only claim to constant action comes from the old school, in the shape of *Hydrobromic acid* and our own *Actaea racemosa* ‖ — both given in much larger doses than we ordinarily care to administer. Dr. Winslow finds drop doses of the former drug sufficient and Dr. Olive has had good results from the 1x dilution of the latter. ¶

---

* HAHN. MONTHLY,. xiii.,89 ; M. H, R., xxii., 625, 591.
✝ See M. H. R., xl., 666 $ B, J. H. xvii., 279. * J.B.H.S., vi, 11
‖ IBID., p. 391. ✝ IBID., viii., 250.

LECTURE XXXIII

DISEASES OF THE DIGESTIVE ORGANS

—o—

THE MOUTH, THROAT- AND OESOPHAGUS

—o—

STOMATITIS—FŒTOR ORIS—GLOSSITIS—ULCERS OF THE TONGUE
—SYPHILIS OF THE TONGUE—CANCER OF THE TONGUE—
TOOTHACHE—GUMBOIL—MUMPS—SALIVATION—RANULA—ANGINA
LUDOVICI—ANGINA FAUCIUM—QUINSY—ENLARGED TONSILS—
CHRONIC PHARYNGITIS—OESOPHAGITIS—SPASMODIC
STRICTURE OF OESOPHAGUS

I begin to-day the study of diseases of the DIGESTIVE ORGANS. This is very comprehensive title : but it enables us to carry our thoughts along the whole alimentary canal, from the MOUTH to the ANUS, taking in also the GLANDS associated with it in function. We begin to-day with affections of the MOUTH and its contents.

And first of the MOUTH itself. Most of the forms of STOMATITIS are diseases of children, and will come for detailed consideration under this heading. I will anticipate their subsequent treatment, however, by saying that they are controlled with us practically by four medicines=**Borax**, **Kali chloricum**, **Mercurius** and **Nitric acid**. These correspond, roughly speaking, to Aphthous, Ulcerative, Scorbutic and Mercurio-syphilitic inflammations of the oral mucous membrane, leaving **Arsenicum** in reserve for the formidable, but happily rare, Gangrenous variety —the "NOMA" or CANCRUM ORIS" of the old Nomenclature. In respect of the first two we are on common ground with our old-school colleagues, and so far as *Borax* is concerned might— at any rate provisionally—have at one time awarded the remedy to them on principle as well as by right of discovery. There was no sufficient evidence that it had ever caused anything like Thrush ; the disease itself appeared to be a parasitic one, the product of the Oidium Albicans ; and any non-irritant Antiseptic seemed as good for it as *Borax*, which undoubtedly exerts such action, and might thus be conceived to effect its cures. So lately as 1895٭ an American colleague, Dr. F. H. Pritchard, has argued the matter in this sense, relating a case which recovered far more quickly when *Boracic acid* (8 grains to the ounce) was substituted for the *Sodic biborate* as the local application. Already, however, I had alleged on the other side ✢ that "small

---

٭ See HAHN, MONTHLY of August in that year.
✢ 'Pharmacodynamics,' 4th Ed. (1880), p. 311.

doses— say grains of the first trituration, given internally, will cure the disease nearly, if not quite as rapidly as when local application is employed" ; and the use of *Borax*, at Sir William Gowers' instigation, as an Anti-epileptic has materially enriched its Pathogenesis, in which we now find sore lips and denudation at points of the epithelium of the tongue.* This is so near to Aphthous inflammation of the continuous lining of the mouth that the possibility of *Borax* being Homœopathic here cannot be denied.

In the case of *Chlorate of Potash*, Homœopathicity ought to be frankly admitted. The drug is "almost a specific" in Ulcerative Stomatitis, writes Mr. Stanley Boyd in Quain's Dictionary but he does not say why ; he does not face the question whether this, like other specifics, obeys the law SIMILA SIMILIBIS, and has been or might have been discovered by means of it. Actually, indeed, its employment in Sore Mouths, so often indicative of depressed conditions of the system, seems to have resulted from Chemical considerations based on the large amount of Oxygen it contains. But the observations of Hutchinson and Trail ✤ soon showed that no such action, nor (as later suggested) any local influence, need be Invoked to account for its efficacy. The drug readily causes Ulcerative Stomatitis when given for other affections : hence its power of curing it when it occurs Idiopathically, "affecting," as Watson argues in favour of giving *Strychina* in Tetanus; "those parts and those functions of the mouth "which are affected in Stomatitis," "and so likely to occasion a morbid action in the mouth" "which would supercede the morbid action of the disease, and yet be less harmful and more manageable. The ONUS PROBANDI of its acting in any other way plainly belongs to our opponents, and they cannot even derive an argument from the dosage required. "It appears that in this affection," writes Still, "the size of dose is not always a measure of its efficacy ; two or three grains, and twenty or thirty grains, in different cases appear to have been equally efficient." ✤✤

Curiously enough, though *Kali chloricum* is thus so highly esteemed and so justly claimed as our own, Homœopathy seems practically to take little account of it. Neither Bahr nor Jousset

---

* Cycl. of drug Path., iv., 519. IBID., iii., 54.

✤✤ Dr. Stille is not so candid as to the other part of the subject. "It is a curious and interesting fact." he writes, "that occasionally *Chlarate of Potash*, produces ulceration of the mouth when administered for diseases in which the buccal mucous membrane is unaffected." After citing authorites, he goes on, "These facts prove that the medicine is a powerful stimulant (!), and that it is curative of the various diseases in which it is administered in virtue of its stimuant power." This is the first time we have heard of ulceration being an evidence that stimulation is being exerted ; nor would the idea have been expressed, I fancy, but for the need of evading the admission of its Homœopathicity.

mentions it among the medicines appropriate to Stomatitis. For myself, in the Ulcerative form I never think of anything else ; and though I should ordinarily depend on *Nitric acid* for the buccal ulcers of Mercury or Syphilis, and on *Mercurius* itself or *Arsenicum* for Cancrum Oris, I should always hold *Kali chloricum* behind these in reserve. In an epidemic of the latter form of the disease which occurred at the Half Orphan Asylum at Five Points, New York, they were losing their cases fast till they began its use, and thence forward had most srtisfactory results.

Chlorate of Potash ought to be acknowledged Homœopathic to Stomatitis, but *Mercury* must be. Yes, our opponents may say, but which of us would think of employing it ? Curiously enough, some of the best observations we have of the value of *Mercury* in Cancrum Oris come from an eminent old school physician, Dr. Duncan, of Dublin. He is himself astonished that the sloughing here, so far from getting worse under the use of the drug, is actually controlled by it ; yet he cannot but admit the fact. *Mercury* is suitable here ; but is no less so in Simple Erythematous Stomatitis. It would be so in the scorbutic form, save that here the proper change of diet is the one important thing ; but it is very useful in conditions of the mouth allied to this, when a low state of system leads to inflammation there, rapidly spreading and readily ulcerating. In such cases there is generally a thickly-coated but moist tongue, fœtor of breath, and perhaps a sweet taste in the mouth. In this it is contrasted with a drug closely allied to it locally, though not possessing its dissolvent and putrefying influence : I speak of *Nitric acid*. This too, even when applied externally only, causes Stomatitis and salivation, but without fœtor. It is thus more suitable still than *Mercury* itself when Syphilis invades the mouth. The tongue indicating it tends to be red and even glazed. Therapeutically, it has shown good power of dealing with the ulcerative phenomena of this and other morbid states ; and though itself has not proved capable of producing such change. the latter has resulted from its combination with *Hydrochloric acid*. "At length," says Scott in describing the effects of prolonged bathing or sponging with this, "little speaks or small ulcerations, quite superficial, are seen on the interior of the mouth and over the tongue, so that some degree of excoriation or rawness is at last produced." The *Nitro-muriatic acid* seems to be quite a TERTIUM QUID. Its value in Oxaluria was substantiated by the older physicians, though - like many other clinical facts—it is being obscured by the newer Pathological doctrines coming into vogue ; and the compound *acid* deserves further proving and testing at our hands.

I have preferred approaching diseases of the mouth from the side of drugs, the more because their Nosology seems hardly

---

* In the Article on the *Oxalic acid* diathesis in Quain's Dictienary, the remedy is not even mentioned.

settled. While with us "Aphthæ" mean the lesions of Thrush, the French Pathologists use the name to denote the minute ulcers resulting from the vesicles of what we call Folicular or Vesicular Stomatitis—the remedy for which, I should say, is *Rhus*. I have used the British phraseology here ; and where I have elsewhere connected the French "Muguet" with anything but Thrush, I must apologise for and withdraw the identification.

FOETOR ORIS may sometimes come before you as the main trouble calling for treatment. If it be flatus or mucus that has the odour, you will think of **Carbo vegetabilis** ; but in default of any such localisation should give your patient the benefit of **Aurum**. You will find cases showing the value of these two remedies in the Second (p. 353) and fourth (p. 331) Volumes of the JOURNAL OF THE BRITISH HOMOEOPATHIC SOCIETY. *Capsicum* and *Arnica* are possible alternatives.

The LIPS present little for medicinal treatment, since Herpes Labialis and Hypertrophy of the Upper Lip are symptomatic affections only. I may mention that the presence of the former is considered both in Intermittent Fever and in common Catarrh (not, I think, in Pneumonia) to call for *Natrum muriaticum*, and that of the latter in Scrofula to indicate *Sepia*. FOETRIS PARIBUS must of course be understood in either case. Cracks in the corners of the lips are often removable by *Cundurango*. Cancer of the lips, which is always of the epithelial variety, and so less intractable, has (as I have mentioned when speaking of the disease in general) been cured by *Arsenic*.

The TONGUE is the seat of acute Inflammation, of Ulceration, of Syphilis and of Cancer. And, first, of—

GLOSSITIS.—This rapid and formidable disease is well under the control of Homœopathic remedies, without the need of the incisions, and of old time leeches, considered indispensable in the old school. A case of Dr. Guinness's in the Fifth Volume of the BRITISH JOURNAL OF HOMOEOPATHY illustrates my statement. The remedies were *Belladonna* 3 alternated every hour with *Mercurius* 5. The description of the patient, twenty-four hours after the initial rigor, is as follows ; "the whole tongue was enormously swollen ; it nearly filled the cavity of the mouth, so that it was quite impossible to see the throat, but the tonsils externally felt enlarged, and were painful to the touch ; face very red and swollen, headache, pulse 100, full ... ... The surface of the tongue was coated white, but the point, and edges, and inferior surface were deep red, glossy, tense, and shining. His skin wcs burning hot, and he had passed a very restless night." Swallowing and speaking were almost impossible through the pain thereby occasioned. Improvement began almost immediately ; and in forty eight hours, hardly a trace of the illness remained. The Homœopathicity of the **Mercurius** here is indubitable ; but in so frankly inflammatory an affection it will generally need reinforcement by **Belladonna** or **Aconite**.

There is an acute œdema of the tongue which is rather urticarious than inflammatory. It is due to the ingestion of some offending article of diet ; and, if the time is passed for an Emetic, might be treated with advantage by **Apis**.

It should also be stated that if Glossitis is the effect of a Burn or Scald, *Cantharis* may be its most suitable remedy.

ULCERS OF THE TONGUE require and yield to the same treatment (*Mercurius* and *Nitric acid*) as that of Ulcers of the Mouth, with which they are Pathologically identical.* I think however, that *Muriatic* is preferable to *Nitric acid* here. A very obstinate form of ulceration of the tonge is one that appears at the tip, and frequently recurs after healing. If the application of *Caustic* is ever necessary it is to these troublesome and painful little sores.

SYPHILIS OF THE TONGUE often appears in the form of superficial ulceration, when there will rarely be need to depart from the *Mercurius*, or *Nitric acid*, or both, already recommended for simple ulcers. The *Bichromate* (or *Chromate*) *of Potash* should be borne in mind in severe or obstinate cases. Another form of Syphilis of the Tongue is the 'Chronic Interstitial Inflammation" described in Quain's Dictionary, presenting deep fissures and hypertrophied papillæ. This condition appears generally to be secondary to gummatous infiltration, and is, consequently treated in the old school with full doses of *Iodide of Potassium*. If Professor Langston Parker is right, however the prolonged used of this drug may bring the tongue into just such a hypertrophied, tender, fussured and lobulated state ; so that we might find benefit from smaller quantities. For myself, taking a hint from a case of Dr. Laurie's in the Twenty-Fourth Volume of the BRITISH JOURNAL OF HOMŒOPATHY (p. 154). I have relied on **Fluoric acid** in this local manifestation of Syphilis.

---

* "Ulcers of the Tongue resulting from the action of *Mercury* are usually associated with similar ulcerations of the gums" (Aitken).

† See EDINB MEDICAL JOURNAL, 1852, p. 379.

TOOTHACHE

CANCER OF THE TONGUE, being also (like that of the mouth) invariably epithelial, ought to be somewhat under medicinal control. I have mentioned, when speaking of **Muriatic acid** some facts pointing in this direction ; and under **Kali cyanatum** have given a long-ago case of Dr. Petroz', where malignant ulceration and induration of the organ got quite well under the *1*st trituration, a grain every fourth day. In the JOURNAL BELGE D'HOMŒOPATHIE for March-April, 1887, Dr. Mersch records a similar case to the last. He alternated with the *Kali cyanatum*, *Muriatic acid* of the same strength, and applied the second trituration of the former to the sore. In a fortnight cicatrization was complete.

I have next to speak of troubles arising from the TEETH. Reserving morbid DENTITION till I come to the Diseases of Children, I shall speak here of TOOTHACHE from its various causes, and of GUMBOIL.

There are FOUR leading forms under which—

TOOTHACHE appears ; and under these heads, I think we may class most of the medicines of real use in its treatment.

FIRST, there is the ache which accompanies Caries of the Teeth. If there is any exposure of the pulp, "stopping" of some kind is of course essential. But with or without this procedure, you will generally (at least that is my experience) earn the thanks of your patient if you give him *Kreosote* in the *12*th dilution to take frequently until he is relieved, and then continue it twice a day or so as a prophylactic. Jahr speaks as highly of **Chamomilla** *30*, by a single dose of which (he says) he has removed the Toothache of a number of persons, the tooth subsequently decaying without a return of the pain.

NEXT, there is the burning, throbbing misery of inflammation of the dental pulp. Here, I think, you will find **Belladonna** specific ; and this also has served me best in the medium and higher dilution.

THIRDLY, there is a "RHEUMATIC" Toothache, apparently situated in the periosteum of the jaws, but produced by cold and without tendency to Gumboil. This is what is commonly called "FACE-ACHE." **Pulsatilla** is the remedy most frequently effectual here ; but *Broynia*, *Mercurius* or *Chamomilla* may be required, and I am myself rather partial to *Rhododendron*.

LASTLY, Toothache may be NEURALGIC. To afford immediate relief, give *Chamomilla* where the patient's nerves seem unable to endure the pain, *Coffea* where there is much temporary relief from the application of cold, *Aconite* when the circulation is excited. In default of these special indications, or where they fail to bring victory, much reliance may be placed on *Pantago*.

There are numerous testimonies to its efficacy. * Three doses of a low dilution, at hourly intervals, are generally all that is required.

An excellent Toothache Repertory is given by Jahr, to which you will do well to refer for more minute symptomatic indications.

By the familiar name of—

GUMBOIL, I understand an inflammation of the alveolar and neighbouring periosteum tending speedily to Abscess. It is generally, if not always, caused by the irritation of a tooth so far gone from its original rightcousness as to be incapable of restoration; and hence the remedy must be the extraction of the offender. But when the inflammation is actually set up, and yet taken early, I think I can promise you that you may cut it short by repeated doses of the first dilution of *Aconite* and *Belladonna*. In circumstances, moreover, where from any cause extraction is undesirable, **Phosphorus** seems to exert a marked effect in subduing the irritation, and preventing the recurrence of the Abscesses.

The SALIVARY GLANDS are so closely connected with the mouth that their morbid conditions must fall to be considered here.

Inflammation of the parotid gland may occur in connexion with Typhus, Scarlatina, or other acute infections. I have mentioned its treatment when speaking of the two diseases named. But it is best known as the primary and principal feature of the curious epidemic and contagious affection we call.—

MUMPS.—It is possible that patients affected with this malady would get well as rapidly without, as with any medicine. Nevertheless, I think that they suffer less if they are kept on **Mercurius** throughout, with *Aconite* if they be feverish. In the so-called Metastasis to the testicles or mammæ, **Pulsatilla** is of decided benefit.

SALIVATION, when occurring as part of the Mercurial Sore-Mouth, now (happily) rarely met with, will demand such antidotes to the metal as **Iodine** and **Nitric acid** rather than the *Chlorate of Potash*. In Idiopathic salivation these medicines,

---

* INTER ALIA, See J.B.H.S., iv., 337; ix., 180.

and **Mercurius** itself, are obviously indicated; and have been known to cure. Hartmann and Jahr speak highly of *Dulcamara* in cases where the affection seems to have been caused by cold; and Jousset gives indications for *Pulsatilla, Euphorbium* and *Sulphur*. The alkaloids *Pilocarpia*, and *Muscaria* are found to be such powerful sialogogues that they ought to be useful in some forms of Ptyalism; perhaps, as they act through the nerves regulating the secretion, they may help us when the affection is sympathetic, as in pregnancy. Dr. Jousset says that he already owes several successes in Salvition to the former of the two.

RANULA must be mentioned here, though it is doubtful whether the forms of it which have been found curable by medicine are connected with Wharton's Duct. A swelling having all the character of Ranula may arise from dilatation a mucous folicle or bursa. But however this may be, Jahr and Kafka speak of success with *Mereurius*, and the latter of similar results from *Calcarea*; while Dr. Gibbs Blake reports a case cured by **Thuja**, and refers to four others.*

ANGINA LUDOVICI is the inflammation, threatening Abscess and Gangrene, of the cellular tissue investing salivary glands, which was first described by the physician after whom it is named. Bahr describes it as "PAROTITIS MALIGNA." The only Homœopathic experience with it known to me as on record is that of Schweickert, who found the ordinary remedies useless in his first case, but cured the next three with *Anthracine*, a preparation made from the pus of Malignant Pustule. I have myself seen one case, occurring in connexion with Syphilitic Angina; it made a good recovery under *Bryonia* and *Hepar sulphuris*.

The next division of the alimentary canal is the THROAT. This is indeed a Pathological, rather than an Anatomical or Physiological entity, comprising as it does, parts so diverse from one another and so blended with their neighbours as the soft plate with the uvula, the tonsils, and the pharynx. The throat, thus understood is liable to be involved in Erysipelas and Variola, and presents special phenomena under the influence of Scarlatina and Syphilis; it is often also invaded by Aphthæ. The treatment of these affections has been or will be discussed under their appropriate heads. I shall here consider Catarrhal SORE-THROAT; QUINSY and ENLARGEMENTS OF THE TONSILS; and CHRONIC PHARYNGITIS. The first I will call—

ANGINA FAUCIUM.—The mucous membrane of the throat

---

* M. H, R., xii., 583.

is frequently inflamed from the usual causes of Catarrh. This is quite a distinct affection from true Quinsy (Amygdalitis), with which it is often confounded. It shows itself under several forms. The membrane may be highly inflamed, without much swelling. Here **Belladonna** displays those wonderful powers which has given it such repute in throat affections, and which are now being rediscovered in the old school of medicine. You have probably already tested its value ; but you may confirm your faith by consulting the authorities collected by Dr. Imbert-Gourbeyre in the Fourteenth Volume of the BRITISH JOURNAL OF HOMOEOPATHY. You will there see, moreover, that it occasionally needs the aid of *Aconite*, when there is much excitement of the general circulation and elevation of temperature.

The presence of ulcers is no contra-indication to this treatment by *Belladonna*, with or without *Aconite*, if they are on an inflamed base and very painful. It is only when the inflammation is of a low grade, with tendency to general ulceration, that **Mercurius** is preferable. For one case in which I see indications for its use, I see twenty in which *Belladonna* is the true simile ; and I do not remember a single one which seemed to call for the routine alternation of the two.

There is yet another form of Acute Sore Throat. When you examine the fauces, you find general OEDEMA of the sub-mucous cellular tissue covering the tonsils, uvula, soft palate, and even the posterior portion of the hard palate. It looks almost as if a bee had flown in and stung the patient there. I am repeating what I have already said under the head of **Apis**, when I tell you that you will find this medicine invaluable here.

Less common forms of Acute Angina Catarrhalis are the Rheumatic, the Pultaceous or Follicular and the Nervous. The first, characterized by much pain and stiffness of the external muscles, calls for **Aconite**, and rarely requires any other medicine. For the third, where the pain (generally of an aching kind) is out of all proportion to the inflammation present I cannot speak too highly of **Lachesis**. The second, in which the mucous crypts of the tonsils pour out their secretion, and whitish patches (often supposed to be Diphtheritic) form on the mucous surface, you may give *Belladonna*, *Apis* or *Mercurius* If the character of inflammation seems to demand it ; but I think you will get still more satisfaction from **Phytolacca**. Where spotty throats occur, with probably much fever and pain in back and limbs, but without the worst symptoms of Diphtheria, *Phytolacca* will verify its repute as an Anti-diphtheritic. I have shown this in my 'Pharmacodynamics' ; and am interested to find, in the Article on Follicular Sore Throat in Quain's Dictionary, the statement—'occasionally this affection appears to be contagious, and to attack one member of a family after another. In such cases examination of the contents of the crypts of the tonsils has revealed the presence of the Staphylococcus or Strepto-coccus Pyogenes.

Gangrenous or Malignant Sore-Throat I apprehend to be always connected with Scarlatina, and I must refer you to what I have said of this malady for suggestions as to its remedies.

In the tonsils we have an element in the throat-structure analogous to the salivary glands in the mouth, and conceivably calling for other remedies when inflamed than those which control the mucous surface. I know that *Belladonna* and *Mercurius* are much used by our practioners in—

QUINSY ; and as the tonsils are largely formed of an involution of the lining membrane of the fauces, there is no reason why these tried remedies for Catarrhal Anginæ should not follow up their seat into these recesses. But the tonsils are something more than this ; and when, as often heppens, the mischief is parenchymatous from the outset, a special class of remedies may reasonably be invoked. The large supply of blood these glands receive, and the high fever which they ordinarily excite when inflamed, show that **Aconite** may profitably commence the treatment of most Quinsies. But if resolution has not commenced within twenty-four hours, I counsel the use of **Baryta carbonica**. If you will look at the the Paper read by Dr. Edward Madden at our Congress of 1890, * and the discussion following, you will find a general cosensus as to its abortive power here when its use is begun in good time. If S. 279 of Hahnemann's Pathogenesis in the 'Chronic Diseases' can be depended on, the action is a demonstrably Homœopathic one ; but even without this the minute doses with which it can be effected strongly is **Guaiacum**. Its claims come from men of the old school, ✝ and there is little in its meagre Pathogenesis to vouch for its being Homœopathic to the malady. The late Dr. Ozanam, however, has shown † covincing evidence that it acts well in throat-inflammations in at least the 1st and 2nd decimal dilutions. His cases were, perhaps, more of general Angina, including the tonsils, ✝ than of primary Amygdalitis itself ; but it is noteworthy that one of his patients, in whom on two occasions he rapidly cured such a throat, had in the interval between them, when out of his reach, an attack apparently of the same kind, which treated by leches and purgatives went on for nine days, and then ended in Abscess.

In acute Tonsillitis, Homœopathy thus comes out triumphant ;

---

* M. H .R., 1891, p. 172. † See Stille, "Therapeutics," sub VOSE.

† Trans. of Int. Hom. Convention, 1886 p. 238. See also Evans in J.B.H.S., ix, 100.

✝ Here Dr. Ivins and Dr. Goodno bear him out (see J. B. H. S., ii, 97).

but it is with more bated breath that she must speak of her power over hypertrophy of these glands.

ENLARGED TONSILS are very resistant to treatment. I agree with Dr. Copper, * that in certain cases there is a history of repeated attacks of inflammation, while in others—perhaps more numerous—the enlargement seems to be a primary hypertrophy : and I go further with him in believing *Calcarea phosphorica* to be a valuable remedy for the latter form, capable of removing also the adenoid growths which often accompany it ⚜ and the Deafness which they and it alike may cause. I hardly think, however, that he has been as happy in his choice of *Iodide of Mercury* in the other variety. The *Biniodide* is, to my mind, preferable ; and the *Iodide of Barium* better still. † When all is said, however, the medicinal treatment of Enlarged Tonsils is a slow affair, and it would argue no lack of faith in the method of Hahnemann if *Caustics* or operative measures were preferred.

Another very obstinate affection is —

CHRONIC PHARYGITIS, the Follicular or Granular Angina of professional, the "Clergyman's Sore-Throat" of popular Nomenclature. Some preparation of **Mercurius** has generally been relied upon in Homœopathic practice for the treatment of this affection. *Cinnabar* has cured it ; but since Dr. G. W. Cook, in America and Dr. Black, in England, published their experiences with the *Iodide, Mercury* has mostly been given in this form, as you may see from a discussion on the subject at the British Homœopathic Society, initiated by Dr. Edward Blake. $ The lower triturations seem most in favour. You will see that *Antimonium tartaricum* and *Kali bichromicum* also are commended.

While with medicines such as these you are exerting an alterative effect upon the morbid mucous membrane of the throat, you may do a good deal with intercurrent remedies to relieve the subjective symptoms which are nearly always present. **Lachesis** is the chief of these, as I have mentioned when speaking of it. Another is **Capsicum**, which is very useful when the throat is red and hot, and much dry cough is prsent.

Where a Chronic Sore-Throat is obviously the expression of

---

* M.H.R., xi., 546. ⚜ See J.B.H.S., ii, 479.
† IBID., iii., 329 ; iv., 128 ; vii., 227. $ B.J.H., xxxii, 287.

an unhealthy state of the general system (Gouty, Hæmorrhoidal, or Herpetic), **Sulphur** is its best remedy; and *Belladonna* may be given with advantage intercurrently, as recommended by Dr. Jousset. There are also other medicines which occasionally find place in the treatment of chronic morbid conditions of the faucial mucous membrane, among which I may mention *Acidum oxalicum*, *Æsculus*, *Alumina*, *Arum* and *Ignatia*. The indications for each are those mentioned in my 'Pharmocdynamics.' *Alumina* should be especially useful in the "rarefing dry catarrh" described by Wendt.* Dr. Dyce Brown, in a Article on "Follicular Pharyngitis" in the MONTHLY HOMŒOPATHIC REVIEW of 1877, give indications and recommendations regarding *Æsculas*, *Hepar sulphuris*, *Lachesis*. and *Kali bichromicum*; and in the same number of the Journal, Dr. Clifton relates a series of recent cases occurring within a few days of one another, in which the first-named medicine proved the specific remedy. Schussler's *Calcarea fluorata* seems to be remedial where plugs of mucus are continually forming in the tonsillar mucous glands. ✢

A very few words need be said on the affections of the OESOPHAGUS. Inflammation of this canal—

OESOPHAGITIS—is of very rare occurrence, save from the swallowing of corrosive substances. There is a case of it in Dr. Hale's "New Remedies," sub voce, *Gelsemium*, and apparently induced by that drug, *Phosphorus* was here curative remedy after *Arsenicum* had failed.

SPASMODIC STRICTURE OF THE OESOPHAGUS.— (appropriately called by Jousset "ŒSOPHAGISMUS".) *Ignatia* would be the most obvious medicine; but I have more than once obtained such excellent results from **Naja** as to be inclined to count it the principal remedy for the affection. Dr. Cartier and others have had success with *Baptisia*. ✢✢ *Belladonna* has cured some cases.

---

*Ziemssen's Cyclopædia, Vol. vii, ✢ J. B. H. S., viii., 155.
✢✢ Ibid., ii., 218.

LECTURE XXXIV

DISEASES OF THE DIGESTIVE OGRANS

(*Continued.*)

—o—

THE STOMACH

—o—

GASTRITIS—ULCER OF THE STOMACH—CANCER OF THE STOMACH—GASTRALGIA—ACUTE INDIGESTION—CHRONIC DYSPEPSIA—PAIN AFTER FOOD—ACIDITY—HEART-BURN—WATER-BRASH—FLATULENCE—VOMITING—HAEMATEMESIS

I come now to disordsrs of the STOMACH, which from the importance of that organ to the nutrition and the comfort of the body, concern the physician to an extent quite disproportionate to its size. That Homœopathy can do much for such disorders when they occur, I shall show immediately; but I want first to emphasize the faet that they hardly ever should occur. The stomach is so situated that it is very little affected by the most common causes of disease—Cold and Mechanical Injury. Its function, the reception and coction of food, is so fully provided for; its capacity is so elastic, its secretory activity and peristaltic movements are so active, that it is equal to all reasonable dcmands upon it. Save when its venous circulation is obstructed, as by Heart Disease, or its physical integrity is impaired, as by ulcer or Cancer, it should carry on digestion regularly, painlessly, thoroughly, absorbing such of the food as will enter its veins and passing on the rest through the pylorus in a proper state, for assimilation or further peptic change, and this with VESTIGIA NULLA RETRORSUM—annoying us with no "returns" of any kind. If it behaves otherwise, it is nearly always our fault; the stomach is disordered only by what we put into it. We have eaten too often, if we are young; too much at a time (that is, for our digestive powers), if we are old; in either case, we have eaten too fast for thorough comminution and insalivation of our food. We have irritated our gastric mucous membrane with Alcohol and pungent condiments; we have over-heated it with scalding drinks or chilled it with ices. These are the confessions we have to make, if we are Dyspeptic; and the conviction of sin in the matter is the first step to loosing from its consequences. It is the first step, and it is the primary requisite. No medication, however carefully chosen will set the stomach right if these errors are persisted in; and on the other hand, if they be corrected, Nature has great power of righting Herself without further aid. The somewhat

THE STOMACH

rigid dietary of early Homœopathic days probably played no small part in the success of the new treatment. It was prescribed with the idea that our delicate medicines might be interfered with by anything but the simplest aliment. We have found them more hardy than we thought; but the rest which our dietetic restrictions imposed was a positive good in itself, and our Dyspeptic patient at any rate benefited by it. It is not written that Carlyle was ever under our treatment : had he been so, his wife and the world at large might have been spared many a growl.

In all affections of the stomach, then, save in pure Gastralgia (of which anon), we must be dieteticians first, drug-givers secondly only. Regulation of the quantity, quality and frequency of meals : directions for sufficient mastication, and—if necessary —for improvement or supply of the teeth wherewith to perform it ; enjoyment of sufficient exercise to promote Oxygenation and moulting of tissue—these are the all-important things for us as for other physicians. But now, when they have received due attention, there are certain remedies with which Homœopathy has done great things in the past. and which are at the present day our cherished heir-looms and instruments. Among these *Nux vomica* is pre-eminent. It is of course especially when the muscular coat of the stomach is involved, making its "churning" movements irregular, inharminous and painful that this drug is indicated ; but its action extends also to Chronic Catarrh of the mucous membrane and to the spasmodic form of Gastrodynia. Its only peer in this respect is *Arsenic*. The power of this poison to set up Gastritis, however it may be introduced into the system, is well-known ; and correspondingly its place in gastric disorder is where the mucous membrane, from irritative hyperæmia, is the chief seat of the symptoms. Like *Nux*, however, it acts also on the muscular fibres and nervous supply of the stomach, taking the whole organ within its remedial grasp. Let these great medicines, I pray you, be your first thought in all grastric cases that come before you. I do not say, your last also. for other remedies may be better-indicated from the outset, as *Pulsatilla* or *Antimonium crudum* when there is much mucous accumulation, *Kali bichromicum* (of which I shall have more to say immediately), when its yellow fur on a red base is displayed by the tongue, *Lycopodium* when atony predominates over irritability. Again, particular symptoms of Dyspepsia may so predominate as to influence the choice of the remedy. Acidity may require *Calcarea*, *Sulphuric acid*, or *Robinia* ; Flatulence may call for *Carbo vegetabilis* or *Nux moschata*. Let their cry be attended to when it is very shrill, and when other complainings are silent ; but remember that a congested or loaded or atonic mucous membrane with deficient gastric juice, a muscular coat inept to perform the digestive movements, will allow the food to ferment in the stomach, to develop Acid and Gas and to cause Heartburn, so that the fundamental medicines of the altered organ may be the best remedies for the separate elements of its disorders.

Let me say a few words upon one of the drugs I have mentioned —*Kali bichromicum* ;—

I suppose that the chief advance of late years in gastric Therapeutics would be reckoned by the observations of Vulpian,* Fraser, † Bradbury ✝✝ and McHardy $ as to the use of the **Bichromate of Potash.** Only the second-named has even hinted his indebtedness for it to Homœopathic literature, in which, nevertheless, it occupied a prominent place before any of the four were known to fame. Struck by its effects on the workmen engaged in the preparation for the arts (which had been noticed in 1827 by Cumin of Glasgow), Dr. Drysdale in 1844 proved it on 11 men and 5 women, besides animals, and published his results, with all other pathogenetic information available, in the BRITISH JOURNAL OF HOMOEOPATHY for that year. ‖ In 1845, the Austrian Society gave it another proving, conducted on 12 men and 2 women, relating their experiments in the OESTERREICHISCHE ZEITSCHRIFT FUR HOMOOPATHIE for 1847. In 1852, Dr. Drysdale contributed to Part I, of the "Hahnemann Materia Medica" a Monograph on the drug, embodying all that had thus been ascertained as to its Physiological action, and appending much clinical observation with it—in which Chronic Dyspepsia played no small part. His re-issue of the Essay in the "Materia Medica, Physiological and Applied" of 1884 brings down the subject to that day. Vulpian, therefore, who wrote in 1883, need not (if he did) have tried the drug in gastric affections merely as an alternative to *Arsenic* which is the only reason he alleges. Dr. Fraser, whose communication on the subject was read at the International Congress held at Rome in 1894, shows by his mention of Drysdale that he was aware of his work on the subject, but gives him no credit for it ; and yet his cases—of irritative Dyspepsia, with pain and vomiting, and of Grastric Ulcer—were just such as corresponded to the condition of stomach induced by Drysdale experimentally and benefited by him therapeutically. Dr. Bradbury, whose naive acknowledgment of ignorance on the subject has been justly satirised in the MONTHLY HOMŒOPATHIC REVIEW ✝ has merely followed Fraser, but has confirmed his results.

These observations, then, have added nothing to the knowledge Homœopathists already possessed and put forward as to the PLACE of *Bichromate of Potash* as a gastric remedy ; but they have done something to increase our sense of its POWER. This is owing, I think, to the stronger doses which have been administered. We have hardly gone below the 1st trituration ;

---

* JOURN. DE PHARM. ET DE CHIMIE, Sept. and Oct., 1883.

† LANCET, April 14, 1894. ✝✝ IBID., Sept. 14, 1895.

$ J. B. H. S, vii., 415.

‖ Not for 1845, as stated by a misprint in my 'Pharmacodynamics.,
✝Oct. 1895, (p. 587).

GASTRITIS

but Vulpian's centigrammes, Fraser's $\frac{1}{12}$th and Bradbury's $\frac{1}{10}$th grain have rarely disagreed, and have enabled the first-named to bring about striking results in very serious disorder of the stomach, simulating, indeed, malignant disease, which itself he thinks may be retarded and relieved by it. We shall be encouraged hereby to prescribe it more frequently, and push it more vigorously in the gastric affections for which it is suitable. It inflames the mucous membrane of the stomach as surely and as specifically as *Arsenic* does, and perhaps in a manner which makes it more suitable for Chronic Dyspepsia having such basis. Its tongue is a coated one, though the organ beneath the fur is red ; while that of *Arsenic* is not only red but over-clean, and inclined to be dry or glazed. This means, according to Dr. Fenwick, that the inflammation caused by the one is catarrhal, that of the latter erythematous ; and it is the former which obtains in the gastric disorder which calls for such remedies.

I will now speak of the separate affections of the STOMACH which come before us in daily practice. After much pondering as to the best plan of arranging my materials, I have decided upon the following order. First, I will speak of the treatment of the organic affections of the viscus—INFLAMMATION, ULCER and CANCER. Then I will tell you what we can do for its nervous derangements. Last, I will discuss the remedies for the various forms and elements of DYSPEPSIA. And, first, of—

GASTRITIS.—There is no doubt that Acute Gastritis, in the strictest sense of the term ("Croupous" form of the Germans,) is, except as a consequence of irritant poisoning, hardly ever seen. I must agree with Dr. Wilson Fox,* however, that "Acute Gastric Catarrh" is a very common affection. It is usually the result of the introduction of offending substances into the stomach ; but sometimes arises from climatic or even epidemic influences. An account of a number of cases apparently springing from the last-named cause is given by Dr. Yeldham in the Sixteenth Volume of the BRITISH JOUANAL OF HOMOEOPATHY.

Now when Gastritis is caused by cold, I must go with Jahr and Hempel in thinking *Aconite* perfectly appropriate to it ; at any rate, as an initial remedy. But when its force is spent, and in all other forms of the disease, there is one medicine, and one only, on which I advise you to rely. The presence of decided symptoms of gastric inflammation should always to your mind indicate **Arsenicum**. Do not give it in too low a potency ; the *6th* or *12th* will, I think, serve you best. Its Homœopathicity to the morbid condition present I need not argue. With the aid of suitable diet, and perhaps a cold compress to the epigastrium, you will need no other treatment.

The following case will exhibit its action, and show the powerlessness of *Aconite* over the local affection. It was contributed by Dr. James Lawrie to the Tenth Volume of the BRITISH JOURNAL OF HOMOEOPATHY.

---

* In Russell Reynold's 'System of Medicine', Vol. ii.

The next case was that of a man between thirty and forty years age, of a pale and sickly constitution, and whose body was much emaciated. He stated that he had been suffering for a number of years from a severe stomach-complaint, that he had consulted a number of medical men, and had taken a variety of medicine with little or no benefit. He had just returned from the country, where he had been ordered by his former medical attendant for the benefit of a change of air, but was obliged to return home on account of the acute and severe pain in the stomach. His pulse was 150, full and bounding ; tongue parched, with a broad red stripe in the centre ; intense thirst ; skin hot ; bowels confined; urine scanty. I gave *Aconitum*, 1st dilution, ten drops to a tumbler of cold water, a tablespoonful every hour and a half ; and ordered a dose of Castor oil to relive the bowels. On calling in the evening the patient was not relieved ; pulse 115 ; fever much higher ; and pain very severe. I ordered the *Aconitum* to be taken every half hour. Next morning I found that he had passed a very restless night. The bowels had acted freely. His pulse was, however, now reduced to 90, and the fever was almost entirely gone, though the pain at the pit of the stomach continued as intense as ever. He stated that he could compare it to nothing but a burning furnace within. I recollected that this was a leading symptom of *Arsenic* and put ten drops of the 6th dilution of *Arsenicum* into a Wine glassful of water, a teaspoonful to be taken every six hours. The first spoonful gave immediate relief ; the patient fell into a profound sleep for four hours ; the second dose had a similar effect, and the next day the man was quite well, and required no further attendence. Nor, to the best of my knowledge, had he any return of the complaint which had so long affected him.

I know that indications are given in our books for many other medicines in this affection—as *Nux vomica, Bryonia, Pulsatilla* and *Ipecacuanha*. Pathogenesy also would suggest the possible place of *Mercurius corrosivus, Kali bichromicum,* and *Tartar emetic* in its treatment. It is but right that I should mention these ; but I repeat that you will seldom, if ever, want any medicine but *Arsenicum*.

It is almost the same with Chronic Gastritis, at least in that form of it in which the tongue is clean, red and glazed.* Only here if your patient should not respond quickly to the higher dilutions I have named, you will do well to go down to the third (or even second) decimal. **Mercurius corrosivus** is another important medicine here ; it is recommended by Dr. Pemberton Dudley (in the same two attenuations) when distension and soreness of the epigastrium are prominent. **Kali bichromicum** comes in (as I have described) when on the ground of the reddened mucous membrane there is formed (as seen on the tongue) a rough yellowish fur. **Iodium**, also should be well considered and proved curative in a case occurring in a child, and accompanied (which is rare) by Bulimia. †

---

* See two excellent cases in the First (p. 71) and the Fourth (p. 255) Volumes of the B.J.H. † See ANNALS, i., 293.

ULCER OF THE STOMACH

No better medicines than these can be given as long as the inflammation is an Endogastritis only. But there are cases of some-standing in which thickening of the sub-mucous tissues occurs, so that the pylorus becomes narrowed, and dilatation of the stomach results. Dr. Jousset has lately shown that we possess in **Nux vomica** a heroic remedy for this condition, which (owing to the pyloric induration) is sometimes mistaken for Scirrhus.* If it should be insufficient, I should suggest the trial of *Phosphorus*, whose power of setting up a "chronic indurative Gastritis, with thickening," we have seen.

There is another chronic disease of the gastric mucous membrane in which the latter medicine may be of service. It is a degeneration of the peptic glands, which from the hæmorrhages which accompany it, and the marked cachexia it induces, may often be set down as of malignant nature. Such a condition I apprehend to have been present in the case reported by Dr. Bolle as Cancer of the Stomach, and which you will find related in the Twelfth Volume of the BRITISH JOURNAL OF HOMŒOPATHY. The curative power of **Phosphorus** in this (at any rate very serious) disease is manifest.

Lastly, there is that Chronic Gastric CATARRH PAR EXCELLENCE, where the tongue is much coated, and much thick mucus (not glairy, as with *Nux vomica*) is formed and vomited. Unfortunately, this condition is frequently symptomatic of organic disease elsewhere, and defies all treatment. The most promising medicine in its treatment is, I think, **Hydrastis** †

I have now to speak of—

ULCER OF THE STOMACH, by which I mean the Round Perforating Ulcer of Cruveilhier, of non-inflammatory origin.

It might be thought that the ready way in which this ulcer often heals under rest, unirritating diet, and hot or cold compresses to the epigastrium, made its medicinal treatment of comparatively little importance. The jubilation, however, with which our old school colleagues have hailed the *Potassic bichromate* we have supplied to them shows that there was still a gap to be filled in their Therapeutics of this disease. By this medicine, by *Arsenicum*, *Argentum nitricum*, the *Sulphate of Atropine* and the *Nitrate of Uranium*, Homœopathy can do and has done great things in Gastric Ulcers. Our choice has hitherto lain mainly between the first three of these medicines. Dr. Pope has suggested (and Pathogenesy bears him out) that **Arsenicum** is most appropriate when the Ulcer is at the pyloric,

L, ART MEDICAL, xli., 241.   † See case in ANNALS, iv., 541.

Kali bichromicum when at the cardiac end of the stomach. **Argentum nitricum** comes preferably into play when the Gastric Ulcer seems connected (as it often is) with a Chlorotic condition.* **Atropinum sulphuricum**, in the 3, dilution, is a valuable and probably Homœopathic palliative for the pains of the complaint; and I generally alternate it with the medicine I select for healing the Ulcer. This I have of late years most frequently found in **Uranium nitricum**. Dr. Edward Blake's experiments (as also Woroschilsky's) with this substance show it to have a specific power of ulcerating the pyloric mucous membrane in animals, and it has more than once been reported as curing the Idiopathic disease. †

Perseverance with the medicine under which the Ulcer has healed appears to be the best way of preventing its recurrence. But we must enquire, before leaving this affection, what Homœopathy can do in its accidents, hæmorrhage and perforation. For the former the remedies I shall speak of when I come to Hæmatemesis —notably *Ipecacuanha* and *Hamamelis*—will probably avail. As to Perforation, the question is whether we are justified in omitting the usual treatment by *Opium*. "The only favourable recorded terminations to this event" says Dr. Wilson Fox, "are those in which the *Opiate* treatment was pursued". Perforation occurred in two cases recorded in our literature—one of Dr. Holland's in the Fourth. and of Dr. Kafka's in the Fifteenth Volume of the BRITISH JOURNAL OF HOMŒOPATHY. In the former, the patient rallied from immediate collapse under *Arsenicom* 30: but the medicine was not continued, the same symptoms returned a few hours afterwards, and she died nineteen hours after she was first attacked. No Peritonitis was found POST MORTEM. In the second case the inflammation was set up; but was controlled by *Belladonna*, and the patient recovered. This is sufficient, I think, to justify a fair trial of our ordinary remedies in Perforation, according to its consequences; but wider experience is necessary ere we can estimate their comparative usefulness.

Next. of—
CANCER OF THE STOMACH.—Can we modify the hopeless prognosis which comes from Old Medicine when she recognises the disease? I have only probabilities to offer you in the affirmative; but, such as they are, they would inspire me with more hope for gastric than for any other form of internal Cancer.

---

* Here also Dr. Goldsbrough's experience with *Ferrum aceticum* must be remembered (J. B. H. S., vi., 291).

† See for all these statementt, B. J. H. iv. 379; xv.. 238; xxiv., 657. xxvii., 307; ANNALS, v., 411; M. H. R., xix., 680; J. B, H. S., vii., 415.

GASTRALGIA

Of the two cases recorded in the BRITISH JOURNAL OF HOMOEOPATHY as supposed examples of the disease, I have already given reasons for relegating one (Dr. Bolle's) to another category. The second, by Dr. Veit Meyer, may be read in the Thirteenth Volume. The patient was desperately ill; and her age (45) favoured the Carcinomatous interpretation of her symptoms, which embraced nearly every feature of the disease, including an undoubted Tumour. She made a complete recovery under *Arsenicum* and *Calcarea*, with *Belladonna* and *Chamomiila* for subjective symptoms. More recently we have had a case of Dr. Kypke's where vomiting and pain at the stomach co-existed with a Tumour in the pyloric region about the size of half an orange. The patient was greatly emaciated, and she was sallow and hollow-eyed. *Bismuth* and *Belladonna* did no good but under *Calcarea fluorata* and *Nux vomica* (6_x) improvement gradually ensued, and went on to complete recovery—the Tumour having disappeared.

I have then to remind you of the testimonies I have collected in my 'Pharmacodynamics' from Friedriech and Nussbaum in the old school, and Fischer in our own, as to the value of *Cundurango*, and the case I have mentioned there under *Hydrastis*—to which I could now add several others.* I think that these facts are sufficient to show that we may undertake the treatment of any supposed Gastric Cancer with **Arsenicum**, **Calcarea** and **Kali bichromicum** with **Cundurango** or **Hydrastis** (not forgetting **Kreosote** for the vomiting), according to the symptoms, with reasonable grounds for hope. Suppose all the cases to which I have referred to have been wrongly diagnosed; they were nevertheless instances of cure of a painful and menacing morbid condition, against which ordinary remedial means were unavailing. The patient committed to our care as the victim of Scirrhus may not be demonstrably so affected; but for all practical purposes he is so, and a cure will be valued accordingly.

Many affections of the stomach, and notably its Round Ulcer, are accompanied with pain; but that is not what we mean when the speak of Cardialgia, Gastrodynia, or (best)—

GASTRALGIA.—We mean pain referred to the epigastrium, without evidence of inflammation or other disorder of the gastric mucosa; recurring paroxysmally, sometimes even periodically; and rather assuaged than otherwise by introducing food into the stomach or pressing upon it from without. Dr. Fenwinck doubts the existence of such a distinct complaint;

---

* See ANNALS, iv., 542; J.B.H.S., i., 178; viii., 27, 52—6.

but Ansite had no such hesitancy, and spoke warmly of the value of *Strychnia* and **Arsenic** in its treatment. We prize the same remedies, only giving the former in the shape of **Nux vomica**, and using much smaller doses than he recommends. We further discriminate,—choosing *Nux vomica* preferentially in robust constitutions, and where the pain is crampoid, as if seated in the muscular coat of the stomach ; *Arsenic* in delicate or worn subjects, and where the sufferings seem Neuralgic.* In slighter degrees of the latter variety we also employ **Bismuth**, as the other school does ; but as a rule we find it active enough in the triturations from the *1st* to the *3rd*. This suggests that its action is Homœopathic, though I confess I cannot prove the point from Pathogenesy. We have other medicines for it too. **Abies nigra** is effective when the pain is as of something sticking in the cardia or gullet. *Anacardium* or *Hydrocyanic acid* should be given when relief by food and return of the pain as soon as this leaves the stomach is very marked, the latter being preferable where there is a distressing sensation of sinking complained of. **Atropinum sulphuricum**, of whose sedative power over the pains of Gastric Ulcer I have already spoken, is useful when these are simulated without the lesion being present ; † and also in the hyperæsthetic form in which the stomach immediately resents by pain and vomiting the introduction of food, this being usually associated with Hysteria, or Spinal Irritation, or both. Dr. Kafka gives two cases of the kind in which a cure took place under doses of the 180th of a grain ✢

There is a general agreement among our therapeutists as to the efficacy of Homœopathic treatment in this disorder, and as to the supreme value of *Nux vomica* and *Arsenicum*. Jahr adds *Ignatia* as a useful medicine when the character of the symptoms indicates *Nux*, but the patient is of the female sex. Dr. H. Goullon relates two cases showing *Graphites* (which he gives in the 3rd trituration) to be a very effective remedy for pure Gastralgia, occurring in Anæmic or debilitated subjects, without any sign of Catarrh of Stomach, and having the pains (which are crampy) rather relieved by eating. ✤

I have thought it better to speak of the various forms of Dyspepsia in a distinct category. The German writers—whether of the old or the new school—consider them as merely so many symptoms of Chronic Gastric Catarrh. But I must maintain that digestion may become difficult, painful, or otherwise

---

* See B.J.H., xxxi., 367.   † J.B.H.S., v., 198.
✢ B.J.H., xv., 242.   ✤ J.B.H.S., v., 195.

perverted from its form without any inflammatory action having occurred ; and the numerous forms it takes require special study and treatment. In this I am in accordance with Dr. Jousset.

The difficulty of classifying the disorders of the stomach is especially felt here. The late Dr. Marston, in a very practical series of "Notes of cases of Indigestion," published in the MONTHLY HOMŒOPATHIC REVIEW for 1867-8, has adopted the plan of running through the list of medicines of service in Dyspepsia, indicating the special place and value of each ; and I am not sure but that this method is the best. You would hardly be content with it, however ; and I must still keep disease in the fore-front, and hang on my medicines to its several forms. I will speak, therefore, first of ACUTE INDIGESTION ; then of CHRONIC INDIGESTION in general ; next of the special elements of the latter—PAIN, ACIDITY, HEARTBURN, WATER-BRASH, and FLATULENCE —each of which sometimes comes before us for treatment as a substantive malady ; and, last, of VOMITING, with HÆMATEMESIS as an appendix.

ACUTE INDIGESTION may be simply the result of the ingestion of improper food. I hope that here your Homœopathic convictions well not be felt as a bar to your resorting to the common-sense remedy of promoting vomiting by the most suitable and least injurious means. Hahnemann, however, has justly pointed out* that this derangement of the stomach is usually of "dynamic" origin, "caused by mental disturbance (grief, fright, vexation), a chill, exertion of the body or mind immediately after eating, often after even a moderate meal." Here, he argues, Emetics are out of place ; while a single dose of the suitable Homœopathic remedy will remove the symptoms in a couple of hours. He mentions **Pulsatilla** as most frequently called for its indications being 'constant disgusting eructations with the taste of the vitiated food, generally accompanied by depression of spirits, cold hands and feet, &c."

When the quantity or quality of the ingesta themselves has been the sole discoverable exciting cause, **Pulsatilla** is still useful if the indigestion has arisen from taking fat or other rich food. The prominence of mucous derangement— white tongue, Nausea with little vomiting, passive Diarrhœa, and absence of much pain—is the symptomatic indication for the drug. When, however, the indigestible substance is such on account either of its bulk, or of its hardness and insolubility, as cheese, white of eggs, and such-like, **Nux vomica** comes into play. Its symptoms are those of violent pain and expulsive action : it is the nervo-muscular apparatus which is here at fault † **Arsenicum** is recommended by Teste as the specific remedy for the disturb-

---

* Organon (Dudgeon's Translation), p. 6, Note.

† "Foreign bodies usually appear to cause pain through excting spasm of the muscular coats" (Wilson Fox, LOC CIT.)

ance of the stomach caused by sour fruits and vegetables, and (Jousset adds) ices : the condition is sub-inflammatory.

CHRONIC DYSPEPSIA generally comes before us as a more or less complex condition ; and requires the full resources of diet and Hygiene to be brought into play for its aid. But over and above these we have medicines of the utmost value in its treatment. It you have read Dr. Chambers' pleasant volume on "The. Indigestion." and have noted his suggestion of the impotence of our remedies in this disease, let me recommend you to weigh especially Dr. Marston's cases, which were published in reply. I cannot refer you morever, in a better account of the place and action of our chief Anti-dyspeptic remedies, though some valuable additions are made by Dr. Jousset, in the Forty-First Volume of L' Art Medical (p. 251) ; by Dr. Clifton in the Seventeenth Volume of the Monthly Homœopathic Review (p. 150) ; by Dr. Dyce Brown in the Thirty-Seventh Volume of the same Journal (p. 519) ; and by Dr. T. G. Stonham, in a Paper on "Simple Dyspepsia," in the Sixth Volume of the Journal of the British Homœopathic Society. I will sketch them in outline here.

Of **Nux Vomica** I have spoken fully when lecturing on that drug. To the symptoms there mentioned as indicating it, I would add craving for food with speedy satiety ; and among the subjects of its influence would include those who take Alcohol largely. In the "Pituitous Dyspepsia," with vomiting of glairy mucus, to which these persons are subject, **Nux** is an excellent remedy. When the symptoms are those of slow digestion (Bradypepsia) Dr. Jousset recommends its alternation with *Graphites*, the one before, the other after a meal.

Pulsatilla expends its influence upon the mucous membrane. The mucus is increased ; hence slow digestion, fermentation of the food, Acidity, Heartburn, foul eructations, bad taste, and Nausea. Rich and fat foods are instinctively avoived. The bowels tend to looseness. It is the Dyspepsia of persons of soft fibre and feeble circulation. Other symptomatic indications may be found in my 'Pharmrcodynamics.'

Bryonia is less frequently indicated than either of the two great remedies now described. Its indigestion is more directly the consequence of an unsuitable diet than of constitutional derangement. I have already, when lecturing upon this drug, cited Trink's graphic description of the cases to which it is suitable. With this Dr. Marston's experience fully coincides. The sense of PRESSURE after food, even as if a heavy stone lay on the stomach, bitter taste and vomiting, and the tenderness of the epigastrium to touch and on movement, especially when making a false step, with Water-brash and Constipation,—are characteristic symptoms for *Bryonia.* I think Dr. Marston has made a very happy suggestion when he points to the muscular coat of the stomach as the part mainly at fault in these cases. The liver is probably also involved. *Bryonia* is a favourite medicine with Dr. Stonham ; and he gives some good cases illustrative of its virtues.

Lycopodium, though not mentioned by D·. Marston, I regard as far superior to any other of the medicines he has used, save only these three. It is in the thoroughly atonic Dyspepsia of weakly subjects, where the digestion is delayed through deficient glandular secretion and muscular energy ; where there is so little nervous force to spare for digestion that during its process an irresistible drowsiness comes on, and the sleeper wakes exhausted ; and where from like causes flatulence collects in abundance, and the bowels are utterly torpid, that *Lycopodium* displays its powers. Farinaceous food is especially ill borne. I have related in my 'Pharmacodynamics' a typical case illustrating the action of the medicine. A copious deposit of red sand or Lithates in the urine is another indication for its choice ; as also is a sense of repletion after taking but a few mouthfuls.

Carbo vegetabilis is often a capital medicine for the Chronic Dyspepsia of old people. Much flatulence, Acidity and Heartburn are usually present, and often frontal Headache and giddiness, but rarely Constipation.

Sulphur and **Calcarea carbonica** are said by Dr. Marston to be often required in obstinate cases and in Dyscratic subjects. The former helps forward the action of *Nux* ; the latter that of *Pulsatilla. Sulphur* is especially suitable to the bilious and sanguine temperament ; and where there is a tendency to Constipation and Hæmorrhoids, and to retarded and scanty Catamenia. *Calcarea* suits children, females, and persons of phlegmatic temperament or Scrofulous diathesis ; and is indicated by the presence of Acidity and the tendency to loosenes of bowels and to Menorrhagia.

These are leading medicines for Chronic Dyspepsia ; and you will seldom have to go beyond their range. If you do, however, I may refer you to the indications given by Dr. Clifton for *Chelidonium, Hydrastis* and *Sepia ;* and by Drs. Jousset and Stonham for *China.* You will find these in my 'Pharmacodynamics ;

and we also learn there of the milk-white tongue indicative of the mucous flux calling for *Antimonium crudum*; of the deficiency of gastric juice which *Alumina* helps; and of the irritative catarrh where *Ipecacuanha* is useful. With these in reserve, and the seven I have specified as protagonists, I think you will be prepared to meet with Dyspepsia as a whole, and will do as well as Dr. Marston, who cured even his dispensary patients in the proportion of 77 per cent.

And now as to the treatment of the different elements of Indigestion which I have enumerated.

PAIN AFTER FOOD may signify either organic disease of the stomach—Inflammation, Ulcer, or Cancer; or one of its Neuroses—the Spasmodic, Neuralgic or Hyperæsthetic forms of Gastralgia. The treatment of these I have already discussed. But there is another not unfrequent variety, in which the pain comes on as soon as the food is swallowed and continues during the whole process of digestion, but is unattended with vomiting, which I cannot refer to any of these morbid states. In some of these cases the patient's history and general condition have disclosed a Rheumatic tendency, which may easily be conceived of as affecting the muscular coat of the stomach. Here I have found **Bryonia** of much service. In others the same muscular coat seems affected with debility, so that its contractions are attended with pain and soreness. Here, besides the obvious tonic measures, **Arnica** may be given with decided advantage.

ACIDITY.—Dr. Chambers has forcibly pointed out how this trouble may arise from deficient vitality of the stomach, allowing the Saccharine and fatty elements of the food to undergo Acid fermentation. But I think he was led away by his theory when he rejected the possibility of hyper secretion of gastric juice, as if it were an excess of vitality, which is impossible. One of his own school, Dr. Inman, took much pains to prove that excessive secretion always implies a depressed condition of the secernent organ of the general system. And I cannot but think, with Dr. Wilson Fox, that Acidity—as with an empty stomach—often depends on hyper-secretion. It is a symptom not easy to remove. Something may be done by careful dieting ; something by giving Lemon-juice, as Dr. Kidd advises in his capital paper on this agent,* two hours after meals. On the whole, I find **Calcarea** the most useful medicine. *Phosphorus. Kali carbonicum* and *Sulphuric acid* also are recommended. The favourite Alkaline palliatives of the old school are quite inadmissible, except as a very rare temporary expedient.

So I wrote in 1878. Since then the existence of Acidity from excessive secretion has been demonstrated, and is now known as "Hyper-chlorhydria." The Acid present in it is the *Muriatic*, whereas in Acidity from fermentation of the gastric contents it is the *Lactic* and *Butyric*. We have hardly yet, perhaps learnt to apportion our antacids to these two forms of the trouble. The *Calcarea* I have so warmly commended probably suits the Hyper-acid form ; and Dr. Coumont, of Verviers, relates a chronic case cured by this drug and *Phosphorus* in alternation, both in the 6th dilution,—a subsequent relapse being speedily checked by the same medicines.† The **Robinia** which America has sent us appears to act in this way, and has been shown by Dr. Kent to act well even when the gastric Acidity is connected with malignant disease of the stomach †† Dr. Goodno finds *Atropinum sulphuricum* relieved the pain often associated with Hyper-chlorhydria as it does that of Gastric Ulcer. $

For Acidity from FERMENTATION, *Sulphuric acid* and *Argentum nitricum*, with perhaps *Sulphur* itself, ‖ are most esteemed ; and if *Bismuth* is to take place among our Antacids it would probably come in here. ↓ The same may be said of *Natrum phosphoricum*, which is indicated (Dr. Neiderkorn says**) where there is a creamy yellow coating of tongue.

HEARTBURN is another troublesome symptom of Indigestion ;—troublesome to bear, and troublesome to cure. When obviously connected with Acidity, the treatment of that affection may be all that is required. Where no symptoms of excess of Acid are present, Dr. Chambers suggests that Heartburn arises from hyperæsthesia of the gastric nerves. It would then be felt soon after a meal, and not, as in the other form, three or four

---

* See B. J. H., xxi., 37.
† JOURN. BELGE D' HOMŒOPATHIE, Nov.—Dec., 1896.
†† J. B. H. S. iii., 830. $ IBID., ix., 182.   ‖ IBID, viii, 356.
↓ IBID., iv., 330.   ** IBID. vii., 416.

nours later. The medicines from which I have derived most benefit in this affection are **Pulsatilla** and **Capsicum**,—the latter at the time of suffering, the former regularly. Dr. Drury recommends *Ammonium carbonicum*.

WATER-BRASH is much more under control, but is proportionately rarely met with. I have seldom failed to remove it pretty rapidly with **Lycopodium** ; and, where this has not hit the mark, **Nux vomica** has succeeded. *Bryonia*, too, has Water-brash so well-marked in its Pathogenesis (including the contractive pain at the lower end of the œsophagus so often felt in connexion with it), that it must not be forgotten. I think that the "Water brash" of sour or foul-tasting fluid mentioned by Dr. Marston as curable by *Pulsatilla* is an eructation from the stomach rather than true Water-brash. Dr. Bayes recommends *Veratrum album* in cases where there is much pain after food, with coldness of the hands and feet.

FLATULENCE, like Acidity, may result from disengagement of gas from decomposing food and so yield to the treatment called for by the primary disorder. It may also arise from a bad habit of swallowing much air with the food. But I cannot help thinking, with Dr. Inman, that the intestine has a property, when in a weakened state, of forming gaseous accumulations. Whence, otherwise, Tympanites of peritoneal inflammation, where there is nothing but the paralysed state of the muscular fibre to account for it ?

We have two primary medicines for this trouble, **Carbo vegetabilis** and **Lycopodium**. Both are suited to the general and intestinal a-dynamia usually present where excessive Flatulence is complained of. The former I think preferable where the stomach and small intestines are the seat of distension, which often keeps the patient awake at night* (as observed by Drs. Chambers and Bayes) ; the bowels are natural, or tend to Diarrhœa. The Flatulence calling for *Lycopodium* seems to be situated in the colon, and is nearly always accompanied by Constipation. Dr. Bayes adds that it is incarcerated ; while for Flatulence, frequently breaking up through the œsophagus he recommends **Argentum nitricum**, an experience I have often confirmed.

With one of these three medicines Flatulence may generally be reduced to such a minimum as to cease to trouble the patient. There are others, however, which may be mentioned

---

* Dr. Cooper prefers here the *Carbo animalis*, in the 2_x or 3_x trituration (B.J.H., xxxvi., 227).

as occasionally helpful. **Nux moschata** and **Apocynum cannabinum** are excellent for the sense of "bloating" after food: the sensation being referred with the former to the epigastrium, with the latter to the abdomen generally. *Lobelia* and *Gratiola* are another pair. **Lobelia** is useful where Flatulence causes oppression with weakness at the epigastrium and a sense as of a lump in the throat-pit, impeding respiration and deglutition. **Gratiola**, a well-proved but rarely used medicine, is commended by Dr. Tessier where, with great distension of stomach, there is afflux of blood to the head, with heat and somnolence especially after meals, when also there is lassitude and constriction of the throat and rectum, with Dysphagia for liquids and Constipation. In such cases, he says, it has rendered him "incomparable service".*

The last of the affections of the stomach of which I shall speak is

VOMITING.—I need not tell you that this is a very common symptom of organic disease of the stomach, of its Neuroses, and of its Dyspepsiæ. Nor need I remind you how frequently it is sympathetic of mischief elsewhere of disease of the brain, ears, heart, lungs or kidneys; of abdominal tumors; even of the presence of the gravid uterus. In all these the main treatment must be addressed to the primary diseases, of which I have spoken or shall speak in their places. But even in disease elsewhere, especially when chronic, you will often want an intercurrent remedy for the Vomiting itself; and this you may find in **Kreosote**, as I learned from the late Dr. Hilbers, or in **Apomorphia**, as I have mentioned in my 'Pharmacodynamics,' *Kreosote* will likewise help the Vomiting of organic disease of the stomach, as Dr. Lambreghts has lately reminded us.✝

The grand remedy for simple Gastric Vomiting is **Ipecacuanha**. I have given as an indication for its use, "the presence of a moderate mucous irritation causing, by reflex excitation, disproportionate muscular expulsive action in the part." This is what we constantly have in gastric cases; and wherever is this Vomiting a prominent symptom you must think of *Ipecacuanha*, as even our old-school colleagues have come to do. As alternatives, I may mention *Antimonium tartaricum* where the mucous disorder is more

---

* Revue Hom. Francaise, Aug., p. 296.

✝ Journ. Belge d' Homœopathic. May—June, 1900.

pronounced, and there is distressing Nausea and prostration ; *Ferrum phosphoricum* where, with little of this, the stomach is utterly intolerant of food ; and *Cuprum* in obstinate cases with much straining.*

The Vomiting of Sea-sickness is not easy to check, as in this "tolle causam" cannot be obeyed—until you get to land. Every now and then, however, a judicious choice of remedy will yield satisfactory results. The motion of the vessel may be felt primarily either in the head or in the stomach itself. In the former case it shows itself either in the giddiness, when **Cocculus** will help, or in Vomiting whenever the head is raised, which will often be checked by **Apomorphia**. When the stomach is the seat of distress, and the head unaffected, **Petroleum** (not stronger than the 3rd) will relieve the Nausea, but generally requires the aid of *Ipecacuanha* to check the emesis. When the Nausea is of the character designated by the word "deathly," *Tabacum* may be preferable ; and when it is the downward motion of the vessel which annoys, *Borax*. †

Vomiting of Blood,

HÆMATEMESIS, whether signifying Ulcer or Cancer, or portal congestion, must be stopped at once. In the first two alternatives, **Hamamelis** is most to be relied on ; in the third **Ipecacuanha**. Either may be given in drop-doses of the 1_x dilution frequently repeated.

The power our medicines have over hæmorrhage is curious, but it is indubitable. Although quite prepared to use the hæmostatics of the old school in case of need, just as I should put a ligature around a superficial artery which had been wounded, yet I have never had occasion to resort to them. This is a point on which beginners naturally need encouragement ; and I am glad to be able to give it to you.

---

* See, for these, Practitioner, iii., 386 ; iv., 61. 1/3 ; J. B. H. S., iii., 327 ; iv., 333 Ibid., ii., 219.

† For these remedies see, besides what I have said of them in my 'Pharmacodynamics, J. B. H. S., ix., 78 ; vi., 228 ; vii., 229 ; v., 193. M. H. R., xx., 766.

LECTURE XXXV
DISEASES OF THE DIGESTIVE ORGANS
(*Continued.*)

—o—

THE INTESTINES
—o—

ENTERITIS—MUCO-ENTERITIS—DUODENITIS—TYPHLITIS—
PERITYPHLITIS—PROCTITIS—ULCERATION OF THE BOWELS—
INTESTINAL CANCER—HAEMORRHAGE FROM THE BOWELS—
COLIC—DIARRHŒA—DYSENTERY.

I must now pass from the stomach to the BOWELS, and treat of the diseases affecting them, beginning with those of an inflammatory character. By

ENTERITIS I mean an inflammation beginning in the intestinal mucous membrane, and either limited thereto, or involving the other coats of the bowels. This gives us one division of the subject, viz., MUCO-ENTERITIS and ENTERITIS proper. Then again the affection takes a special form according to the portion of the tract affected; and so we have to distinguish for treatment—DUODENITIS, TYPHLITIS, and PROCTITIS; I will endeavour to give you some Therapeutic hints as to each of these,

1. Acute MUCO-ENTERITIS has for its two most common forms – inflammatory Diarrhœa (the Acute Intestinal Catarrh of the German authors) and the "Gastric Remittent Fever" of young children. Both these will be considered in their proper places. I hardly know it otherwise, but the chronic form not uncommonly comes before us as substantive ailment. It also has two forms, the Erythematous and the Membranous. The former is generally associated with Gastritis, and evidenced by the pathognomonic "beefy" tongue. It is so often indicative of profound exhaustion of the system that it is not a hopeful condition. **Arsenicum** is its one medicine. *Mercurius corrosivus* and *Oxalic acid* are locally Homœopathic, but hardly correspond to the constitutional state. You will do well here to call HYDROPATHY to your aid, in the shape of a continual abdominal compress.

Another form of Muco-enteritis is the PSEUDO-MEMBRANOUS, generally paroxysmal and recurrent. Several communications upon this malady have lately been made to our Journals. Dr. T. K. Cocke relates a case, where the presence of the false membrane was established by microscopical examination. Before passing it, severe attacks of Colic were experienced, which *Colocynth* 2x relieved. The curative treatment consisted of

Mercurius corrosivus 3_x and *Nux vomica* 2_x. Under these remedies the attacks became fewer and slighter, and soon ceased altogether.* Dr. Pritchard sends a similar case in which, after several remedies had been given in vain, *Argentum nitricum*, in the $6x$ trituration effected a rapid cure. † Dr. Julia Haywood has seen five cases. Two were secondary to Cancer of the stomach and Pulmonary Tuberculosis respectively, and a third proved dependent on an intestinal parasite. The remaining two were cured medicinally—one with *Iodide of Mercury* (and flushing of the colon), the other with *Kali bichromicum*. ††

2. True ENTERITIS, distinguished from Muco-enteritis by its severe Peritonitis-like pain and its Constipation would be admirably met by **Mercurius corrosivus** or **Colocynth** if in the large intestine. The latter would be preferable to the former, if there were much Colic, and if the rectum were involved. **Aconite** might advantageously precede or be alternated with either. In true Enteritis of the small intestine, however, I cannot indicate a remedy with precision. *Podophyllum* is the only poison which inflames the mucous membrane of this portion of the tract ; and I have no evidence of its action reaching down to the PERITONEUM. I should trust to *Aconite* rather than to any other medicine ; and Hartmann speaks in strong terms of its sufficiency in all cases to True Enteritis. Of intestinal inflammation, obstruction, and Intus-susception, I shall speak further on.

3. DUODENITIS usually comes before us as the basis of a form of Dyspepsia, acute or chronic. In the former the catarrhal process is apt to extend along the biliary ducts, and to cause Jaundice. Here **Podophyllum** will be found specific. Nor will it fail to help in Chronic Duodenitis, though I think you will sometimes have to fall back upon **Arsenicum**. **Kali bichromicum**, which acts so specifically upon this part of the intestine, is most valuable in the "Duodenal Dyspepsia" of authors, where its bitter taste of food, thickly coated whitey-brown tongue and pale stools are present. $

4. In time past we, in common with others, have had to deal with what we have called TYPHLITIS and PERITYPHLITIS ; and

---

* J.B.H.S., i., 91.   † IBID., p. 474.   †† IBID., ii., 102.

$ It is not my province in these pages to speak of diet ; but I must mention here the obvious indication in duodenal disorder of giving the part rest by making the food mainly animal, so that the stomach may deal with it. In a case of this kind occurring in a cobbler (qy ? from the pressure of his last), his (old-school) attendant had kept him for eleven weeks almost entirely upon farinaceous diet. No improvement whatever ensued and he came to see what Homœopathy could do for him. He got *Arsenicum*, 3rd dec. and was ordered an animal diet. The pain subsided in a few days , and the only return he had of it (I kept him under observation for three or four weeks) was after pertaking of rabbit-pie, and, eating the crust rather freely with the meat.

have found them fairly amenable to our remedies,—of which *Lachesis* and *Arsenicum* in the former, * *Belladonna* and *Mercurius corrosivus* in the latter, may be taken as typical. During the last few years, however, it has increasingly become the opinion that inflammations in the right iliac region nearly always begin in the appendix vermiformis cæci, and have a mechanical origin —as from fruit stones, impacted fæces, and the like ; that they are thus the subject rather of the surgeon's than of the physician's art, and in the great majority of cases require the knife for their aid. Consentaneously with this idea, the disease has either occurred more frequently or been more frequently diagnosed. "Appendicitis" has become a familiar term with nurses and patients, and even in society ; and the operation for removal of the offending diverticulum has been so often performed as to have led to a new classification of mankind. The penultimate division was into those who have translated Homer and those who have not : this is unto those who have or have not undergone "Appendectomy."

There have of course been extremes and extravagances here ; but I think that both surgeons and physicians are now settling down to the golden mean. The Article on "Perityphlitis," by Mr. Treves and Dr. Allchin, in the New Edition of Quain's Dictionary, and the papers and discussions on Appendicitis which have appeared of late years in the CLINIQUE of CHICAGO (Nov., 1893, March and may, 1894) † and the JOURNAL OF THE BRITISH HOMŒOPATHIC SOCIETY (Oct., 1894) breathe a like spirit and give similar counsels. It is fully recognised that many of these inflammations will recover under medical means alone—ours being, by unanimous consent, the internal use of *Belladonna, Bryonia,* and *Mercurius corrosivus,* according to the indications. But the Pathology of the appendix which has of late come to the light is not to be forgotten. It must urge the physician to associate a surgeon with himself in every serious case of the kind, so as to be alert for the first opportunity when manual aid should come in.

5. PROCTITIS, in its acute form, would require **Podophyllum** or **Aloes** —the latter in preference when the tenesmus is great. Chronic Proctitis is nearly always associated with ulceration within the rectum ; but whether with or without this condition, is wonderfully amenable to the influence of **Phosphorus**, as I have mentioned when lecturing upon that medicine. For Acute Periproctitis threatening Abscess and Fistula, I should recommend *Mercurius,* as in Perityphlitis.

---

* See B. J. H. v., 40 ; ix, 330.

† In these Journals 18 cases are related, in one of which only was an operation performed, and that one died. Of the remaining 17, treated by medical means only, 16 recovered. (See also J. B. H. S. v.. 102.)

ULCERATION OF THE BOWELS also requires its medicinal treatment to be modified according to the portion of intestine affected. When occurring in the duodenum, it appears to be of the same non-inflammatory character which we have seen in the Round Ulcer of the Stomach. It is, as you know, especially apt to follow upon burns of the surface. **Kali bichromicum** has been found curative here ; * and *Uranium nitricum* must not be forgotten. The former medicine will often do great things for Chronic Catarrhal Ulceration of either small or large intestine, as in some excellent cases communicated by Dr. Hilbers to Dr. Drysdale's Article on it in the "Hahnemann Materia Medica." **Mercurius corrosivus**, however, is no less in place here, and **Sulphur** is in considerable repute. "If there are signs of Ulceration in the Intestines," writes Bahr, "we have to think in the first place of *Sulphur*."

In the ileum, Ulceration constitutes the well-known lesion of Typhoid Fever ; in both ileum and colon obtains to a large extent in Phthisis Pulmonalis and Tabes Mesenterica ; and in the colon accompanies the Dysenteric process. Of all these in their place, I will only add here that, when Ulceration is seated in the rectum, you may hope for good results from **Phosphorus**.

INTESTINAL CANCER.—Of this affection we have, alas ! neither record nor promise holding out any hope of benefit to be obtained from specific medication. We shall at least refrain from aggravating our patient's suffering by purgatives ; and if *Opium* in full doses promotes his well-being, as Dr. Habershon's cases seem to show, ✢ we may not refuse him the benefit of it.

HÆMORRHAGE FROM THE BOWELS, when not resulting from ulcer or Cancer, or occurring as a portion of Purpura, is (I suppose) Nature's rough way of relieving portal congestion. You will of course attend to the cause of the engorgement, which may be hepatic, splenic, pulmonary or cardiac. But the hæmorrhage itself, whatever be its origin, needs active remedies ; and these I think you will find (as in the corresponding affection of the stomach) in **Ipecacuanha** and **Hamamelis**.

COLIC (ENTERALGIA or ENTERODYNIA) is to the intestine what Gastralgia is to the stomach. It is rarely, however (at least to my thinking), Neuralgic ; but is ordinarily seated in the muscular coat of the bowel, which may be irritated by worms or unsuitable ingesta, over-distended or fretted into spasm by Flatulence,

---

* See J. B. H. S., vii., 415   ✢ "On Diseases of the Intestines."

or Rheumatically affected by cold. Its remedies must be chosen accordingly. For Worm-colic. **Cina** is excellent. For pains in the bowels induced by indigestible food **Nux vomica** is as useful as in corresponding symptoms in the stomach. Flatulence may cause pain, as I have said, either by over distending some portion of the intestinal tube, or by inducing spasm. **Belladonna** has been commended here, and is said to be especially indicated when the transverse colon is so puffed out as to project like a pad. I have myself, however, more confidence in **Chamomilla**, which in this affection I prefer in the MOTHER TINCTURE. When Colic is distinctly traceable to cold (and under these circumstances it is especially apt to occur during the warm days and cold nights of Autumn, as Bahr points out) there is no remedy so effectual as **Colocynth**, though we may follow Hempel in premising a few doses of *Aconite*.

With such remedies you will rarely fail to relieve the paroxysms of Colic. But you will often have to treat cases where the attacks are liable to recur on the least provocation. If it is to variations in diet that the intestines are so morbidly sensitive, a course of *Nux vomica* will be very helpful; and it does hardly less for habitual 'Spasms' *i. e.*, Flatulent Colic. For recurring Rheumatic Colic **Veratrum album** is often curative, as Hahnemann has taught us. *

There is another form of Chronic Enteralgia which seems to own no such exciting causes and which we can only consider as a Neurosis of the abdominal nerves. For this **Plumbum** is, as its pathogenetic effects would suggest, a most excellent remedy. You would not, moreover, pass by this great medicine even in an acute case where its characteristic symptoms of Constipation, retracted abdomen, and scanty urine were present.

When Lead itself is the cause of colic, **Opium** seems not so much Anodyne as specific, for it soon gives relief even in the attenuated doses used in our school. Cases illustrative of this statement may be found in the Third Volume of the BRITISH JOURNAL OF HOMŒOPATHY (p. 213) and in the Fourth Volume of the ANNALS (p. 287). * There is of course no reason why warm baths and enemata should not expedite your patient's solacement.

I have said nothing of **Dioscorea** in the treatment of Colic, because I really do not know to which of the categories of the affection to refer it. The "Bilious colic," for which it was first recommended, would seem to be the pain attending the passage of Gall stones, which is not in question here. However, as the drug caused decided umbilical pain in its provers, it is probable that it will find a place in the treatment of true Colic; and it may well be held in reserve for a nonplus. Dr. Clifton thinks

---

* LESSER WRITINGS p. 605 (Dudgeon's Translation).
† See also L'ART MEDICAL, xliv., 338.

that it is Flatulent Colic which calls for it, * and others describe its pains as recurring at regular intervals, and often associated with similar sufferings in other parts.

I next proceed to speak of the morbid fluxes of the intestines. Of these, Cholera has already come before us among General Diseases, and "Cholera Infantum" will have to be considered among the Diseases of Children. We shall treat in this place only of DIARRHŒA and DYSENTERY. And, first, of.

DIARRHŒA. — I have not to speak now of this malady as it occurs in children, nor of its appearance as a complication of general disorders, as fevers, or as a symptom of intestinal disease, as ulceration. I shall confine my remarks to those cases in which Diarrhœa, Acute or Chronic, comes before us for treatment as a substantive ailment.

In suggesting medicines for its various forms, I must guard you against supposing that I mean that these are the only, or even the best remedies you can use. No pathogenetic effect of drugs is more common than purging ; and it is probable that every substance in Nature which by specific affinity, and not merely by local irritation, causes Diarrhœa, has some corresponding variety of the idiopathic disorder for which it is a remedy better than any other. Indeed, you cannot no better than refresh your memory from time to time as to the characteristics of the action of your former friends, the cathartics, if you would be thoroughly fitted to deal with Diarrhœa. You would do well, too, to possess yourselves of Dr. James Bell's "Homœopathic Therapeutics of Diarrhœa, &c.," from which you may often derive help in peculiar or difficult cases. In a work like this such minute detail is impossible. I can only tell you what medicines myself and others have found most useful in the leading forms which the malady presents.

1. Unquestionably the most frequent cause of Acute Diarrhœa is elevation of the temperature. All through the Summer we are being called upon to treat it. In my own experience the history of the malady and its treatment has been in most years as follows, In June and July there has been a simple increase in the fluidity, frequency, quantity of the stools, with griping pains, more or less severe, in the abdomen. The medicine I have found specific for such a Diarrhœa has been China, in the 1st dilution. Giving a drop or two at once, and repeating the dose after each relaxed motion, it is rare that more than two or

---

* M. H. R. xxi., 473.

DIARRHŒA

three administrations are requisite. The pain yields almost immediately. Sometimes the stools are more watery, and expelled with more violence, but with less griping ; and the whole attack is ushered in by a sudden burst of vomiting. Here **Veratrum album** acts even better than *China* ; and may itself be superseded by **Croton** if the stools are very sudden and copious, streaming from the patient as if propelled from a hydrant. As we get into August and September vomiting and purging go together throughout the attack, and the ejecta are largely admixed with bile. This is the Diarrhæa which in its severer forms is known as "CHOLERA NOSTRAS." I believe its specific remedy to be the **Iris versicolor**, which I give in drop doses of the *1*st dilution every hour or so.

I have been obliged to put my own experience in Summer Diarrhœa prominently forward, as it is too common a disorder for cases of it to appear in print. So far as I know of the practice of my colleagues, *China* and *Veratrum* are with them as with me its leading remedies ; and Dr. Lade has published * results similar to those I have myself obtained with *Iris* in English Cholera. A corresponding experience with these remedies is pretty generally expressed in the papers and discussion on the subject in the Sixth Volume of the JOURNAL OF THE BRITISH HOMŒOPATHIC SOCIETY (p. 196). As regards authors, more stress seems to be laid on co existing gastric troubles than my observations in this country would warrant, so that *Ipecacuanha* and *Pulsatilla* play a prominent part among the medicines recommended. *Dulcamara*, moreover, seems highly esteemed when alterations in temperature are the exciting cause.

2. Acute Diarrhœa from improper food of course but a further manifestation of Acute Dyspepsia. and requires the same treatment—with *Nux vomica*, *Pulsatilla*, or *Colocynth* (the latter taking the place of *Arsenicum*) according to the nature of the offending ingesta, and temporary starvation.

3. Diarrhœa from noxious effluvia is probably salutary, and at any rate requires no other treatment than the **Baptisia** you will give to prevent or remove any other results in the system at large.

4. Inflammatory Diarrhœa is a kind of intestinal Coryza, and is a step in the advance from simple Diarrhœa to Muco-enteritis and Dysentery. *Aconite* alone is often sufficient to arrest it ; but, if necessary, may be reinforced by *Bryonia* when the weather is hot and dry, *Dulcamara* if it is damp.

5. Chronic Diarrhœa is generally a symptom of some deeper mischief, intestinal or general. But cases do occur which are

---

* M. H. R., x., 28,

Diarrhœa and nothing more. Of this nature is the "White Flux" of the Indian and the "Camp Diarrhœa" of the European and American soldiers—the result of continued heat on the one hand, of bad diet, exposure, and fœtid exhalations on the other. I cannot say whether improved hygenic conditions are as indispensable as they are desirable for these patients. I can only tell you that we have in **China** and **Arsenicum** two most valuable medicines for them. *China* is most suitable where the affection is simple, passive and painless ; *Arsenicum* where the intestinal alterations seem more deeply seated. A friend of mine in the Peninsular and Oriental Company's service had several opportunites of treating soldiers invalided for Chronic Diarrhœa with this medicine ; and he tells me that one of his colleagues said to him —"Well ; I know nothing of Homœopathy but I certainly believe in *Arsenic* for Chronic Diarrhœa." I give *China* in the first centesimal dilution, *Arsenic* in the third decimal trituration.

In another form a Chronic Diarrhœa the persistence of the complaint—probably acute in its origin—seems dependent upon Nervous Debility. **Phosphorus** and **Phosphoric** acid take the place of *Arsenicum* and *China* here, having the same differential indications. Sometimes, when the Diarrhœa occurs only early in the morning, it will be well to substitute a medicine having this feature among its characteristics. Such are *Sulphur, Podophyllum, Apis, Aloes, Nuphar lutuem,* and *Rumex crispus* : the indications for each you will find in my ,Pharmacodynamics' under the several medicines. When, moreover, the motions consist largely of shreddy muçus, *Colchicum* seems an efficient remedy.

I have next to speak of—

DYSENTERY.—It seems very doubtful whether true Dysentery is ever seen in its acute stage in this country, save under exceptional circumstances, as in the Milbank Prison Epidemic of 1874. By true Dysentery, I mean a specific febrile disease, having the same relation to the solitary glands of the large intestines as Typhoid Fever has to the agminated glands of the small. The nearest approaches to the disease we have in England are (1st) Dysenteric Diarrhœa, where a flux primarily

---

* J. B. H. S., vii., 84.

fæcal becomes sanguino-mucous, attended with tormina and tenesmus ; and (2nd) Muco-Enteritis of the colon and rectum. In both these conditions **Mercurius corrosivus** is our great remedy. Hahnemann was the first to recommend it, saying (in 1830), "A very small part of a drop of the *15*th, better of the *30*th, dilution I have found almost specifically curative in the common Autumnal Dysentery, giving only one dose ; the efficacy of Homœopathic treatment is here most satisfactorily displayed." It is evident, indeed, that in the *Corrosive sublimate* we have an exact simillimum to all the essential features of an ordinary attack of Dysentery ; and all subsequent observers have confirmed Hahnemann's estimate of its value, though generally giving it in somewhat lower dilutions and more frequent repetition. If the temperature is much elevated, and the patient is thirsty and and restless, you may premise *Aconite* ; but I think it is rarely required.

There are some other remedies occasionally useful in such sporadic Dysenteries, of which I must make some mention. *Mercury* itself has always a Dysenteric tendency in its Diarrhœa, and is preferred by some practitioners (in the *solubilis* or *vivus* form) for children and in the less painful and non-sanguineous variety ("Dysenteria Alba") of adults. On the other hand, when the Colic is unusually severe. *Colocynth* may sometimes advantageously reinforce or even replace the *Corrosive sublimate* and the same may be said of *Aloes* when the tenesmus is very distressing. The latter remedy, however, is more effectual when the tenesmus continues after the inflammatory symptoms have subsided. When the hæmorrhage is considerable, *Arnica* aud *Ipecacuanha* deserve consideration : the former, moreover, has considerable power over the tormina, and the tenesmus is somewhat under the control of the latter. *Hamamelis*, also, may be useful. An Indian practitioner, named Baptist, finds it (in the 1x dilution) not only to arrest the hæmorrhage but to asuage the other symptoms also. * *Capsicum* is praised by Jousset as the principal remedy for Dysentery in its stage of full development ; I have no other knowledge or it here. If the mischief is from the first confined to the rectum, and Prolapsus occurs at every stool, *Podophyllin* may be a better medicine than any ; it certainly is so with children. If you see the case only when it is far advanced, and prostration is extreme, *Arsenicum* must first be prescribed.

Now I see no reason why these remedies—especially *Mercurius corrosivus*, *Arnica* and *Arsenic*—should not be found effectual also in Epidemic and Tropical Dysentery ; but here there is a primary stage in which *Aconite* and N*u*x vomica are indicated. There is a lack of experience on record ; save that Bahr mentions an Epidemic in 1846, where Dr. Elwert, of

---

* J. B. H. S., vii., 330.

498 DISEASES OF THE DIGESTIVE ORGANS

Hanover, treated nearly 300 petients without a single death, the old-school mortality being more 10 to 20 per cent. He does not specify the remedies used. In America, where Dysetery probably stands midway between ours and that of the Tropics, they report very satisfactory results from treatment. I hope that ere long some more of our East Indian practioners will tell us what they do in the affection as seen there ; and whether they can do better than old-school practitioners with their large doses of *Ipecaeuanha* powder. *

Three special varieties of Acute Dysentery must be noted here as requiring their own remedies. In the Scorbutic form there is general assent as to the virtues of *Rhus* (though *Arnica* must not be forgotten), and in the Malignant or Typhoid form to those of *Arsenic*. When the symptoms intermit and return periodically, you must treat the case as if it were one of Ague, *i. e.*, with *Cedron* or *Quinine* unless the symptoms point definitely to any other medicine.

And now a word about Chronic Dysentery, which not unfrequently comes before us for treatment, especially in returned Anglo-Indians. A capital case is reported in the First Volume of the ANNALS of the British Homœopathic Society, as treated at the London Homœopathic Hospital by Dr. Hamilton. *Mercurius corrosivus*, followed up by *Nux vomica* and ultimately *Phosphoric acid* were the curative medicines,—all in medium dilutions. Cod-liver Oil was also given.—the emaciation being great ; and milk only allowed for food. I would add **Sulphur** and **Nitric acid** to the list of remedies. Of the former Jahr writes :—"If in spite of all treatment various single symptoms remain, such as tenesmus, slimy discharges with or without pain ; or if blood reappears in the discharges from time to time, there is no better remedy than *Sulphur*, which should be resorted to in every case if the disease, after the first violent outbreak is subdued, threatens to run a protracted course." As regards *Nitric acid*, we have Rokitansky's statement that "the Dysenteric process offers the greatest analogy to the corrosion of the mucous membrane produced by a *Caustic acid*" ; and in the present instance we have evidence that the action is not local only. Stille mentions a case (you may read it in the 'Cycolopædia of Drug Pathogenesy') fatal on the eighth day after the ingestion of a teaspoonful of strong *Nitric acid*, in whlch the usual lesions were found in the mouth, fauces, œsophagus, and stomach, but the small intestine was sound. The colon, nevertheless, was "intensely and deeply ulcerated."

---

* I have discussed this medication in my 'Pharmacodynamics,' and am unable to claim it for Homœopathy, or to deny its efficacy. The question between it and our own remedies must be a comparative one.

LECTURE XXXVI

DISEASES OF THE DIGESTIVE ORGANS
(*continued*)
—0—

THE INTESTINES,
—0—

CONSTIPATION—INTESTINAL OBSTRUCTION—HERINA—CHRONIC CONSTIPATION—HAEMORRHOIDS—FISSURE OF THE ANUS – PROLAPSUS ANI—FISTULA IN ANO—WORMS —PROCTALGIA—PARESIS-ANI.

From the Diarrhœa and its congeners I pass to the opposite condition of the bowels, and shall begin the present Lecture by discussing.

CONSTIPATION and some of its offshoots. The way in which we behave towards constipation, and in regard to the action of the bowels generally, affords one of the most obvious points of difference between the new school and the old. Purgation by various means constitutes at least one half of the ordinary practice of physic ; and 'aperient medicines" from the staple alike of the apothecary's stock-in-trade and of the family medicine chest. Conceive, then, the revolution which ensues when Homœopathy is adopted, whether by physician or patient. With fear and trembling at first the treatment of cases is conducted without the customary "unloading of the bowels." But as time goes on we come to see that our patients do all the better without having an artifical Diarrhœa added to their other troubles. We find that daily defæcation is by no means an essential of health ; that the bowels are a part of the whole organism ; that their inaction, if obviously morbid and injurious, is a disease requiring specific treatment, and not an obstruction to be overcome by temporary expedient. Instead of "clearing out the alimentary canal" with drugs which act like brooms and shovels, we became convinced that Nature is her own scavenger. Remove the morbid condition which hampers the intestinal action, and the bowels will act of themselves. See how it is in acute febrile disorders. The Constipation which obtains here is of the same nature as the anorexia on the one hand, and the scanty secretion of urine on the other. You would not dream of whipping up the appetite by bitters, or stimulating the kidneys by diuretics. You know that both the gastric and the renal inaction depend upon the fever and will depart with it. You have only to apply the same principle to the bowels. If you will just leave them alone, and apply yourself to the fever, they will give you no trouble, Three, ten, fourteen days may pass before they act, but no inconvenience will result; and at last they will be opened as naturally as though they had been so the day before. As it is with fevers, so it is with other diseases, both acute and chronic. The Constipation is but one element in the whole morbid condition. It should be taken into account, often into special account. It may guide us to medicines like *Sulphur, Nux vomica* and *Lycopodium* in preference to *Calcarea, Pulsatilla* and *Carbo*. But it would be unscientific to go out of our way to treat it independently,—still more to do so with purgatives. In chronic disease accompained with Constipation, the bowels will often begin to act regularly under a medicine having no special relation to the intestines, but which is influencing the whole organism for good.

I am not denying that Constipation, both acute and chronic, may come before us as a substantive and primary intestinal disorder. Indeed it is my object at present to tell you how to treat it when so occuring. Without further preface, then, we will proceed to our subject.

CONSTIPATION in its acute form may be said to be present when the bowels become temporarily inactive in consequence of a sudden change from active to sedentary habits, as at the beginning of a sea-voyage, or of the confinement necessitated by a fracture or other accident; also sometimes from change of air, and (in women) from marriage. But this is no disease, it generally rights itself, and hardly calls for specific medication. You may give your *Nux* or *Opium* if you like; or, if inconvenience is caused, you may let the patient use an Enema, or take a *Seidlitz powder* or a dose of *Castor oil*. The temporary trouble is removed by temporary means; and then all will go on as before.

But the true disease in which Acute Constipation occurs as a substantive malady is—

INTESTINAL OBSTRUCTION, the ILEUS or PASSIO ILIACA of the old writers. I need not remind you how large an addition to our power of diagnosing this malady has been made by the researches of the late Dr. Brinton. Nor can we do better than follow his guidance in the management of these cases as regards the limitation of the ingesta and the maintenance of rest. We need not, but we are glad to, agree with his injunctions to refrain from purgative medicines. And the use of Enemata, of insufflation, of Electro-magnetism, and of Surgical procedures is common ground between us; the only difference being that the medicinal remedies we possess make us to a large extant independent of these aids.

For practical purposes, the important diagnosis is between cases of Simple OBSTRUCTION and cases of STRANGULATION, the latter of course including INTUS-SUSCEPTION. That simple Obstruction, without special tendency to inflammation, may exist, is I think abundantly evident if we look over any collection of cases of this kind. It has its parallel in incarcerated Hernia. If fæcal accumulation can be detected, the explanation is evident; and not less so the indications for treatment. **Opium** is the medicine called for, as sluggishness of the peristaltic action must have preceded the accumulation; and Enemata, manipulation and Electro-magnetism are available auxiliaries. Where such mechanical obstacle exists, I take it that partial Spasm or Paralysis is at the bottom of these cases. I commend to you here the steady use of **Plumbum**. It has hardly been given with the confidence it merits; but it has played an important part in the treatment of several cases of Intestinal Obstruction. * As to its perfect Homœopathicity I need say nothing.

When the symptoms of Obstruction are attended with those of local inflammation, we have to fear Intus-susception in the child, internal Strangulation (more commonly) in the adult. In the former case, the Hippocratic inflation of the intestines with air seems the most reasonable mechanical remedy for the mechanical disturbance; while **Belladonna**, † **Nux vomica** and **Aconite** may help to correct irregular and excessive peristalsis, and to obviate inflammation. A case of Dr. Morgan's in which the two latter remedies proved curative, seems to have been an instance of this form of Obstruction in the adult. ✢ If internal Strangulation, as by bands, adhesions &c., external to the intestine, be satisfactorily diagnosed, I can suggest no better medicines, but I could not hope much from their action. If were myself the suffer, I do not think I should hesitate to have my abdomen opened with a view to having the Strangulation relieved. The chances of recovery from the operation would be materially enhanced by our possession of such remedies as *Aconite, Arnica, Belladonna* and *Mercurius corrosivus* to obviate its evil consequences.

There is pretty general agreement among our Therapeutic writers as to the value of the remedies I have mentioned, especially as to *Nux vomica* and *Belladonna*. $ Jousset agrees with me about *Plumbum* and *Opium*; but Jahr says that he has never seen any great effect from these medicines' and Bahr denies the Homœopathicity of *Plumbum*, because in Obstruc-

---

* See B.J.H., xvi., 76; xxxi., 376; M.H.R., ii., 66.

† In the form of *Atropine*, given in about milligramme doses, this medicine has triumphed single-handed over disperate cases (see J. B. H. S., viii., 251; x, 112). ✢✢ See M.H.R., ix , 100.

$ I may refer also to a Paper by Dr. Drysdale, in Vol. xxxv. of the M. H. R., (p. 1), with the discussion which followed its reading.

tion of the Bowels the abdomen is distended, whereas in Lead Poisoning it is hard and contracted. Such an objection hardly seems to me to carry weight.

It is obvious that if our medicines can give this help in Intestinal Obstruction, they should not be less serviceable in —

HERNIA.—I do not mean that they can cure a rupture of any standing ; although such an accident in young children, having evident connexion with ome constitutional fault, might not unfairly be expected to yield under treatment. Dr. Guernsey says that "the properly selected Homœopathic remedy is always sufficient to cure" such cases. Dr. J. F. Baker even goes further. In some "Lessons from Forty Years' Practice" which he put fourth in 1867, in the HAHNEMANNIAN MONTHLY, he speaks of having cured in all about twenty cases of Hernia in the adult. *Lycopodium* is his chief medicine against Inguinal Hernia (espeeially, he thinks, when occurring on the right side) ; *Nux vomica* or *Cocculus* for the Umbilical form. I was thinking, however, of the accidents of Hernia—its incarceration or strangulation. Here it is certain that we may do much with medicines to effect spontaneous reduction, or to turn a previous failure of the the taxis into success. In incarceration, **Opium** ; in strangulation, **Aconite**, **Belladonna** and **Nux vomica** have been used with frequent triumphs over the Obstruction. Thus, our eminent surgical representative in Berlin, Dr. Mailander, says :— "Since I have practised Homœopathy not a single case of Strangulated Inguinal Hernia has come within my experience, in which spontaneous reduction was not effected within at most four hours when *Belladonna* 2 and 3, and *Nux vomica* 3-6, had been administered in frequent alteration." Dr. Baumann confirms from his own experience the value of the remedies, but considers that in **Plumbum** we have yet another remedy which may obviate the necessity of resorts to the knife. He gives two cases of strangulated Femoral Hernia in which the last medicine proved very effectual.

And now, of =
CHRONIC CONSTIPATION.=I have alluded to the frequent occurrence of this condition as one element of the complex morbid states which come before us in practice ; and have said that in this case it must only be given its due weight among the other somptoms of the patient. If he improves as a whole under the treatment prescribed, his bowels also will act more easily. But

CHRONIC CONSTIPATION

it is hardly credible to old-school practitioners how many patients come to us whose sole or at least central and fundamental malady is Constipation itself. The refusal of the bowels to perform their duties spontaneously and naturally is the plague of their lives, and is a source of numerous other troubles. This condition, moreover, can nearly always be traced to the practice of taking aperients whenever the evacuations delay. Nature's work is thus done for her, and a morbid habit set up which at last become settled. It would not be easy to estimate the many thousands of persons who—in this country at least—never get an action of the bowels save from purgative medicines. Hence the enormous sale of the patent pills destined to achieve this purpose, and—of late years—of the aperient bitter waters.

Now it cannot be too widely known that Homœopathy has means which, in the great majority of cases, will CURE this condition, so that the bowels shall resume their normal function henceforth. Of course every wise physician, whatever his therapeutic creed, will prescribe certain hygienic and regiminal measures adapted to improve the intestinal inaction present. But I can tell you also of some capital medicines for it, out of which you will generally be able to select one which will prove beneficial. These are *Sulphur, Hydrastis, Opium, Plumbum, Nux Vomica, Lycopodium, Graphites* and *Natrum muriaticum.*

With **Sulphur** the treatment of Chronic Constipation may generally be advantageously commenced, if the patient's history is one of bad constitution and frequent ill-health ; a tendency to Piles confirms us in its choice. The bowels will generally improve immediately under its action ; but, curiously enough, if it be continued, they will almost as certainly relapse into their original condition. This, at least, is my experience. I never persevere with it longer than a week, and then either discontinue all medication, or change to one of the other remedies I shall name. I have always given the *12th* dilution.

Hydrastis has in my hands, been curative of Constipation more frequently than any other remedy. It is of most value in constitutions otherwise normal, but whose function of defæcation has been spoiled by the abuse of aperients. The mode of administration, I find most effectual, is to give a drop or two of the mother-tincture in water once daily before breakfast, and after a week or so gradually to decrease the frequency of the doses.

Opium is of great value in Constipation connected with sedentary habits and head work, where there is an absence of the symptoms of which I shall immediately speak as indicating *Nux vomica.* Its motions are of large size.

Plumbum is invaluable in the more obstinate cases of the kind which indicate *Opium,* when the lack of intestinal secretion is so great that the stools come away in small, hard balls, and especially when Colic and retraction of the abdomen are present. In patients with much rigidity of fibre, *Aconite* (as Hahnemann himself recommends) may advantageously reinforce *Plumbum* ; you may give the one in the morning, the other at night.

Nux vomica is indicated under the same circumstances as those mentioned under *Opium*, when the patient has the general condition characteristic of the drug and when—instead of torpor—there is ineffectual urging to stool. The co-existence of Dyspepsia and Hæmorrhoids are additional indications for this medicine. It often acts well after *Sulphur*.

Lycopodium is good where much Flatulence and other signs of impaired intestinal vitality are present.

Graphites is indicated by large, knotty stools ; and by a tendency to cutaneous disorder and (in women) Amenorrhœa.

Natrum muriaticum should be given when the patient has the thin, dry state of the system and the sallow complexion characteristic of the drug. It will then give every satisfaction.

Of the remedies last named *Opium* and *Plumbum* seem to have acted well in all potencies, the rest mainly in the higher.

There is a purely Rectal Constipation—the lower bowel seeming unable to expel its contents—which requires its own special remedies. When it is connected with a congestive condition of the part, as shown in Piles, **Collinsonia** is very useful. When it depends on simple Paralytic interia - as from the abuse of Enemata—**Veratrum album** and **Alumina** are good medicines.

I have given you in these remarks very much what I wrote on the subject in my 'Therapeutics' of 1878, Since then, Dr. Arthur Clifton has read a paper upon it, at our Congress of 1885, reminding us of the importance of taking into account the whole Pathological condition of our patients, when there is one, and prescribing mainly for this, when any intestinal torpor there may be present will improve of itself. In this way, in his experience, a number of medicines not generally thought of as regulators of the bowels may become so ; he cites *Berberis, Chelidonium, Phytolacca, Mezereum, Agaricus, Zincum, Ferrum, Guaiacum* and *Staphisagria*. I advise a study of this paper, and of the discussion which followed it, to any one who has a difficult case of Constipation to treat.

Another valuable contribution to this subject has been made by Dr. Conrard Wesselhœft in some papers published in the NORTH AMERICAN JOURNAL OF HOMŒOPATHY, during 1895. The medicine on which he seems chiefly to rely is *Strychnine*, which he gives in the 3_x dilution. With what he says about the frequent harmlessness of temporary delay in the evacuation of

---

* See Annals, viii., 438 for other indications and examples of its efficacy.

the bowels, however prolonged, I fully agree ; but I think he minimises too much the evil of habitual Constipation. A specimen exhibited before the BRITISH HOMŒOPATHIC SOCIETY some years ago showed such unmistakable ulceration at the spots where hardened fæces had lain PERDUS in a case of the kind, that the local possibilities of prolonged inaction became manifest. Sir Andrew Clark, moreover, was surely not wrong in his conviction that Anæmia in young women, otherwise healthily surrounded, is frequently due to this cause. The shrewd and successful physician I have named is the more to be heeded as he was not an advocate of purgatives. His instructions for the management of Costiveness are extant, and are almost entirely hygienic. A few laxative drugs are mentioned at the end, but quite as an occasional and even DERNIER RESSORT. We, availing ourselves of the general measures common to him and to us, have special medicinal resources of which he had no knowledge. By their additional aid, I hope that more and more it may be said of Homœopathy that, though it does not use aperients, it cures Constipation.

I proceed now to speak of the morbid states of the LOWER BOWEL so far as they come within the sphere of medicinal treatment. These are HÆMORRHOIDS, FISSURE, PROLAPSUS and FISTULA. And, first, of —

HÆMORRHOIDS.—Here again it cannot be too widely or too clearly known that Homœopathy possesses medicines for Piles which in the great majority of cases render unnecessary the knife, the ligature or the application of *Nitric acid.* If it had done nothing else for the art of healing, it might base on this alone its claims to the gratitude of mankind.

I distinguish three conditions under which Piles my occur.

1. They may be the expression, in the primary radicles and lawest gravitating point of the abdominal venous system, of impeded circulation higher up The obstruction may be portal, abdominal, or pelvic. Since all the veins of the intestinal canal pass by the vena portæ through the liver, this latter organ is very often saddled with the main responsibility of Piles. I doubt if the reproach is generally merited. There is no disease in which the portal circulation is so obstructed as Cirrhosis of the Liver ; yet this malady is rarely associated with Piles. I incline to think that in most cases of portal obstruction ths overloaded veins relieve themselves by Diarrhæa and serous effusion, as in Cirrhosis, or —more commonly—by gastric or intestinal hæmorrhage. I would not deny, however, that the impediment to the circulation, of which Piles are a symptoms does sometimes consist of an engorged liver. In such cases **Podophyllum** or **Hepar Sulphuris** will be indicated, the latter especially where clay-coloured stools are present. More frequently, according to my experience, the delay of the venous current is on the hither side of the portal vein. This is the "Abdominal Plethora" of the old writers, showing itself by

weight, fulness and heat in the bowels, with slow digestion, delayed stools and scanty and pale urine, The Piles accompanying it are of the "Blind" character ; they bleed little, but are very annoying by their fulness. It is here that **Sulphur** and **Nux vomica** display their great Anti-hæmorrhoidal virtues. They seem to act better conjointly (*i. e.*, in alteration) than when either is given separately. Pelvic congestion is of course more common in women than in men. For Hæmorrhoids thus arising the classical and truly Homœopathic remedy is **Aloes**. But it has recently found a rival in one of the indigenous American medicines, the **Collinsonia Canadensis**. Both from the proving of this drug and from its Therapeutic reputation, it appears that congestive inertia of the lower bowel is the condition to which it is specially related. In Constipation and Hæmorrhoids resulting from this cause —as in Pregnancy - I myself prefer *Collinsonia* even to *Aloes*.

2. The most common of all causes of Piles is, I think, Constipation. It is rare that Hæmorrhoidal sufferings are absent when this condition is of long continuance. These too are of the "Blind" variety, and cause more pain then bleeding. The means whereby we remove the primary Constipation are often sufficient to cure also the resulting Hæmorrhoids ; but in many cases the trouble is too inveterate to disappear with its exciting cause. Here, if **Sulpnur** has not already been used in the treatment of the Constipation, it may by given with benefit, as it has a decided influence upon the rectum. But I have rarely seen *Sulphur* cure these cases. They find, I believe, their best remedy in the **Æsculus hippocastanum**. Dr. Hale has narrated several cases illustrating the action of this medicine in the Article on it, in the Second Edition of his 'New Remedies'. I cannot resist giving here a case of my own, which I first related in the BRITISH JOURNAL OF HOMŒOPATHY in 1865. I give the narrative in the patient's own words :—

"I first began to suffer when thirteen years old (being now forty-eight) ; I fancy from being one of a great number of girls, with small accommodation, hence waiting and Costiveness, the bowels only relieved once a week or so. I should say that Constipation is hereditary on both sides. For a few years I was constantly taking medicine to relieve the bowels. The pain was nothing particular, and there was but a small protrusion. Matters grew worse from the age of twenty five to that of thirty four when I was attacked with the first dredful very dreadful pain. I could not sit, stand, or lie ; the only possible pasition was kneeling. This lasted for many weeks in the Winter ; in the Summer it was, as always, better, For about two years the pain was bad' off and on. I then used leeches. which eased the severe pain ; but still it was bad. The next very severe attack was in 1862 ; it lasted for weeks, and returned again in 1863. The pain was like a knife sawing backwards and forwards, almost a martyrdom for agony. I took *Belladonna, Pulsatilla, Aconite* and *Mercurius*, with no benefit ; was recommended some stuff to apply, which relieved a little. Again in 1864 things became very bad, much pain, the bowels always wanting to be relieved."

In the November of that year, I was consulted by this lady. I prescribed *Æsculus*, in the 2nd centestimal dilution, three drops to be taken in a wineglassful of water, morning and evening. Here report continues :

"I then took the *Æsculus*. At the end of one week I was a degree better, after another better still, and so on for a month. At the end of this time I was wonderfully better. The medicine seemed to relieve the bowels, and cause the protrusion to be the soft. I left it off for a time, and when the pain returned again at all badly, took the medicine and became relieved. I have taken nearly a bottle (two drachms) since November, on and off. I only take it when I am bad, and cannot sleep for pain. The protrusion always remains. I feel so grateful to you for the advice and relief given me."

I wrote to recommend her to take the medicine regularly. She next reported, "I have not taken the *Æsculus* as before for another month, and may fairly call myself well. I have no pain, and the protrusion is nothing but a flabby piece of skin."

This was in 1865, and the following, dated Nov., 1868 completes the history.

"I had no return of them till February last, when I had a severe attack. I took *Æsculus* for a fortnight, and it did no good. You came to see me, and finding that the bowels were loose instead of confined told me to take *Hamamelis*. I did so, and was very soon well again. Since then I have not suffered at all, and have only a few pieces of skin hanging which cause no pain.

I recommend the *Æscutus*, also, in those cases where a few days Constipation will bring on Hæmorrhoidal symptoms often of long duration. Two of such I have given at p. 485 of the same Volume of the JOURNAL. One of them is worth citing here.

"Mrs, F—, æt 60, years ago a martyr to Hæmorrhoids. Each attack would last from six to ten months, during which time she rarely leave the recumbent posture. Since adopting Homœopathy, the bowels had acted with much greater regularity, and the Hæmorrhoids attacks had been absent. On May 22nd, 1865, I was called to see her. I found her in bed, suffering intensely from several large Piles, which seemed quite to block up the rectum. The bowels had been confined for several days in the preceeding week ; and on the 20th old Hæmorrhoidal symptoms had supervened, and were increasing in intensity. There was little or no bleeding. She anticipated many weeks of suffering. I gave her a drop of *Æsculus* 3 every four hours. Next morning there was improvement rather than the reverse. On the 24th she was decidedly better. She said, 'Are you giving me an aperient ? The bowels are acting so comfortably. On the 25th she was well and about the house ; and I took my leave.

3. Lastly, Hæmorrhoids may be idiopathic. Without portal, abdominal, or pelvic congestion, and without Constipation, Piles may be present. I believe this form of Hæmorrhoids to be a

true Varicosis; and it is sometimes associated with the same morbid condition of the veins elsewhere. The Hæmorrhodis thus caused bleed very freely; they are the "Bleeding Piles" of the popular phraseology and the amount of blood lost at each evacuation is often considerable. We have one grand remedy for them, and that is Hamamelis. I have now in my mind at least half-a-dozen cases in which this medicine has proved curative. It would be useless to detail them, as they tell but one story,—Hæmorrhage, more or less profuse, occurring with every evacuation for months or years, with other symptoms of Piles; and rapid improvement and complete cure under the use of *Hamamelis*, generally in the 2nd centesimal dilution. I do not remember a case in which it failed.

Dr. Ringer tells us that he gets corresponding results from *Hamamelis* in one or two minim doses of the tincture; and Sir Lauder Brunton has recently echoed his experience. Dr. Jousset begins one of his LECONs with a narrative of a chronic case cured by it, in the 3rd dilution : and goes on to speak fully of Piles and their treatment. Returning to the subject in L'ART MEDICAL for December, 1900, Dr. Jousset says he esteems it so highly that if it fails to arrest the loss of blood, he infers that there must pretty certainly be Cancer of the rectum. While generally giving fractional doses of the tincture, sometimes he finds the 3rd dilution preferable. From his statements here, and in his 'ELEMENTS DE MEDICINE PRACTIQUE', it appears that he considers these excrescences to be manifestations of a general Hæmorrhoidal diathesis. To this he would refer, not only the general Varicosis of which I have spoken under *Hamamelis*, but also the abdominal congestions and the Constipation which I have suggested as ultimate causes of the appearance of Piles He may well be right; and, indeed, if we study *Æsculus*, a close resemblance appears between its Pathogenetic effects and the symptoms of the Hæmorrhoidal diathesis which Dr. Jousset describes. It too, therefore, and still more *Nux* and *Sulphur*, may act as constitutional remedies in the cure of Piles.

An interesting Paper on Hæmorrhoids was contributed to the World's Homœopathic Convention of 1876 by Dr. Minor, of New York, and may be read in its 'Transactions', His indications for the six leading remedies, which he counts *Æsculus, Collinsonia, Aloes, Acidum muriaticum, Nux vomica* and *Sulphur* to be, are very clear and full. He does not attach the same importance to Constipation as an indication for *Æsculus* as I have been led to do; and indeed prefers under such circumstances to give *Collinsonia*. A sense as of a foreign body in the rectum, with dryness and fulness, indicate these medicines. *Aloes* takes their place when Its characteristic Diarrhœa is present. and *Muriatic acid* when the Piles are of large size and very tender. Here, probably, would come in the *Hypericum* which Drs. Rohrig and Ussher so commend.* *Nux* and *Sulphur* are indicated by the general symptoms of the patient.

---

* J. B. H. S., viii., 188, 189.

PROLAPSUS 509

I have only to add that when the Piles become much inflamed *Aconite* is indispensable ; and when they project externally may be applied locally with benefit.

FISSURE OF THE ANUS is another local trouble which Homœopathy has found means of reaching through the constitution. It has several times been cured without operation by our medicines. There is a case by Hahnemann himself in the Seventh Volume of the BRITISH JOURNAL (p. 496), and several by Dr. Perry of Paris and one of the editors in the Eighth. In all these **Nitric acid** was the curative remedy, in high dilutions. *Ignatia* also was of service. I must add the following case of my own, which seems to have been one of Fissure ; though, from the patient's delicacy, I forebore an examination.

Miss W.—æt. 40 consulted me Sept. 26th, 1865. She had been suffering for two months with hæmorrhage and pain after stool The bowels were moved every other morning ; the bleeding was considerable, and the pain intense, gradually subsiding afterwards but not leaving her until the evening. She felt much weakened, and was beginning to suffer from neuralgic pain in the face.

Regarding the hæmorrhage as the more important symptom, I prescribed *Hamamelis* 2, a drop three times a day.

Sept. 30th.—The bowels have been twice moved without any bleeding, the pain was intense as ever. *Æsculus* 2, a drop three times a day.

Oct. 3rd—The last evacuation was painless as well as blodless. Continue.

7th—No pain or bleeding since. The Neuralgia troublesome. *Arsenicum* 6. twice a day.

14th.—The Neuralgia much better, and no pain after stool, but some return of bleeding. *Hamamelis* 2. twice daily.

21st.—No bleeding since the 16th ; much better and stronger, Omit.

I saw this lady again in 1867, and found she had no return of her troubles.

Dr. Jousset speaks very highly of a little-known remedy which he confesses he uses empirically only, *Sedum acre*. Of Dr. Allen's use of *Ratanhia* here I have spoken in my Pharmacodynamics'. His indication for it, that the pain is worse after, than during stool, has lately been confirmed by another cure. *

PROLAPSUS ANI is generally cured with little difficulty in children, as I shall have to state hereafter. It is, however. a difficult matter to overcome in adults. There is a case in the Fifth Volume of the BRITISH JOURNAL in which **Arnica** in mother-tincture seems to have been curative, and I have myself

---
IBID., ix., 180.

some good results from it. *Aloes* in the same strength, and *Ignatia* also recommended.

FISTULA IN ANO you would hardly expect to be reached by internal remedies ; and I am not confident that it would be so cured without local applications being employed. But, with the **Calendula** and **Hydrastis** of our own Materia Medica thus applied, we have several cures to report. You may read a case by Dr. Eadon in the Ninth Volume of the MONTHLY HOMŒOPATHIC REVIEW (p. 350), in which *Calcarea Phosphorica*, with injections of *Calendula* and the steam-douche, proved curative ; another by Dr. Clifton in the Twelfth Volume of the same Journal (p. 408), *Causticum* with *Calendula* locally, being the remedies ; and a third from America in the Twenty-Sixth Volume of the BRITISH JOURNAL (p. 664), where *Nux* and *Sulphur* were given with injections of *Hydrastin*.

I have now a few words to say about the Homœopathic treatment of intestinal parasites, generally known as—

WORMS. — In recommending specifically-acting remedies for the various forms of Helminthiasis, I must not be supposed to doubt the parasitic nature of Worms, or to adhere to the exploded theory that they are products of the morbid intestine. I make no question but that it is very good practice to expell the Tape-worm with oil of male fern and the Round Worm with *Santonine*-lozenges, and to exterminate Thread-worms by injections *Quassia*, *Salt*, *Iron* or *Sulphuric ether*. I should have no hesitation in using such measures did I find it necessary. But, explain it how we may, there is no doubt that Homœopathic remedies given in the usual manner. have singular power of abolishiug the troubles caused by Worms and often of effecting their expulsion. Thus, in cases of Tape worm, repeated drop-doses of *Oleum filicis maris* and of dilutions of *Mercurius corrosivus*, of *Stannum* or of *Cuprum aceticum* will often free the patient entirely from all Worm-symptoms, even though joints continue to pass away by stool. The same may be said of *Cina*, *Spigelia* and *Santonine* where Lumbrici are present ; and here a cure may often be effected by the expulsion of the Worms. Ascarides offer more resistance to treatment. *Cina* and *Santonine* are good here also ; ✢ but my favourite remedy is *Teucrium*, in the first decimal dilution. Under its use quantities of Worms are usually expelled and all morbid symptoms disappear. Two of the medicines we have seen acting upon the anus — *Æsculus* and *Ratanhia*—seem to have a similar power, especially over the

---

* See J.B.H.S., ii., 216.
✢ See Dr. Hamilton's case in Vol. xiii., B.J.H. p. 254.

irritation.* In obstinate cases, I have sometimes found the course of medicine recomended by Teste effective ; viz. *Lycopodium 30* for two days, *Veratrum albnm 12* for four days and *Ipecacuanha 6* for a week. Dr. M. M. Gardner and T. L. Bradford have recently † written to commend this medication, giving lower dilutions, and adding *Santonine* 1_x to the series, by which they include Lumbrici among its benefits. I have tried the *Stannum* and *Viola odorata* recommended by Teste for the last-named without perceiving any benefit. The irritation in the anus set up by Ascarides especially at night causes the patients to put their fingers to that part often unconsciously in their sleep. The eggs attach themselves to the fingers and get under nails. If the patient has the bad habit of putting his fingers in his mouth or biting his nails the eggs find their way to the stomach and bowels, where they are hatched into ever fresh broods of Thread-worms It is therefore absolutely necessary that the patient should give up this bad habit, otherwise the cure is difficult or impossible.

A word now upon—
PROCTALGIA.—Pain in the rectum is generally due to one or other of the disorders of that part we have had before us. Dr. Conrad Wesselhœft, however, has written an excellent essay in the NEW ENGLAND MEDICAL GAZETTE for 1897 upon a form of it which he describes as truly Neuralgic. In his first case the pain seemed to have been brought on by the use of *Croton oil* as an habitual aperient, aed several of the subsequent ones illustrate the Homœopathic application of this experience. He gives **Croton** in the 3_x dilution. His other remedies are the *Sulphate* of *Strychnine* and *Atropine*, generally in the same potency.

Lastly, of—
PARESIS ANI.- Loss of power of the anal sphincter, causing incontinence of fæces, is a distressing affection. I have more than once found it amenable to **Causticum** in the 3rd dilution. In troublesome cases, you may think of *Phosphorus 4-30*, and of *Ergotin* 2_x, cures with which have been reported.†† *Aloes* also, has proved effectual, according to its old repute, when the sphincter of the bladder has been affected with a like uncertainty of tenure. $

---

* J. B. H. S., i, 281 ; iv., 338 ; vi., 392.   † IBID., ix., 287.
†† IBID., vii., 220 ; ix., 102. $ IBID., xii., 322.

LECTURE XXXVII
DISEASES OF THE DIGESTIVE ORGANS
(continued)
———o———
THE PERITONEUM, PANCREAS AND LIVER
——o——

PERITONITIS—ASCITES—PANCREATITIS—HEPATIC CONGESTION —HEPATITIS—ACUTE ATROPHY OF THE LIVER—CIRRHOSIS OF THE LIVER—FATTY LIVER—WAXY LIVER—PIGMENTARY DEGENERATION—CANCER OF THE LIVER—JAUNDICE —GALLSTONES—FUNCTIONAL DERANGEMENTS.

I must not leave intestines without noticing the morbid conditions of the PERITONEUM. And, first of—

PERITONITIS. I do not speak here of the acute Puerperal, or of the chronic Tubercular form of this malady. The former belongs to the disorders incident to pregnancy and its termination; the latter to the diseases of childhood. I have here to speak of Simple Acute Peritonitis, as excited by cold or medicinal injury, or by extension from inflammation of the organs enveloped by the membrane. In diffuse inflammation of the peritoneum excited by cold, **Aconite** is indispensable, and may single-handed accomplish all that is required. More frequently, however, it will have to be followed up by **Bryonia** as the primary fever relaxes, and effusion threatens. In the rare case of the effusion being plastic, **Sulphur** is required, as in Pleurisy. In the Peritonitis lighted up by mechanical injury, as wounds and operations upon the abdomen, *Bryonia* should be given from the commencement, or— which I think better still—**Mercurious corrosivus** The tendency to purulent effusion always present in these cases supports the indications for the latter medicine. Whether it would prove sufficient when the inflammation resulted from extravasation of the gastro-intestinal contents is a question. I have not met with such a case, nor do I know any on record. In the most severe instance I have seen the mischief was set up by mesenteric Tubercle; it was the analogue of the intercurrent Pleurisy of Phthisis The patient rapidly recovered under *Aconite* and *Mercurius corrosivus.*

Peritonitis, by extension from the abdominal organs covered by the membrane is of a more circumscribed character. It never requires *Aconite. Bryonia* is sometimes useful for it; but a still better remedy is **Colocynth** which with Dr. Jousset entirely takes the former's place.* Colicky pains are of course a special indication for it, but their presence is not essential.

---

* Dr. Galley Blackley entertains a similar opinion (J. B. H. S., vii., 146.

The foregoing remarks represent all that I knew of Acute Peritonitis in 1878. I have nothing to withdraw from them; and the case reported by one of our Spanish colleagues, as translated in the Second Volume of the JOURNAL OF THE BRITISH HOMŒOPATHIC SOCIETY (p, 497), shows how rapidly a well-marked case of the kind will decline under *Aconite* and *Mercurius corrosivus*. Pathology, however, has modified its views about Peritonitis very considerably during the last two decades. The present-day doctrine is well set forth in the Paper read by Dr. Burford and Mr. James Johnstone before the BRITISH HOMOEO. PATHIC SOCIETY in 1199, and published in the Seventh Volume of the JOURNAL just-named ! and yet more fully by Dr. Burford singly in two post-graduate lectures on the subject which you may read in the MONTHLY HOMOEOPATHIC REVIEW for 1896. Primary Acute Peritonitis, we are told, does not exist. Peritonitis is always secondary to some extra-peritoneal lesion of organ or tissue. The link between the two is septic production and invasion. Inflammation of the serous membrane, when it occurs, is an effort of Nature to fortify it against its enemies; and the most dangerous cases are those in which the septic hosts, while producing the symptoms of Peritonitis, do not really excite that process, and the patient dies overwhelmed and exhausted by the onslaught.

I can give no opinion upon these views; but they seem well-supported. The sole question for us here is how far they ought to influence the Therapeutics of the disease. Our authors agree that though the inflammation here is of conservative intent, it must, when established be controlled and reduced by the remedies I have mentioned (among which they would replace *Aconite* and *Belladonna*); so that there is no change required here. But where rapid pulse-rise, without corresponding temperatures, and persistent vomiting indicate the septic to predominate over the inflammatory condition, they advise in preference such medicines as *Crotalus*, *Lachesis* and *Rhus*; and they there make a valuable contribution to our means of dealing with the malady.

ASCITES is never a condition of importance QUA peritoneum, save in Chronic Tubercular Peritonitis, of which I shall speak among the Diseases of Children. It thus hardly comes before us here. As occurring in connexion with Cirrhosis of the Liver, I shall speak of it further on in this Lecture. When part of a general Dropsical condition resulting from cardiac or renal disease, its treatment is that of the primary affection, as illustrated by a recent case reported by Dr. Vincent Leon Simon, in which it yielded to *Digitalin*.* His father before him had made a

---

* J.B.H.S., iv., 344.

collection of the older cases of cure by Homœopathic rumedies, which you will find in the Ninteenth Volume of the BRITISH JOURNAL OF HOMOEOPATHY. They are too brief to be instructive ; but they show that Ascites, especially when occurring as a SEQUELA of exhausting disease, like Ague, Dysentery or Typhus, is fairly amenable to such medicines as *Arsenicum*, *Apocynum* and *Apis*. In an instance of it, in a girl of 18, apparently due to Amenorrhæa and Chlorosis, the abdomen being as large as that of a woman at term, the Ascites and all other symptoms subsided under the persistent use of *Senecio aureus*. 1$_x$*

I have now remaining only the glands subsidiary to the digestive process. Of these the salivary have already come under our notice ; and in the present Lecture, after saying a few words upon the pancreas, I shall devote myself to the DISEASES OF THE LIVER.

Of the diseases of the PANCREAS, the only one I can specify is simple inflammation of its substance.

PANCREATITIS.—Rademacher has described this disease as occurring in both an Acute and a Chronic form, and states that its "organ-remedy" is **Iodine**. There is no doubt as to this medicine being Homœopathically indicated here. as also are **Mercurius** and **Iris**. I should prefer the two latter in Acute, the first in Chronic Pancreatitis. I have had several obscure cases which I have traced to this organ, and where the persistent use of *Iodine* has effected great improvement. (For one of these see the MEDICAL ERA of January, 1891. The disease had been set down as malignant.) Bahr has recorded a sub-acute case of some standing, in which, after *Iodine* had failed, improvement set in under the *Sulphate of Atropia*. Jahr has never seen the idiopathic disease ; but mentions one occurring from *Mercurial*-poisoning, in which *Kali iodatum* 12 and *Carbo vegetabilis* seemed to be curative.

You will remember the possible origination of Diarrhœa Adiposa in the pancreas, and here *Iodine* may fairly be expected to prove serviceable. Dr. Horace Dobell's views, moreover, as to the part played by the pancreas in the development of Phthisis are worthy of consideration. and confirm the indication for *Iodine* in this complaint.

For Cancer of the Pancreas I have no suggestion to offer.

The diseases of the LIVER constitute a wide field for study, and present many difficulties in the way of classification, I

---

* J.B. H. S. v., 98.

HEPATIC CONGESTION.

think I shall best present the Therapeutics of the subject to you, if I consider hepatic maladies under the headings of congestions, inflammations, and degenerations, ending with Jaundice and Gall-stones.

HEPATIC CONGESTION.—The treatment of this affection will necessarily vary according to the forms under which it presents itself.

1. There is the excited state of the liver which shows itself in increased secretion of bile, familar to those who practise in warm climates, and not unknown to us after a hot summer. I have already spoken of this among the forms of Diarrhœa, and indicated **Iris** as its specific remedy. When the "Bilious" symptoms are more pronounced, and patient and physician concur in talking of an "overflow of bile" (Polycholia of Frerichs), **Podophyllin** is better still. Sometimes, especially if there is much soreness of the head and eyeball, **Leptandra** is preferable.

2. A more common variety of hepatic Congestion is the passive or venous form. The engorgement may be seated either in the hepatic vein, as from valvular disease of the heart; or in the potal vein, from the habits which induce abdominal plethora. In the former case the liver can hardly be aided by specific remedies and the cause must receive our chief attention. In the latter, **Sulphur** is a remedy of great value, supposing that the patient will modify in the right direction his way of life. **Hepar Sulphuris** is highly commended here by Dr. Bayes especially when Hæmorrhoids result; and he concurs with Dr. Pope in praising **Lycopodium** which the latter places next to *Sulphur*.

Another form of passive Hepatic Congeston is that which occurs in women in connexion with imperfect performance of the uterine functions. **Sepia** is here an excellent remedy when the patient is at the Climacteric age, and **Magnesia muriatica** under other circumstances. I must refer you to my 'Pharmacodynamics' for the special indications for these medicines, as for those of *Lycopodium* and *Hepar sulphuris*.

Yet again, a Chronic Congestion of the Liver of this kind may be met with as a sequal to Malarious Fever. Dr. Jousset has recorded such a case in one of his LECONS CLINIQUES. It was cured by *Vipera*, which he esteems highly in such conditions. Dr. Majumdar writes that he has seen a good many cases of this affection in India among children. *Calcarea arsenicosa* 30 and the abandonment of milk are the main features of this treatment, which he claims as satjsfactory. *

3. In neither of these forms of Congestion is there any tendency to inflammation; save that interstitial Hepatitis some-

---

* J. B. H. S. v., 208

times supervenes upon the chronic mechanical engorgement incident to cardiac disease. But there is a Congestion of the liver which is obviously sub-inflammatory. It is most frequently the result of cold, when **Bryonia** will prove its most efficient remedy. If, however, it be caused by excess of stimulating food or Alcohol, **Nux vomica** will be preferable ; and if a fit of anger has provoked it, **Chamomilla** is its standard remedy.

There may be cases requiring *Mercurius, Chelidonium,* or *Sepia* ; but here more or less Jaundice will probably be present and I shall speak of them when I come to that affection.

Inflammation of the liver is described by Frerichs as circumscribed, tending to suppuration, or diffused, going on either to Softening and Atrophy, or to Induration. I shall limit the term Hepatitis to the first of these, considering the other two under the headings of Acute Atrophy and Cirrhosis respectively.

HEPATITIS, in its simple form, is rare in this country. In the only case I have seen, *Bryonia* and *Mercurius solubili*s, each in the 3rd decimal potency, rapidly removed the symptoms. I see no reason why the same medicines should not prove serviceable in the malady as met with in India and other hot climates. The former would correspond best where the surface (and therefore, in Peri-hepatitis), and the latter where the parenchyna was most affected. Dr. Gerson thinks *Calomel* the best *Mercurial* preparation in this disease. Whether we can check suppuration by such treatment, I know not ; when once established, I should expect more benefit from **Hepar sulphuris**. But I fear that such cases escape from the domain of medicine into that of Surgery.

Of Abscess of the Liver not dependent on inflammation, but occuring in connexion with Dysentery or Pyæmia, we have no experience on record ; and I have no medicinal suggestion to make regarding it.

In 1894, Dr. Dyce Brown read an interesting Paper on Acute Hepatitis before the BRITISH HOMOEOPATHIC SOCIETY, which you may read in the Third Volume of its JOURNAL. He was able to relate three cases which had recently come under his notice, and accounted for their comparative frequency by ascribing them to an Influenzal origin. Of the ordinary remedies, *Hepar sulphuris* was the only one which showed any marked effect and in both instances in which it did so the advanced stage of the malady and the persistence of the symptoms suggested that Abscess was threatening. Similar improvement under similar threatenings has been obtained from *Mercurius solubilis,* * but it had little effect in Dr. Brown's cases. I suggested, in the

---

* J. B. H. S., vii., 419.

CIRRHOSIS OF THE LIVER.

discussion on his Paper, that *Chelidonium* promised more than any of the medicines which had been mentioned if Hepatitis should be seen in its early stages; and I adhere to my recommendation.

Of Chronic Hepatitis I shall speak under the head of Cirrhosis of the Liver.

ACUTE ATROPHY OF THE LIVER, as frequently forming (or seeming to form) the Pathological basis of the "Malignant Jaundice" of the old writers, has given rise to some of the most interesting investigations of recent medicine. Is it not remarkable, moreover, that no sooner has it been distinctly recognised than its pathogenetic analogue appears in the shape of **Phosphbrus**? The symptoms of actute poisoning by this drug are those of Malignant Jaundice, and we have Frerichs own authority for the statement that the Pathological state induced is identical with that of the Acute Atrophy he has so well-studied. I have gone much into this subject when lecturing on *Phosphorus*; at present I have only to mention the medicine as a promising, and indeed the only promising remedy for this disease. Bahr, indeed, suggests *Digitalis* in the incipient stage; but I can hardly see the grounds of his recommendation. I know of only one recorded instance in Homœopathic literature in which this malady has been satisfactorily diagnosed and treated, and here the patient died, *Phosphorus* having played but little part in her treatment.* In Quain's Dictionary we read: "A few cases, in which the diagnosis of Acute Yellow Atrophy has been thought justifiable, have recovered; and these have been treated with the mineral acids and saline purgatives, *Aconite, Quinine* and *Camphor*." I hope our one remedy may be found at least as effectual.

In
CIRRHOSIS OF THE LIVER, *Phosphorus* is no less Homœopathic and has proved more curative. I have stated, when lecturing on this drug, that Wcgner had found that while acute poisoning with it caused a diffused inflammation like that of Acute Atrophy, its gradual administration sets up an interstitial Hepatitis, in which the organ was hard, enlarged at first but subsequently atrophied, and then presented a granular appearance. All this is the Pathological history of Cirrhosis; and we find associated therewith several of the clinical features belonging to the disease as observed in the human subject—icterus, Ascites, and such like. Aufrecht indeed maintains that Cirrhosis of the

Liver is the result, not of interstitial inflammation, but of that process in the glandular cells of the peripheral acini. As, however, he gives a similar account of it when occurring from slow *Phosphorus* poisonnig, we are not concerned, therapeutically, with the question at issue. **Phosphorus** is evidently a true simile to the disease before us. Dr. Salzer, of Calcutta, communicated a study of its possible remedies to our Convention of 1876, in which he mentioned some experience of his own with the drug. He speaks of its "great curative power in this otherwise unmanageable disorder." "When," he says again, "we see that a man, in spite of moderation in diet, has been for months going from bad to worse, and that after he began to take *Phosphorus* he began to gradually to rally, we may fairly ascribe the improvement to the curative action of the drng administered. And this is what I have seen, in a few cases." Physicians from India, from England, and from Belgium, have recorded similar benefits from the drug.*

After *Phosphorus*, the most promising remedies are **Iodine**, **Aurum** and **Lycopodium**. For the first we have the suggestion of a case of poisoning cited by Christison, where the leading symptoms were pain in the region of the liver, loss of appetite emaciation, Quartan Fever, Diarrhœa, excessive weakness, and after the emaciation was far advanced a hardened liver, could be felt. The patient appears to have died of exhaustions. "From this case," he says, "and another of which the appearances after death will be presently noticed, it is not improbable that *Iodine* possesses the power of inflaming the liver." *Aurum* is said to have cured hepatic disease with Ascites ; and its repute (especially with Dr. Bartholow) in affections of the testes, kidneys and ovario-uterine organs points to some power over chronic indurations. It would probaly act best in cases having a Syphiltic origin. *Lycopodium* is considered by Bahr to be "particularly adapted to the treatment of Cirrhosis ; and Jahr speaks very highly of it in Chronic Hepatitis "of whatever nature it may be." A case has been put on record by Dr. Childs, of Pittsburg, † which was presumably one of Cirrhosis, though the only physical description of the liver speaks of its enlargemeut. The patient, however, had great Ascites, for which he was tapped sixteen times in a twelvemonth, yielding altogether 1,020 pints of fluid. He was kept nearly all this time upon *Lycopodium*, in the 30th and higher attenuation, and after the last operation seemed to have regained his health.

There are two other drugs whose pathogenesis shows them to act upon the liver, and which have found place among the remedies of Chronic Hepatitis. These are **Ptelea trifoiiata** and **Carduus marianus**. To the credit of the former we have only

---

*J. B. H. S , iii., 210 ; v , 104 ; vi., 103.

† See Hahnnmannian Monthly, xii., 334.

FATTY LIVER

one case as yet; but here a long-lasting enlargement of the liver with emaciation, sallow pallor, and other symptoms of impaired health, took on (Dr. H. K. Leonard says) a marvellous change for the better under this drug in mother-tincture. * A yet more potent "organ-remedy" for the liver we seem to have in *Carduus marianus*. Cirrhosis, with Dropsy, is among the hepatic affections it has cured; and the three cases reported by Dr. Proll in 1894 ✝ show its great power over serious chronic diseases of this kind.

It is to illustrate the use of remedies of this kind that Dr. Burnett published his BROCHURE on "The Greater Diseases of the Liver" (1891). *Cardaus* is one of his chief medicines: he thinks its action to be upon the left lobe of the liver, and that it is specially indicated when there is a patch of eruption over the lower end of the sternum, and when any enlargement present is horizontal. When it is perpendicular he prefers *Chelidonium*. *Hydrastis*, *Myrica* and *Cholesterine*—as used by him—will come before us in reference to other affections of the organ.

Recently, quite fresh ground has beed broken here by the use of *Calomel*—our **Mercurius dulcis**, not as a cholagogue, but in small non-perturbative doses. Commenced in the old school, ✝ it has been taken up in our own by Dr. Jousset. This physician, experimenting with the drug on rabbits in the laboratory of the Hospital St. Jacques, has found it set up a condition of liver precisely resembling the initial stage of Cirrhosis. It is especially in the hypertrophic form of the disease that this medication has proved effectual. ✝✝

The Ascites of Hepatic Cirrhosis is of course secondary to portal obstruction, and can only be permanently removed by striking at its cause. It may sometimes be reduced meanwhile by the *Apocynum cannabinum*, given in teaspoonful doses of a strong infusion or concentrated decoction. When it fails to yield readily, I am much in favour of an early resort to paracentesis. The continued presence of the fluid is a serious hindrance to our endeavours after the control of the disease which causes it.

The DEGENERATIONS OF THE LIVER which are of practical import are the FATTY; The AMYLOID, WAXY or LARDACEOUS; the PIGMENTARY; and the CANCEROUS. THE

FATTY LIVER, if its possessor will abstain from following voluntarily the habits practised against their will by Strasburg geese, ought to afford another opportunity for **Phosphorus**; and Dr. Bayes speaks of having derived unequivocal benefit from it.

---

*J. B. H. S., vi., 104.   ✝IBID., ii. 480,
✝See M. H. R., xxxvii., 490.   ✝✝ J. B. H. S., ii. 365. viii., 79, 159; ix., 282.

Dr. Buchman says that he has "completely cured the Fatty Liver of a Scrofulous girl, æt 4, the border of which extended as far as the navel, with accompanying icterus, in six weeks, by three doses of six globules each of *Chelidonium* 3."

WAXY LIVER has been cured, in old-school practice, by *Nitric acid* * and by the *Chloride of Gold*, ✝ of course in somewhat material doses. I cannot think of any Chemical action as being exerted by **Acidum nitricum** here, and must conclude that the specific influence which it undoubtedly has on the liver (as shown by Scott's experiments) was called into operation in the instance recorded. The same influence may be claimed for **Aurum**; and either would be appropriate when Syphilis was the exciting cause. In cases occurring independently of this taint, and due to chronic bone disease or to suppurations, *Calcarea* and *Silicea* would be the most promising remedies.

PIGMENTARY DEGENERATION appears to be the process which takes place sooner or later in the enlarged liver left behind by Malarial Fevers. I have spoken of some remedies for this enlargement under the head of Chronic Congestion of the organ. Dr. Maclean, in Russel Reynolds' "System of Medicine," speaks so warmly of the inunction of the *Biniodide of Mercury* here; both elements of the compound have such an irritant effect on the liver; and the quantity of it which can be absorbed from the ointment applied is so minute, that we can hardly regard the cure as otherwise than Homœopathtc. Dr. Salzer spekes highly of *Argentum nitricum*.

CANCER OF THE LIVER is but little under the control of medicine. Dr. Mohr, however, reports a ease in which all sufferings were eharmed away by *Nitric acid* 3 ✝ and Dr. Burnett has obtained some unexpectedly favourable results from *Cholesterine* in the 3 or 6 trituration.

I have now to speak of a condition which, though often symptomatic of the various disorders of the liver, sometimes appers without evident hepatic complication, at any rate merits separate Therapeutie consideration. I mean—

JAUNDICE—I have gone rather fully into the Pathology of this malady, and the medicines which claims Homœopathic rela-

---

* See B. J. H., xxi-, 672,
✝ See Bartholow's 'Materia, Medica,' Sub Voce. ✟ J. B. H. S.. vi.,298

tionship with it, in an Article in the Twenty-Second Valume of the BRITISH JOURNAL OF HOMOEOPATHY. Were I rewriting it now, I should only have to follow Dr. Murchison in suggesting that the hæmatic forms of Jaundice may sometimes depend upon arrested destruction of the bile in the blood ; and to add to the drugs which have caused it—*Chelidonium, Leptandra* and *Myrica cerifera*, to those which have cured it—*Chamomilla, Podophyllum* and *Hydraṣtis*. In this place I may sum up the indication for the use of remedies as follows ;—

1. RECENT JAUNDICE - excluding its presence as a mere feature of hepatic inflammation or congestion (where it is seldom complete), or as a sequel to the passage of a biliary eoncretion, in which cases it needs no special treatment—commonly occurs in one of the two ways. It may supervene rapidly upon a fright or fit of anger ; or it may develop after premonitory symptoms of Gastro-duodenal Catarrh. In the former case, **Chamomilla** is in high repute and evidence of a direct action exerted by it upon the liver has accumulated of late. Dr. Jousset accounts it with *Nux vomica*, the principal remedy in what he calls "Ictere Essential." The second variety seems due to an extension of the catarrhal process along the bile-ducts, causing obstruction and re-absorption of the secretion. **Mercurius** is often quite sufficient here. Bahr would supplement it when necessary with *Nux vomica*, and Jahr with *China* ; other physicians have found benefit from *Polophyllum, Digitalis, Hydrastis* and **Chelidonium.** I have several times used the last named with advantage in cases owning neither a psychical origin nor catarrhal prodromata. A somewhat similar remedy is *Chionanthus*, which Dr. Morrow praises highly, *and the *Myrica cerifera*, which in Dr. Burnett's hands has several times acted curatively.

2. Sometimes Acute Jaundice takes on a MALIGNANT character, being accompanied with hæmorrhage and cerebral disturbance, and threatening speedy death. This condition is a regular part of Yellow Fever, and may supervene in the course of other toxœmic disorders ; it may also be connected with Acute Atrophy of the Liver. Where hypochondriac pain and tenderness indicated the presence of the diffused inflammation with which the latter malady sets in, I should rely upon **Phosphorus**. When the Jaundice originates in the blood, the *Serpent poisons* —especially **Crotalus**— are indicated, as in Yellow Fever itself. Dr Jousset says that he has known some cases of cure of Malignant Jaundice by the mother-tincture of *Aconite.* There is certainly evidence that this drug in one case of poisoning (SECUNDUM ARTEM) caused Jaundice ending in death.

J, B. H. S., iv, 404. ✢ If the itching of the skin often caused by the presence of bile in the blood should need a special remedy, you may find it in the *Dolichos pruriens*. of which I shall speak under Prurigo (J.B.H.S.. i., 177, 272).

3. Where Jaundice comes before us in a CHRONIC form, and there is no evidence of mechanical obstruction to the flow of bile, *Phosphorus* and *Iodium* should be considered. Two striking cases of cure by the latter medicine have been put on record* : it was given in low attenuation. Dr. Burnett relies here upon *Chelidonium*, in the mother-tincture, and gives several good cases illustrating its efficacy.

Of the affections on the GALL-BLADDER I shall speak only of—

GALL STONES.—The presence of these calculi is generally first announced by their passage along biliary duct, and the pain and vomiting thereby occasioned. Several of our ordinary medicines are recommended here in the text-books — as *Belladonna*, *Chamomilla*, *Colocynth*, *Digitalis* and *Arsenic*. My own experience was that of Bahr, that no degree of evident success was to be obtained by such means : and I was in the habit of resorting to the inhalation of *Chloroform* when Dr. Drury's recommendation led me to try **Calcarea** 3J. The effect of this remedy in the next case I had, was something marvellous ; and it has never failed me since : Drs. Bayes and Dudgeon have also borne testimony to its efficacy. Should it disappoint you in any case, I may mention **Berberis** as possibly playing the same part here as we shall see it doing in the passage of urinary Gravel. In a mild attack of the kind I once underwent in my own person, this medicine —prescribed by my colleague, Dr. Edward Black— was of decided service ; but on a second occasion *Calcarea* relieved me much more quickly. *Berberis* seems to act best in the mother-tincture, and where Gall--sand passes rather than forming Calculi, ✝ Dr. Burnett does not mention this medicine, and relies during the passage of the calculus on H*ydrastis*, which he gives in similar form, carrying the dosage sometimes up to ten drops every half-hour. Perhaps (as Dr. Galley Blackley suggests) it may be the *Berberine* contained in *Hydrastis* which does the work.

The treatment of the tendency to Billiary Calculus is mainly dietetic and regiminal. But I may draw your attention to the experience of the late Dr. Thayer, of Boston, as to value of **China** in such cases. He states that with this medicine, given in the 6th dilution (probably decimal) at increasing intervals he had far more than twenty years treated patienrs subject to the passage of Gall-stones, and had never failed to obtain a radical cure. Sometimes, he says, its first effect seems to be to expel the Calculi more rapidly ; but after this the attacks cease to recur. Dr. Claude, of Paris, has confirmed this experience ; ✝ while Dr. Amberg has shown that if the tendency has been

---

* Se B. J. H., xxii., 357 ; xxxiv., 381.   IBID.. xxxlii., 345.
BULL. DE LA SOC. MED. HOM. DE FRANCE, Vol xx,i

recently acquired it may be stamped out with *Chelidonium*.*
Dr. Bourzutscky speaks no less warmly of *Carduus marianus*

An interesting Paper was read before the British Homœopathic Society in 1894, by Dr. Wolston, of Edinburgh, entitled "Gall-stones and their Vagaries."✝✝ In the discussion which followed you will find several useful bits of experience as to the efficacy of *Hydrastis*, *Gelsemium* and *Belladonna* in the attacks of Calculus, of *Berberis* and *China*, and also of *Olive oil* ** and the Ems waters, in the intervals.

These are all the substantive affections of the liver of which I have to treat. But Dr. Murchison has thrown fresh light upon this department of Pathology by calling our attention to the

FUNCTIONAL DERANGEMENTS of the organ, and pointing out that in thinking of these we are not to limit our view to the secretion of bile. Besides this office, the liver is an important blood-gland, having much to do both with the formation and with the purification (by destruction) of the vital fluid; so that its functional derangement may lead not merely to alteration in the quantity and quality of the bile, but to various disorders of nutrition and elimination—such as Diabetes, Lithiasis and Gout, these in their turn inducing many derangements and even diseases of particular organs. These are important considerations in many ways and have also a strong bearing upon our special subject.

Following the maxium of prescribing upon the totality of the patient's symptoms, both past and present, we should look out for a history of hepatic disorder in cases of the maladies specified, and should be guided in our prescriptions accordingly. When Diabetes can be traced to the liver, Dr. Sharp has shown us ‖ the value of **Chamomilla**, which in such cases might take the place of the *Uranium* or *Phosphoric acid* we should otherwise prescribe. When "Lithæmia" is present by itself, or associated with symptoms specially called "Gouty", an hepatic origin would suggest **Lycopodium** and **Sepia**, both of which have the Congested Liver and the loaded urine in their symptomatology.

When functional derangement of the liver simply shows itself by excess or deficiency of bile, **Podophyllum** or **Leptandra** in the former case, and **Mercurius** or **Chelidonium** in the latter, will be suitable.

---

*J. B. H. S., v., 89 ✝ Ibid., ix., 282.   ✝✝ See Ibid., ii., 371.

**A more agreeable, and apparently equally effective, substitute for *oil* is *Glycerine*. M. Ferrand extols it highly in "Biliary Lithiasis," saying that in a dose 20—30 grms, it makes an end of the calculous attacks, and in daily quantities of 5—25 grms averts their repetition (L' art Medical, June 1894).

‖ Essays in Medicine, p. 791.

LECTURE XXXVII

DISEASES OF THE RESPIRATORY ORGANS.

––––o––––

THE NOSE,

––o––

RHINITIS—CORYZA—OZAENA—HAY FEVER—EPISTAXIS—
POLYPUS NARIUM—SNEEZING.

The Diseases of the Respiratory Organs (to which I now come) play, in this climate, a large part in the work of every practitioner of medicine; and it is of the utmost importance to enquire if Homœopathy can do much for them. The answer to the general question can be given in the affirmative with the greatest assurance. Our Statistics, in respect of such of these affections as threaten life, have always been most favourable ; and our text-books show a confidence in their treatment which is eminently satisfying. This happy state of things arises from our exclusively possessing, or alone adequately using, certain patent medicines, of which I would specify *Aconite* and *Bryonia*, *Antimony* and *Phosphorus*, *Iodine* and *Sulphur*. Let me say a few words on each of these.

1. *Aconite* is known and valued chiefly for its action on the Circulation at large—for the power it has over Fever. But we must remember how Fletcher has shown—as Fordyce, according to Dr. Sharp, had suggested before him—that Inflammation is locally what Fever is in the general system ; so that *Aconite* might be expected to do in the microcosm of any organ somewhat of that of which it accomplishes in the organism as a whole, It does so, but with this limitation, that it is effective only in the primary, congestive stage of Inflammation, before exudation has taken place : that is, while the local circulation is the offending mechanism, and the extra-vascular tissues are comparatively untouched. This corresponds with a well-established symptomatic indication for it, and one which constantly calls for it in the disorders we are considering, viz., that its troubles are such as arrive from DRY COLD. This NOXA acts on the blood vessels, while irritants begin their operations upon the living substance outside them ; and in inflammations owning the latter origin *Aconite* plays little part.

In Active Congestions, then, of the respiratory tract from the nose to the air-cells, especially when traceable to breathing cold air or receiving its impact too harshly upon the surface, *Aconite* is our prime resource, and no other remedy should be so much as thought of until the patient has had the benefit of it. In the

DISEASES OF THE RESPIRATORY ORGANS. 525

common "Cold in the Head"—little cared for in ordinary practice, but a cause of wide-spread inconvenience and often a beginning of worse things—we should depend upon it perhaps more than we do. *Camphor* precedes it when we have only a suspicion that we have taken a Chill—which suspicion it generally dissipates; but when this is converted into a certainty, and the well-known "stuffy" feeling indicates commencing congestion of the nasal passages, *Aconite* should be at once resorted to and continued until this is resolved. Still more is this so in those painful cases where the Catarrh affects the posterior nares, or the ethmoidal cells and the frontal sinus.

The medicine is no less serviceable for an incipient Cough, when pain is caused by it or soreness is felt in the larynx, trachea or large bronchi. Where one would poultice externally, one should choose *Aconite* for internal administration. *Bryonia* may come in excellently afterwards : but *Aconite* should be given first. This canon holds good in one of the affections of the larynx which causes the liveliest concern - the Catarrhospasmodic "Croup" of Childhood. *Spongia* is a tried remedy for it, but *Aconite* should begin and will often end its treatment, and parents should be instructed to begin its administration before they send for the doctor. The same thing is to be said of Bronchitis itself. If you can catch it in the forming stage when dry rhonchus is the respiratory sound and the Cough also is dry or brings up but a scanty and perhaps blood-stained sputum, *Aconite* is most important, and will alone do much if not all that is needed. It does as much for Acute Congestion of the Lungs themselves, where the pulmonary artery is the seat of the vascular disorder. Whether it exerts any control over true Pneumonia is a more doubtful question. I shall discuss it when I come to that disease, and you will see that I lean to the negative side in the controversy. But when there is any uncertainty as to the diagnosis, and simple Pulmonary Congestion is possibly present, no harm can be done in beginning with *Aconite* until the condition be clear.

In some of these affections, we may find the "anxious impatience, the unappeasable restlessness, the agonized tossing about" which Hahnemann specified as leading indication for the choice of our present remedy. In proportion as we do so, it will be the more precisely suitable, and may be given in more attenuated form. But we must not wait for these. They, as also the thirst and the rapid pulse which he mentions, may be absent, and yet it shall be the proper remedy, acting locally upon local mischief. It is, I think, a too great reliance on such indications which has given *Aconite* a place unworthy of its merits in Dr. Goodno's Treatise. He prefers *Gelsemium* in acute Nasal Catarrh and Schussler's *Ferrum phosphoricum* in simple Bronchitis—assigning in the latter case the reason that "there is an absence of the restlessness, irritability and asthenic symptoms of *Aconite*." Such absence may be a bar to its action in the higher infinitesimals, but it will not prevent the dilutions from the 1st to the 3rd decimal doing excellent work. I know that this has not been Dr. Goodno's hindrance, but it is that of many of the so-called "Hahnemannian" party among us; and I have seen it boasted in print by one of them that he very seldom had occasion to use the drug which his acknowledged Master hailed as the great substitute for the Antiphlogistic apparatus of his day, the specific remedy for acute Inflammation and Inflammatory Fever.

For the place *Aconite* holds in this country we are much indebted to our Liverpool colleague, Dr. Hayward. In his little book called 'Taking cold: the Cause of half our Disease," which I am glad to see in a Seventh Edition, he shows exellently the way in which a Chill to the surface sets up Fever and Inflammation, and the supreme place which *Aconite* holds among the remedies for ill-effects. It is interesting to compare with his Treatise one of the latest utterances of the late M. Dujardin-Beaumetz, an acknowledged leader in French clinical medicine. He, too, has discovered * that *Aconite* is abortive of acute Catarrhs, Nasal and Bronchial, but supposes that for this purpose massive doses of the tincture (15-20 drops) must be employed; and, recognising that but few patients can take these with impurity, would limit it to their circle. He denies it, accordingly to children, and warns against continuing its use longer than eight days for fear of accidents. To such inanity is traditional therapeutics reduced, when it shuts its eyes to the discoveries of Hahnemann and the experience of Homœopathists !

2. It is in virtue of its action on the Blood-vessels that *Aconite* modifies disorders of the respiratory organs; but **Bryonia** is a pure irritant to their tissue. The kind of irritation it sets up, moreover, is shown by its full development in the rabbit which M. Curie poisoned slowly with the drug, after whose death a firm pseudo-membraneous tube was found, extending from the larynx to the third ramifications of the bronchiæ. *Bryonia* becomes thus a remady for Membranous Laryngitis, Plastic Bronchitis, Croupous Pneumonia and Pleurisy with fibrinous effusion. But it is also valuable (generally after *Aconite*, and sometimes in alternation with it) for dry catarrh of the primary bronchi; accompanied by an irritative shaking Cough] As this is the form usually taken by a "Cold on the Chest." it is not surprising that *Bryonia* and Cough have become so associated in the lay Homœopathic mind that one rarely occurs without the other being used as its remedy, and often with advantage.

3. Antimony—I speak mainly of its *Potassio-tartrate*, the

---

* SREE JOURN, BELGE D' HOMOEOPATHIC, Vol. ii., No. 5. p. 349.

well-known "**tartar emetic**"—is the precise opposite of *Bryonia*, not in the seat but in the character of the inflammation it sets up. Its tracheo-bronchial exudation is abundant and mucous; its effusion into the air-cells is serous instead of fibrinous. In poisoning by it, moreover, the lungs are not affected primarily, as they are by *Bryonia*; the inflammation is found only in the respiratory passages if the animals are killed early enough, and later works thence down to the air-cells. *Tartar emetic* thus becomes the typical medicine for Broncho-pneumonia in all its stages; and for Simple and even Capillary Bronchitis where free exudation exists from the first, or has supervened. In the last-named formidable disorder—the "Suffocative Catarrh" of the old Nosologists—I have found it a potent remedy. I have always given it here in the 1st trituration, and Dr. Goodno says that he has repeatedly observed success follow this preparation after smaller doses had failed. This physician also has much faith in the *Iodine* of the metal, at the same strength, in both Acute and Chronic Bronchitis with heavy yellow muco-purulent expectoration and tendency to hectic. When the sputum is mucous only it can be much diminished in quantity in the most chronic cases by the steady use of the *Potassio-tartrate*.

4. In our use of *Antimony* we are on common ground with the other school, though we employ it to reduce rather than to favour expectoration; but **Phosphorus** as a respirtory medicine is all our own. It stands as an irritant about mid-way between *Bryonia* and *Tartar emetic*, and has the lungs themselves—the area supplied by the pulmonary artery—for its special seat. *Phosphorus* is therefore precisely suited to the form of Pneumonia most frequently encountered occuring, as I have said, "in delicate persons, with lowered health, or secondarily to such blood-infections as Typhoid and Scarlet Fever, and, as I would now add, Influenza. The exudation here would be corpuscular rather than fibrinous." Fleischmann's use of it as a specific for Pneumonia in his Hospital (Gumpendorf) at Vienna was thus justified by the result, his low rate of mortality being one of the first palpable evidences of the value of Hahnemann's method in acute disease. We may discriminate more closely, and with advantage; but we must always associate Pneumonia and *Phosphorus* together in our minds.

In such discrimination, the distinctive characteristics of the action of *Phosphorus* as drawn for us by Dr. Allen in one of his instructive lectures on Materia Medica, may well be borne in mind.* The presence of hæmorrhages in its inflammations, the absence of nervous and circulatory excitement, the aggravating effect of hot weather, the softness and compressibility of its pulse, the mental apathy and indifference and the sense of general oppression as from an external weight,—these are the leading features on which he dwells, and which—without insisting on their presence—we should seek to find in order to perfect its Homœopathicity to a given case of pulmonary inflammation.

5. **Iodine** is an undoubted irritant, pathogenetically, of the respiratory organs. The Coryza of common Iodism is well-known; and provings and poisonings exhibit a similar influence exerted lower down the tract. -In the larynx and trachea," I have written in my 'Pharmacodynamics,' "we may have Hoarseness, Aphonia and chronic inflammation, even simulating Laryngeal Phthisis ; and while the bronchi are but moderately affected, the lungs show the influence of the drug by congestive oppression, Hæmoptysis and even Pneumonia." The apparent exception I have made now falls under the rule ; for in the first case of poisoning in the Cyclopædia of Drug Pathogenesy we find in the narrative of the autopsy—"The whole of the bronchial tubes down to their finest branches inflamed and covered with viscid mucous; the mucous membrane swollen and injected." In Ricord's account, moreover, there cited, of his early experiences with *Iodide of Potassium*, we read —"The bronchiæ were sometimes found to be affected. The symptoms were those of simple Bronchitis : the expectoration ended as it had begun, without ever becoming purulent." So also Sir Lauder Brunton writes of Iodism —"Not unfrequently the bronchial mucous membrane becomes congested, there is cough and pain in the chest."

The false membranes often manifested as a local effect of *Iodine* (some of which are mentioned in the case of poisoning I have just referred to) led to its earliest application in the respiratory sphere among Homœopathists,—Koch (OUR Koch) in 1841 advocating its use in preference to *Spongia* for Membranous Croup, and Elb a little later verifying and extending his experience. Still later, Kafka—inferring that what was good for Croup could not be amiss in Croupous Pneumonia—tested it in this latter disease, and found that administered when the physical signs first appear it will arrest the progress of localisation and abort the whole disease. The practice has of late been much adopted in America, and excellant results have been reported, especially when the right lung is the seat of the inflammation.* Dr. McMichael speaks of it here as being "as nearly specific as may be," and Dr. H. K. Leonard as supplying "one of the few almost certainties in the practice of medicine." It will of course be in the class of cases in which we have hitherto given *Bryonia* that it will play its part. Then Dr. Nicholson has shown us how well the *Iodide of Potassium* will act when Bronchial Catarrh similar to its Coryza is set up, especially when compli-

---

*See N. A. J. H., June-July. 1 95.
†See IBID., Aug , 1893 ; N. ENGL, MED. GAZ., July, 1893 ; MED, CENTUARY, Aug., 1895.; J. B. H. S., v., 92.

cated with Asthmatic dyspnœa; * and in Coryza itself, when the phenomena are those which it causes in the healthy, it is highly esteemed amongst us.

Besides these applications, *Iodine* has played a large part in respiratory affections, in the compounds it forms with other elements. We have just heard Dr. Goodno on *Iodine of Antimony*. Dr. Youngman has lately tested the *Iodide of Tin* to see if the well-reputed action of *Stannum* in chest disease could be enhanced by the combination, and has had very favourable results with its 3rd deci-trituration in chronic pulmonary affections simulating Phthisis. It appears to reduce especially the profuse secretion and expectoration. ✢ De. Nankivell's reports, as to the value of *Iodide of Arsenic* in Phthisis ✢† are familiar to us all, and have established this drug as perhaps our fundamental remedy in dealing with such cases. In all these instances, the *Iodine* seems to intensify the action of the other element of the compounds; but has this additional advantage, that besides its local influence it corresponds to the state of general health usually associated with chronic chest affections. The emaciation of Chronic Iodism, with its rapid pulse and sweating, forcibly suggests the Phthisical condition; and in the Marasmus of childhood I have constantly used the analogy to advantage. I have no less confidence in it in those cases which Dr. Cartier calls "Bronchite Suspecte", where grave Bronchitis or Broncho-pneumonia manifests Phthisical tendencies. He relies here upon one of the *Tuberculin* products, $ but I have been so satisfied with *Iodine* that I have found no need of any Nosodes for its reinforcement. =

6. In our use of **Sulphur** as a medicine having specific influence on the respiratory organs we stand quite alone. I know that the Sulphureous waters of the Pyrenees have been used, INTER ALIA, for chronic bronchial and pulmonary affections; but it was rather with the idea of the drug acting as an "alternative," and indirectly benefiting the morbid state through the system at large. Now, indeed, a physician of the Eaux Bonnes has recognised their local affinity, and explains their action by the theory of "substitution". They cause a "congestive POUSSEE towards the respiratory organs," bring on Hæmoptysis even in healthy persons, "create artificial Asthma," and so on.

It is in the deeper and graver disorders of this region that *Sulphur* plays so prominent a part in our hands. I have shown in my 'Pharmacodynamics,' from Wurmb and Caspar and also from Bahr, what it can do in Pleurisy and Pneumonia; from Russell, its power over Asthma; from Meyhoffer, its value in

---

* M. H. R., Sept,. 1894. ✢ HAHN. MONTHLY, Jan., 1896, ✢ B. J. H., xxx., 515. $ See Transactions of the International Homœopathic Congress of 1896. = Bahr, and our American collegue, Dr. W. T. Laird, confirm this experience. See also a case of Dr. H. K. Leonard's in J. B. H. S., vii., 221.

DISEASES OF THE RESPIRATORY ORGANS

Chronic Bronchitis due to some morbid diathesis like Gout. Some of the older Homœopathists, like Jahr, considered it the leading remedy for Pneumonia when *Aconite* had spent its force ; and the physician named defended its use as against the *Bryonia*, *Phosphorus* and *Iodine* now generally employed in Homœopathic practice.

We proceed now to consider in detail the morbid states of the RESPIRATORY ORGANS. The NOSE, as being the commencement of the true air-passages, will have its diseases rated in this category ; and we shall then go on to those of the LARYNX and TRACHEA, the BRONCHIAL TUBES, the LUNGS and the PLEURA. I shall not, however, as in the alimentary canal, consider each region separately ; since so many respiratory affections—*e. g.*, Influenza, Hay-fever, Broncho and Pleuro-pneumonia—involve more than one of these.

RHINITIS.—The nose, like the eyelids and the ears, may be inflamed without, as well as within ; and the inflammation in the former case partakes of the character of Erysipelas. When acute, **Belladonna** with or without *Aconite* will be necessary. But I have generally seen Rhinitis as a sub-acute and tardy inflammation, which has found its effectual remedy in **Sulphur.** *Aurum* also is Homœopathic, and might help in case of need ; as it did in a patient of Dr. Kranz and his son at Wiesbaden, whose story you may read in the Sixth Volume of the JOURNAL OF THE BRITISH HOMOEOPATHIC SOCIETY. Here the Rhinitis was chronic, exacerbating with every pregnancy. Steady treatment with *Auronatrum chloratum* 5_x effected a cure.

Internal nasal inflammation is NASAL CATARRH, or—

CORYZA.—This is one of the minor but daily ills of humanity, for whose treatment the blunderbuss of ordinary medicine is worse than useless, but which the Homœopathic arms of precision often enable us to strike and conquer. It is everything to attack a "Cold" while yet it is incipient. Here we have two potent weapons against it, **Camphor** and **Aconite.** I have already indicated their distinctive spheres of action. *Camphor* will soon dissipate that chilly feeling which with most persons is the precursor of a 'Cold in the head'. *Aconite* is required in its stead, when the chilliness is evidently the first stage of Catarrhal Fever, and the temperature is already rising. Such a Cold is a true Catarrhal Fever ; and *Aconite* is its remedy throughout. Sometimes, however, especially in old people the symptoms resemble those of Gastric Fever, and here **Baptisia** is preferable ; while even in younger subjects the fever may be of such a type as to call for **Gelsemium** rather than *Aconite*.

When once established and localised, the cure of a Cold is not an easy matter; but a good deal may be done to relieve its symptoms and to shorten its duration. In the "Running Cold" or Fluent Coryza, **Mercurius**, in medium potencies, is the established remedy, and Bahr advises its use unless the discharge is such as to call for *Arsenicum*; but I have myself a special favour for **Euphrasia**, with which I have arrested many a Catarrh of this kind. Jahr goes with me in favouring this remedy. **Arsenicum and Kali bichromicum** and **Iodatum** are also thoroughly Homœopathic, and are sometimes preferentially indicated :—the first when there is prostration like that of Influenza, and the flux is copious. thin and acrid; the second when a foul tongue indicates the involvement of the digestive mucous membrane, the third when the nose is red and swollen externally, the discharge being cool and unirritating. For the "Stuffy Cold." I think (herein again coinciding with Jahr) that Nux vomica is the specific. Dr. Jousset would have us use this remedy also in the incipient dry stage of Fluent Coryza; and says that by giving a dose of the 3rd dilution every hour he has often arrested the malady by the end of its first day. I confess I prefer *Aconite* here : and still more when the congestion, the stuffiness, implies and invades the higher ramifications of the nasal mucous membrane.

When Nasal Catarrh has passed into its third stage of thick and bland discharge, and is inclined to linger, **Pulsatilla** is the medicine best calculated to hasten its departure; and may be relied on no less in Chronic Coryza, of simple character, and without constitutional taint. It will cure even when the flux is so profuse as to deserve the name of Rhinorrhœa ; I have recorded a case of the kind in the Thirty-First Volume of the BRITISH JOURNAL OF HOMOEOPATHY (p. 370). I assume that the discharge is thick : if it is thin, *Kali iodatum* is preferable. But it is seldom that a Chronic Nasal Catarrh is of so simple and limited a character. It is generally connected with systemic disorder, and requires careful treatment with remedies of profounder action. That such treatment, however, will repay the pains you may take, I can give you every assurance ; and you will find it quite unnecessary to resort to the local astringent and other applications of the ordinary practice, which are always unpleasant and often hurtful.

In undertaking the management of a case of this kind you may derive greatest assistance from a little Monograph, 'ON NASAL CATARRH', by Dr. Lucius Morse, Memphis, U. S. A. He gives a series of clinical illustrations of the disease, showing the action of its various remedies ; and then comments on them SERIATIM. He shows that sometimes most good is effected by such constitutional remedies as *Alumina, Calcarea, Lycopodium, Sepia,*

Silicea and *Sulphur*. Of the more locally-acting medicines he has especial confidence in *Arsenicum iodatum, Aurum, Graphites, Hydrastis, Kali bichromicum* and *Sanguinaria*. His indications for each are those which I have given in my Pharmacodynamics ; but I may briefly summarise them here.

Arsenicum iodatum : delicate, Tuberculous subjects ; discharge acrid : burning in nose and throat.

Aurum : discharge offensive ; bones of nose sore ; spirits very depressed. In Mercurialised and Syphilitic subjects.

Graphites : catarrh extending to Eustachian tubes and middle ear : tendency to eruptions on skin.

Hydrastis : tenacious stringy discharge : constant dropping down of mucous from posterior nares.

Kali bichromicum : yellow or stringy (white) discharge.

Sanguinaria : sensation of stinging and tickling accompanied with irritative swelling of the parts, either with or without free discharge.

Besides the medicines now specified, Jahr mentions *Cyclamen* as very effectual if the patient sneezes a good deal, and complains of Rheumatic pains in the head and ears ; and Bahr thinks *Iodatum* especially deserving of attention. I may also refer you to an Article on "The Nasal Passages", by Dr. Allen, in the Fifth Volume of the AMERICAN HOMOEOPATHIC REVIEW ; and to papers on nasal discharges by Dr. Vincent Green in the Seventh and Ninth Volumes of the JOURNAL OF TNE BRITISH HOMOEOPATHIC SOCIETY. Dr. Cooper has introduced a new remedy for Chronic Nasal Catarrh in *Lemna minor*, the common duckweed. His success with it has been endorsed by Drs. Burnett and Clarke. *

OZÆNA is now described as "Chronic Atrophic Rhinitis" ; so it must be included among the inflammations of the nose. It is a very intractable disease. I speak not only of that essential form which Jousset describes as existing without a lesion, characterized only by the execrable odour which proceeds from

---

* J.B.H.S., iii., 101.

the patient, and which he himself (deprived of the sense of smell) alone is unaware. This can but be palliated by deodorising injections, unless Dr. Cooper's *Lemna minor* should prove effective in it. Dr. Shearer describes its action as "wonderfull" ; and adds that it must not be administered in too low a dilution as it then causes a sense of intense dryness in pharynx and larynx. * Nor do I include under the head of Ozæna cases of mere Chronic Catarrh with some occasional fœtor about the discharge. To be a true instance of the disease, even in its more amenable form, fœtor must either be a constant attendant upon the habitual flux, or must accompany the formation of the "plugs" which the patient brings down from time to time.

The medicine most in repute for this disease is **Aurum** ; and the following case of Dr. Chalmers' will show what it can sometimes do.

A married lady, suffering from great general debility and loss of appetite, complained chiefly of heat and burning pain in the nostrils with great pain over the frontal sinus. There was obscure vision and pain in the eyes, which were much inflamed, with profuse discharge of sero-purulent matter, gluing the lids together. She had a copious discharge of yellowish-green pus from the nostrils, of a very fœtid odour, and she soiled five or six handkerchiefs daily. All the lining membrane of the nose was red, much swollen, and had many small ulcerated points on it, especially along the septum on both sides · she could not breathe through the nostrils.

This state of matters had been going on for several months, during which she has had various local and general applications without relief, and she is now almost sick of existence from the discharge and smell, &c. I gave her *Fowler's* A*rsenic* in two drops, twice daily, which was continued throughout January, with no relief as far as the nose was concerned but eyes are much improved as well as the general health.

Feb. 1st,—*Aurum met 2*, gr. 1 morning and evening.

Feb. 14th.—Is now considerbly better in health, and the discharge from the eyes and nose is much diminished, especially so from the former ; from the latter there is still abundant fœtid discharge ; she eats better, and the pain in frontal sinuses is removed.

Continue *Aurum* nightly.

23th—Eyes are quite well, being free of redness or discharge ; vision is quite well ; discharge from the nose much diminished in quantity, and is now pure pus, with little or no fœtor. She has a good appetite and looks fresh and well, and has no complaint if the nose were but right.

Continue *Aurum* every second night.

March 14th.—Still improving, and the discharge from nose almost gone ; the redness, swelling, and ulceration quite so, and she now breathes comfortably through the nostrils.

Aurum every third night.

31st.—She is now quite well, and has no discharge from nostrils for a week past.

---

* HAHN. MONTHLY, Aug., 1895, 55k. ✝ M.H.R., xii., 539.

I am mentioning two other cases also. Dr. Amberg had one of Chronic Nasal Catarrh with purulent fœtid discharge; the nasal mucous membrane was red and swollen. *Kali bichromicum* and *Pulsatilla* did no good; but *Aurum metallicum* 3 removed the trouble in a fortnight.* Dr. Delap reports a case beginning with a common Cold from exposure, but going on to Necrosis of the Bones. There is no Syphilitic history. Cleansing local applications were used, and *Aurum muriaticum* 2 given internally. A severe Headache which was present, greatly aggravated by stopping, yielded rapidly to the medicine. Dead bone came away. and the patient became quite well. ✢

Perhaps none of these cases would be ranked under "Atrophic Rhinitis, but they were certainly examples of Ozæna. *Aurum* would not be less suitable when the disease was of Syphlitic origin; though under these circumstances Jahr speaks highly of *Nitric acid*, especially if much *Mercury* has been taken. *Kali bichromicum* must not be forgotten, when the discharge is tenacious; though it has yet to win its spurs as curative of true Ozæna.

The nose is thus liable of several inflammations; it has only one Neurosis.

HAY-FEVER.—Such a description of it may be questioned. Is it not —some may ask—the direct result of the inhalation of the pollen of certain plants? None should acknowledge this more readily than Homœopathists: for it was a respected member of their body—Dr. C. H. Blackely—who discovered the fact now mentioned, and obtained for it, by his admirable experiments and resonings, universal recognition. †✢ But it is not all people —it is only a very few—who suffer from Catarrh or Asthma or both in

"The golden hour
When flower is feeling after flower."

It requires a predisposition as well as an exciting cause; and such predisposition, besides its definite response to pollen shows itself in hyper-sensitiveness to dust and similar irritants, even to bright sunshine, or merges into the "Paroxysmal Coryza" which Ringer has described so well, where without provocation of any kind, and in one season as much as in another, violent sneezing aud nasal defluxion are apt to occur. Such a tendency must be reckoned a Neurosis, and must be dealt with accordingly.

In true Hay fever, however, where a special and material CAUSA OCCASIONALIS has been traced, our principles would lead us to remove it if possible. This may be done either by keeping

---

* J. B. H. S.. v., 103 † IBID., i., 276.
✢✢ See his "Experimental Researches on the cause and nature of Catarrhus Æstivus (Hay-fever or Hay-asthma)". 1873.

out the pollen from the nostrils (for which Dr. Blackley has devised an ingenious apparatus); by destroying its vitality with a spray of a solution of *Quinine* (two grains to the ounce), as Binz advises, or by temporarily deadening the sensibility of the mucous membrane to its tormentors by the use of *Cocaine*, which Dr. Theodore Williams considers the best plan. But, while we do this, can we not as Homœopathists administer similarly-acting drugs which shall neutralise the susceptibility to the irritant, or, where the affection is a pure Neurosis, modify this in the direction of health?

We can; and the medicines APROPOS of which Dr. Ringer discusses "Paroxysmal Coryza" *Arsenic* and *Iodine*, warrant the affirmative reply, for both cause the symptoms he vouches that they cure. Given separately, or in combination as *Arsenicum iodatum*, they play a prominent part in our treatment of Hay-fever proper, and *Chininum arsenicosum* is sometimes a better compound still. Among other testimonies in favour of *Arsenic* I may cite that of Dr. J. E. James, of Philadelphia. He says of the disease —"I believe we have its remedy in *Arsenicum* 2 or 3. It has in my hands cured effectually several cases. . , . The first season I gave it about half the time, the second season for about a week, and the third for a day or two; and the attack did not recur. These cases were all of long-standing when they came under my care". Dr. Ivins, in a very practical paper on the subject presented to the International Homœopathic Congress of 1891, confirms the good that has been said of *Arsenic* and its *Iodide*, but reports yet more favourable results from *Allium cepa* where the flow is profuse, *Naphthalin* where Asthma predominates over Coryza, ✢ and *Arum triphyllum* where the latter is excoriating. His prognosis of the disorder is too encouraging to be omitted. "While I do not think every case curable," he writes, "or even capable of permanent amelioration, I do feel that cure is a frequent occurrence, permanent palliation the rule, temporary relief the exception and irremediable cases practically unknown,"

If you have to look further for your remedies, I would refer you, for coryzal cases, to what Dr. Bayes has said about *Sabadilla*, as quoted by me when lecturing on that medicine; and for Asthmatic ones to the striking parallelism of the effects of *Ipecacuanha* on certain susceptible subjects. As an alternative to the latter, I may add *Aralia racemosa*, for which see what I have said in the appendix to my 'Pharmacodynamics'. Mr. Dudley Wright, in a very practical paper on the disease in the Forty-Second Volume of the MONTHLY HOMOEOPATHIC REVIEW, commends *Euphrasia* very warmly in the actual coryzal attack, while relying mainly on *Arsenicum* for prophylaxis.

---

* HAHN. MONTHLY, xii., 21.

✢ Drs. Terry and Pope highly commend this drug, in the 1_x trituration for the Asthmatic attacks (see M. H. R., xiii., 252).

536 DISEASES OF THE RESPIRATORY ORGANS

Dr. Jousset regards Hay-fever as a manifestation under the influence of a special irritant, of what he calls "Gouty Coryza",—an affection characterized by paroxysms of nasal flux and repeated sneezing, which he has never seen save in Gouty and Hæmorrhoidal subjects. He finds *Kali Chloricum* 6 very beneficial in its treatment ; but says that *Arsenic* and *Nux vomica* are preferable in some cases. Dr. Ringer also has (as I have said) noticed this "Paroxysmal Coryza", praising *Arsenic* and *Iodide of Potassium* for it as internal remedies, and *Camphor* and *Iodine* by inhalation. I have lately had a case of the kind where the discharge was thick to indicate any of the these remedies, and where—after *Pulsatilla* and *Hydrastis* had failed—I was led by the excessive sneezing to give Dr. Bayes' *Sabadilla ;* and the patient got steadily well. He was certainly a HAEMORRHOIDAIRE. In another, where the discharge was thin and acrid, a cure seems to have resulted from *Arsenicum iodatum* ; the patient was a boy, and had a tendency to Asthma. In neither of these instances was there any susceptibility to such vegetable emanations as are encountered in the Spring and early Summer. As an alternative to the last named remedy I should mention *Euphrasia*. A cure of a case of ten years standing with the mother-tincture is reported in the NORTH AMERICAN JOURNAL OF HOMOEOPATHY for May, 1895 (p. 310).

EPISTAXIS, to which I come next, is rarely sufficiently severe or obstinate to require medical treatment. The usual domestic expedients generally suffice to arrest it. If, however, you are sent for to check one that has defied these measures, you cannot do better than mix a few drops of **Hamamelis** 1_x in a wineglassful of water, and give a teaspoonful every five minutes till the flow stops—which it will do pretty rapidly. I have formerly given indications for *Arnica*, *Millefolium*, *Belladonna*, *Nux vomica* *Bryonia* and *Aconite* in such an emergency, but in practice they all yield to *Hamamelis*. It is otherwise when you are consulted on account of the frequent recurrence of the hæmorrhage, whether in young subjects or old. Here **Ferrum phosphoricum**, as long ago recommended by Dr. Cooper, has often served my turn, and never disappointed me. I give it, as he did, in the first trituration.

POLYPUS NARIUM deserves mention here, because it has not unfrequently been cured by the internal administration of

Homœopathic remedies, especially **Teucrium** and **Calcarea carbonica**. As you may feel somewhat sceptical about this, let me read you a case of Dr. Goullon's :—

A married woman, aged 46, still menstruating, subject to Prosopalgia, got a polypus on the left side of the nose, which grew apace, and had already almost reached the level of the nostril. By its pressure on the septum narium it stopped up not only the left, but also the right nasal cavity, so that she could only breathe through her mouth. She was about to undergo an operation, when I requested her to make a trial of Homœopathy. She took twelve doses of *Calc. Carb. 30* without change ; then eight of *Calc. Carb, 18* in the same way ; thereafter *Calc. Carb. 9*, and thereupon diminution and shrivelling up of the Polypus began and went on so quickly that fourteen days after taking the last dose nothing was to be seen but a large fold of mucous membrane ; the nasal passages were quite free, and have remained so ever since, now two years.

Turn now to Vol. VIII of the MONTHLY HOMOEOPATHIC REVIEW, and consider the four other cases from our literature which Dr. Lippe has summarised there, in which a cure has followed the exhibition of the same drug in similar potencies. I think you will then feel no doubt about my assertion, at least, so far as *Calcarea* is concerned. The evidence in favour of *Teucrium* is hardly less convincing ; it must be given, however, in low potency, even, to the tincture. It suits the purely mucous Polypi, the product of chronic Catarrh. We have also two medicines whose general relation to these growths indicates them, and from which success has every now and then been obtained ; I speak of **Phosphorus** and **Thuja**. The former would be suitable when the growths bleed readily. Lastly, Dr. Eubulus Williams advocates the use of *Mercurius iodatus*, in the 3x trituration. He learned its value from the late Dr. Black, and reported at a meeting of the Western Countries Therapeutic Society ✝ that he had used it for twenty-one years, and had cured at last two dozen cases.

SNEEZING is sometimes so troublesome as to demand a special remedy. This you may find in Jahr's *Cyclamen*, already mentioned, or in the *Senega* and *Asafœtida* which has been reported as curative. ✝✝ On pathogenetic grounds I should prefer *Ipecacuanha*.

---

* B.J.H., xi. 484. † See M.H.R., xxxix., 426. ✝✝ J.B.H.S., vi. 400.

LECTURE XXXIX
DISEASES OF THE RESPIRATORY ORGANS
— o —

THE LARYNX AND BRONCHIAL TUBES.
— o —

LARYNGITIS—OEDEMA GLOTTIDIS—APHONIA—BRONCHITIS
—BRONCHIECTASIS—EMPHYSEMA PULMONUM—ASTHMA.

In coming to the disorders of the air-tubes proper, I must say at the outset how much use I shall make of the "Chronic Diseases of the Organs of Respiration" by my late friend, Dr. Meyhoffer. This accomplished physician, born a Switzer, practising in Italy, while Nice was Italian, writing almost equally well in French, German and English, published in 1871, in the last-named language, the First Volume of his Treatise, containing the diseases of the larynx and the bronchial tubes. It is full of the original work which his capacity, knowledge, and extensive opportunities in Riviera practice enabled him to carry out, and is as practical as it is scientific. It is to our discredit, as well as our loss that the Second Volume on diseases of the Lung's still remains in MS., for the lack of a publisher. The first should be in the library of every Homœopathic practioner, and will bear repeated perusal.

We begin to-day with the LARYNX.
LARYNGITIS is not with us the dreaded disease it is under the old system. We do not say, as Aitken does, if inhalation, leeches, and fomentations fail, 'tracheotomy ought not to be delayed." I will refer you to some cases in the MONTHLY HOMŒOPATHIC REVIEW for 1866, by Dr. Meyhoffer himself. You will see that we have capital medicines in specific relation with the larynx and its inflammatory states. Aconite seems indispensable at the commencement, and is sometimes sufficient for the cure. **Spongia, Kali bichromicum, Bromine** and **Hepar sulphur** stand next in order of requirement. The first two have most experience in their favour. *Hepar* is most suitable when the cough has become loose, but hoarseness remains. Should Œdema Glottidis supervene, repeated doses of Apis would give the best chance of averting tracheotomy.

A more superficial form of Laryngitis may be called "LARYNGEAL CATARRH." Under this title there is a good Article by Kleinert, in the Twentieth Volume of the BRITISH JOURNAL. He seems to have had much experience among professional singers, who indeed in all places are found to resort in preference to Homœopathic advice. You will profit much by a perusal of his remarks and cases. **Causticum**, *Bromine* and *Selenium* with *Aconite*, in recent cases, and **Carbo vegetabilis** in those more chronic, appear to be his especial remedies. The first and last are those which my own experience leads me to commend.

For Chronic Laryngitis we have the advantage of Dr. Meyhoffer's experience in the shape of a series of chapters in his book. He speaks first of the catarrhal variety, illustrating the effects of *Kali bichromicum*, *Tartar emetic*, *Kali iodatum*, *Hepar sulphuris*, *Manganum aceticum*, *Carbo vegetabilis* and *Phosphorus*. The first is indicated by glutinous, the second by copius and easy expectoration; *Kali iodatum*, *Manganum* and *Phosphorus*, where the larynx is dry and irritable; *Hepar sulphuris* where, while the expectoration is like that of *Kali bichromicum*, the patient's organism is more unhealthy; and *Carbo* "in long-standing Catarrhs of elderly people or in persons whose vitality is reduced to the lowest ebb, by insufficient nourishment rather than by disease, with venous capillary dilatation of the pharyngo laryngeal parts, and prevailing torpor of all the functions." Dr. Wurmb's experience at the Leopoldstadt Hospital in Vienna is confirmatory of the value of the last-named medicine. * Dr. Meyhoff adds *Causticum* and *Lachesis*, the former to restore power, the latter to diminish irritability. He then speaks of a more obstinate form of Chronic Laryngitis—the Follicular: pointing out that this is generally primary, while the Catarrhal variety is usually the sequel of a series of acute attacks. *Iodine* and its compounds with *Potassium* are his chief remedies here; and he finds its local application necessary in most cases, if a speedy cure is to result. Where the follicular throat is the manifestation of a morbid condition of the general system, apt to show itself by cutaneous eruptions (the "herpetic" or "dartrous" diathesis of tbe French), he finds *Sulphur* of the utmost value—sometimes in the Homœopathic attenuations, sometimes in the thermal waters of the Pyrenees. Dr. Meyhoffer next passes to the more profound alterations to which the larynx is liable—Hypertrophic Laryngitis, inflammation of the vocal cords, and Perichondritis Laryngea. For all these he deems local treatment indispensable, and Homœopathy has little to say for them. It is otherwise, however, with that more serious affection still—Tuberculous Laryngitis (Laryngeal Phthisis). Here although he thinks the conjoined, direct and indirect administration of the suitable remedy the best practice, he is satisfied as to the efficacy of the latter even when employed singly. The medicines from which he has derived most benefit are *Acidum nitricum*, *Argentum nitricum*, *Arsenicum iodium* and *Seleniate of Soda*—the first and last suiting more recent cases, the other those of longer-standing. Laryngeal Syphilis, again, hardly requires local

---

* See J. B. H., xxii.

treatment at all. When occurring in connexion with secondary symptoms, *Mercurius corrosivus* and *Nitric acid* are its remedies —the former when Ulcers, * the latter when mucous patches and Condylomata constitute the lesion. In Tertiary Syphilis of the larynx he finds *Mercurius biniodatus* and *Iodide of Potassium* answer every purpose, and does not think it necessary to give large doses of the latter. When the skin is very eruptive, he often gets the best results from *Cinnabar*—in the third or higher triturations.

I have dwelt thus fully on Dr. Meyhoffer's recommendations because his position gave him unusual opportunities of studying this class of affections, and because of the thoroughly scientific and satisfying character of his communications on the subject. Of our other therapeutists Jousset touches only the Tuberculous (or, as he would call it, Scrofulous) form ; he adds *Drosera* and *Calcarea* to the medicines suitable for it, the former when cough is frequent and violent, the latter when ulceration is present. Bahr's indications for remedies, so as far as they go, are mainly the same as Dr. Meyhoffer's though he attaches more value to *Manganum*. Kafka's only special point is the recommendation of *Atropia* (in drop doses of the first dilution of the *Sulphate*) when the Cough sympathetic of laryngeal ulceration is very distressing.

I would add two cases more recently put on record. One, from Dr. Bartus Trew, was diagnosed Tubercular by its former old-school attendants, but got well in his hands under *Cansticum* 6 and *Calcarea* 30 The other is reported by Dr. Speirs Alexander, and the laryngoscopic evidence given. It practically recovered under *Arsenicum iodatum* 3_s and *Causticum* 30. *

Besides the laryngeal troubles of childhood, of which I shall speak in their proper places, I have yet to mention two other morbid states incident to the part, which may or may not be connected with its inflammations. These are ŒDEMA GLOTTIDIS and APHONIA.

---

* Mr. Dudley Wright sent to the MONTHLY HOMOEOPATHIC REVIEW of April, 1894, a case of ulceration, presumably Tubercular, which recovered under *Kreosote* 1. Subsequently he found that the subject was a Syphilitic one (J.B.H.S., viii., 227).

† J.B.H.S., vii., 90 ; viii 223.

ŒDEMA GLOTTIDIS.— I think that the best advice I can give you as to the treatment of this dangerous condition, under whatever circumstances it may occur, is to trust to **Apis**,—which, if necessary, may be given subcutaneously as in a striking case recorded in the NORTH AMERICAN JOURNAL OF HOMOEOPATHY for June, 1895. Since this remedy has cured it even in its most fatal form, viz , that which occurs in children which after drinking from the spout of a tea-kettle, it will probably be competent to deal with all other forms of the malady. Should it ever fail you however, you may (before thinking of Surgical measures) consider the claims of **Sanguinaria**, as illustrated by the Second Part of the Fourth Edition of Dr. Hale's "New Remedies."

AHHONIA, when dependent upon substantial changes in the organ of voice, has obviously no Therapeutics of its own. When, however, in Simple Laryngeal Catarrh, Acute or Chronic, the weakness of vocalisation is out of the usual proportion **Causticum** is nearly always a helpful remedy. For Hysterical Aphonia I know no medicinal means which can compete with localised Galvanism, though Jousset speaks well of *Nux moschata*, *Platina* and *Ignatia*. Dr. Meyhoffer agrees with me here. In Paralytic Aphonia which is not of this character, and which is not traceable to compression of the recurrent nerve by Tumours or Aneurisms, **Phosphorus** would seem the most hopeful remedy, but *Silicea* has actually proved curative.

Gelsimium has cured WEAKNESS OF VOICE coming on at each menstrual period, ✝ and *Antlmonium crudnm* is said to be beneficial when it occurs every time the patient is exposed to heat. ✝✝,

A lesser degree of Aphonia is HOARSENESS, and this may generally be dispelled by one of the remedies already mentioned—*Causticum*, *Manganum*, or *Carbo vegetabilis*, to which may be added *Kali bichromicum* and *Hepar sulphuris*. An old-school physician is cited in L'ART MÉDICAL for October, 1897,

---

* See N. A. J. H., Dec., 1895, App., p. 96.

✝ See Meyhoffer, LOC. CIT, p. 230.

✝✝ Dr. Pearsall reports to the NORTH AMERICAN JOURNAL OF HOMOEOPATHY of June, 1893, two cases of Aphonia, with flabby relaxed condition of the laryngeal mucous membrane and imperfect approximation of the vocal cords during phonation. *Arsenicum iodatum*, given in one case in the 30*th*, other in the 2 proved curative.

as calling attention to *Erysimum* (he does not say which species of the genus so named, probably the *officinale*). Its efficacy has given it the title of "Herbe aux chantres." and this Dr. Herbary says he has been surprised by the rapidity of its action in the cases in which he has tried it.

I come now to the BRONCHIAL TUBES, and take up the large subject of —

BRONCHITIS.—A Paper on this disease, which I read before the British Homœopathic Society will be found (with the discussion following it) in the Fifth Volume of its ANNALS. Of that paper my present remarks will contain the substance, though in a somewhat different arrangement.

I shall speak here of SImple ACUTE BRONCHITIS, of CAPILLARY BRONCHITIS, of TOXAEMIC BRONCHITIS and of CHRONIC BRONCHITIS.

1. For Simple ACUTE BRONCHITIS in the fairly healthy adult, it is rare that any medicine but **Aconite** is required, if the case be taken in time. It must be remembered, however, that this medicine attacks inflammation through the blood-vessels, and not—like a specific irritant of the part—by influencing the inflamed tissue itself. It is only because in a Catarrh like this, the tissue is so lightly affected that I believe *Aconite* is capable of breaking up the disease. Should the inflammation have thoroughly established itself, we cannot expect *Aconite* alone to cure it. But even here it is a most useful auxiliary; and a few introductory or alternating doses will greatly help the specific irritant of the tissue to effect a cure.

Of the medicines falling under the latter category I shall speak of *Bryonia*, *Kali bichromicum* and *Ipecacuanha*.

In our domestic treatises, **Bryonia** generally heads the list of Bronchitic medicines. I think, however, that too extensive claims are made for it. It unquestionably produces inflammatory irritation of the trachea and largest bronchii, but there is no evidence that its influence goes further than these. I have argued this point in my paper, and you will see from the discussion that my colleagues share in my dissatisfaction with its action in most cases of Bronchitis. Good for the common "Cold on the Chest"—*i.e.*, where the catarrh invades only the trachea and largest bronchi—it is of little use beyond.

In animals poisoned by **Kali bichromicum** it is noted that the bronchiæ were inflamed as far as their ramifications could be traced; and symptoms of the disease are manifest both in the provers and in Chrome-workers. My own experience with it is that in most cases of Simple Bronchitis, if after *Aconite* has expended its action, any other medicine is required to modify the condition of the inflamed tissue, *Kali bichromicum* will do it. It is also very effectual in the Bronchitis of Influenza. We have here a general condition which demands, not *Aconite* and cold water, but *Arsenicum* and *Champagne*. When the Influenzal Catarrh runs down into the bronchial tubes, *Arsenic* will not follow it ; and here *Kali bichromicum* comes in most usefully. There is one symptom often present in these cases, which is especially characteristic of the remedy now under notice. This is a thickly-coated tongue, which, with loathing of food, indicates that the catarrh has involved the alimentary passages.

Every now and then a case will occur whose symptoms remind you of the phenomena which in susceptible persons, follow the inhalation of ipecacuanha. One such instance I have recorded in my paper. In these attacks—midway between Bronchitis and Asthma, half Neurosis and half Phlogosis—the power of *Ipecacuanha* is very great.

2. CAPILLARY BRONCHITIS, as constituting one of the pulmonary affections of childhood, will come under our notice later on. At present I shall consider it, as it occurs in old persons,—the "PERIPNEUMONIA NOTHA" and "SUFFOCATIVE CATARRH" of the older writers. The grand remedy for this dangerous disorder is **Tartar emetic**. Perfectly Homœopathic to both the local and the general condition, I have almost invariably relied upon it single-handed, and have seen desperate cases recover under its use. *Arsenicum* is often recommended ; but I cannot see its Homœopathicity, and have never used it. On the other hand **Carbo vegetabilis** can be unreservedly commended when the general symptoms (Collapse, Cyanosis, Coldness, &c.) predominate over the local. * One danger in these subjects is from Paralysis of the Lungs. I would refer you to the remarks I have made in my 'Pharmacodynamics' upon Solanine, the Alkaloid of *Dulcamara*, as suitable to such a condition. I have reason to feel much confidence in it. Dr. Cartier has communicated a striking case in which *Bacillinum* 30 obviated this danger. †

3. TOXÆMIC BRONCHITIS is liable to be set up by the specific poisons of Measles, of Typhus and Typhoid Fever, and of Gout, and by the excess of urea in the blood which obtains in Chronic Bright's Disease. Of the first I have already spoken, and I speak again. The Bronchitis of fever generally calls for *Bryonia* or *Tartar emetic*. In that which occurs in sufferers from Chronic Bright's Disease, I would suggust *Mercurius corrosivus*,

---

* Sec. M. H. R., xxxvli., 227, 354. † J. B. H. S., ii., 217.

which is Homœopathic to the primary malady, and in a case of poisoning by which, recorded by Dr. A. Taylor, the bronchial mucous membrane was found inflamed throughout its course. The connexion of Bronchitis with Gout has been insisted upon by Dr. Headlam Greenhow. If the disease proved obstinate in a patient owing to this diathesis, I should be disposed to give him the benefit of the as yet mysterious powers of *Colchicum*.

4. CHRONIC BRONCHITIS presents itself under such various forms, that it is well-nigh impossible to lay down any general laws for its management. Each case requires to be studied as an individual, and to be treated on its own merits. But I will make an attempt to classify its leading varieties, and to suggest their most suitable treatment. I will base my classification on the Pathological character of the expectoration,—viz., whether it is Mucous, Purulent or Fibrinous.

a. In CHRONIC BRONCHITIS with MUCOUS EXPECTORATION, the choice generally lies between two great mediines,— the determining symptom being the CONSISTENCE of the mucous. If it comes up in lumps, be easy to detach and expel, or difficult only because of the muscular debility present, **Tartar emetic** is usually the remedy. But where the sputa are difficult and tenacious, and come up in long strings of opaque white mucus, the preference should be given to **Kali bichromicum**. This indication for the latter medicine which has been verified over and over again, we owe to Dr. Drysdale.

b. Chronic Bronchitis with PURIFORM EXPECTORATION is a very serious matter. In cases of moderate severity, I have seen **Mercurius** in the medium dilutions of great service. Probably **Silicea**, which Teste commends highly in Chronic Bronchitis, may find its place here. *China* will at all events be useful in sustaining the constitution.

c. If you meet with the rare form of Chronic Bronchitis, in which semi membranous expectoration (bronchial polypi) occurs, M. Curie's experiments would point to **Bryonia** as its most Homœopathic remedy, though *Kali bichromicum* is hardly less so.

In all forms of Bronchitis, but especially in the influenzal and the senile varieties, the cough is sometimes violent, quite out of proportion to the local affection. We have here to call in the help of the neurotic drugs, the chief of which are **Senega Hyoscyamus** and **Conium**, *Hyoscyamus* is generally a capital medicine for such a cough occurring in Influenza—the characteristic indication being aggravation on lying down. In old persons, where the cough is harassing, I have much confidence in *Senega*. These neurotics may be given at the same time with the more strictly curative remedies, either in alternate doses, or (which I think better) the one by day and and the other by night.

Sometimes, both in Acute and Chronic Bronchitis, we have to depend upon the neurotic in preference to the tissue-irritant medicines. I have already spoken of *Ipecacuanha* in the acute disease; and not uncommonly in chronic "Winter Cough" you will find no medicine so efficacious as Nitric acid. This remedy, long a favourite with me, has found still further employment in my hands since Dr. Dyce Brown's communication on the subject; * and I owe to it many most gratifying successes.

So far I have been doing little more than epitomizing a paper of the date of 1886, which itself was almost limited to the results of my own experience. I have been content to do so, as all subsequent observation on my part has confirmed the rules of conduct I there proposed. But I must say a few words upon the treatment recommended by our Therapeutic writers.

Jousset and Jahr agree with me in urging us to commence our medication with *Aconite*; and although Bahr gives the preference to *Belladonna*, his reason seems to me mainly theoretical. There may well be cases, however, in which its substitution would be appropriate. In the treatment of the more advanced stage, *Mercurius* occupies with Bahr and Jahr the place I have given to *Kali bichromicum*—which they hardly know. In Capillary Bronchitis Jousset speaks in high terms of the value of *Ipecacuanha* and *Bryonia*, given alternately, each in the 12th dilution, to arrest the malady in its early stage, † Later on, he advises *Arsenicum, Carbo vegetabilis* and *Tartar emetic*,—Jahr also commending the two former, and Bahr the third-named, with *Veratrum album*. You will bear these suggestions in mind in case of need, or as alternatives to the remedies I have myself put forward.

For the treatment of Chronic Bronchitis we have again the benefit of the experience of Dr. Meyhoffer, who has devoted to this disease the second half of his Volume. He makes three divisions of my first variety of the disease. viz., that with mucous expectoration. The first is the "Catarrh Sec" of Laennec; it is situated chiefly in the smaller bronchial tubes, and from its locality and the tenacious character of its sputa causes violent and prolonged coughing, producing venous engorgement of the face, and not uncommonly Emphysema Pulmonum. When more acute bronchial irritation supervenes, the dyspnœa is such as to give the condition the name "Asthma Humidum." For this he recommends *Aconite* and *Bryonia* at the outset, followed up later by *Iodine* or *Sulphur* according to the patient's constitution, or by *Arsenicum* if Emphysema is present. In attacks of "Humid Asthma", he has

---

* M.H.R., xviii., 422·

† Another French prescription is Dr. Leboucher's of *Calcarea* and *Nitric acid*, 6 or 12 (REV. HOM. FRANCAISE, Oct., 1895).

546 DISEASES OF THE RESPIRATORY ORGANS

obtained great benefit from *Cannabis Indica*, in the 1st decimal dilution. Dr. Von Grauvogl has some interesting remarks upon this condition, which he describes as occuring in a chronic form, —the physical signs simulating the presence of much mucus in the chest, which however post-mortem examination proves to be absent. He tested in a case of this kind the validity of the ancient doctrine of "signatures", by giving a first centesimal trituration of dried fox's lung : and with brilliant success. * A preparation of this kind is now sold by Homœopathic chemists as "*Pulmo vulpis*." This is the form of the malady for which I have mentioned *Kali bichromicum* as most suitable, and I think that Dr. Meyhoffer has rather underrated its efficacy here. My second form he classes as "Bronchorrhœa" including under that term the cases in which the bronchial secretion is purulent. For this, besides my *Tartar emetic* and *Silicea*, he praises *Lycopodium* very highly, and, when the disease occurs in delicate leuco-phlegmatic children, *Calcarea*. † He then describes a third form, in which the expectoration is sero, mucous, viscid, stringy, and transparent — coming up (often in large quantities) after long and violent paroxysms of coughing. The mucous membrane seems here little altered. He names as remedies for it *Carbo vegetabilis*, *Lycopodium*, *Silicea* and *Sulphur*. I should add *Arsenicum*. My "Plastic" variety does not appear to have come under his notice.

Besides these more definite species of Bronchitis, Dr. Meyhoffer calls attention to its frequent occurrence in connexion with diseases of other organs (as of the heart) and with general constitutional disorder, as Lithiasis, Rheumatism, Gout, Herpetism, Scrofula, Rachitis and Senile or Anæmic Debility. His recommendations as to the treatment of these conditions, and illustration of the same by clinical cases, are full of instruction. There is no book, moreover, in which so much information is given as to the mineral baths and waters appropriate to the patients under consideration.

Of our other Therapeutists, Bahr has given a separate and well-wrought section to Chronic Bronchitis, which he divides much as I have done. In his indications for remedies he mostly agrees with Dr. Meyhoffer, adding *Spongia* to those for the "Catarrh Sec" and speaking in warm praise of *Silicea* (in the higher TRITURATIONS) for Bronchorrhœa with tendency to suppuration, seen in stone-cutters and others who inhale an

---

* Text-book of Homœopathy, i. 170.

† He might have added *Kali carbonicum*. Dr. H. C. Coburn relates a striking cure with this medicine, given in the 2_x and 3_x trits. The case was of long standing, and had been under eight old-school physicians. Patient was discharged, after two months' treatment, and went on gaining weight up to twenty-four pounds. The profuse expectoration was the leading feature of the case (J. B.H.S., ii., 485).

irritating atmosphere. Jousset and Jahr give us no special assistance.

Under the name of—

BRONCHIECTASIS I propose to speak of those cases of Chronic Bronchorrhœa in which dilatation of the bronchial tubes may be presumed to be present. The most obvious sign of this lesion is fœtor of the expectoration. Dr. Meyhoffer makes a special class of this "Putrid Bronchitis," and speaks well of *Sulphur, Calcarea* and *Stannum* in its treatment. I suppose that Pathologically this dilatation is the same lesion as Emphysema, only seated in the air-tubes instead of the air-cells. I have only seen one case of it; it ended fatally in Gangrene. I must agree with Bahr that the only prospect of benefit is from treatment of the co-existing catarrh, which may best be carried out by the remedies mentioned above, with, possibly, the aid of deodorising inhalations.

EMPHYSEMA PULMONUM.—There seems no doubt that Emphysema of the common lobular variety, and with a history of gradual invasion, whatever be its exciting cause, has for its basis a primary degeneration of the pulmonary vesicles, constitutional and hereditary, often appearing to be a manifestation of Gout. If we only knew further what was the nature of the degeneration,—whether fatty, fibroid and so on—we might find specific remedies for it, and so at least prevent the further yielding of the cell-walls. The hypothesis of Fatty Degeneration is supported by Rainey, Williams and Chambers; but Dr. Waters' more systematic investigations do not sustain it. It is a pity; for in that case *Phosphorus* would have bid fair to help us greatly. But if we are driven back upon simple functional debility of the elastic fibres which conserve the diameter of the air-cells, then morbid Anatomy will not help us to the remedy. Symptomatology is equally at fault as regards the parmanent dyspnœa; but for the occasional Pseudo-asthmatic attacks

which harass the Emphysematous patient, it has given us an excellent remedy in Lobelia. Dr. Vawdrey says that the *"acetum"* of this drug, given in 3—5 minim doses three times a day for a month at a time, will give marked relief in the chronic complaint. *
A good deal, moreover, can be done towards diminishing the Bronchial Catarrh which always plays some part in the history of the complaint. For occasional attacks supervening in the course of its progress the symptoms nearly always call for **Tartar emetic**, and in no form of Bronchitis is its action more satisfactory. There is, however, in most Emphysematous patients a chronic condition of slight Bronchorrhœa with glairy, white-of-egg-like expectoration ; for this condition a steady course of **Arsenicum** is most beneficial. When the mucus is profuse, *Carbo vegetabilis* may be preferable, as recommended by Bahr.

By such remedies a good deal of help can be given to patients labouring under this otherwise irremediable malady. They can also be aided by removing some of the incidental symptoms which harass them as by **Lycopodium** when intestinal catarrh with Flatulence and Constipation is developed, by **Digitalis** and **Phosphorus** when a weak heart adds to the dyspnœa. For suggestions in this direction I would refer you to an able paper on the disease by Dr. Edward Blake, which you will find in the MONTHLY HOMŒOPATHIC REVIEW for 1877.

I am thus brought to—

ASTHMA.—In my callow days, in the First Paper I read before the BRITISH HOMŒOPATHIC SOCIETY, I remember maintaining that Asthma was essentially a tonic spasm of the muscles of respiration—a kind of Bronchial Tetanus ; and that our remedies for it should accordingly be such as have a direct excitant influence on the motor centres, of which the chief are *Strychnia, Aconite* and *Hydrocyanic acid.* I remember the Vice-President, then in the chair,—the wise old Dr. Chapman saying in the discussion which followed :—"Dr. Hughes has stated that Asthma is under the control of *Strychnia, Aconite* and *Hydrocyanic acid.* There were, unfortunately, cases of this distressing complaint which were not relievable by these drugs." I need hardly say that I have found this only too true ; and have had to look much further afield for its remedies, finding them rather in such drugs as *Arsenic* and *Sulphur* than in the more obvious analogues to the paroxysms I then selected. These have their places ; but the others, hardly less demonstrably Homœopathic, go more to

---

* M. H. R., xxxvii., 35.

ASTHMA

the root of the matter, and give better aid and actual approach to cure.

I of course limit the name Asthma to the true idiopathic paroxysmal dyspnœa, and do not include under its heading the varities of difficult breathing which are sometimes miscalled "Asthmatic". Yet I cannot distinguish it as "Spasmodic Asthma," for I think it has yet to be proved that spasm is the essence of the affection. I know few more interesting pieces of Pathological reasoning than Dr. Russell's argument that the dyspnœa of Asthma is a morbid exaggeration of the normal BESOIN DE RESPIRER and that no real Asphyxia is present or imminent. I am referring to his discussion of this disease in the Ninth and Tenth of his Clinical Lectures. He goes on to study the remedies most suitable to meet it; and if to his remarks you will add the paper of Dr. Blundell in the Second Volume of the ANNALS, with the discussion following, you will have got the substance of English experience in the treatment of Asthma. Jahr will then supply that of the older Homœopathists and Bahr and Jousset that of the modern school in Germany and France respectively.

First, what can we do in the paroxysm? Have we any medicines which give speedy relief? Or must we resort to the *Stramonium*-smoking or inhalation of the fumes of *Nitric*-paper in vogue in the old school? The latter at least, is harmless enough if it is needed. But very often our remedies act with great rapidity. If you are called to a patient during an attack, ascertain first whether the exciting cause has been atmospheric, as fog, or cold dry air. If it is so, give him **Aconite** in repeated doses. If on the other hand, the stomach seems to have given the provocation, administer **Lobelia** in the same way,—not as an emetic or depressant, but from the second to the sixth dilution. If no exciting cause can be traced, **Ipecacuanha** (mother tincture or first decimal trituration) should be administered when Bronchitic symptoms co-exist. **Cuprum** or **Hydrocyanic acid** when the attack seems purely nervous (as when *Chloroform* and other sedatives will at once arrest the paroxysms). If you have reason to think that the curative treatment of the case will have to be conducted by *Arsenic*, you will do well to try it as a remedy for the paroxysm, in which as Bahr says, it "sometimes exerts a magical effect." To leave no possible aid unnoticed, I will add that Jousset has had good results from **Sambucus** 0 when the obstruction of breathing was very pronounced. The cases published by Dr. Percy in the NEW ENGLAND MEDICAL GAZETTE for 1891 enhanced my esteem for it, and I have of late made it my standard remedy for the Asthmatic attack. Hahnemann himself recommended the mother-tincture of the drug for ordinary use.

When by such means you have got your patient through his paroxysm, you will have to consider the best means for

550 DISEASES OF THE RESPIRATORY ORGANS

obviating the tendency to its recurrence. The chief medicines I shall mention under this head are *Nux vomica, Arsenicum* and *Sulphur*.

Nux vomica is about the best curative medicine we have for Simple "Spasmodic" Asthma where there is no bronchial lesion, but a standing reflex excitability of the pneumogastric to impressions from without or through the stomach. One of the early cases which made Hahnemann famous was of this kind ; and the *Nux* was given in material doses. Dr. Kidd, also states that he considers it our best Anti-asthmatic. While giving you confidence in the medicine, his testimony may also suggest the doses in which you should use it. * You may often, indeed, get all the good effect of *Nux* in this malady from its alkaloid *Strychnia*.

Arsenicum is placed by both Bahr and Jousset at the head of our remedies for Asthma. Symptomatically, it is indicated by the supervention of the attacks towards midnight, by the severity of the patient's sufferings and his distress at the time and prostration afterwards, while the susceptibility to exciting causes is not so marked as in the cases calling for *Nux vomica*. Dr. Russell esteems it most highly where Bronchitic Asthma tends to become, or has become chronic ; and furnishes several illustrations of its efficacy. It is also obviously indicated by the co-existence of Emphysema or cardiac disease. But *Arsenic* is not less valuable when Asthma presents itself to us as a pure and typical Neurosis, hereditary (without the intermediation of Gout), and interchangeable with other forms of the nervous disorder. The growing favour in which it is held in ordinary therapeutics under such circumstances is but a reflex of that which it has long enjoyed in the school of Hahnemann. Dr. Goodno prefers it in the form of *Cuprum arsenicum*, which he thinks "a remedy of exceptional value in the ordinary type of Bronchial Asthma."

In a great number of cases of Asthma you will discover on inquiry Gouty inheritance or proclivity, or some form of cutaneous disease alternating with the dyspnœa ("Asthme Dartreux" of the French). In these cases (though in the second alternative *Arsenic* may do well) you will get most satisfactory results from **Sulphur**. You may send your patients to a Sulphureous spring, as Dr. Russell recommends ; but I think they will often do nearly if not quite as well at home under the usual potencies of the drug, of which here I prefer the lowest.

---

* I can confirm the following remark of Dr. Russell about this drug. "After paroxysm subsides, it leaves a condition of the digestive organs for which *Nux vomica* is the great remedy. The tongue is coated with a thick yellow fur ; there is often slight nausea, flatulence and constipation. Besides, the breathing is seldom quite right ; generally there remains a sort of physical memory of the struggle. The patient feels that no liberties must be taken, either of diet or exercise. Out of this secondary state of bondage nothing will liberate so effectually as *Nux vomica*."

There is another classic medicine which must not be ignored in the treatment of Asthma, and that is **Iodine.** I have formerly spoken of the old-school use of *Iodide of Potassium* in this complaint as growing in favour. It is not made much of, however, in the Article upon Asthma in the Second Edition of Quain's Dictionary, which is by Dr. Theodore Williams, "In more chronic instances, where some thickening of the walls of the larger bronchi and enlargement of the bronchial glands exist, *Iodide of Potassium* in doses of gr. v. to xv, or *Iodide of Sodium* in doses of gr. v., or a combination of both the *Iodides*, has been found very beneficial when persisted in for long periods." This is all he says, and it represents the drug here only in its old capacity of a liquefacient and absorbent. Bahr, on the other hand, calls attention to the frequent occurrence of Asthmatic symptoms in slow poisoning by this Halogen. "In the DEUTSCHE KLINIK of 1856" he writes "three cases of Iodine-Asthma are recorded, which are of considerable interest : the Asthma set in after a protracted use of the drug." Dr. Nicholson of Clifton, adducing similar pathogenetic evidence, which, however, included acute dyspnœa, went on to test the drug in the Asthmatic paroxysms, giving two grains every three or four hours : and found it very effective. When he read a paper on the subject, he found several in the discussion which followed who could corroborate his experience. *

I can only give a passing mention to *Blatta orientalis*, † *Grindelia robusta*, †† *Naja tripudians* $ and *Natrum sulphuricum*, ‖ as having gained praise as Anti-asthmatics ; but must give a fuller account of a recent candidate for the post in the shape of the South American plant *Quebracho*. It has been found to have an influence, uncertain but sometimes pretty speedy, over the symptom dyspnœa as such, from whatever cause arising ; and as it causes dyspnœa in dogs, the action seems Homœopathic. A preparation of the alkaloids found in it, under the title "*Aspidospermin*" is in the markets ; and Dr. Halbert reports a case of Asthma rebellious to other medication in which this drug in the 3_x trituration, proved of great value. σ

---

* See M. H R., xxxviii.. 534.
† HAHN, MONTHLY, July, 1895.
†† J. B. H. S., vi., 300.
$ IBID., iii., 329.
‖ IBID , iv., 228.
σ CLINIQUE, October, 1900.

LECTURE XL

DISEASES OF THE RESPIRATORY ORGANS
—o—

THE LUNGS (*continued*).
—o—

PNEUMONIA—ABSCESS OF THE LUNGS—GANGRENE OF THE LUNGS—PULMONARY CONGESTION—ŒDEMA PULMONUM—HÆMOPTYSIS

Having now finished the consideration of the diseases connected with the bronchial tubes, we come to those of the pulmonary parenchyma, *i.e.*, the AIR-VESICLES themselves. Of these we will first discuss—

PNEUMONIA, by which I mean the true primary inflammation of the lungs—the "Croupous Pneumonia" of the German Pathologists. The treatment of this disease has been one of the great battle fields of Statistics. The orthodox treatment by blood-letting, *Calomel* and large dose of *Tartar emetic* resulted in a mortality from 20 to 30 per cent; and this was long regarded as the normal fatality of the malady. When, therefore, Homœopathic treatment showed a death-rate of some 6 per cent only, it was thought a remarkable triumph of the new system. But then expectancy stepped in, and demonstrated that a considerable proportion of the usual number of deaths was due to the treatment employed: for when nothing was done a much smaller percentage of patients succumbed, very nearly in fact that which appeared in the Homœopathic Statistics. The latter were accordingly considered to be no more than the result of letting the patients alone, and the triumph of Nature over Art in the cure of disease was thought to have found a striking exemplification. Already, however, Dr. Henderson was able to show that average duration of the disease was materially less under Homœopathic than under expectant treatment; * and the subsequent result of the do-nothing plan in the hands Dietl and others made it evident that his first percentages were unusually favourable. Dr. Jousset shows † that, taken altogether, they make the mortality of expectancy nearly 19 per cent; while that of Homœopathy rarely reaches to 6. He also disposes of the astonishing results claimed by the late

---

* See his Article on the whole subject in Vol. x. of the B. J. H.
† LEÇONS DE CLINIQUE MEDICAL, p. 400.

Dr. Hughes Bennett, by pointing out that he has excluded certain complicated cases which, if reckoned with the rest, would have made his mortality 25 instead of 3·10 per cent. It is now recognised on all sides that no uncomplicated case of Pneumonia in a fairly healthy person at either extremity of life ought to be fatal. The cases presenting complications constitute the real danger ; and a just comparison between rival methods must include these in the general mass.

One of the latest developments of old-school treatment in Pneumonia is that expounded by Jurgensen in Ziemssen's 'CYCLOPÆDIA'. It consists of cold baths and *Quinine* to reduce the fever, with Alcohol to neutralise the depressing effects of the former and the intoxication liable to be induced by the latter in the large doses in which it is given. Under this eminently scientific and pleasant treatment he can only claim to have reduced the fatality of the disease to 12 per cent, which is still at least double that of Homœopathy.

Dr. Jousset, in another of his lectures, points out a further proof of the difference between Homœopathic and purely expectant medication. Under the latter, as is well-known, a sudden defervescence is wont to occur somewhere about the seventh day of the malady, while the physical signs persist for some time longer. Under Homœopathic treatment, on the other hand, the fever diminishes gradually and the pulmonary mischief PARI PASSU with it, so that after a few days there is little trace left of either.

What, then, are the remedies with which these favourable results are obtained ? They are happily as few as they are effective. I shall speak of them one by one. Let me say, however before going further, that besides the references I have already made you will find valuable information on the Homœopathic Therapeutics of Pneumonia in articles on the disease by Dr. Russell in the Ninth Volume of the BRITISH JOURNAL OF HOMŒOPATHY, and by Dr. Clotar Muller in the first Volume of the VIERTELJAHRSCHRIFT ; in Bahr's section devoted to the subject ; and in Tessier's CLINICAL REMARKS CONCERNING THE HOMŒOPATHIC TREATMENT OF PNEUMONIA,' translated by Dr. Hempel.

The first question concerns the value of Aconite. It would seem obvious that if you saw your patient early, while the temperature was high and the signs of exudation slight, you would be doing right in at least beginning his treatment with this great Anti-Pyretic. You would be acting in accordance with the modern view of the Pathology of the disease, which regards it as a specific fever out of all proportion to the local inflammation (which is only its expression), and running an independent course of its own—defervescence occurring at or even previous to the height of the consolidation,

It would seem possible to anticipate this crisis by our *Aconite*, and so to be rendering an unquestionable benefit to our patient, whose distress depends far more on his general than on his local symptoms. If moreover, Drs. Stokes and Waters be right, that there is a stage of Pneumonia prior to that of engorgement, characterised by dryness and intense arterial injection of the pulmonary membrane, and revealing its presence to the ear by a harsh, loud, puerile respiratory murmur in the spot where dulness and crepitation are afterwards discovered—if, I say, these ovservers are right—*Aconite* might fairly be expected to extinguish the whole morbid state unaided.

I think, nevertheless, that if you expect much from *Aconite* in Pneumonia you will be disappointed. Given in substantial doses, indeed, as an "arterial sedative," it may do something, and hence perhaps Bahr's commendation of it in the earliest period of the disease. But if you will read Tessier's cases you will see that in Homœopathic attenuations it had little effect ; and Jousset entirely omits it from his list of remedies. Still more decisive is Kafka's experience. "Croupous Pneumonia," he writes "always begins with a chill, more or less violent, followed soon by febrile symptoms, for which Homœopaths prescribe *Aconite*. We used to follow this plan ; but *Aconite*, that often heroic remedy, has NEVER given us any results in these cases. In Catarrhal and Rheumatic inflammations it has a powerful and rapid action, but in the fever accompanying Croupous inflammations we may say that its influence is negative ; not only is the temperature not lowered, but the pulsations of the heart do not diminish in frequency, there is no perspiration, and the febrile heat becomes still stronger and more dry."

I believe, indeed, that we have in Pneumonia a disease which is inflammatory from the very outset, and in which the fever is so high simply because of the intensity of the local process. I follow Henderson in ascribing the early and rapid defervescence to the self-limiting character of the disease—the pulmonary exudation, when at its hight, extinguishing the inflammation by the pressure it exerts, just as the surgeon endeavours to cure an Orchitis by strapping the testicle.* Hence *Aconite*, which has no power of inflamming the lung, has little influence over the fever which accompanies that process when ideopathically occurring. You cannot, indeed, do any harm by giving a few initial doses if the symptomatic features are present which indicate the drug ; but even here I think you will generally find that the patient's anxieties depend upon the distressed state of his chest ; and is best relieved by the medicine which touches the local inflammation. This will usually be found in either *Bryonia* or *Phosphorus*.

---

* See B, J, H, xxxiv., 308.

PNEUMONIA

The claims of **Bryonia** on our notice are very strong. The hepatised lungs found in the animals poisoned by it, the Croupous exudation it has produced in the bronchi, and the short, quick and oppressed breathing with heat and pain in the chest, fever and bloody expectoration experienced by its provers show its perfect Homœopathicity to the essential elements of the disease. Not less weighty is the clinical evidence in its favour. Tessier found it already in high repute in Homœopathic practice, and his records of its action gave it the support of scientific and trained observation. He frequently reinforced it with *Phosphorus*, giving the one by day, and the other by night ; but Dr. Jousset generally finds *Bryonia* alone to suffice. Both of these physicians have preferred it in the dilutions from the 11th upwards. Bahr speaks no less highly of it, but would restrict its use to the period when defervescene is setting in and the lung is thoroughly hepatised. The symptomatic indications for *Bryonia* are the severity of the pains in the chest (and therefore any pleural complication which may exist), and the causation of the attack by dry cold winds : Pathologically it corresponds to the most thoroughly fibrinous nature of the exudation.

Phosphorus was first brought into notice as a remedy for Pneumonia by Fleischmann of Vienna, who was always fond of single specific remedy for definite types of disease. This he considered he had found in the present instance ; and he was able to report (in 1844) 377 cases of Pneumonia treated by *Phosphorus* alone, with only nineteen deaths, *i. e.*, 5 per cent. His last seventy eight cases had all recovered. The Homœopathicity of *Phosphorus* to true Croupous Pneumonia is hardly so demonstrable as that of *Bryonia*, though it unquestionably irritates and congests the lungs. Our present knowledge of its Pathogenesy would rather lead us to limit its use to Catarrhal Pneumonia, or to the true disease when occuring secondarily, as in Typhus. Experience, however, has shown that it is difficult to define its sphere of usefulness, and that it may either come in (as Jousset recommends) to reinforce *Bryonia* when that medicine is not telling, or from the outset when the latter is not especially indicated, with the utmost advantage, The comparative delicacy of the patient, with the absence of the atmospheric exciting cause and the severe pains of *Bryonia*, have been to me sufficient indications for the drug. It would probably suit an inflammation having a less fibrinous and more corpuscular exudation. *Phosphorus* seems to act equally well in the 24th dilution of Tessier and Jousset, and the 3rd decimal of Fleischmann and Bahr.*

---

* The older attenuations of *Phosphorus* were generally made from the primary solution as a zero. Since this is itself of about a one-in-a-thousand strength, the 3_x would evidently correspond to our present 6_x — stronger than which I doubt the wisdom of giving the drug in Pneumonic conditions.

Dr. Kafka would (as I have said) have us abandon both *Phosphorus* and *Bryonia* in the earlier period of Croupous Pneumonia in favour of **Iodine**. The former medicines, he considers, only moderate the intensity and shorten the duration of the disease, while *Iodine* arrests it then and there. "Often," he writes, "after the fifth or sixth dose" (of the first, second or third decimal dilution, repeated every hour or so) 'the dyspnœa, the oppression and the pain diminish, the cough becomes easier, the fever abates : after six or ten hours the pulse falls from 120 —112 to 100—92, very often a slight moisture is perceptible, and the patient feels better .. ... On examination of the chest, we ascertain still all the objective symptoms of Pneumonia, but it is arrested in its evolution, and we soon see the period of resolution set in ; expectoration is easy, thin, rarely puriform ; it diminishes rapidly to such an extent that, twenty-four hours after the exhibition of *Iodine*, the cough and expectoration have completely disappeared." The use of *Iodine* here is borrowed from its employment in Croup ; and, as in that disease, **Bromine** is sometimes found preferable. I have no experience as to this treatment ;† I must limit myself to bringing it under your notice. But that Pneumonia may be arrested at its commencement I fully agree with Dr. Kafka, for I have more than once seen it done by *Bryonia* — which, however, I have always given in the first decimal dilution.

Another important remedy in Pneumonia is **Tartar emetic.** You know its reputation in old-school practice ; and have read in my 'Pharmacodynamics' the demonstration of the Homœopathicity of its action, which is also evidenced by the small doses (gr. $\frac{1}{4}$ to $\frac{1}{16}$) in which it is found curative by Hughes Bennet and Waters. In Homœopathic practice it is considered especially indicated in the second stage of the malady, when resolution is taking place but is ill-supported, oppression and prostration occurring. Here its action is unanimously commended. It is also praised by Drs. Wurmb and Caspar ✢✢ when Œdema of the lungs occurs. It would seem especially suitable to the Pneumonia of Influenza and of Delirium Tremens.

I have last to speak of **Sulphur.** Jahr recommends our reliance upon this medicine as soon as *Aconite* has done all it can accomplish ; and Wurmb and Caspar think it the most effective means for promoting resolution after defervescence has occurred. Bahr praises it when the second stage draws to its close in uncertainty—whether re-absorption or purulent dissolution is about to take place.

---

* I once, however had a case, lobular in seat but Croupous in quality, recurrent and persistent, where other remedies failed to operate but *Iodine* in the 3_x dilution at once laid hold of the morbid process and led to a speedy recovery. For testimonies as to its value in ordinary Lobar Pneumonia, see references on p. 528.

†✢ See B.J.H., xi., 389.

PNEUMONIA

The last condition—the "yellow" or "gray hepatisation" of the morbid Anatomists, which used to be so frequent and so much dreaded in the days of heroic treatment, plays little part in the clinical history of pneumonia now. When it does occur and *Phosphorus* has not been given before, it may check the supervention of the suppuration. Should it have fully set in, *Carbo vegetabilis* is praised when great prostration is present, *Hepar sulphuris* and *Sanguinaria* when the constitutional symptoms are chiefly those of hectic. Of circumscribed Abscess of the Lungs I shall speak presently.

I have said that when the exudation is slow in being absorbed *Sulphur* will quicken its departure. When, however, you meet with Pneumonia already in the Chronic condition, I think you will get most benefit from *Lycopodium*.

Of Catarrhal Pneumonia—where the inflammation runs down the bronchial mucous membrane into the air-cells—I shall speak among the diseases of childhood, to which stage of life it almost exclusively belongs. I may just say again, however, that in its occasional occurrence in old people it finds its best remedy in *Tartar emetic*.

In the foregoing remarks I have done little more than echo what I had written in my 'Therapeutics' of 1878. I find particularly nothing therein to alter; but there are several additional points to be made.

1. Pathologists are more emphatic still than before as to Pneumonia being the local manifestation of a primary and essential fever; and they have even assumed, on the strength of some cocci they have discovered POST MORTEM, that this is of bacterial origin. The writer on the disease in Quain's Dictionary (Dr. T. H. Green) draws the logical inference that, now that we know the true nature of the disease and its "rational therapeutics", becomes possible, its mortality ought to diminish. He wrote, in 1894, "has diminished"; but alas for his assumption ! Drs. Osler and Talamon in 1900 have to publicly confess * that they cannot reduce the mortality below the 25 per cent. of their fathers. As I have already shown, the death-rate under Homœopathic treatment averages less than one-third of this figure.

2. The question as to the value of *Aconite* continues to be a moot one. The following testimony from an old-school practitioner bears out the views regarding it, which I have just brought before you. "Some years ago," he writes, "I gave a trial of *Aconite*, and for long time I treated every case of Acute Pneumonia, that I met, in this way; one drop of the tincture was given every ten minutes for an hour, and then the same dose was given every hour for twenty-four hours. By

---

* M.H.R., xiv., 379.

this means I succeeded, certainly, in controlling temperature ; but I failed to observe any control over the disease. All I could claim was that I had introduced irregularities into the temperature charts —an exploit that I have no ambition to repeat." * On the other hand, *Aconite* will be invaluable in the condition in which venesection is again being called upon ; where the intense engorgement is threatening obstruction of the circulation.

3. In a paper presented to our Matlock Congress of 1883, † Dr. Bryce commended to our notice the action of *Digitalis*, given in about half-drop doses of the mother-tincture, in Pneumonia. Dr. Jousset had already, in his communication to the World's Congress of 1876, pointed out its applicability to Pneumonia occurring in the aged ; but this is a different matter. It is not easy to see how it acts but his cases certainly seem to show it is hastening defervescence and promoting resolution. They will encourage us to rely upon it, perhaps single-handed, in those menacing cases where the heart's action flags, and in which the ordinary practice can do nothing but pour in Brandy, at the expense of the inflamed lung and the feverish body.

4. I have spoken of *Sulphur* and *Lycopodium* for slow resolution and chronic hepatisation respectively. I have nothing to say here in derogation of these well-tried medicines, but I would commend *Iodine* to you as perhaps excelling either. Dr. H. K. Leonard relates a striking case of Pneumonia, where the exudation under old-school treatment remained unresolved, and the patient presented all the appearances of Acute Phthisis. Forty drops of the ordinary tincture of *Iodine* were put into a gobletful of water, and a teaspoonful given every two hours. "The patient simply raced his way to recovery." †† Repeatedly, too, I have seen chronic coughs, with physical signs and general symptoms strongly suggestive of Phthisis, clear away under this potent drug.

---

* PRACTITIONER, July, 1894.
† See M. H. R., xxvii., 605.
†† MED. CENTURY, Feb., 1899.

GANGRENE OF THE LUNGS

I have now to discuss some less frequent or important affections of the lungs—Abscess, Gangrene, Congestion, Œdema and Hæmorrhage. Of Emphysema Pulmonum I have already spoken, as although involving the air-cells, its clinical relations are with Bronchitis and Asthma; and Phthisis Pulmonalis I must reserve for my next Lecture.

ABSCESS OF THE LUNGS—I mean of course Non-tubercular in nature—I believe to be more common than is usually supposed. I have myself seen seven well-marked cases of it, mostly beginning as a result of Croupous Pneumonia invading an unhealthy subject and then becoming chronic. I consider suitable climatic conditions to be the most important element in the treatment of such cases; without these, medicines are of little avail. When such can be secured, **Hepar sulphuris** (of whose efficacy Bahr relates a striking instance) and **Silicea** may be of service; and **China** is always helpful to sustain the patient's strength.

GANGRENE OF THE LUNGS is also liable to occur as a sequel of Pneumonia in debilitated subjects, but also in connection with Bronchiectasis and putrefactive processes elsewhere. Disinfectant inhalations would, I should think, be indispensable for its treatment, which by their aid is far from being wholly unsuccessful. Whether we can add to their efficacy by our internal remedies, I cannot say. The only one of our Therapeutists who devotes any special consideration to the subject is Kafka. *Arsenicum* and *Carbo vegetabilis* are recommended by him in common with the others—he adding *Secale and Kreosote* and Jousset *Lachesis*. The occurrence of the disease as a secondary process would certainly indicate the last-named medicine.

Drs. A. K. Wright * and R. D. Hale † have each put on record a case of Gangrene of the Lungs going on to recovery. The remedy to which the former ascribed his success was *Capsicum*; the latter relied upon *Arnica*. Either was guided in his choice by symptoms in Hahnemann's Pathogenesis of the drugs (*Arnica* 319, *Capsicum* 199 and 200) which speak of foul air being expired from the lungs. It seems to me, however, that this experience on the part of provers could hardly mean that Pulmonary Gangrene, however slight, had begun in them; and in the absence of such condition their fœtid breath (which might arise from other causes) would have no real parallelism with that observed in the patients in question.

---

* Trans. of N. State Hom. Society, x., 123.
† ANNALS, ix., 374.

Another case has since been reported, * by Dr. C. N. Hart of Denver, where both lower lobes and part of the left upper lobe were solid, and Gangrenous lung-tissue was found in the profuse and offensive expectoration. *Lycopodium* 200, effected prompt improvement going on to complete recovery. There is no fœtor of breath in the Pathogenesis of this drug.

PULMONARY CONGESTION is a frequent and not unimportant affection, having quite a different clinical history from Pneumonia, with which its acute form is too often confounded. It is the ramifications of the pulmonary artery, not the bronchial, which are involved ; and the mischief if not relieved goes on to serous rather than lymphous exudation. It is, as Bahr trully says, of two kinds,—an active hyperæmia caused by afflux of blood to the lungs or passive engorgement resulting from an obstructed efflux of blood from the lungs. It is active Pulmonary Congestion which most commonly comes before us, and it is no uncommon cause of death in this country in the Winter and Spring months. There are two great remedies for it. **Aconite** and **Phosphorus** The former is all-sufficient when the case is taken early enough ; the latter comes in aid when the vascular turgescence has been sufficient to allow œdema to occur. Here *Ferrum phosphoricum* may also come in. † Chronic Congestion of the Lungs is mostly passive and mechanical, arising from some cardiac obstruction, in dealing with which as best we can its treatment will consist. It is described, however, as occassionally occurring under the same circumstances as other congestions, and requiring *Belladonna, Ferrum, Nux vomica* or *Sulphur* for its removal.

---

* J. B. H. S., iii., 334.
† See J. B. H. S., vii., 86.

ŒDEMA PULMONUM—I have spoken of the supervention of this condition in Congestion of the lung, and of the power of **Phosphorus** over it. Kafka and Bahr unite in praising the action of this medicine whenever an Acute Pulmonary Œdema occurs in connexion with Pneumonic or other diseases of the respiratory organs. "This remedy sometimes has a brilliant effect"- says the former "it is possessed of extraordinary curative powers against Œdema," is the testimony of the latter. Wurmb and Caspar speak equally well of **Tartar emetic.** "We have only twice this year," they write, "met with this dangerous complication of the Pneumonia, but on both occasions we were surprised at the beneficial action of this remedy. Both times the bronchial tubes were filled with a quantity of fluid ; the breathing was very difficult ; the patient sat upright, and was in constant dread of suffocation ; there was Cyanosis, audible rattling and snorting, etc. On both occasions the symptoms disappeared in a few hours after the administration of *Tartar emetic.*" I have myself more than once seen Œdema of the Lungs occuring in the course of general Dropsy, subside entirely under the use of the same medicine

Dr. Dills, in a discussion on **Apis,** mentioned a case of Œdema of the Lungs where it effected a cure He was guided to its use by the symptoms "he feels as though every breath would be his last."[*] I have seen a number of chest cases during the Influenzal epoch of the last decade to which I could only give this name. They have all recovered, but I confess I could not trace any brilliant results of the medicines I have administered. Their list, besides those just named, has included *Kali carbonicum, Sanguinaria* and *Arsenicum* ; and I think that from the last. given (in the 6th dilution) from the analogy of its usefulness in fluent Coryza, I have seen most marked benefit.

An interesting and anomalous case of Pulmonary Congestion and Œdema, which I had the opportunity of seeing with Dr. Meyhoffer at Nice, may be read in the Tenth Volume of the ANNALS (p. 5). Since Influenza has been with us, I have seen a good deal of Œdema of the Lungs, as I have mentioned when speaking of the epidemic disease, and have found it very amenable to medicines,

---

[*] J. B. H. S., ix, 175

562 DISEASES OF THE RESPIRATORY ORGANS

HÆMOPTYSIS – Under this term I include (though not very correctly from an etymological standpoint) Hæmorrhage from the chest of all kinds, whether there be blood-spitting or not. When this occurs from mechanical violence or strong physical exertion, *Arnica* is obviously indicated; and when it appears periodically as a vicarious menstruation, *Bryonia* is said to be efficacious in restoring the menstrual hæmorrhage to its proper place. The Hæmoptysis of cardiac disease is either the result of over-action of the heart or of mechanical embarrassment of the circulation : in the former case *Cactus* will help, in the latter *Digitalis*. "Help," I mean, to check recurrence; it is rare that any remedy is required at the time. We thus have left for consideration one only, but the most important and frequent variety of this Hæmorrhage,—that occuring in connexion with Pulmonary Tubercle.

In sanguine temperaments, when the pulse is full and bounding, and signs of local hyperæmia are present, Aconite is dispensable, and may do all that is required. I myself have never had occasion to use it. The two medicines on which I have learnt to rely are Millefolium and Hamamelis. The former is most suitable when blood is florid and frothy, *Hamamelis* when the flow is more passive and like that of venous hæmorrhage; with neither is there much cough. When the last-named symptom is present, and there is much tickling in the chest behind the sternum, Ferrum aceticum may replace *Millefolium*, and Ipecacuanha, *Hamamelis*. With these remedies, and with the obvious adjuvants of rest, silence and cold, you will be able to arrest or prevent nearly every Pulmonary Hæmorrhage which may come before you.

I have no experience of *Ledum* in this cases ; but it has caused Hæmoptysis and Drs. Drury and Jousset speak highly of it in its treatment—the latter indicating it in the more profuse hœmorrhages we sometimes encounter.

If inflammatory symptoms should supervene upon Pulmonary Hæmorrhage, *Phosphorus* should be administered.

LECTURE XLI

DISEASES OF THE RESPIRATORY ORGANS
(*continued*)
——o——

THE LUNGS (*contd.*), PLEURA. DIAPHRAGM AND THORACIC WALLS.
——o——

PHTHISIS PULMONALIS—PULMONARY SYPHILIS PULMONARY CANCER—PLEURISY—HYDROTHORAX—DIAPHRAGMATITIS—ACUTE RHEUMATISM OF THE DIAPHRAGM—PLEURODYNIA

In my present lecture I have first to speak of the Therapeutics of the graver diseases of the LUNGS —TUBERCULOSIS, SYPHILIS and CANCER. I will begin with —

PHTHISIS PULMONALIS —It is not my intention to enter into the controversy which has been carried on regarding the Pathology of Tubercle, and the relation of Pulmonary Phthisis to it. The only important bearing it has on Therapeutics is that the views of Niemeyer and those who think with him appear to coincide with that which clinical experience has long established, *viz.*, the existence of two forms of the disease. Whatever may be their Pathological unity, their history, prognosis and behaviour under remedies are very diverse. The type of the one is what is now called "Acute Miliary Tuberculosis," which is to the lungs what Acute Hydrocephalus is to the brain, and—like that—is almost always fatal. When occuring in chronic form it is characterized by insidious course, by debility, emaciation, shortness of breath and fever out of all proportion to the physical signs ; and has as nearly certain an issue. On the other hand, we not uncommonly see cases which trace their commencement to one or more inflammatory attacks ; where the signs of Chronic Pneumonia are evident, and the fever and general symptoms correspond therewith. Here, under favourable circumstances, a great deal can be done by treatment, and cure is not uncommon. To call these ''Pneumonic Phthisis" and the other "Pulmonary Tuberculosis" is at any rate, convenient for clinical purposes ; and I shall, without prejudice to the unity of the disease, venture to do so. Both, I should say, are pre eminently affections belonging to the Scrofulous diathesis.

And now, speaking of the Therapeutics of Phthisis, I desire to yield a hearty and ungrudging testimony to the advance which old Medicine had made in the treatment of this disease,

564 DISEASES OF THE RESPIRATORY ORGANS

There is no doubt that the mortality is less, and the duration of life greater, in Phthisis than it was fifty years ago : and it has been a genuine triumph of scientific investigation. The unanimous consent of all the teachers of the present day as to the principles of treatment to be observed in Phthisis is worthy of admiration and commends the method to us with unwonted force.

When we examine the method in question, however, we find it to be purely regiminal and dietetic,—the Iron and Cod-liver Oil which are the only "medicines" given, falling under the latter heading. And herein is illustrated that which Dr. Madden has insisted upon*,—that the recent advances made in the old school are on the common ground of Hygiene, and no relation to the administration of the drugs. We can thankfully recognise and adopt them ; while in our own department of specific medication we still, unhappily, stand alone. Some day we hope that prejudice will no longer.

> "To the marriage of true minds
> Admit impediments."

Let it be fully understood, then, that the basis of the treatment of Phthisis must be with us, as with others Hygienic. Let us nourish our patient well and wisely ; let him always breathe fresh air, and take plenty of exercise ; choose his climate for him if possible ; and give him Cod-liver Oil and perhaps—save in the rare "Phthisis Florida"—chalybeate food. But Homœopathy will enable you to do more than this. It will enable you to keep down pulmonary inflammation without lowering the system. It will give you "cough medicines" which will not spoil the stomach, "alteratives" free from the poisonousness of *Mercurials*, acid remedies for Diarrhœa which do not constipate. It has even means of no slight energy for modifying the Tubercular diathesis itself. Let me tell you all I know about the medicines which are useful in Phthisis.

1. And, first, as to the premonitory symptoms—the "Pre-tubercular stage," as it has been called. The most recent researches "leave very little room for doubt that the bad habit of body in Scrofulous affections associated with the growth of tubercle-matter must be established in the first instance through the digestive processes, as first described by the late Dr. Tweedy Todd under the name of STRUMOUS DYSPEPSIA, and which has been since so fully described by Sir James Clark, Bennett, Hutchinson and others."—So writes Aitken. The characteristic features of this Strumous Dyspepsia are dislike to and difficulty in the assimilation of fats, "biliousness." Heartburn, Flatulence, and – above all – acid eructations after talking food, for such a Dyspepsia, as well as for the Strumous diathesis which underlies it, we have (as I have pointed out in my Pharma-

---

* See the Articles on "The Renewal of Life" in the MONTHLY REVIEW for 1867-8.

codynamics') a most promising remedy in **Calcarea carbonica**; and upon it I should advise you to rely if the incapacity to use fatty food shows itself in the above symptoms, and the patient is otherwise fairly nourished. *Pulsatilla*, also, might be helpful. There are cases, however, in which the difficulty seems to lie not so much in the digestion as in the assimilation of fats, and to point to the pancreas and perhaps the mesenteric glands as at fault. I mean, where loss of flesh is the earliest sign of anything being wrong. It is here that **Iodine** first begins to play the important part it occupies among the Anti-phthisical remedies. It will, as Dr. Nankivell has said, enable milk or Cod-liver Oil to be taken with comfort and advantage. With one of these medicines, and suitable diet and Hygiene,—testing your patient's progress by his weight and temperature rather than by the sounds of his chest, and paying more attention to his chylopoietic viscera than his lungs, you may do much to avert a threatened Consumption.

2. I will now follow up the line of what I have called the true Tubercular cases. The most serious form which these can assume is the "Acute Miliary Tuberculosis" of the present Nomenclature. Whether we can hope to avert the usually fatal issue here, I cannot say. Of our hopes from *Tuberculin* I shall speak later on Dr. Pope mentions one case, presumably of this nature, in which *Arsenic* and *Calcarea* given alternately produced a most rapid and unexpected change, resulting in complete recovery. † I have myself had another, where the physical sighs were only those of a diffuse Bronchial Catarrh, but where the rapid pulse, high temperature, profuse perspirations and emaciation made the presence of Miliary Tubercle exceedingly probable. Here, when *Phosphorus* was doing nothing, *Iodine* - in the 3_x dilution—made a speedy change in the patient's condition (she was a child), and led to an entire restoration to health.

When a patient comes to us with the signs of Tubercular deposit already existing having a bad family history and a considerable amount of debility, wasting and dyspnœa, I fear that we can do little to stay the course of the disease. You would of course put the whole Anti-Phthisical regimen into operation, and would especially bring mountain air into play where attainable. If there is any medical help to be obtained in such cases, it is from **Sulphur**. It is especially useful when the patient or his parents are otherwise unhealthy—have what Hahnemann called a "Psoric" constitution, as manifested by cutaneous eruptions. It should be given (as Dr. Jousset recommends) in the higher dilutions, and not too frequently. Sometimes, moreover, the constitutional symptoms may be notably ameliorated for a time by *Iodine*, given in the same way.

---

* M. H. R., xvii, 632. † B. J. H., xx., 36.

If softening has begun in such a case, the treatment is that which I shall recommend for the other variety of the disease; but it is palliative only.

3, When our Phthisical patient has a distinct history of inflammation of the respiratory organs as initiating his malady, and the general symptoms are not out of proportion to the local changes, we may treat him with fairer prospect of success. Here, too, the disease may appear in an Acute or a Chronic form. The first is that known as "Phthisis Florida", or 'Galloping Consumption." In one such case, occuring in an adult man, I have succeeded in arresting the symptoms by giving *Arsenicum* 3 and *Phosphorus* 2 on alternate days; and upon these medicines I should be disposed to rely, save in those cases where our late colleague Clotar Muller so justly recommended *Ferrum*.* Frequent Hæmoptysis is the great indication for it; and, where this symptom was present, I should substitute it for *Arsenicum*.

In the Chronic form of Pneumonic Phthisis, *Arsenic* and *Phosphorus* † are still our leading remedies,—the former for continuous use, the latter for intercurrent attacks of inflammation. Dr. Nankivell—whose position at Bournemouth gives him ample opportunity of seeing Phthisical cases has a high opinion of *Arsenic* in the form of the *Iodide* (2_x to 6_x trituration); and has communicated some excellent instances of its efficacy. †† When lecturing on *Arsenic*, I have mentioned the repute it is obtaining in the old school as an Anti-phthical remedy. and have shown its Homœopathicity at least to the general condition present. The presence of *Iodine* in this compound probably counts for something, and from this drug itself beautiful results may often be obtained in the present malady. Rapid emaciation and pronounced hectic are here— as elsewhere—its chief indications. I prefer (within Bahr) the lower decimal dilution. The only rival to *Arsenic, Iodine* and *Phosphorus* in this form of the disease is Lycopodium. It suits cases of a more chronic and passive character, and is, I think, especially useful when Phthisis occurs in young men. In such patients, moreover, *Calcarea* may again be suitable; and Dr. Nankivell prefers the *Phosphate* (which is much commended by Dr, Verdi).* the *Iodide* and the *Arsenite* of *Lime* to the *Carbonate*. Dr. Martiny of Brussels, medicates all his Phthisical patients with *Arsenicum iodatum* and *Calcarea phosphorica* on alternate days, and gets good results, which Dr. Marc Jousset confirms $

---

* See J.B.H., xviii. 79. † It is curious that while Consumptive patients look Anæmic enough, their blood when tested is found with corpuscles and hæmoglobin up to and even above the normal Acute *Phosphoric*-poisoning presents the same peculiar quality of blood. (See N.A.J.H., Nov., 1898).

†† See B. J. H., xxx., 515; and M.H.R., xviii., 629. $ See B. J. H., 751.

So far I have been speaking of treatment which may POSSIBLY, be curative. Too often, however, the Therapeutics of Pulmonary Phthisis must be palliative only ; and it is important to know what we can do to moderate the symptoms and check the accidents of the disease.

a. The FEVER of Phthisis will rarely need any special medicine in the early stage of the disease. It is otherwise, however, when softening has set in and puriform expectoration has brought hectic in its train. I have been accustomed to prescribe China for such patients ; but though it supports them, I cannot say that it displays any striking antipyretic properties. The Late Dr. Mitcell of Chicago, called our attention to the value of Baptisia here. He speaks of seeing it 'reduce a pulse from 120 or 130 to 80 or 73, change a steep temperature curve to one comparatively smooth," and therewith "reduce profuse purulent expectoration almost to nothing, and nearly banish cough". If it can do this, it will be of great assistance to our Consumptive patients ; and it has often acted thus in my hands.

b. COUGH is among the earliest, the most constant, and the most troublesome symptoms of Phthisis. After Softening has set in, it is the inevitable effort required for expulsion of the sputa, and can only be eased by reducing their quantity. This may sometimes be effected, as we have seen, by *Baptisia*. When the fever which indicates this drug is insufficient to call for it, we may often get good results from Stannum, less frequently from Kali carbonicum Cough in the earlier stages of Phthisis means, if excessive, either unusual implication of the air-passages in the morbid process or increase of reflex excitability. In the former case I think we get most benefit from *Phosphorus*. In the latter, several medicines may be considered, as *Ipecacuanha*, *Lobelia*, *Lachesis* and *Crotalus*, and *Corrallium rubrum* ; but the most important is *Drosera*. The great indications for this remedy are tickling in the larynx and vomiting of food with the cough ; when these are present, Dr. Jousset tells us that we may relieve or remove the cough in nearly every case. The possible relation of *Drosera* to Tubercular deposition itself (which I have mentioned) strengthens the indications for it here : though I cannot yet recommend it with any confidence as a fundamental remedy for the disease.

c. Of the DIGESTIVE DISTURBANCES of Phthisis I have to speak of two,—VOMITING and DIARRHŒA. The former, when connected with the cough, will generally prove amenable to *Drosera*, which may be reinforced if necessary with Ipecacuanha. If it occur independently it will usually yield to Kreasote, which also has (so Dr. Hilbers used to think) a supporting and restorative influence over the whole system in Consumption. Of the Diarrhœa of

---

* REV. HOM, FRANÇAISE, Feb., 1899,

Phthisis my experience has been that *Arsenicum*, in the 3rd decimal trituration will often check it ; but that if it fails to benefit no other medicine will succeed. The frequent dependence of this symptom upon Tubercular Ulceration of the Bowels explains its obstinacy.

d. Laryngeal symptoms supervening during the course of Phthisis are frequently Cattarhal only, in which case they will yield to **Spongia**. Of Tubercular Laryngitis I have spoken under the head of that disease itself.

e. PERSPIRATIONS, often colliquative, are a great source of weakness to the Consumptive patient. When they are nocturnal only, and from one stage of the patient's hectic, their excess may be greatly moderated by *Iodine*. Later on they occur whenever he falls asleep, and simply evidence great debilty. The *Stannum* you may give for the profuse expectoration, will often help the patient here ; but **Phosphoric acid** will generally do most, and is altogether beneficial in presence of the numerous fluxes, which at this time, drain the strength of the sufferers. *Jaborandi*, also, must not be forgotten here ; and, should Homœopathy fail us, we have an axactly Antipathic remedy, and one often palliatively effectual, in *Atropia*.

The foregoing was what I had to say about the Homœopathic treatment of Phthisis when I revised my 'Therapeutics' in 1878. During the twenty-three years which have passed since then, what changes we have seen ! The BOULEVERSEMENT which former doctrines on the subject have undergone during these years has been something marvellous. The Strumous diathesis itself, in its two forms, you have heard graphically described by Miller, is no longer recognised ; the Pre-tubercular stage of Phthisis, apparently established by a number of competent observers, is ignored ; everything is made to depend on the reception of the Bacillus Tuberculosis which Koch has identified and cultivated and tested. Any predisposition to Phthisis which is more than depressed health generally or embarrassed lung-action locally is denied ; and heredity itself is well-nigh dispossessed in favour of infection. In fact, our present-day Pathologists are very much in Hahnemann's position, when he had evolved this theory of Psoric miasm as lying at the root of all genuine chronic disease which was non-venereal. The Itch was so essential a part of the doctrine, that every patient had to be questioned as to his having at some time incurred it, and inheritance was put out of court with quite Weismannic thoroughness. And so it is here. That the patient should have Consumptive relatives is a small matter in comparison with the chance of dried sputa having being inhaled or Tuberculous meat or milk ingested.

In Tuberculosis, therefore, as in the infectious febrile maladies dynamic constitutional remedies would seem out of court, and germicides should be the only aid which medicine can bring to Hygiene. But here again, after a brief, spell of fashion, the measures which seemed theoretically so well indicated have proved fallacious, and the old ones have re-asserted themselves. "It cannot be affirmed," writes Dr. Theodore Williams in Quain's Dictionary, "that any form of antiseptic treatment has succeeded in destroying the bacillus, or in counteracting the effect of the Ptomanies which it is supposed to propagate; and far better results have been obtained by constitutional measures which render the patient less vulnerable to bacillar attack." And once more, while Art has outrun Science, Science has come to substantiate Art and prove it reasonable. The very researches which have shown us the "bacillar attack" have revealed to us also the phagocytic defence. The "giant cell," so long deemed an essential element of the noxious Tubercle, now seems a massing together of healthy leucocytes to resist the invaders, a forming square to receive cavalry. Our wisdom is not to open with grape upon the clashing MELEE, risking injury to friend as well as foe; but to support the defenders with food and drink and pure air to breathe, and to hearten them with timely stimulus.

Of the advances made in the former direction I have not to speak here. The "open air" treatment of Phthisis with its conjoined active feeding, is a great step in the right direction and has the sympathies of all of us. What I have to enquire is: Has any corresponding advance been made in the direction of stimuli—of specific stimuli, *i. e.*, medicines? It thinks it has; and would first speak of the use of *Iodide of Arsenic*, on which I have already touched more than once in this and a foregoing lecture.

We owe, it would seem, the first proposal of the use of this remedy to the late Dr. Hempel. In his "Materia Medica" of 1859, pointing out that *Arsenic* excites in the respiratory organs a process similar to Phthisis, and should therefore be of use in many cases of the disease, he suggests that in the Tubercular form the *Iodide*, 2nd or 3rd trituration, may be substituted for *Arsenious acid*. The hint remained barren, however, till Dr. Herbert Nankivell acted upon it. His position at Bournemouth gave him large experience in Phthisical cases; and he found that in those which Niemeyer classes as Non-tubercular, "Pneumonic Phthisis", *Arsenic*, especially in the form of the *Iodide*, and occasionally in that of the *Arsenite of Lime*, has a very considerable sphere of cure. In a paper before the BRITITH HOMŒOPATHIC SOCIETY in 1872. * he broached the subject and related a series of cases bearing out his thesis; and he followed it up by another presented to our Congress of 1873, † in which he gives the later history of his former cases,

---

*See J. B. H. S., xxx. 515.   † See M. H. R. xvii., 620.

and relates new ones. He has generally given the 3x trituration.

Dr. Nankivell has not written further on the subject, but in his speech at the International Congress of 1896, it appeared that he continued to be well-satisfied with this medicine in the class of classes now specified. **Arsenicum iodatum** has certainly become the standard medicine for Phthisis in British Homœopathic practice, and we are all well-satisfied with it. Every now and then moreover, we get testimonies in its favour from abroad. Dr. Kroner of Potsdam, has published a series of cases of incipient and even advanced Phthisis, in which its action was all that could be expected ; * and warm appreciation of it is expressed by Dr. Carb Crisard in the NEW ENGLAND MEDICAL GAZETTE of May, 1899. In twenty-eight cases of pulmonary disease coming under his care, all in which Tubercle bacilli were absent, recovered under it, and three out of seventeen in which this feature appeared were alive and well at the time of his report. He gave the low triturations in increasing doses ; Dr. Kroner prefers a second decimal solution made with Absolute Alcohol and a little Ether.

To all appearance, however a yet further step has been made in the employment against Tuberculosis of the product of its own bacillus. This was the claim made by Koch in 1890, on the strength mainly of some experiments on animals. You know what occurred in consequence—the mad rush of doctors and patients to Berlin, the high hopes raised, the State aid and honours given to the supposed discoverer ; then the disappointment, the disasters, and finally the relegation of the new treatment to the limbo - already too full of medical illusions. Homœopathy, however, has sought by its better methods to evoke the "soul of goodness in things evil" which may exist here as elsewhere. Even an old-school practitioner was seen that insufficient reduction of dosage might be the cause of failure. The late Dr. Sinclair Coghill of the Ventnor Consumptive Hospital, obtained arrest of disease in eight cases of Phthisis, six of whom, four years later, were enjoying excellent health ; and he "mainly attributes the exceptional success of the treatment in his hands" to his adapting the amount of *Tuberculin* so as to obtain merely an indication of reaction— Koch not being content unless this was quite pronounced. † The disciples of Hahnemann at once perceived that a substance which introduced into the healthy organism, caused fever and cough ; and which, in the strength used by Koch, set up in Phthisis cases fresh inflammation and softening might, whatever its source, be of the nature of a SIMILE to the bacillus Tuberculosis, and should do something—its virulence being subdued by our processes of attenuation—to control the ravages of that

---

* See J. B. H. S., iii., 203. † LANCET, Nov. 16, 1895.

microbe. Dr. Clarke took a leading part in so arguing in the Journal he edits—the HOMŒOPATHIC WORLD, collecting in the No. of April, 1891, all the pathogenetic effects of *Tuberculin* which had up to then been put on record. The most decisive evidence of this conclusion being sound has come from Dr. Bernhard Arnulphy. In the MEDICAL ERA of October, 1892, and the CLINIQUE of March, 1894, he has reported five cases of Acute Phthisis treated by it in the 3_x—8_x trituration, with four recoveries, describing it as having, "the most wonderful remedial action he has ever seen." In Chronic cases he had at first but indifferent success with it; but later could write: * "Since I found out that *Tuberculin* is capable in inhibiting the development of Tubercle, provided, it be given early enough, and persistently enough, incipient Phthisis has lost almost all its terrors for me." He conjoins with the internal treatment inhalations of super-heated air medicated with some antiseptic like *Thymol* or *Guaiacol*. Still later, he reports the result of raising the drug to the 12_x and mostly the 30_x degree of attenuation. "The change was attended in the main," he writes, "with very gratifying result." It enabled him to give *Tuberculin* in all stages of the evolution of the Tubercular deposit, without risk of aggravation, and in most cases with certain signs of improvement. Of twenty-five cases advanced beyond the incipient stage, and thus treated, five only died while under treatment; seven were lost sight of after some measure of improvement has been obtained; and the remaining thirteen seemed to have recovered – the lesions being quiescent, and the rational symptoms absent. Of eighteen incipient cases sixteen had been brought to a similar standstill; the other two had failed to report. †

These results were obtained with Koch's preparation (which seems to be a pure solution of the toxin generated by the bacilli, these being filtered out of it), and were due to his initiative. But about the end of 1890 there had appeared a little Brochure by Dr. Burnett, entitled "Five years' experience in the new cure of Consumption by its own virus, illustrated by fifty-four cases." He reminded us that a *"Tuberculinum"* was among the isopathic remedies brought forward some time ago by certain members of our school, and that some recoveries from Tuberculosis had been reported from its use. It had the rather unsavoury origin of Phthisical sputa; and he states that he had substituted for it a preparation of Tubercle itself, triturated with Spirit, which from the chemist who made it he would call *"Tuberculinum Heathii,"* or more briefly—bacilli having been found in it—*Bacillium*. † With this substance he had, since 1885, been

* CLINIQUE, July, 1894.   † IBID, Dec., 1895
† I have ascertained that this is a mistake of Dr. Burnett's, see Appendix to this Lecture.

treating every presumed Tuberculous case that came under his care, and with a very large measure of success. Dr. Burnett wrote AD POPULUM rather than AD CLERUM, and his cases often fail to bear close analysis. Physical examination of the chest is rarely noted, microscopical investigation of the sputa never; and there is no record of temperature, pulse and respiration. He confesses (pp 114, 184) that he has written CURRENT CALAMO, and the book bears too strong evidence of it. Nevertheless, it is impossible to read his fifty-four narratives, and those additional from himself and others in the Third Edition which the Book has now reached, without being impressed with the real curative properties of *Bacillinum,* and feeling that they far exceed those of other remedies reputed in Phthisis.

All this, it must be confessed, is isopathic rather than strictly Homœopathic treatment, though the two probably move on the same lines. Dr. Burnett's use of the Nosode is frankly of this kind. Whenever he has reason to think a patient's illness to depend upon Tubercle, present or threatening or even far back in the past, he puts in his *Bacillinum* ; and whenever an outlying symptom, *i. e.*, Ringworm, yields to *Bacillinum*, he sets it down as of Tubercular origin. There is, of course, a Homœopathic action of *Tuberculin.* Drs. Arnulphy and Mersch have made a beginning of this in respect of Broncho-pneumonia but its chief advocate and expositor is Dr. Cartier, of Paris. He would explain thus what it does in Tubercular Phthisis ; "I consider." he writes (I quote from his excellent Haper presented to the International Congress of 1896), "*Bacillinum* a powerful moderator of the muco-purulent secretion of Consumption. While diminishing the secretion it modifies the auscultation ; there is less fluid sputum, the cavities are drier, the Peri–tuberculous congestion less intense. The clinical symptoms follow those of the auscultation ; as the patient expectorates less, he is less feeble. coughs less, gains strength and regains his spirits ; but the Tubercle remains untouched. It is as one may observe with the naked eye when Koch's lymph is employed in the amelioration of Lupus. The Peri-tuberculous inflammation disappears ; the skin seems healthy ; but the yellow Tubercle remains as it was, and the patient is uncured. Such are the limits I assign to *Bacillinum* in its action on Consumption."

PLEURISY 573

PULMONARY SYPHILIS is described as occuring in two forms. It may be a Chronic Bronchial irritation, with the general symptoms of Phthisis, complementary to the secondary cutaneous syphilides ; or it may consist in the deposit of Gummatous Nodules, which sometimes soften like Tubercle (Syphilitic Phthisis). In the former variety the *Iodides of Mercury* would probably prove curative ; in the latter I cannot suggest any improvement upon the ordinary employment of *Iodide of Potassium.*

PULMONARY CANCER must be named here, for the sake of completeness ; but I have no information to give or suggestions to make as to its treatment. In the only case I have seen, *Hamamelis* checked the hæmorrhage ; and this was all I could do.

To complete the diseases of respiratory organs we have yet to discuss the affections of the PLEURA and DIAPHRAGM, and those of the THORACIC WALLS.

Of the PLEURA—

PLEURISY is a disease the Homœopathic treatment of which is as well-established as that of Pneumonia. The remedies indicated by Wurmb thirty-five years ago (I refer to his excellent Monograph on the disease, translated from the Twelfth Volume of the HYGEA in the first of the BRITISH JOURNAL) continue to be those on which nearly all of us rely at the present day. We have, moreover, a confidence in our power of controlling Pleuritic inflammation without heroic measures which does not seem to exist in the old school in the present day. Fraentzel, the writer on the subject in Ziemssen's 'CYCLOPÆMIA,' after speaking of the "infinite mischief" which expectancy has wrought when applied to Pleurisy, counsels a return to the experience of our predecessors, viz., "a severe Antiphlogistic treatment, combined with means which promote absorption," and failing these measures, to Throacentesis. On the other side, Behier and Peter report that the mortality among Pleuritics in the Paris Hospitals during the six years 1871-7 has doubled, so that the more recent French views on the subject do not seem to lead to very successful results.

In SIMPLE ACUTE PLEURISY, arising from exposure to Cold, in a healthy person, and connected with distinct fever, **Aconite** is confessedly the one sufficient medicine. The pleura is among the few parts to which it is a specific irritant, and hence it covers the whole disease. When the patient's condition is that which indicates this remedy, it may cure very quickly and in the most minute doses;—"the whole trouble," as Jahr says, "is sometimes removed as if by magic within twenty-four or forty-eight hours by means of *Aconite 30*, given every two or three hours." As a good illustration of its efficacy, I may refer you to the case related by Dr. Hayle at our Bristol Congress. * It seems to have occurred ("many years ago," he says) before the days of thermometry, or even of physical diagnosis ; but I think there can be no doubt of its having been one of incipient Pleurisy aborted by *Aconite 30*.

But I think you will agree with me that this typical Pleurisy is seldom seen. Without speaking now of the occurrence of the disease as a secondary lesion, it commonly sets in after a more insidious manner, with no distinct rigor, and with early fibrino-serous effusion. Hence our great Anti-pleuritic is the remedy for this variety of the disease—*Bryonia*. You will remember my citations from Trinks as to the place of this medicine in all serous inflammations. † Consider, in addition, the Reports of the Leopoldstadt Hospital, in which it stands from year to year at the head of the remedies for Pleurisy ; and you will see that an almost invariable use of it, in the form and stage of the disease I am now considering, is well-warranted. *Bryonia* is also recommended to follow *Aconite* when the latter has failed to arrest the progress of the malady ; and I myself habitually rely upon it in the circumscribed plastic Pleurisy which we not uncommonly encounter, and which, if not recognised, becomes the seat of very injurious adhesions.

Dr. Jousset is the only therapeutist (to my knowledge) who does not rely upon *Bryonia* in ordinary Pleurisy. He replaces it, as soon as effusion has set in, by *Cantharis*, as I have mentioned when speaking of that drug. He admits that it sometimes fail (in one case *Apis* superseded it with advantage) ; but as a rule recommends its steady continuance, reminding us that the changes in Pleurisy are gradual ones. ‡

Other remedies may be required by peculiar features of individual cases. If the exudation should be mainly plastic, and slow to disappear, *Sulphur* is eminently calculated to promote its absorption. Still further off from the primary disorder, *Hepar sulphuris* is strongly recommended by Wurmb to remove the lingering deposit of lymph ; and a good case in point may be read in the Eighteenth Volume of the BRITISH JOURNAL OF HOMŒOPATHY. The same authority speaks warmly of

---

* See M. H. R., xx, (71. † 'Pharmacodynamics', SUB VOCE.

‡ See J. B. H. S., i., 93.—Dr. Jousset continues to rely on *Cantharis* as the chief Anti-pleuritic, and can adduce good proof of its efficacy (see L'ART MÉDICAL, Oct., 1892).

Arsenicum when the serous effusion of Pleurisy is unusually rapid or copious. "*Arsenic*", he says, "is especially indicated in serous Pleurisy, and our confidence in it is so great, that we wholly despair of the possibility of curing a case of serous Pleurisy in which *Arsenic* has produced no beneficial change at all, as in the art-defying hæmorrhagic effusion. The first good effects of the remedy are manifested by the alleviation of the painfully Asthmatic respiration ; after this, the Dropsical swellings abate, the febrile attacks become less frequent, and at length the absorption of the effusion takes place. *Arsenic* is also one of those medicines which do good speedily, if they are to do good at all." * He also (with Fleischmann and Bahr) recommends Digitalis for this "Pleuritis Serosa." Latter experience has added Apis as an excellent medicine when serous exudations into the pleura remain too long unabsorbed.

When pleuritic effusion undergoes the purulent metamorphosis, and empyema is present, it is very doubtful whether we can do anything without evacuating the fluid. If the symptoms are not urgent, we may try (as Bahr recommends) to check the change with *Mercurius*, or promote the absorption of the pus with *Hepar sulphuris* ; † but as a rule I think it the best practice to let out the matter, and endeavour by means of Silicea to prevent its fresh formation. You might inject a solution into the cavity of the pleura, besides giving the drug internally. You will of course remember the power of *China* over the hectic which drain of pus excites.

SECONDARY PLEURISY, when calling for special attention, is to be treated upon the principles already laid down. If it supervene upon Acute Rheumatism, you will continue your *Aconite* and *Bryonia* : If it occur in connexion with Pulmonary Tubercle, *Bryonia* may suffice ; but it is here that Kali carbonicum has gained too much repute. The Pleurisy incident to Bright's Disease would probably be helped by *Arsenicum* in preference to any other medicine.

---

* For some cases illustrating the value of *Arsenicum* here (whether *album* or *iodatum*), See J. B. H. S., iii., 201.   † See IBID., ii., 259.

This brings us to—

HYDROTHORAX, which name I take the liberty of using to signify a collection of fluid in the pleural cavity, however originating. It may therefore be either the effusion left behind by an inflammation, or a secondary Dropsy. In the former case, we may proceed to treatment with a very fair prospect of success, and need only tap the chest when the amount of fluid is excessive. If the inflammatory attack have been tolerably recent, good results may often be obtained from Apis. But our great medicine here is **Sulphur**, I may refer you to the testimony in its favour by Dr. Cate of salem, U. S. A., in a thoughtful Paper on Hydrothorax contained in the transactions of the American Institute of Homœopathy for 1868. Alike in Pleuritic effusion failing to be re-absorbed, or that which comes on insidiously from the first, "I know," he writes, "of no remedy so efficacious as *Sulphur* ....These forms of Hydrothorax I have frequently cured with the continued use of the tincture of *Sulphur* three or four doses a day at first, but. as the improvement continues, one or two doses a day. Under the use of this remedy I have had the satisfaction of seeing the effusion diminish steadily from day to day, until it was all gone. When the fluid was gone, I have found that the spots of induration and thickening give way also, and the health becomes fully restored by the continued use of the same remedy. For this purpose I have continued its use for several months at a time, and in some cases for even a year and a half." He also finds considerable effect from it in cases where adhesions have formed "By its continued use the adhesions are gradually absorbed, the chest expands, and the crippled lung resumes, to some extent at least, its former size and action."

When Hydrothorax is a Dropsy (and to this form of it strictly the name should be confined) the possibility of removing it by medical treatment must depend upon its cause. When it is of mechanical origin, connected with pulmonary obstuction or insufficiency of the right heart, *Digitalis* or *Arsenicum* might sometimes improve the cardiac condition, and much temporary relief may often be given (as Dr. Cate has shown) by acting on the engorged lungs with *Tartar emetic* and *Phosphorus*. But the affection is practically incurable. When Hydrothorax is part of a general Dropsy having its root in the kidneys, it may often be removed by the measures we adopt to improve the state of these organs and the impoverished blood.

PLEURODYNIA

Of PNEUMO-THORAX I have nothing here to say, as it is obviously out of the range of medicinal influences.

Of the maladies of the DIAPHRAGM we know very little, either Pathologically or Therapeutically. Kafka is the only one of our authorities who gives us any information regarding them. Its inflammation.

DIAPHRAGMATITIS—is always an extension of Pleurisy or Peritonitis to its serous covering, and requires no special treatment, unless it be for the spasmodic condition into which the muscle is thrown. When this is continuous, causing contractive pain encircling the body like a hoop, *Cactus* or *Cuprum* would be indicated. Sometimes (Kafka says) it may cause spasmodic laughter, when he recommends the latter medicine, with *Belladonna*, *Hyoscyamus* and *Ignatia*. Still more frequently it manifests itself in HICCUP, which may be relieved (he says) by the same remedies, giving *Sulphate of Atropine*, if *Belladonna*, though indicated, fails. I suppose that HICCUP is always a clonic spasm of the diaphragm; and it sometimes comes before us as a troublesome symptom incident to other affections, or apparently of Idiopathic nature. In such cases I would commend **Cicuta** to you; and, where it is connected with exhaustion (as in the last stage of Phthisis), **Moschus**. *

I have seen one case of Acute
RHEUMATISM OF THE DIAPHRAGM. It yielded very nicely to *Bryonia*.

The THORACIC WALLS are the seat of—
PLEURODYNIA—I include under this heading every form of pain occuring in the chest walls. Pleurodynia, in this extended application, may be either a Rheumatism, a Myalgia, a Neuralgia or a Neuritis.

1. In RHEUMATIC PLEURODYNIA you will give **Aconite** in repeated doses of a low dilution, if the attack be recent, especially if fever is present. But unless speedy relief is obtained, you will do well to substitute remedies having more local affinity with

---

*Hiccup has yielded to *Zincum valerianicum 1*, to *Sulphuric acid 1* and *2* (frequently), and to *Magnesia phosphorica* 3 (J. B. H. S., ii, 366; v., 201; viii., 82).

the thoracic walls. **Bryonia, Actæa, Racemosa, Ranunculus bulbosus** and **Colchicum** are all more or less Homœopathic and curative. I should choose the first when the Rheumatic diathesis was marked ; the second for women ; the third where the pain was very intense, so that the patient dare not move ; * the fourth where a gouty as well as a Rheumatic tendency was present.

2. MYALGIC PLEURODYNIA had also found its remedy in *Ranunculus,* as in some cases by Dr. Strong in the Tenth Volume of the MONTHLY HOMŒOPATHIC REVIEW. But its chief medicine is **Arnica**.

When it resembles Pleurisy so much as to render diagnosis very difficult ("Spurious Pleurisy"), a few doses of this drug will often clear up the question by extinguishing the symptoms.

3. NEURALGIC PLEURODYNIA (Intercostal Neuralgia, Inframammary Pain) appears under two leading forms. First, in young women otherwise fairly healthy, where it is Hysterical, or otherwise symptomatic of deranged uterine function. Here **Actæa racemosa** is specific. Secondly, as an Idiopathic Neuralgia in Anæmic or debilitated subjects. In these **Arsenicum** or **Ranunculus** again will relieve the pain ; but its return must of course be guarded against by measures suited to build up the system at large.

4. It is not often that Pleurodynia comes before us as a Neuritis ; but, should it do so, I would remind you of the remarkable effects of this kind observed in poisoning by *Sulphuric acid,* and recorded in the First Volume of the Cyclopædia of Drug Pathogenesy' (p. 744).

This has been my own experience with Pleurodynia, but I must add Dr. Jousset's contributions to its Therapeutics. He speaks under this heading only of what I have called the Rheumatic form *i. e.,* that which results from exposure to cold or wet. He recommends *Nux vomica* in preference to *Bryonia* where the patient cannot lie on the affected side (the opposite symptom indicating the latter medicine) ; and *Actæa racemosa* where *Bryonia,* thought well-indicated, has failed, especially when its characteristic sinking at the stomach is present. For Intercostal Neuralgia in Hæmorrhoidal subjects, he speaks of *Nux vomica* as a very sure remedy ; and praises *Pulsatilla* in subjects appropriate for that medicine when the pain becomes easier every time the patients change their position.

---

* See Dr. Dudgeon's case in Vol. xxxiv, of the B. J. H., p, 160

APPENDIX TO LECTURE XLI 579

I would add a few words as to the preparation of *Tuberculin* we should employ. Two are at present in the field.

a. Koch's *Tuberculinum* is "a *Glycerine* extract from a pure cultivation of the Tubercle bacilli." He found that its effects — tuberculisation of healthy animals, improvement even to recovery of those already tuberculous—followed equally whether the injected fluid contained living bacilli, or whether these had been previously killed by heat, cold or Chemical means. They were due, therefore, not to a multiplication of the bacilli in the system, but to some specific poison formed by them. Dissolving this in *Glycerine*, and filtering out the dead bacilli, he obtained his pure solution,—using it in a strength about equivalent to our third centesimal attenuation. It was this, raised by trituration to a 6_x-12_x potency, which Dr. Arnulphy has employed. Dr. Burnett, also, states that he has used it, in a 5th dilution and has satisfied himself that it "is a good Anti-tubercular remedy but nothing like so good as *Bacillinum*."

b. This, as I have told you is the name he has given to what others have called *Tuberculinum Heathii*, from the well-known Homœopathic chemist of Ebury Street who first prepared it. Dr. Burnett tells us nothing more of this than that it is triturated in Spirit, and that bacilli were proved to be in it by an expert in Practical Bacteriology. I therefore enquired of its maker, who kindly furnished me with the following statement, "in the Westminster Hospital in 1883 was a man in the last stage of Phthisis. The substance I used was taken from this man, and consisted of a mass of gray and yellow Tuberculous matter, containing the Bacillus Tuberculosis, pus, blood, ptomaines, & c, Patients in this stage of Phthisis often bring up suddenly, without effort, almost solid lumps; such a lump was my *Tuberculin*."

Now I think it will be agreed that the latter preparation possesses no advantage over that of Koch, * and that this is far superior to it in cleanliness and—the bacillary origin of Tubercle being granted—scientific precision. It has the merit, moreover (in the eyes of most of us), that it need not be carried to unimaginable heights of attenuation to make it effective without being harmful.

---

* I am bound to say, however that Dr. Heath considers his preparation superior to Koch's, as being the whole product of Consumption,—not a selection of one element only; and I must admit that the facts about Sreptococci which have come to light in respect of the Antitoxin treatment of Diphtheria bear out the importance of these secondary factors of the disease.

LECTURE XLII

DISEASES OF THE CIRCULATORY SYSTEM

―o―

THE HEART

―o―

GENERAL AFFECTIONS—PALPITATION—HYPERTROPHIA CORDIS—DILATATIO CORDIS—ADIPOSITAS CORDIS—PERICARDITIS—ENDOCARDITIS—VALVULAR DISEASE OF THE HEART—CARDIAC DROPSY—ANGINA PECTORIS.

Instead of passing from the respiratory organs to the next great tract of mucous membrane—the genito-urinary, I shall first review the Disorders of the Circulatory System, with which the former are both Anatomically and Physiologically so closely connected. Under this heading I shall consider the Diseases of the Heart, of the Arteries and Veins, of the Lymphatics and Lacteals, and of those ductless glands—notably the Spleen and Thyroid—which belong functionally to the blood and its circulation.

I take first the Diseases of the HEART. In their discussion I shall follow closely in the footsteps to Dr. Russell, who in his Papers on Cardiac Disease in the Twelfth Volume of the BRITISH JOURNAL OF HOMŒOPATHY and in his Clinical Lectures, did so much for this subject.

Our text-books—among which Dr. Goodno's may be given no mean place—devote large space to their consideration. We now have in addition, a careful study of some of the leading cardiac medicines from the pen of Dr. Meyhoffer, in a Paper presented to the Paris Congress of 1878, which you will find translated in the Thirty-Eight Volume of the BRITISH JOURNAL OF HOMŒOPATHY (p. 158); and also, from this country and from America respectively, two Monographs on the subject. Ours is from the pen of Dr. Clarke; * on the other side of the Atlantic the work has been done by Dr. E. M. Hale. ✝ The latter, in the Third Edition to which his Treatise has now attained, gives a full conspectus of the present-day literature of the subject, drawing alike from Homœopathic and from old-school sources; and advocating a somewhat eclectic treatment. Dr. Clarke's book is rather a record of individual experience. It is apparently intended, like Dr. Burnett's similar publications, for the lay reader as well as the medical;

---

* "Diseases of the Heart and Arteries", Gould & Son. 1895.
✝ "Lectures on Diseases of the Heart", 3rd Ed., Boericke and Tafel, 1825.

THE HEART

but the way in which physical diagnosis is handled shows that we can depend upon his having had realities to deal with. I must only caution you about his quotations of symptoms under the heading of particular diseases. He tells us (p. 142) that these are to be understood as "taken direct from the Materia Medica"—that is, as Hahnemann and his disciples have always employed the term, the record of the effects of drugs in the health. Frequently, however, you will come across symptoms which are obviously clinical—such, that is, as have disappeared rather than appeard under the action of the drugs ; * so that Dr. Clarke's must have been a Materia Medica "Impura" instead of the "Pura" which was Hahnemann's ideal.

With the circulatory, as with the respiratory organs, we will begin by considering some of their special remedies. The curative power of Homœopathy depends partly on its fuller development of old medicines, partly on its addition of new. Among the former I would speak here of *Aconite* and *Arsenic* ; among the latter of *Cactus* and *Spigelia*.

1. That we should employ *Aconite* in all cases of over-activity of the heart may be thought natural, but hardly Homœopathic, since it is supposed to be Physiologically a cardiac depressant. I have shown in my 'Pharmacodynamics', however, that this supposition is unwarranted, based only upon the exhausting effects of poisonous doses and contradicted by the results of gentler and more careful experimentation—both on men and the lower animals. *Aconite* is truly Homœopathic, as I have said in "all diseases of the heart characterized by increased action, especially when the left side is chiefly involved" ; and acts here in doses far too small for any Physiological influence to be exerted. So witnesses Dr. Meyhoffer. "We find in *Aconite*," he writes, "the remedy PAR EXCELLENCE for Palpitations of the Heart in adolescents and plethoric adults : it is not less potent in insufficiency of the aortic valves, with a strong and abrupt pulse, throbbing of the peripheric arteries and dilatation of the capillary network. The transmitted diastolic bruit in the carotids, when existing, sensibly diminished, by it, becoming sometimes scarcely perceptible after the patient has taken three or four doses. By dose I mean one or two drops of the first or second decimal dilution."

One of the great recommendations of *Aconite* in cardiac disorder—sometimes so painful and distressing—is the rapidity of its action. The way it once relieved for me a Spasm of the Heart was recalled by a narrative of Dr. Clarke's. A lady who had suffered from Sciatica suddenly, one day, felt the the pain cease in the limb, and strike to her heart. "Happening to be calling at the very time of the attack," he writes, "I found her in a most perilous condition. She was cold and livid. The pain

---

* See, for instance, the last but one of *Iodide of Potassium* on p. 166.

which was of a stitching kind, was so intense, that she dared not take a breath, and was gasping when I found her. The heart's action was tumultuous and violent, with an extraordinary sharp clapping sound audible at several feet distant from the patient. She felt she was dying. I gave her a dose of *Aconite* 3 immediately, and repeated it until she came round, which, happily, she did after one or two doses more." The attack proved to be the beginning of Influenza.

But *Aconite* does more than irritate the heart's action; it inflames its membranes. This has not been actually ascertained as regards the pericardium, though the analogy of the pleura and peritoneum—which it has so affected—raise a probability that it might so act. In the endocardium, however, and especially in those folds of it which constitute the mitral valve, inflammation was plainly manifest in four out of six rabbits slowly poisoned with it by Dr. Jousset. * This interprets the painful palpitation and præcordial anxiety, alternating with articular sufferings, experienced by one of the Austarin provers of the drug; and shows that in Endocarditis *Aconite* may be relied upon, not marely as an antipyretic and cardiac sedative, but as a specifically-acting local remedy. It may do something even for the generally fatal ulcerative form of this disease. Tessier and Jousset have gained unexpected successes from it in what they have considered "Idopathic Pyæmia," but which probably depended on this then unknown lesion; and Dr. Byres Moir, giving it in the last of a series of five cases treated in our London hospital—the account of which you may read in the First Volume of its "Reports," had decided success for a time, though the patient died four months later. Since then a real recovery has been recorded, † and here *Aconite* played an important part in the treatment: so that Dr. Moir concludes that we may look to it as the remedy most likely to be of service. It must be given here, it seems in the mother tincture.

2. About *Arsenic* as a heart-poison I do not think I have anything to add to what I have written in my "Pharmaco-dynamics", basing myself on Dr. Imbert Gourbeyre's instructive Treatise. I have summed up its action in the words of Trousseau and Pidoux: it "abolishes the heart's contractility and often inflames its tissue." In the former it is opposed to *Aconite*, though the distress occasioned very similar with the two drugs: it is thus indicated when the suffering organ is feeble rather than over-active. "It is the remedy," writes Meyhoffer, "for the incipience of the cardiac cachexy. The heart grows feeble, the pulse begins to show irregularities, the nights are troubled by oppression and anguish, œdema of the feet appears and disappears. The fear lest Fatty Degeneration should have begun to invade the heart is a further indication for the choice of this mineral. *Arsenic*,

---

* See Cycl, of Drug Pathogenesy, i., 116. † LANCET June 20, 1891.

by its profound influence on nutrition, is capable for a long time of holding in check passive Dilatation of the heart, and maintaining the equilibrium of the circulation." To the same effect writes Professor George Balfour, in his book on "The Senile Heart"; "Most excellent results occasionally follow the prolonged use of almost infinitesimal doses. I well-remember one old gentleman, exceedingly sensitive to the action of drugs, to whom the $\frac{1}{50}$th of a grain of *Arsenious* acid was quite poisonous, but who could tolerate the $\frac{1}{100}$th without difficulty. After taking this minute dose daily for two or three weeks, and nothing else, for a dilated and hypetrophied heart beginning to fail, he said to me, "I can go upstairs much easier than I used to do." As an irritant, it resembles *Aconite* in inflaming the serous membranes, but does so after a slower manner. It thus takes the place of the other in Pericarditis with copius serous effusion, and in chronic inflammations of the endocardium.

If the whole range of the usage of *Arsenic* in the old schoo! were not surprising—obvious similar as it is at every point—it wold be curious to see how Homœopathic is their employment of it here. Dilatation and valvular mischief are the conditions regarded as calling for it ; and by the French clinicians it seems preferred .in the form of *Arseniate of Antimony*. The reason for this is not very obvious ; and Dr. Clarke seems to have better warrant for urging the claims of the *Iodide*. It was in doing this that he first came forward * as a special student of cardiac disease, and in his present work he relates how he came to use the compound in question. Observing marked improvement in the heart symptoms of patients suffering from both pulmonary and cardiac disease, when he had been led to choose the medicine from the pulmonary symptoms alone, he went on to follow up its indications of the latter kind, and with most satisfactory results, "It seems" he seys "to act on the heart muscle, arresting degenerations and restoring vitality" Dr. Clarke has of late years taken ground in what I have called the extreme left of our school, but his dosage of *Arsenicum iodatum* remains at its old point—the 3rd decimal trituration or dilution.

3. The use as a medicine of the night-blooming cereus, *Cactus grandiflorus*, was initiated in 1862 by the late Dr. Rubini, then practising Homœopathically at Naples. He proved it on himself and his wife in ten-drop doses of the tincture made from the flowers and tender branches. It produced such distress at the heart as in the female prover to cause weeping aloud and lively terror, and they had neither of them courage to push their experiments further. Dr. and and Madame Rubini must have been

---

* See B. J. H., xlii, 383.

unusually susceptible to the drug's action, as it has since been proved in such larger doses without such result. In the quality of its effects, however, their experiences are well borne out. It has been found to act as a stimulant on the ganglionic centres in the cardiac walls (perhaps also on the sympathetic nerves going to the heart), causing prolonged and more energetic contractions, with raised arterial tension. Such an influence, in sensitive subjects, might well be felt as pain, — especially such pain as if the heart were constricted with an iron band, which was noted by both the provers, and has generally been found a valuable indication of the medicine in practice.

I make the remarks, because of a friendly controversy waged between Dr. Conrad Wesselhœft and myself in the NORTH AMERICAN JOURNAL OF HOMŒOPATHY for 1895. Dr. Wesselhœft has been testing our published pathogeneses for recurrence and congruence ; and tried by this test, found the *Cactu*s symptoms of the Rubinis' untrustworthy. Unfortunately, however (as I pointed out), he took as material for his analysis the presentation of the drug in Allen's "Encyclopædia." Here the complete symptom-list originally published by Dr. Rubini is reproduced, clinical ones and all, although forty of them were very obviously of the latter character. If he had referred to the 'Cyclopædia of Drug Pathogenesy', he would have found in the Appendix to the First Volume a presentation of the truly Pathogenetic part of Dr. Rubini's Pamphlet, based on information supplied by the author himself, in which also Madame Rubini's symptoms are separated from her husband's, and those of either are arranged according to the time of their occurrence (when this is specified). In the body of the Volume, moreover, besides the four other provings collated by Allen, we have given a later experience much more in harmony than these with the effects first ascribed to the drug.

Cactus has now been taken upon by the other school ; and experiments. Pathogenetic and Therapeutic, have been made with it upon a considerable scale. The whole literature bearing upon it has been collected by Dr. de Moor in the first two Volumes of the JOURNAL BELGE D' HOMŒOPATHIE ; and there is a valuable store of information on the *Cactaceæ* generally from the pen of Dr. E. M. Hale, in the Transaction of the American Institute of Homœopathy for 1890 (p. 180). In ordinary practice it is of course used Antipathically, as a "cardiac tonic" ; and that it has virtues of this kind which MAY profitably be exercised appears from the experience of one of our own practitioners, Dr. Snader of Philadelphia. * Giving the drug as he does, in five-drop doses of the first decimal dilution or mother-tincture, he misses its Homœopathic action ; and accordingly notes that in two out of the only three cases in

---

* See HAHMEMANNIAN MONTHLY, Sept., 1895.

which he met with the "iron band" symptom, he failed to remove the sensation with it. On the other hand he gets "tonic" effects from it. They are trady and mild, he allows, as compared with those of *Digitalis*, but there is less exhaustion of irritability, and no cumulative phenomena manifest themselves. It thus acts best in the incipiency of cardiac incompetence ; and, not materially increasing arterial tension, may be safely given when Sclerosis and Atheroma are present in these vessels. Very different are the results obtained by Meyhoffer, for whom "one or two drops of the second decimal dilution" were a sufficient dose. It is when "exaggerated action" of the heart is the evil that he considered it indicated, and so in hypertrophy and excessive compensation. "*Cactus* does not," he writes, "augment the power of the heart, but it moderates and regulates its actions, and thus economises its force. It produces no effect on an enfeebled heart." While the former action of the drug is available for us as for others, the latter is all our own ; and am I need not say, that which we should mainly cultivate.

4. The remaining one of the heart medicines I have mentioned not only was, but is, peculiar to us. That *Spigelia* irritates the heart was a natural inference from the cardiac symptoms of Hahnemann's proving (which was an unusually heroic one),—these being great pressure on the chest, shooting pains through it and down the left arm, and voilent palpitations. It was a bold step, however on Fleischmann's part to rely on it in consequence in all Rheumatic inflammations of the heart ; yet his confidence was justified by the results. In 1855 he was able to report that he had treated fifty-seven of such cases with but one death ; and *Spigelia* was the only medicine employed. * Most of our later authorities agree as to the high, though not perhaps the sole, place it occupies here ; and Dr. Goodno echoes their praise, at least as regards Pericarditis. "Of all the medicines which have been recommended here," he writes, "*Spigelia* has given me the most favourable results. I hasten to give it as soon as the diagnosis is clear, if another medicine is not indicated. It is remedy PAR EXCELLENCE during the painful period, and until liquid effusion is pronounced."

In Dr. Clarke's Book the sharp pain caused by *Spigelia* in the heart is so emphasized, that the drug seems hardly regarded as indicated unless this is present. I cannot assent to such limitation ; but this symptom nevertheless, gives the remedy a place quite its own in the treatment of cardiac pain, pure and simple, such as is often met with from the abuse of Alcohol or Tabacoo or both, such as is incident to hearts damaged from Rheumatism and especially in Angina Pectoris. Whether this affection is always a Neuralgia is still uncertain, but there can be no doubt that it is very often such ; and, while we must not forget the

---

* See B. J. H., xiv., 28.

claims of *Arsenicum* and *Cuprum*, *Spigelia* should always be (as Jousset maintains) our first thought, and when its keen stabbing pains are present should have the preference over every other remedy.

Coming now to particular cardiac affections, I will, with Dr. Russell, begin by speaking of—

PALPITATION, including under this heading the various forms of cardiac disturbances classed by Dr. Hale as "Functional Disorders of the Heart."

Dr. Russell divides the cases of this disorder into those in which the primary evil is 1st, in the heart itself, 2nd, in the blood and 3rd, in the stomach.

1. The heart becomes liable to Palpitation from any cause which weakens its nervous or mascular energy. The former is impaired by great mental exertion, anxiety, or emotional tension of any kind, masturbation or excess in venery, abuse of Tea, Coffee, or Tobacco, and such-like causes. To relieve an acute attack of this kind, I know of nothing equal to **Moschus**, which is also the best remedy (at the time) for the Palpitations of Hysteria. The chronic tendency may be obviated, if the exciting cause can be removed, and suitable regimen carried out, by such medicines as *Coffea, Iodine, Nux moschata* and *Phosphoric acid.* **Coffea** is most suitable for Palpitation resulting from physical causes, unless the patient has been accustomed to drink much of it. in which case *Nux vomica* would be preferable. **Iodine** may be given in similar cases, where the whole nervous system is much depressed, and there is tendency to Melancholia. Thus the Palpitation of Hypochondriasis calls for it. **Nux moschata** is very useful for the cardiac disturbances of Hysteria. **Phosphoric acid** has in my hands proved invaluable for disorder of the heart's action resulting from sexual excess. Bahr recommends **Digitalis** here ; but I am rather disposed to consider this medicine as suitable where the muscular tissue of the heart is itself enfeebled. *Tabacum* (in non-smokers) is also useful here. Such Palpitations often alternate with fainting attacks. Palpitation brought on by excessive Tea-drinking may be removed by *China*.

The action of *Atropine* in paralysing the vagi, and so allowing a rapid action of the heart, ought to be utilised in Simple Nervous Palpitation ; and perhaps *Muscarine*, which produces an opposite effect, might find place as an Antipathic palliative. *Glonoin*, and probably the *Serpent poisons* act like the former, and have some repute against Palpitation ; *Jaborandi* and *Physostigma* resemble *Muscarine*.

2. The blood induces Palpitation either by its excess or defect, or by the presence of the Gouty poison in it. When Plethora or Anæmia is the cause, the cardiac disorder is best treated by the measures necessary to improve the patient's

whole condition, but Aconite and Cactus in the one case, and Pulsatilla and Spigelia in the other, are useful adjuncts. For Gouty Palpitation I cannot suggest anything beyond the treatment of the diathesis, but it may be here that what Bahr says of *Sulphur* is true, that it is "eminently useful in obstinate cases, where it often effects a radical cure."

3. Dyspeptic Palpitation is often nothing but Gout. When it owns no relationship to that diathesis, you may with advantage remember what Dr. Elliotson says of **Hydrocyanic acid**, that it is good for "those disorders of the stomach which, in some of their symptoms, resemble affections of the heart." The *Prunus Virginiana* (Wild Cherry) mentioned by Dr. Hale probably owes its virtues to this constituent of it. A similar reflex disturbance may result from Worms or uterine disorder. Besides attending to the cause, Spigelia may be given in the former case, and **Lilium tigrinum** in the latter.

Passing now from the functional to the organic diseases of the heart, I will take first those of its muscular substance, beginning with—

HYPERTROPHIA CORDIS—In the acute attacks of Palpitation incident to this disease, **Aconite** takes the place filled by *Moschus* in Nervous Palpitation. It will also relax the Spasm of the Heart which sometimes occurs. The continued use of the same medicine I have found very serviceable in relieving the permanent distress of these sufferers. A still higher value in this direction is assigned by Dr. Russell to **Naja** and Drs. Rubini and Meyhoffer* to **Cactus**. A good case is given by the first-named illustrative of the value of his favourite medicine. † But whether with this or any other medicine you can actually REDUCE an hypertrophied heart is another question. The change is often a necessary and a compensatory one, and you would do no good by opposing it, even were you able to do so. The only form of the disease in which such a result may fairly be excepted is, I think, that which results from violent excercise, as rowing. Here I may remind you of the curative effects which Drs. Madden and Bayes have obtained from **Arnica**.

The above remarks apply to Hypertrophy, whether accompanied with Dilatation or not. But we have now to consider—

DILATATIO CORDIS by itself, *i. e.* where there is no thickening of the cardiac walls. I have nothing to say against the usual

---

* Chronic Diseases of the Organs of Respiration, i., 352. † B. J. H., xii. 543. ✝ Pharmacodynamics, SUB VOCE.

prescription of *Iron* in this condition. I suppose it to act dietetically, and to be a suitable adjunct to the nourishing regimen you will prescribe. Nor can I claim for Homœopathy the action of the Nauheim waters, or the influence exerted upon the dilated heart by *Apocynum*, according to the observations of Dr. Glinski. * I must do so, however, with regard to **Digitalis**, so far as its so-called "tonic" action is concerned. In lecturing upon this plant, I have adduced good reason for believing it to be, pathøgenetically, direct paralyser of the muscular substance of the heart. Therapeutically, then, it should be a true tonic here ; and any action it exerts in the 1st and 2nd decimal dilutions, and even in one to three drop doses of the tincture must surely be of this kind.

As medicines promising, from their effects in health, to be serviceable here I may mention *Gelsemium*, *Physostigma* and *Tabacum*. The first is recommended by Dr. Hale when the patient fears every movement, lest the heart should stop beatings ; the last by Dr. Edward Blake, when Sleeplessness co-exists. Two fresh cardiac remedies which have lately come to the fore seem to find their places here. One is the common White Bean, *Phaseolus nanus*, so much affected in Boston as an edible. Dr. Cushing, of Springfield, has found this to have a potent action upon the heart. Weakness and irregularity of beat : fluttering Palpitation, with feeling as if the heart would stop—these are his indications for it. As it acts well in the medium dilutions it would seem to be Homœopathic. † This can hardly be said of the other member of the pair now under consideration—the Hawthorn, *Cratægus oxyacantha*. It was introduced as a heart remedy by an Irish practitioner named Greene ; and he gained a great success and reputation from its use. An American one, Dr. M. C. Jennings, communicated what he had learnt of Greene's practice to the NEW YORK MEDICAL JOURNAL of October 10th, 1896, giving cases which showed it, in crude dosage, to have great power in restoring failing compensation. It soon made way in our school across the Atlantic, and numerous testimonies to its efficacy were borne. ✢ It seems to do, in about five drop doses of the tincture (which is made from the fresh berries) all that, *Digitalis* in much larger quantities can accomplish. The following case will illustrate its power :

"Dec. 3rd 1899, I was called to visit Mr. H. æt. 38, who had been afflicted with Heart Disease for many years. I found the patient cyanotic, his limbs enormously swollen ; almost complete suppression of urine ; a very rapid intermittent, irregular, and at times almost imperceptible pulse. He was not able to raise himself in bed without immediate symptoms of collapse appearing ; he spoke with great difficulty, and in fact presented a perfect

---

* M. H. R., xxxix., 461,   † J. B. H. S., v., 199, 289.
✢ See J. B. H. S., vi., 299 viii., 78, 355 ; ix., 100. Also, for recognitions of its value on this side, see M. H. R., xlv., 555.

Picture of approaching dissolution from the heart failure. An examination of the chest showed in enormously enlared and dilated heart with leakage regurgitation of aortic and mitral valves. It is just in such cases as these that I have seen *Cratægus* exerts its wonderful powers. The patient received it in the useful dose"—five drops of the tincture —"every three hours, night and day for four days. At the end of this time he was sitting up in bed, Dropsy having entirely disappeared, urinary secretion restored and pulse fairly good." No relapse had occurred up to April.

ADIPOSITAS CORDIS presents itself in two forms. In the first, the fat is deposited upon the heart, and only causes Degeneration of tissue when it is also infiltrated among the muscular fibrils ; in the second, there is a Fatty Degeneration from the outset. The treatment varies accordingly. Patients of the former class have to be urged to a diet and mode of life calculated to avoid obesity, and *Digitalis, Phaseolus* and *Iron* may be given to strengthen the loaded muscle. The medicines suited to the variety are studied in an interesting Paper by Dr. Drury in the Nineteenth Volume of the BRITISH JOURNAL OF HOMŒOPATHY. **Arsenicum** and *Phosphoric acid* are the medicines he most favours ; and the former, being now known to be capable of setting up Adipose Degeneration in the heart and elsewhere, has a strong claim on our notice. Dr. H. C. Clapp, from an experience including thirty cases, has no doubt of the benefit it causes. It does not, of course, cure ; but it stays the onward march of the process, and tones up the unchanged muscular fibres to greater strength and activity. *
Still more potent is the action in this direction of **Phosphorus** ; and it seems likely to take the first place among the remedies for Fatty change.

Arnica is much recommended by Kafka and Liedbeck as giving relief to the dyspnœa attendant on fatty heart. It may even do more, so strengthening such a heart that diuresis is established and œdema removed. †

I will now speak of the inflammatory affections of the heart beginning with that of its investing membrane—

PERICARDITIS—The idiopathic form of this disease is rarely witnessed, and so little is known either to Pathology or Therapeutics of its Pyæmic, Hæmorrhagic or Tubercular varieties that I shall speak of its treatment only as accuring in connexion with Acute Rheumatism and in the course of Bright's Disease of the kidney.

If in the progress of a case of Acute Rheumatism a double-friction sound begins to be heard, and the other symptoms of Pericarditis are setting in, you can nearly if nor quite always arrest them in twenty-four hours by giving your **Aconite** alone

---

* See NEW ENGLAND MED. GAZETTE. Dec., 1893.
† See J. B. H. S., v., 192.

in sufficient strength and frequency (a drop of the 1st decimal dilution every hour or so), and covering in the heart with a hot Linseed-meal poultice. EXPERTO CREDE. * But you are not always fortunate enough thus to catch the disease at its first breaking out, and must be prepared for its treatment in its several stages. You will begin by reading the cases narrated by Dr. Drysdale in the Twelfth Volume of the BRITISH JOURNAL OF HOMŒOPATHY (P. 557), by Dr. Laurie in the Fifth Volume of the same Journal (p. 310), by Dr. Kidd in the Thirteenth Volume (p. 198), and by Dr. Russell in the Clinical Lectures. You will find that (after *Aconite*) *Bryonia*, *Colchicum*, *Spigelia* and *Arsenicum* are in the highest favour. **Bryonia** has never been trusted to alone, but always in the alternation with *Aconite* and *Spigelia*. I think the distrust only natural, and always suspend its administration in Rheumatic Fever in favour of other medicines when cardiac mischief sets in. **Colchicum** has no A PRIORI evidence in its favour ; but its action in Dr. Kidd's and one of Dr. Laurie's cases was not a little remarkable. † **Spigelia** has the highest reputation, and has in its favour the testimony already cited of by Fleischmann, who used no other medicine. The presence of much pain would here, as elsewhere, be a main indication for it. **Arsenicum** is preferable to it only when serous effusion into the pericardial sac is considerable. It is noted here by more than one observer that it frequently relieves the anxiety and oppression some time before the physical signs announce the re-absorption of the fluid.

Armed with these medicines, you may with much confidence encounter the Rheumatic form of Pericarditis. In that which occurs in Bright's Disease *Colchicum* and *Arsenicum* are the only members of the group likely to be called into requisition.

I may add a brief account of the Therapeutic instructions of our systematic writers on this point.

Jousset seems hardly to speak from the experience we should expect : he recommends *Aconite* at the outset, *Apis* and *Cantharis* subsequently, and *Arsenicum* at a later stage still, if the amount of effusion causes Orthopnœa and tendency to Syncope. Jahr agrees with me as to the general sufficiency of *Aconite*, but finds the 30th dilution efficacio is. Bahr treats of Pericardial, Myocardial and Endocardial Inflammation together under the general heading of "Carditis" He also maintains that "in every Pericarditis, whether primary or secondary, *Aconite* is the first and most important remedy whenever the inflammation sets in with febrile phenomena : we consider also," he add, "this remedy

---

* The experience I spoke of in 1878 was with others ; but since then I have had an attack of Plastic Pericarditis in my own person, and the effect of the treatment I have sketched above was most satisfactory.

† See also J. B. H. S,, vii 100 ; and a case of Hydropericardium in which it was equally successful in Vol. iii., p. 453.

indicated even if the fever is moderate or is altogether wanting. *Aconite* is not only indicated at the commencement of the disease, but in many cases during its whole course, more especially in Rheumatic cardiac inflammations, as long as the organic alterations do not result in Paralytic or Cyanotic symptoms." When the affection sets in insidiously, and there is free effusion of serum, he recommends *Digitalis*. *Spigelia* he regards as suitable only to Plastic Pericarditis and for lingering cases of this kind he commends **Sulphur**. "In a case of Peri carditis," he writes, "where uncommonly loud friction-murmurs and a rubbing of the pericardial surfaces against each other — that could even be felt by the hand, had already existed for upwards of three months, the symptoms disappeared entirely after *Sulpur* had been given for a fortnight." The resolution in my own case was obviously aided by this remedy. Dr. Hale follows pretty closely in Bahr's footsteps, though he attaches more value to *Bryonia* in the Plastic form, and mentions *Asclepias tuberosa* as an analogous remedy with which he has obtained good results.

ENDOCARDITIS, which, in its acute form, may for all practical purposes be considered exclusively in its connexion with Rheumatism. You will find a capital case by Huber in the Twelfth Volume of the BRITISH JOURNAL (p. 562), where *Aconite I* was the only medicine given; and another in the Eleventh Volume of the MONTHLY HOMŒOPATHIC REVIEW (p. 355), where *Spigelia*, in Dr. Bayes' hands, proved equally effectul. These cases very fairly illustrate the accepted Homœopathic treatment of Endocarditis. **Aconite** and **Spigelia** are the great remedies for inflammation of the lining as of the covering membrane of the heart, as might indeed be expected, when we consider the close similarity of the two textures, and the identity of the usual exciting cause. They are, moreover, manifestly SIMILIA to the affection. We have seen this of the former; and the pathogenetic effects of the latter point to endo rather than to pericardial irritations. The great success Fleischmann obtained with it by giving it indiscriminately in all Rheumatic inflammations of the heart may well have been due to the fact that of these, Endocarditis is by far the most frequent.

Dr. Arnulphy would extend the action of **Naja** in Chronic Endocarditis, of which I shall speak directly, to the Acute affection. "It is not only in the later stages of mitral disease" he writes,* "that *Naja* does its work. In alternation with *Aconite*, at the commencement of acute articular Rheumatism. I have seen it speedily abort Endocarditis which was developing. As a curiosity, I will quote a case of facial Erysipelas in an

---

* See M. H. R., xiv., 83.

elderly Sioux woman whom I had under my care at Hahnemann Hospital, Chicago, who exhibited at one stage alarming symptoms of Malignant Endocarditis with peripheral embolism. *Naja* and *Rhus* acted promptly, and the old Indian made a complete recovery. I will mention also three cases of serious Endocarditis supervening on acute non-articular Rheumatism of Gonorrhœal origin. It is well known how rebellious such cases of Endocarditis are, and how often they prove fatal. I am convinced that it is to *Naja* I owe the recovery of these three patients."

These last two experiences would lead one to think that we may have in *Naja* a remedy for the dreaded "Ulcerative Endo-carditis," of the use of *Aconite* in which I have already spoken. We want a supplementary medicine; and I had formerly suggested that this might be found among the *Serpent-poisons*, though then giving to *Lachesis* the preference. Dr. Byres Moir, in a later paper than that to which I previously referred, * reports two cases of recovery, and *Naja* played some part in the treatment of both.

VALVULAR DISEASE OF THE HEART is either a SEQUELA Endocarditis, or a manifestation of the disease actually existing in a chronic form. Our hope of modifying it to any extent must depend upon which of these alternatives is present. As long as inflammation exists, we can control it: but if we have to deal with the damage it has done, when the fire has burnt itself out, our aid can be palliative only. From Dr. Russel's experience (which I have frequently verified) it seems that **Naja** should always be given during the convalescence from an acute endocardial attack, and has great power of ensuring complete recovery. Dr. Arnulphy endorses these statements. Dr. Jousset has had similar results from **Aconite**, when the mischief was localised at the aortic orifice, and occurred in children. You will remember, also, Dr. Well's communication about the use of **Spongia** here, and his special indication for it — "starting from sleep at night, with fear of suffocation." With one of these remedies, steadily continued, the disastrous after-effects of an Acute Endocarditis may often be obviated. Then, again, there seems little doubt but that endocardiac inflammation may be chronic from the first, under the influence especially of Gout and Alcohol, and possibly of chronic Nicotonic intoxication and even of simple old age. Thus valvular disease may originate without the history of any acute affection. Here we require deeper acting remedies, and find them, I think, in **Arsenicum** and **Plumbum**. The action of *Arsenic* upon the heart has been thoroughly studied by Dr. Imbert Gourbeyre. ✝ It is evidently exerted upon the endocardium as well as on

---

* J. B. H. S., vi, 336.
✝ De A' action De L'arsenic sur le cæur. Paris, 1874.

other parts, and the results obtained in France with the *Arseniate of Antimony* in chronic cardiac disease leave no doubt of its efficacy. It has long enjoyed high repute here in the school of Hahnemann. Still more perfectly Homœopathic is *Plumbum*, in slow poisoning by which (as Jousset says) there is produced a Chronic Endocarditis and Endarteritis. We have as yet, however, no experience of its value.

The palliative treatment of chronic valvular disease may either be conjoined with that of a curative kind, or may—where permanent organic change exists—be pursued alone. The *Aconite* and *Naja* already mentioned are often useful under the latter circumstances. Where there is much Hypertrophy and excited action of the heart, **Cactus** may often replace *Aconite* with advantage; and **Spigelia** should be steadily given where there is much pain.* The acute paroxysmal attacks incident to valvular disease, and implying embarrassment of the cardiac circulation, are generally relieved by *Aconite*, but sometimes, (as found by Dr. Russell) by *Camphor*; and sometimes, especially when they take the form of "Cardiac Asthma," they find their best palliative (as Mr. Spencer Cox has well shown†) in *Glonoin*.

I have not spoken of *Digitalis* here, as its sphere is found only where the embarrassed circulation of valvular disease has led to—

CARDIAC DROPSY, which is a sufficiently important feature of chronic disease of the heart to merit special Therapeutic attention. Whether Homœopathic medication is adequate to deal with it, is a very important question. The answer must depend, in the first instance, upon the nature of the condition. If it be purely mechanical, from obstruction of the return of the venous blood, it would be inconceivable that dynamic measures could help it; and the only rational course to pursue would be the draining off of the effused fluid through the kidneys, through the bowels, or (by punctures) through the skin. But it is now generally recognised that this—save in the rare cases of primary disease of the right heart—is not the Pathology of Cardiac Dropsy. It is the lack of arterial tension from the embarrassment of the left heart which leads to overfilling of the venous system, and to such deficiency of blood-pressure in the kidneys as to make their secretion scanty. Hence excess of water in the blood and its extravasation into the tissues. It is obvious, therefore, that any drug which can restore the lacking tension to the arterial system will, temporarily at least, relieve the Dropsy; and that this may be done in two ways,—either by strengthening the heart-substance itself, or by stimulating the vaso-motor nerves. In **Digitalis** we have a medicine which unites both these properties, though in different ways. It

---

*See ANNALS, iii 30. † J. B. H. S., 69.

strengthens the cardiac muscle Homœopathically, for it weakens and even kills it in health; and hence, if the weakness of the heart's action which lead to Dropsy be curable, *Digitalis* may permanently remove the effusion by striking at its cause, and here need only be given in our usual doses. But too often it is not so. The left ventricle cannot fill the arteries, not because its own life is feeble, but because through alterations in its valves it is embarrassed in its work; and these alterations are irremediable. Our only resource in this case is to stimulate the vaso-motor nerves, which act directly on the arteries as well as on the heart itself. This, too, we can do with *Digitalis*; but it must be by inducing its primary, Physiological action, which—as we have seen—is to excite the sympathetic supply of the circulation, and increase arterial tension. Larger doses are here required, and an infusion or decoction of the leaves seems the most effective preparation. The inhalation of compressed air has a similar effect,—this also heightening the arterial tension; but it is found of less lasting influence than *Digitalis*.

I do not think that you can improve upon this plan by any more Homœopathic measures. Dr. Jousset indeed, who concurs in recommending it, seems to consider it as conforming to the Law of Similars, because *Digitalis* in excessive doses causes a condition of "Asystolia" very like that which is present. But this is only its secondary effect and the sign of consecutive exhaustion; and if when it is present you induce the opposite condition by doses sufficient to cause it in the healthy body, you are evidently practising Antipathically and not Homœopathically, and should recognise the fact. Bahr and Jahr writing from a strictly Homœopathic standpoint, speak very hopelessly of the treatment of Cardiac Dropsy,—with which view my own experience accords; while Dr. Hale's recommendations are as eclectic as they are theoretical.

I need not tell you that in exerting this action upon the circulation, and so dispelling Cardiac Dropsy, *Digitalis* does not stand alone. It is the type (though it is the prince among them) of a number of plants, of which—besides the *Cactus* which has already come before us—I may mention the *Adonis vernalis*, the *Apocynum cannabinum*, the *Convallaria majalis*, the *Erythrophlœum guinense* ("*Caoca*"), the *Oleander* and the *Strophanthus hispidus*. The alkaloid of Coffee, *Caffeine*, has been found possessed of similar powers (Dr. Meyhoffer speaks warmly of it); and possibly this may be so with the *Theobromine* we obtain from Cocoa, as in the form of a *Salicylate* it has become a patent medicine of some renown under the name of "*Diuretin*." Certainly the *Cytisus scoparius*, which as "Broom-tea" is an antihydropic of old repute, has in a glucoside it contains, to which the name of *Spartein* has been given, a substance of like action with the foregoing. Of all these, Dr. Hale has given an account more or less full in his book—to which we can not do better

ANGINA PECTORIS

than refer whenever a Cardiac Dropsy seems to require any other remedy than the *Fox-glove*. Perhaps the most frequently chosen alternative is *Strophanthus*. This is distinguished by having far less action on the arteries than *Digitalis*. Now there are some cases in which arterial contraction is undesirable, and where *Trinitrine* is used in conjunction with *Digitalis* to obviate this effect of it, *Strophanthus* would here be a TERTIUM QUID which might well take the place of the two.*

ANGINA PECTORIS.—There can be no doubt, I think, that this affection is essentially and always a Neurosis of the Cardiac nerves. That it is sometimes associated with organic change in the heart or aorta, while it gravely affects our prognosis, does not alter its nature or affect our treatment of it. It must not, of course (as Eulenberg points out), be confounded with the attacks of "Sthenocardia" which are liable to occur in every case of chronic cardiac disease with embarrassment of the circulation of the organ.

Our treatment of Angina Pectoris resolves itself into two departments:—What aid can we give during the attacks? And, what can we do to check their recurrence.

For both these purposes I think that two forms of the disorder must be recognised, in one of which SPASM is present causing oppression, while in the other pain is the single feature of the distress. In the former, I must recommend an Anti-pathic-palliative medication. The inhalation of *Amyl nitrite* gives such rapid and certain relief that I should be loth to risk the prolongation of my patient's sufferings by trying any similarly-acting remedy. Where spasm is absent, this substance is useless, and ordinary treatment has nothing of a brillant kind to offer which should lead us away from Homœopathy. Jahr mentions a case in which the attack was on every recurrence, relieved almost immediately by a dose of *Arsenicum* 30; and no better medicine could be given when (as in his case) the anxiety is accompanied by prostration and threatened Syncope. When the circulation is more active, *Aconite* (perhaps best given as *Aconitine*) might be helpful.

There is much more to be done in the way of preventing the recurrence of the paroxysms. Arsenicum is the leading remedy here, in both forms of the disease, when the symptoms of attack call for this remedy. It is commended as warmly by Hartmann and Bahr in the higher Homœopathic attenuations as by Anstie in the substantial doses of *Fouler's solution* administered in the old school. If other remedies are needed.

---

* Exceptionally, of course, Cardiac Dropsy may subside under other medication as from *Arsenicum iodatum* 3_x (J. B. H. S., v., 192) and from *Lycopus Virginicus* (IBID., viii., 357).

you will think, in the spasmodic form, of Hydrocyanic **acid and Cuprum**,— the former in recent cases, the latter in those more advanced ; and, in those purely Neuralgic, of **Spigelia**. To the favourable experience of Drs. Bayes and Kendall with this drug (which I have mentioned in my 'Pharmacodynamics') I may add that of Dr. Jousset. "*Spigelia*" he writes, "is the principal medicine for Angina Pectoris ; it corresponds to the anguishing sub-sternal pain radiating to the neck and arms. The irregularity of the pulse, the tendency to Syncope, the palpitations, the aggravations by the least movement, fix the choice of *Spigelia*. I am accustomed to begin with the 3rd dilution, three or four doses a day ; I descend to three drops of the mother-tincture, or mount to the 6th, 12th and 30th, according to the susceptibility of the subject. I can reckon many cases in which this remedy has given me a lasting cure or amelioration of long-continuance."

I may add *Digitalis*, with which Bahr cured the only case he had to treat ; *Nux vomica*, which Jousset ranks second to *Spigelia*, and gives in preference to Gouty and Hæmorrhoidal patients ; and *Naja*, which achieved a cure in Dr. Bradshaw's hands.* It is also well to remember M. Beau's observation of the frequent supervention of Angina Pectoris upon excessive smoking, and the inference thence resulting that we should prohibit Tobacco where it is used by sufferers from this malady, or prescribe *Tabacum* when otherwise indicated, to those not addicted to it.

The chief old-school advance which has been made since the foregoing was penned in 1878, has been along the lines of the use of *Amyl nitrite* already mentioned. Its own action is too temporary to induce lasting changes ; but *Trinitrin*e—under which name our *Glonoin* has been introduced into ordinary Therapeutics—while slower in giving palliation, is more effective towards cure, and not unfrequently (it is said) achieves one. As its action here must be acknowledged Antipathic, we can but make our colleagues a present of it ; and can the better afford to do so, as the *Cuprum*, I only causally mentioned formerly has become in our hands a more and more trusted resource. † You must think of *Cratægu*s, also, when the heart's action is weak and irregular.‡

---

* ANNALS, i., 296. † See J. B. H. S., iii., 374 ; M. H. R., xl, 599,
‡ J. B. H. S., vi., 299 ; viii., 78 355

APPENDIX TO LECTURE XLII

As my explanation of the action of *Digitalis* in Cardiac Dropsy, made in the foregoing lecture, hardly receives the general endorsement of my Homœopathic colleagues; I put in an Appendix a further development of the argument, with a reply to certain objections advanced against my position, which I contributed to the Fifth Volume of the LONDON HOMŒOPATHIC HOSPITAL REPORTS (1885).

THE TREATMENT OF CARDIAC DROPSY.
BY RICHARD HUGHES, L. R. C. P., M. R C. S.

In the course of Post-graduate Lectures of Homœopathic Therapeutics which I lately, delivered at the Hospital, I had to deal with "Homœopathy in Diseases of the Heart. I began by an account of what we can do here with four leading drugs—*Aconite* and *Arsenic, Cactus* and *Spigelia*; and then proceeded to speak thus :—

"With these great medicines, then, aided here and there by others of lesser range but as true aim, we can treat with confidence most of the diseases to which the heart is liable. Were I to enumerate the latter, however, I should not include Cardiac Dropsy among them; and you may have noticed that *Digitalis* has found no place in this Lecture among the leading heart-remedies of Homœopathy. It is nevertheless mainly by the use of the *Foxglove*, in substantial doses, that our brethren of the old school can do so well here, that a leading man among them Dr. Howship Dickinson has lately written : 'There is nothing I like better to treat than Cardiac Dropsy.' Homœopathists, if confining themselves to their usual resources, would have to make a confession in precisely the opposite direction ; as indeed Bahr and Jahr do explicitly, and Dr. Clarke—by his significant silence on the subject—implicity. Jousset uses other language, but then he relies on *Digitalis*.

"I know that some of us and Dr. Jousset himself is among them—maintain that in spite of its dosage, *Digitalis* is Homœopathic here. They point to the Asystolio induced in poisoning by excessive or too prolonged administration of the drug, and ask whether it is not therefore a similar to such condition when occuring idiopathically, and allowing of engorgement of the venous system, depression of the action of the kidneys, and unabsorbed effusion of serum into the tissues. Dr. Piedvache is unable to follow his master in Paris when so arguing ; * and I must continue, as I have always done, to side with him as against

---

* See L'ART MEDICAL for June, 1895, and Dr. Jousset's reply in the July No.

a corresponding contention here, I have, both in my 'Pharmacodynamics' and my 'Therapeutics', gone fully into the action of *Digitalis*, pathogenetic and curative. I have recognised, indeed maintained, that its direct influence on the heart-muscle in health is that not of a 'tonic', but of a poison; that it is therefore truly Homœopathic to Cardiac Debility, and will benefit this in small doses; and that if by giving tone to the heart the kidneys could be induced to act and the Dropsical fluid could be absorbed, we should not have to look further. The dosage, however, which suffices for the one will not be effective in the other; * and when we raise it to the standard required, we are administering quantities capable of inducing an excitant influence on the nervous supply on the heart, both pneumogastric and sympathetic. Through the one the heart is retarded; but through the other it is stimulated to beat forcibly, and would beat fast if the inhibitory influence of the vagi would permit. Therewith (the excitation coming from the vaso-motor centre at the base of the brain) the whole arterial system thrown into a state of tension, the vessels themselves are contracted,✝ and the blood-pressure raised. This is a condition precisely opposite to that which obtains in Cardiac Dropsy; and if you give doses which can induce it, and on its induction find Diuresis set in and œdema disappear, I think you must not claim your results for Homœopathy. Nor should you wish to do so. What you are aiming at here is palliation not cure. The valvular disease on which, ultimately, the Dropsy depends, remains untouched, and sooner or later the Anasarca which dogs it, is sure to recur. For such almost mechanical consequences of organic alteration Homœopathy, whose aim is cure, has no remedies; but Homœopathists may be thankful that medicine, in the larger sense of the term, is not without resources for the purpose. Though the disease may be incurable the patient's life may be prolonged, and that in tolerable ease. Those of you who have read Dr. Kidd's, "Laws of Therapeutics' may remember a severe case of Cardiac Dropsy there related, ✝✝ in which the primary attack and two relapses yielded to *Digitalis* with certain adjuncts. This patient—in the care of whom I have had the pleasure of being associated with Dr. Kidd for a long time past—went for twenty years without another attack, in fair enjoyment and adornment of life; and when, in 1894, a fourth occurred, similar treatment restored her to practical health. It is because of such positive results, only to

---

* Balfour (Clinical Lectures) reckons the "tonic" dose of *Digitalis* to be 1 grain of the leaves taken twice daily; whereas to remove Dropsy the equivalent of 40 grains or more has usually to be (gradually but rapidly) given, and saturation to be effected.

✝ Dr. Snader, of Philadelphia, in the excellent Article on *Cactus* in the HAHNEMANNIAN MONTHLY for Sept., 1895, to which I have already referred, speaks of *Digitalis* being given (in old-school treatment) "until the arteries are like pulsating cords of steel."

✝✝ At p. 180 of the Second Edition.

be in this manner obtained, * that I have, here and elsewhere, spent so much argument on the subject."

Since delivering the lecture, from which the foregoing is an extract, I have had the pleasure of reading the following recognition of the thesis for which I have contended from the pen of one of our American colleagues, Dr. W. A. Boericke, of San Francisco, Professor of Materia Medica and Therapeutics in the Hahnemann Hospital College of that city. "What physician," he asks, "will not avail himself at times of the direct action of *Digitalis*? I am well aware of Hahnemann's special warning against it, and yet there are times when a heart-tonic and powerful stimulant of the pneumogastrics is needed. You do not expect to cure permanently that failing heart, with its frequent feeble pulse, its full veins, its insufficient diastole. It is an overworked, over-worried, starving heart, whose career is soon to be ended; but a Physiological dose of *Digitalis* will work definite and remarkable and beneficient changes. It will quiet it, produce a long diastole and powerful systole; and a great wave of blood is sent through the arteries cleansing, feeding, enlivening. You get the re-assuring full strong beat of the pulse; and the machinery, at least for the time being, is in better running order, and every individual function responds." † Dr. Boericke's point of view is not quite the same as my own; but I welcome his support to what seems to him a self-evident assumption—that the good *Digitalis* does in incurable cardiac disease, is derived from its direct, primary action, and can only therefore be obtained from Physiological doses.

At a recent meeting, however, of the British Homœopathic Society Dr. Dyce Brown directly challenged the views I have expressed, both in my published works and in my hospital lecture (which he had heard) on this subject. He did not quarrel with my practical conclusion as to full dosage, but explained its necessity otherwise; differed widely from me as to the MODUS OPERANDI of the drug, both Physiological and Therapeutical. His paper appears in the forth Volume of the Society's JOURNAL; and I trust I shall be found doing justice to its statements and arguments, even though (as I must do) I traverse them.

1. Dr. Brown accepts my view that *Digitalis* acts on the heart through its pneumogastric and sympathetic nerve-supply, and thus also on the arteries. He questions, however, the direct influence on the cardiac muscle I postulate. He would explain

---

* I of course recognise (and in my lecture went on to speak of them) that there are other drugs—alike *Adonis*, *Apocynum*, *Convallaria* and *Strophanthus* which may in certain cases be substitued for *Digitalis*. But their Physiological action, with whatever minor variations, is essentially the same and so—accordingly—must be their MODUS OPERANDI.—I am glad to receive herein the support of Dr. Cowperthwaite.

† PACIFIC COAST JOURN. OF HOMŒOPATHY, Dec., 1895

all symptoms of debility of the heart-walls by nervous exhaustion consequent on over-stimulation : and reckons among these the slow pulse of the drug, noting that not uncommonly the heart's action is at first quickened. Dr. Brown surely forgets that slowness of pulse, if induced through the vagi, implies their stimulation, not their depression. The latter corresponds to their experimental division, and thereupon the heart starts off on a rapid course, it palpitates and does not drag. Retardation is the effect rather of their excitation, as by Galvanism. But what we have to do in unravelling the confessedly complex state brought about by *Digitalis*, is to account for the loss of power in the heart-muscle (as shown by the great quickening of the pulse on the assumption of the erect posture) while the retarded beat and raised arterial tension show that the nervous supply of the organ is still excited. If (as I have brought other evidence to prove) the drug is a muscular poison, affecting the heart earlier than any other muscle, the difficulty is solved. We can thus, moreover, best account for the faintness and even mortal Syncope *Digitalis* is apt to induce. I must stand to my point that no exhaustion of the nervous supply of the heart can bring this about, is the organ itself if healthy. Dr. Brown urges that, "nervous shock, mental or physical, can and does kill the heart, when there is no evidence of the heart itself being diseased." Yes ; but surely in such cases the shock is of a stimulating rather than exhausting kind. It passes down the vagi from the emotional centre in the brain, and inhibitis the heart's action, as a flash of lightning or a too strong Galvanic current might do. ✳

So much for Physiological ; now for Therapeutical action. In looking through the treatment of *Digitalis* in the successive editions of my 'Pharmacodynamics,' I am struck by seeing the gradual way in which, thought and experience have brought me to my present position about it. At first, I tried to account for its usefulness in heart disease by supposing that it acted as a cardiac tonic here, being a depressant of the organ in health. I soon found, however, that this would not account either for the benefit obtained or for the dosage required ; that the primary excitant action on the cardiac nerves had to be invoked ; and that in Cardiac Dropsy this alone was effective. Dr. Brown is too good a practical physician to question the facts which have led me to this conclusion. He fully recognises that Cardiac Dropsy is "the effect of a low arterial tension and a dilated weak heart," and that *Digitalis* removes it by strengthening the heart-beats

---

✳ In such a case heart would stop in diastole : whereas if it were directly poisoned by the drug it (or at any rate its left ventricle) might well be found in systole. Dr. Brown's own citations show that either alternative may obtain. But if his view of nervous exhaustion being the cause of death in *Digitalis*-poisoning were correct, the heart ought always to be flaccid POST MORTEM.

and raising the tension of the vessels—as it does in health. But he maintains that this is to be called Homœopathic action, not Antipathic; because if such stimulation be too strong, or be carried on too long, it results in exhaustion. If then the secondary depressant effects of *Digitalis* be taken as our guide, SIMILIA SIMILIBUS would lead us to give it analogous states of circulatory depression in dosage sufficient to exert its stimulant effect and no more. "If by *Digitalis*," he writes, "you produce a state of increase of power of the heart-movements, and develop a state of increased tension, short, be it observed, of over-stimulation, and by so doing you remove the Dropsy, then, I maintain, it is unmistakeably Homœopathic in its action." Again, as to dosage, he says,—"Whatever the size of the dose, be it drop-doses of mother-tincture, or 5 drops or even 10 drops of it, or one or two teaspoonfuls of the infusion, provided we get the desired result of stimulation, the normal point, or as near to it as possible, and provided that we do not develop the over-action, and so make the patient worse, that dose is Homœopathic." If this is Homœopathy, what is Antipathy? I confess, I do not know Hahnemann's method in Dr. Brown's putting of it. The Master said, SIMILIA SIMILIBUS CURENTUR; and he bade us seek this similarity mainly in the primary effects of drugs. Dr. Brown would limit us to their secondary effects; it is here, he says, that we must find our parallels, and then by inducing the primary influence of the medicine we shall counteract the morbid condition present. On this mode of proceeding, *Strychnia* would be Homœopathic, not to Tetanus but to Spinal Paresis; *Stramonium* would be selected for Dementia rather than for Mania; and as induction of primary effects, opposite to the condition present, generally requires substantial dosage, infinitesimals would find little, if any, place in Homœopathic practice.

And there is yet more to be said. I have explained why the Antipathic action of *Digitalis* has to be resorted to in Cardiac Dropsy: it is because palliation is all that can be aimed at, and CONTRARIA CONTRAIIS is generally our guide towards this end. It is no argument against such a view to point, as Dr. Brown does, to the twenty years for which—in case instanced by me—the palliation (*i.e.*, the absence of the Dropsy) lasted. Longer or shorter, the effect obtained by *Digitalis* here in the essence palliative, because it is the removal (generally temporary) of the result of an incurable cause. It must be remembered that the cardiac weakness which leads to Dropsy is not primary; it is secondary to valvular disease,—often, indeed, it is insufficient compensation only, there is a left ventricle of ordinary power when we want and hypertrophied and forceful one. Simple debility of the heart, as in exhausting disease and in old age, may cause some œdema of the feet; but real Dropsy does not occur from it.* *Digitalis* may remove such œdema. Homœopathically, by strengthening (as I conceive, by direct action) the organ it weakens in health; and for this purpose the ordinary dosage practised in our school will suffice. When, however, the thing we have to do is to assist Nature in her effort to establish, or to restore compensation, it is a stimulant rather than a tonic we want; we are seeking to exaggerate the heart's force that it may overcome an obstacle. Our aim is palliative; we seek a Physiological effect, and must use Physiological quantities. In my lecture I used the considerations to explain and justify our resort to the Antipathic action and dosage of *Digitalis* in Cardiac Dropsy. I now adduce them as supporting my contention that we are proceeding Antipathically in so prescribing it.

Let us look at the picture as it is carried out by our old-school colleagues, who, by virtue of it have "nothing they like better to treat than Cardiac Dropsy." I will take as a leading exponent of it Dr. Balfour, of Edinburgh, in the Fourteenth of his "Clinical Lectures on Diseases of the Heart and Aorta" (2nd Ed.). He describes *Digitalis* as "a tonic and stimulant of the heart," and speaks of the "almost marvellous result which follows its bold and judicious employment." Its tonic dose equals about a grain of the leaves twice daily. But, he writes, "when we wish to remove Dropsy, or contract a dilated heart, *Digitalis* should be given at much shorter intervals and the more urgent the case, the shorter should be the intervals and the larger the dose. The equivalent of rather more than 40 grains may usually be given before saturation occurs,...but nothing but good will follow provided we stop the moment the urine falls, the pulse slows, or nausea occurs." Marked results will not be usually found to occur till a certain amount of saturation is attained. From one to three days subsequently, in cases of Dropsy the full effects of the drug may be expected, the urine will rapidly rise to about 200 oz. in the day, and will in favourable cases continue to flow till all the cavities are emptied." *Digitalis* is FACILE PRINCEPS in its own domain—"the removal of serum accumulated in the body through defective mechanical power in the circulatory system."

How can such practice with any plausibility be described as Homœopathy? Are we not prejudicing our appeal for a hearing on the part of the profession by so claiming it? So far as they have any method at all, they induce the Physiological action of the drugs they use. If this be done in the part affected (affected, of course, in the opposite manner) the practice is Antipathy, or Enantiopathy; if elsewhere it is Allœopathy (now less correctly called Allopathy). So Hahnemann taught, and I see no escape from the position. If we begin adopting the former, on the

---

* It was justly pointed out in the discussion on Dr. Brown's Paper that Dropsy is unknown as an effect poisoning by *Digitalis*.

plea of its being Homœopathic when the secondary effects of drugs only are taken into account, and proporation our dosage accordingly, our opponents in the other camp will have a potent weapon to use against us. We say,- you are taking our similar remedies, small dose and all, and refusing to acknowledge the Law under which they act, using them empirically, or explaining away their apparent Homœopathicity. They will say in return,—you are taking our contrary remedies, full dose and all, under a plea which to us at least is transparently futile.

We shall be weakening our case apologetically ; and we shall be impairing the success of our practice when we have such cases to treat. If our students and begininners are assured that in using *Digitalis* for Cardiac Dropsy they are practising Homœopathically, they will naturally be led to do so with the dosage in which they are accustomed to see other similar remedies act. They may be told that the drug does best here in the mother-tincture ; but they will suppose that this means in one or two drop doses of the same, beyond which they are rarely led to go. Now this is utterly insufficient, and will lead to failure and disappointment. They will run the risk of finding themselves superseded by a man who knowing that he has to induce the Physiological action of the drug, will push it in the Balfourian way, and will be rewarded by seeing the kidneys acting and the waterlogged tissues clearing. * It is painful experience which has taught me this, and I would spare others the necessity of learning it in the same way ;

"Non ignara mali, miseris succurrere disco."

It is because of these disastrous consequences - to our conception of Homœopathy, to our attitude as before the profession, and to our conduct at the bedside, that I have felt the present question of so much importance. If it were one of theory only, interesting as it might be, I should not have entered the lists upon it, and still less when the champion against whom I must tilt is an esteemed friend. I can only ask his pardon for the buffets I have had to deal him with lance and sword, and leave the decision between us, when any counterstroke of his has been displayed to the spectators of the combat.

---

* "The ancient wisdom has said, with reason, that when we cannot cure we should relieve. A fact in my practice illustrates this. It was in 1856, when I was full of illusions, now wholly dispersed, I attended a patient the subject of Asystolia, Anasarcous, and with a dyspnœa which did not allow of his lying down. I prescribed persistently, but unsuccessfully. The patient got no better but rather worse. He betook himself to the practitioners of the neighbourhood, who gave him an infusion of the leaves of *Digitalis*. The urine flowed freely, the œdema disappeared, and some days after the sick man could sleep in his bed. Naturally I lost my patient but I did not lose the lesson his case taught me" (Jousset, REVUE HOM. FRANCAISE, March, 1900).

LECTURE . XLIII

DISEASES OF THE CIRCULATORY SYSTEM
—o—
THE ARTERIES, VEINS, LYMPHATICS AND BLOOD-GLANDS.
—o—
ARERITIS—ANEURYSM—ARTERIAL DEGENERATION—PHLEBITIS—
VARICOSIS—LYMPHANGEITIS—LYMPHADENOMA—LEUCÆMIA—
ADDISON'S DISEASE—BRONCHOCELE—MYXŒDEMA—
EXOPHTHALMIC GOITRE.

I am now going to approach a class of diseases most of which once obscure Pathologically, were still less known to Therapeutics. These are the diseases of the BLOOD-VESSELS ; of the LYMPHATIC and LACTEAL SYSTEMS ; and of the VASCULAR GLANDS ; there is much more to be said about them now.

As diseases of the ARTERIES I will consider ARTERITIS, ANEURYSM and ATHEROMA.

ARTERITIS, if ever diagnosed as occuring in an acute form would probably be met by the treatment suitable to Endocarditis, viz., **Aconite** in low dilution and repeated doses. Such an affection, however, must be extremely rare ; and it is with chronic inflammation of the arteries alone that we are practically concerned. Of general Chronic Endarteritis I will speak under the head of Atheroma ; in this place I shall only mention two localised forms of the malady. The first of these is CHRONIC AORTITIS of which we owe a full account to Tessier and Jousset. *Arsenicum* (especially in the form of the *Arsenite of Antimony*) has been the medicine which has given the latter most result ; he administered the lowest triturations. *Spigelia* he finds helpful for the pain like that of Angina often associated with the disease, and *Cuprum* for its attacks of dyspnœa. These were his Therapeutics formerly. Now he seems to have followed Huchard in abandoning the *Arsenite of Antimony* for the *Iodide of Sodium* of which he gives 20 centigrammes daily ; and for the dyspnœa relies upon *Glonoin* 1. * Dr. Goullon relates a case treated by correspondence, in which anginose symptoms have been diagnosed by distinguished old-school physician as dependent on Aortitis. He sent *Aurum* 6 which was continued for three months with progressive improvement ; and at the end of this time all symptoms had disappeared, and the physician—ignorant of what had been taken—expressed his astonishment, and said there were merely some traces remaining of the lesion. ✝ We have thus in *Aurum* (the dyspnœa of

---

* See J. B. H. S., ii., 364 ; iv, 334.   ✝ IBID„ vii., 419.

which is very marked, and unaccountable for by pulmonary disorder) an alternative to *Arsenic* and *Iodine* in this disease; and an experience of Dr. Edmond Piedvache's shows that *Strophanthus* may sometimes take the place of *Cuprum* and *Glonoin*.*

The second form in which Endarteritis comes before us for treatment is as the morbid process in the arteries (usually of the lower extremities) which results in Gangrene—symmetrical or senile. In the former the mischief hardly goes beyond spasm (this is what is called RAYNAUD'S DISEASE) ; in the second it is obstructive. In either instance, Secale is obviously Homœopathic, and in the senile form Dr. Jousset has been one and Dr. L. B. Wells ✝ three cases recover under it. Symmetrical Gangrene has been cured by *Ferrum phosphoricum I* and by *Lachesis* 6. †

When writing in 1878 about—

ANEURYSM, beyond a passing good word for *Lycopodium*, the only hope I could hold out for the medicinal treatment of this affection lay in the direction of *Iodide of Potassium* which though sometimes useful in small doses (as in a case of my own, mentioned in my 'Pharmacodynamics'), had—I was obliged to admit, generally to be given in large ones. We can now do better. In 1879 Dr. Flint, of Scarborough published in the MONTHLY HOMŒOPATHIC REVIEW for June and the PRACTITIONER for July a case of abdominal aortic Aneurysm, where striking remedial effects, almost amounting to a cure, resulted from the administration of the *Chloride of Barium* (our *Baryta muriatica*) in doses of one-fifth and two-fifths of a grain. He was led to try the drug by the evidence in Ziemssen's 'Cyclopædia' of the great power of *Barium salts* in increasing the blood-pressure and of their analogy in this respect to *Iodide of Potassium*. His experience was not allowed to stand alone. In 1882, Dr. Torry Anderson treated a similar case at our London Hospital, with most beneficial results, by three-grain doses of the 3_x trituration of the *Carbonate* ; × and in 1884 Dr. Clarke had another—the record of which is given in his book—in which the same *salt* and in like strength was employed. Dr. Howitt, of Toronto, reported in 1885 another, where practical cure ensued under the lx dilution of the *Muriate*. ‖ Dr. Byres of Moir, also, has reported favourable results. ✝ These facts will suffice to show that in the *Baryta salts* we have a probably Homæopathic and certainly curative agent in this very serious disease—one, more-

---

* REV. HOM. FRANCAISE, April 1900 (p. 445).
† U. S. MED. INVESTIGATOR, Oct. 1, 1890.
✝ J. B. H. S., vi., 110, 226. × ANNALS, x., 256.
‖ M. H. R., xxix, 669. ✝ J. B. H. S., iv., 216,

over, which will act in the small and non-perturbative doses we affect. In connexion with this I may call your attention to the mineral waters of Llangammarch in Wales as containing an appreciable though small quantity of *Barium chloride*. One of the affections in which they have been found useful is Dilatation of the Heart.

While this affords our most favourable outlook in the direction of Aneurysm, we must not forget *Lycopodium*. In Dr. Majumdar's hands an enlargement of this kind in the right carotid disappeared under it, flatulence and acid eructations combining with the lesion to call for remedy.* Sometimes too, other mineral salts may help us. Dr. H. S. Fuller communicates two cases, both in the neck, in one of which (a boy of 15) complete disappearance of the growth took place under *Calcarea phosphorica* 2_x. In the other, where the patient was a woman of 45, *Calcarea fluorata* 3_x, but especially 12_x and 30_x caused subsidence of the pains, which were severe, and a shrinkage of the Tumour by one-half; so that she became able to walk any distance and attend to her domestic duties.

As regards these pains, I suggested *Aconite*,—which, and also *Glonoin*, Dr. Lambert has found useful. † Dr. Molson exhibited on a "consulation day" at the Hospital a case of pulsating Tumour in the right neck. It was improving under *Baryta carbonica*; but an interesting point was that the patient had applied for intense and constant pain in the right shoulder, going down the arm, which had lasted for six months, and that this had been completely removed by *Kalmia* 1_x.

ARTERIAL DEGENERATION used to be ranked as ATHEROMA, but is now known also under the form of Sclerosis. In either case it often depends on a Chronic Endarteritis, in which case I should think *Plumbum* eminently suited to it. Dr. Arnulphy, however, considers this medicine more effective in true Atheroma which is a primary Fatty Degeneration; and follows Huchard in preferring the *Iodide* in Sclerosis. ‡

The diseases of the VEINS we shall have to consider are PHLEBITIS and VARICOSIS.

PHLEBITIS, in its most familiar form of Phlegmasia Alba Dolens, will come under our notice among the diseases of women. When occuring under other circumstances, and presenting the ordinary sub-acute, "ADHESIVE" form, you will find two excellent medicines for it in **Pulsatilla** and **Hamamelis**. I scarcely know how to distinguish between them, or to which to give the palm. Perhaps you can hardly do better than follow Jousset's example

---

* J. B. H. S., iv., 231. † IBID., p. 217. ‡ IBID., vi., 107, 301.

is prescribing *Pulsatilla* at the outset, and substituting *Hamamelis* it its effects are not so rapid as you could desire. Where burning pain is very marked, Dr. Cartier prefers *Arsenicum*. In Suppurative Phlebitis, **Lachesis** would take the place of either, and what it can do in such cases is illustrated by the three, mentioned by Dr. Dunham which I have cited in my lecture on the *Serpent-poisons*. In the cases of Acute Phlebitis recorded by Mr. Ayerst in the Fifteenth Volume of the BRITISH JOURNAL OF HOMŒOPATHY, *Lachesis* seems to have been the most efficient among the several medicines used. For the painful Thromboses which occur in the course of a vein after Phlebitis, Dr. Ord recommends *Arnica* 1_x. *

In Chronic Phlebitis *Pulsatilla* (best, I think, in the dilutions from the 6th upwards) is of eminent service. ✝ Dr. Espanet alternates *Mercurius* with it, and finds these two remedies sufficient for all Phlegmasiæ of a venous character such as Chilblains) occuring in organs on which they have an elective action. He gives the 6th dilution of each.

In

VARICOSIS—ordinary practice has for its sole resource mechanical and too often surgical measures. It will be of no small comfort to patients, and surely some honour to the Art of Medicine, if Homœopathy can teach us to cure it in a more excellent way. I think it can do so, and mainly by means of two potent medicines – *Hamamelis* and *Flouric acid*.

1. The story of **Hamamelis**, as I have told it in my 'Pharmacodynamics,' is a very interesting one. You see the drug gradually creeping on in our knowledge – at first an empirical and local remedy, then found to act in like manner internally, then proved a similar to the condition it relieved, then ascertained to remedy morbid states of other veins than those of the rectum ; finally standing out as our great venous medicine, good for Phlebitis, Varicosis, Piles (especially the bleeding ones) and passive hæmorrhages. All this was effected some forty years ago, but to this day *Hamamelis* reigns supreme in Homœopathic practice wherever veins are inflamed or painful or dilated or giving way under the blood pressure.

2. Of **Flouric acid** I said in the First Edition of my book (1867), that under it, among other things, "Varicose Veins have shrunk to half their size." I derived my information from a clinical symptom inserted in a Pathogenesis of the drug published by Constantine Hering in the First Volume of the Transactions of the American Institute of Homæopathy. The statement I

---

* M. H. R. xii., 527   ✝ See B. J. H., xxiv., 496.
‡ See BULL. DE LA SOC. MED. HOM., DE FRANCE, Vol., xix.

made about it has twice fallen as seed in good ground. Dr. Burnett, who has devoted another of his little books to 'Diseases of Veins,' tells us how his mind was exercised by the claim put forward ; how he tested it, in a, by no means, favourable case ; and how, finding it fully vertified, he went forward with confidence in the medicinal treatment of the other venous affections to his great satisfaction. I can heartily commend this BROCHURE of his, as containing much practical information, and exhibiting actions of *Ferrum* and *Rhus* (among other medicines) on the veins which are not generally recognized. Later, Dr. Washington Epps, moved by the same statement, was led to give *Flouric-acid* a wider testing in the Varicose Veins and Ulcers which throng the out-patient rooms of our hospital as they do those of similar institutions elsewhere. You will find his results in a valuable Paper contained in the Third Volume of the JOURNAL OF THE BRITISH HOMŒOPATHIC SOCIETY—a paper which has been widely copied and translated, and is indeed most instructive and encouraging. The *acid* has rarely been used below the 6th dilution, and Dr. Epps gets his best results from the 12th and 30th ; so that infinitesimals come in for some of the credit, its successful use has won.

If you have to look further, I may mention that we hear from America that *Carduus marianus* is "as near a specific for Varicose Veins as one could wish." The deeper-seated, and the more knotted and twisted they are, the better.

Staphisagria is recommended by Bhar, and Dr. Cartier praises *Zincum* 6 where the veins are painful.

Of the disease of the LACTEALS nothing is known, but we have something to say about the LYMPHATICS. Leaving the Scrofulous affections of the mesenteric, bronchial and cervical glands till we come to the Diseases of Children, I shall speak here of LYMPHANGEITIS and LYMPHADENOMA.

LYMPHANGEITIS—in its most familiar form, in such as we see when the lymphatics of the arm inflame after a poisoned wound, and the axillary glands follow suit. **Belladonna** and **Mercurius** cover the whole mischief here, if it has not gone too far, and if the general system is unaffected. Jousset considers their alternate use to constitute THE internal treatment of the malady. Where there is fever with great restlessness, **Rhus** may be better, as is proved in two cases of Dr. Waszili's. ✢ When the local symptoms are of a vicious character, and there is constitutional depression, **Lachesis** would supersede one and all.

---

* J. B. H. S., viii., 355 ; see also ix., 282. ✢ IBID., iv., 327.

LYMPHADENOMA

Bahr describes a peculiar form of Lymphangeitis as occuring more particularly in the case of women, and about the head. "With this inflammation," he writes, "a violent fever breaks out very suddenly, accompanied by tearing pains in the scalp and nape of the neck. The abatement of these pains is attended with the simultaneous appearance of several nodes and hard cords about the head, which, however, seldom remain longer than twenty-four hours. After a short interval of ease, another attack takes place, and things may be going on in this manner for several weeks." In this conditon he found Apis rapidly curative.

LYMPHADENOMA is that multiple, spontaneous and painless enlargement of the lymphatic glands which, from the physician who first described it fully, is known as "HODGKIN'S DISEASE." "Of its internal remedies," writes Sir William Gowers in Quain's Dictionary, "*Arsenic* incomparably the most potent. It should be pushed to the largest doses the patient can bear, such as fifteen minims of the *Liquor arsenicalis* three times daily. It often causes some pain in the glands, followed by their diminution in size, and even, in a few recorded cases by their complete disappearance." This dosage is curious, as the drug seems Homœopathic to the disease, miners with it getting Sarcoma of the bronchial glands ; and prolonged medicinal use having caused a similar condition of those of both chest and abdomen. * I should think the *Iodide* a better preparation, and should try this in smaller doses. In the only successful experience with the disease I know of in Homœopathic literature, this drug, with the *Iodides of Barium* and *Iron*, was curative. † Dr. Galley Blackley records three cases in the Sixth Volume of the LONDON HOMŒOPATHIC HOSPITAL REPORTS (p. 19) which he ascribes to this disease, but in none of them was there any improvement under treatment. I once had a case in which a number of the cervical glands enlarged after Influenza. Glandular medicines, like *Conium* and *Iodine*, did nothing : but under constitutional treatment with *Calcarea* and *Thuja* they slowly subsided. I cannot say whether this was the beginning of Lymphadenoma.

The glands subservient to the circulatory system are, besides the lymphatic and the mesenteric already mentioned, the spleen, the supra-renal capsules and the thyroid.

---

* Cycl, of Drug Pathogenesy, SUB VOCE (ii., 73 and note.)
† CLINIQUE Jan, 1897.

The SPLEEN has hitherto come before us therapeutically, almost entirely in the form of the Hypertrophy ("Ague-callo") which follows Intermittent Fever, and may also develop in the inhabitants of Malarious districts where no Ague-paroxysms have occurred. It is then generally associated with a corresponding enlargement of the liver, and the two Hypertrophies form part of the Malarious cachexia. This must then be treated as a whole, by such remedies as *Calcarea arsenica*, *Ferrum arsenicosum* and *Natrum muriaticum*, according to the indications given elsewhere ; and the splenic enlargement will subside with the other symptoms. Where it stands by itself, however, it requires its own organ-remedies ; and until lately we have not known of any drug having the relation to the spleen, which, for instance *Chelidonium* bears to the liver. We seem to have found one now in the **Ceanothus Americanus**. I have told in my 'Pharmacodynamics' how in the Third Edition of his "New Remedies," Dr. Hale cited an old-school testimony to its value in inflammation and enlargement of the organ ; and called attention to the statement made by its employer that "in chronic cases, where the organ is no longer tender, under the use of the tincture it soon becomes tender and painful, and then sinks rapidly to its normal size." This was sufficient to suggest its Homœopathicity, and led Dr. Burnett to give it in some cases of splenic disease which happened to come under his notice, and with most satisfactory results. Since that time (1881) our knowledge of the remedy has undergone considerable enlargement. On the one side Dr. Fahnestock has proved it upon himself, and found, it causes sticking pain in the spleen followed by enlargement of the organ. The pain was worse on motion, and there was inability to lie on the affected side. Following this came similar symptoms in the liver. On the other hand confirmations of the Therapeutic value of the drug have been repeatedly furnished to our journals, and *Ceanothus* has taken quite the chief place in our practice for enlargements of the spleen, both Malarial and Non-malarial ; as also for Splenitis and Splenalgia. * In 1887, moreover, Dr. Burnett collected his own experience with the drug into one of his little volumes, ✞ adding a good deal of interesting talk about the spleen, its diseases and remedies. Should you meet with any case in which *Ceanothus* disappoints you, you cannot do better than consult his treatise. This remedy itself he recommends whenever there is complain of deep seated pain in the left side, even when no tenderness or enlargement of the spleen can be made out ; and he had found consentaneous affections, such as Leucorrhœa, disappear under its use with the pain itself. This has been verified, as regards Leucorrhœa, by Dr. Fahnestock. ⚵

---

* See J. B. H. S., iii., 207 ; iv., 131, 349 ; v., 194 ; H. W., xxxv., 437
✞ "Diseases of the spleen." London : James Epps and Co,
⚵ J. B. H. S., ix., 282.

LEUCÆMIA

In connexion with the spleen I will speak of LEUCOCYTHÆMIA, or—as it is at present generally but less correctly called—

LEUCÆMIA—This disease is an Anæmia in which there is an absolute and often very great increase of the white corpuscle of the blood. By Hughes Bennett it was supposed to be a primary disorder of the circulating fluid ; but Virchow, noting its frequent association with enlargements of the spleen, or the lymphatic glands, or both, supposed it to be secondary to derangements of the blood-making glands. Still more recently, a peculiar change in the marrow of the long bones has been observed in connexion with it, in cases where neither the spleen nor the lymphatic glands were affected ; and so we hear of a Leucæmia Lienalis, a Leucæmia Lymphatica, and a Leucæmia Medullaris. Observations seem multiplying, however, of the existence of these local changes without Leucæmia, and of Leucæmia whithout them, so that the set of opinion at the present day seems in favour of Bennett's original position.

If this be sound, and at any rate in instances where Leucæmia is present without organic change, we have a promising remedy for it in **Picric acid**, which Erb has found to produce a condition in dogs which he himself calls an "Artificial Leucocythæmia." *
But where Lymphatic or splenic hypertrophy is present, remedies suitable to such glandular changes must be sought ; and here the views of Grauvogl demand attentive consideration. This profound scholar and thinker has pointed out that the glandular enlargements and accompanying cachexia described by Virchow were familiar to the older physicians under the name of "Sycosis," which diathesis had in their view a much wider range than that given it by Hahnemann, who recognized it only as an infection of the system by the virus of Gonorrhœa and its accompanying Condyloma. Grauvogl would admit this as one of its exciting causes ; but believes the essential condition to be one in which the blood contains too much water. In it there is a tendency to profuse mucous secretions, and to gelatinous exudations (no pus or fibrin forming) in parenchymatous organs. The patients feel worse in cold, damp weather, and in rain ; and their complaints are aggravated by everything which increases the proportion of water in the blood, as bathing, eating fish, drinking much fluid, and so forth. †

Whatever you may think of these views (and his exposition of them is well worth reading) they seem to have led him to some excellent remedies for the morbid state before us. Where there is a Gonorrhæl anamnesis, he recommends Thuja to be,

---

* Dr. E.R. Johnson, encountering a case of the Anæmia Pseudo-leucæmica Infantum, so constantly fatal, treated it with *Ferrum picricum* 3_x five grains PER DIEM, and was rewarded by complete recovery (N. ENG. MED. GAZ., Nov., 1900).

† See "Text-Book of Homœopathy," s 295-300, 329-339.

given; and where the patient's susceptibility to cold and damp is very marked, **Aranea diadema** and the alternate use of **Nux vomica** and **Ipecacuanha** are much prized by him. But his chief constitutional remedy is **Natrum sulphuricum**, of which he gives about five drops of the third decimal dilution several times a day. Numerous illustrations of the effects of such treatment are related by him, and give a very clear view of the malady he is characterizing.

Dr. Lilienthal in a study of Leucæmia in the Twenty-Fifth Volume of the NORTH AMERICAN JOURNAL OF HOMŒOPATHY, and Dr. Goullon in his prize-essay on *Thuja* therein translated, go largely into this subject in Grauvogl's wake. They concur in thinking *Thuja* best suited to Leucæmia Medullaris, and *Natrum sulphuricum* to the splenic and lymphatic forms. Dr. Lilienthal further recommends the study of *Natrum muriaticum*.

I have little to add to the foregoing deliverance on the subject, which dates from 1878. Two additional points only I would make.

1st. No use for *Myrrh* has yet been found in Homœopathic Therapy. Now that it has been ascertained, however, that its use may quadruple the number of white corpuscles in the blood, it ought to find employment in the form of Leucocythæmia which seems primarily hæmatic, herein reinforcing *Picric acid*.

2nd. The good which has resulted, in the splenic form, from reducing the size of the organ, especially by Voltaic Electricity, suggests that the power *Ceanothus* undoubtedly has in this direction might hopefully be invoked here.

The only affection of the SUPRA-RENAL CAPSULES of which we know anything is—

ADDISON'S DISEASE—Drs. Wilks and Greenhow have shown that there is one special form of the disease of the adrenals with which the bronzed skin, Anæmia and Asthenia described by Addison are connected. This is analogous to the Scrofulous enlargements of the lymphatic glands; "the morbid process in the capsules consists, primarily, in their infiltration by an inflammatory exudation of low type, which destroys the natural structure of the organs, and finally itself undergoes caseous degeneration." * The general symptoms of the malady probably depend upon the relation of the organs to the Ganglionic nerves — those in the neighbourhood being generally involved in the morbid process. Were we to treat the disease as a whole, and symptomatically, **Arsenicum** would seem indicated; and in the case recorded by Dr. Gibbs Black in the Thirty-Fifth Volume of the BRITISH JOURNAL OF HOMŒOPATHY the disease may have

---

* Greenhow; Croonian Lectures on Addison's Disease. 1875.

been induced by this poison, as the bedroom and sitting-room of the patient were found to be lined with green paper, containing *Arsenic* in large quantities. In the only case of the disease I have seen, however, this medicine was not of the least avail. A more hopeful method of treatment might be to attack the Scrofulous process in the capsules as if lymphatic glands were in question, for which purpose *Iodine* might come to our aid. Perhaps something might be done for the vomiting as with *Kreasote* or *Apomorphia* ; though the former failed in my case and the latter was of only temporary benefit in Dr. Blake's.

Jousset has nothing but Anti-scrofulous remedies to suggest for this malady, and Bahr and Jahr do not mention it. Dr. Payr has given a study of Addison's Disease in the ALLGEMEINE HOM. ZEITUNG for 1870, * and Dr. Lilienthal another in the Twenty-Fifth Volume of the NORTH AMERICAN JOURNAL OF HOMŒOPATHY. The latter suggested *Argentum nitricum* as a promising remedy, and mentions a case treated by it in the Ward's Island Hospital where great benefit resulted, though the malady was too far advanced for cure. Later experience has brought us little further aid here. Dr. T. E. Gilman reports a case, apparently of this malady, in the CLINIQUE of July, 1898, in which recovery sets in, when the patient was at a very low ebb, after a critical and most offensive exhalation from the surface. This supervened on the administration of *Hydrocyanic acid.* *Arsenicum iodatum* and some of Schussler's *Salts* were later of value. Dr. Beclere presented to the Societe Medicale des Hopitaux, an undoubted case of Addison's Disease, in which a definitive cure of three years' standing had been effected by hypodermic injection of a fluid extract of the supra-renal capsules themselves. Ingestion of these as fresh food had been previously tried without success.

As diseases of the THYROID I shall speak of the simple hypertrophy, which we call BRONCHOCELE, and of the results of insufficient or excessive action of the gland—MYXŒDEMA and EXOPHTHALMIC GOITRE.

And first of—

BRONCHOCELE —By this name, I say (as by its equivalents GOITRE and DERBYSHIRE NECK), I understand SIMPLE HYPERTROPHY OF THE THYROID, excluding all cystic and other growths within it, which latter are in the province of Surgery. The leading

---

* Translated in Vol. xviii, of the N. A. J. H.
† See L'ART MÉDICAL, March, 1898, p. 216.

feature of the Therapeutics of this disease is obviously the use of **Iodine**. I have gone fully into the question of its relation to thyroid enlargement in my lecture on the drug, and have come to the conclusion that in all recent and soft Goitres, *Iodine* is Homœopathic, and may succeed in small and even infinitesimal doses ; while when the Tumour is hard and knotty, it acts by its liquefacient properties, and must be given in substantial quantities or applied externally (best in the form of an ointment of the *Biniodide of Mercury*).

But *Iodine* will not succeed in every case of Goitre ; and Homœopathy has other remedies upon which to fall back. I refer to **Spongia** and **Calcarea**. Of the former also I have spoken in my 'Pharmacodynamics.' Dr. Jousset habitually use it alternately with *Iodine*, month by month about ; commonly employing the 6th dilution of each. It, too, given in substance, and applied locally, can melt down an old and hard Tumour, as may be seen from one of the cases reported by Dr. Barlow in the Twenty-Sixth Volume of the BRITISH JOURNAL OF HOMŒOPATHY (p. 670). In another of these, indeed, the Tumour is described as ' lumpy, irregular, hard," and was of three years' standing ; but *Spongia*, in the *3*rd and *12*th dilutions, cured it in ten weeks. Dr. Midgley Cash reports a case where *Iodine*, locally and internally, seemed rather to irritate, but *Spongia* 3 cured in two weeks. *
For the action of *Calcarea* in Goitre I would refer you to the valuable 'History of Calcareous Preparations, by Dr. Imbert Gourbeyre, translated from L'ART MEDICAL in the Thirty-Fourth Volume of the BRITISH JOURNAL. It had a great reputation of old in the form of powdered egg-shells ; and it is the belief of many observers that Endemic Goitre and Cretinism are traceable to the use of drinking-water containing Lime in excess. Here, of course, you would not give *Calcarea* ; but in cases otherwise originating it may prove a useful adjunct to our remedial means.

A new and enhanced interest in Thyroid Disease has been awakened during the last decade. Gull and Ord have described, under the name of "MYXŒDEMA," a previously unrecognized form of disease in which a mucous exudation invades the body, causing a Pseudo Anasarca of the surface, clogging the muscles and dulling the mental faculties. It was soon ascertained that in these cases the thyroid gland was greatly atrophied or completely absent ; and experiment proved that a similar condition could be induced in animals by ablation of the organ. Myxœdema was a Cachexia Strumipriva. Then occurred the happy thought of treating the subject of the disease by administering healthy

---

*M. H. R., xxxix., 73,

thyroids taken from animals, whether as medicine or as food. This was done with brilliant success. The large doses, however, in which the glandular substance was at first administered were found to produce evils of their own, and the morbid state induced was essentially that present in Grave's (or Basedow's) disease, where — as its present name "Exophthalmic Goitre" indicates—the thyroid is enlarged and presumably over-active.

I must not follow up the bye-paths, Physiological and Pharmacological, into which these facts invite us, but must confine myself to their Therapeutic bearing. For—

MYXŒDEMA we probably have no remedy which can take the place of thyroid feeding as a rapid restorative of healthy function. It acts like Lemon-juice in Scurvy and *Iron* in Anæmia. Nevertheless it is a continuous palliative rather than a curative agent; and our aim should be to awaken the dormant activity of the patient's own thyroid, and not leave him for the rest of his life dependent on that of animals. That this can sometimes be done, Dr. Clarke has shown us by his case recovering under *Arsenicum*; * and where any such deep-acting medicine is indicated by the symptoms, as this was here, we may surely prescribe it with advantage. In connexion with this I may recall Dr. Guggenbuhl's experience with Cretinism—a morbid state closely allied to Myxœdema, and like that connected with obstruction or atrophy of the thyroid gland. When to the Hygienic advantages he at first afforded the subjects of this disease he added Homœopathic medicine, he found a perceptible acceleration of their improvement. ☥
I am not sure, moreover, that the last word has been spoken about thyroid medication as distinct from alimentation. A series of experiments were made on eight subjects of mental disease, each taking from one to three five-grain doses daily of the fresh gland. The experimenter observed emaciation, Tachycardia, cardiac weakness and mental or motor excitement in all; but two presented also a generalised infiltration analogous to Myxœdema. Conversely, Dr. Mersch had a course where the symptoms of Exophthalmic Goitre were accompanied with Myxœdema of the lower extremities. Lower triturations of *Thyroidin* aggravated the cardiac and nervous symptoms; but when higher dilutions were given, not only did the Tachycardia subside, but the Myxœdema disappeared also. ⚵

EXOPHTHALMIC GOITRE, with its associated Palpitation of the heart and protrusion of the eyeballs, is a very interesting

---

* H. W., 1892, p. 443.   ☥ See B. J. H. xii., 696.
⚵ Journal Belge d' Homœopathie, March—April, 1898.

disease. In the Thirty-Third Volume of the BRITISH JOURNAL OF HOMŒOPATHY you will find three typical cases of it related by Dr. Wheeler at a meeting of the BRITISH HOMŒOPATHIC SOCIETY, with the discussion which followed. His treatment in all three involved the continued use of substantial doses of *Iron,* much Anæmia being present; as it was also in the case reported by Dr. Ker in the Twenty-Sixth Volume of the same Journal and here too **Ferrum** was the main remedy. Dr. Wheeler also gained much benefit from remedies calculated to quiet the excited cardiac action, especially **Cactus.** I ventured to say however, that I thought we should look deeper for a single remedy controlling the whole series of morbid changes involved in the malady; and that we might find this in **Belladonna.** Dr. Kidd long ago put on record, a cure effected by this medicine, * and you will see several others mentioned in the discussion which took place at the Society. Dr. Jousset also writes —*"Belladonna* is the remedy for Exophthalmic Goitre." He gives the dilutions from the 6th to the 30th. Its use is being adopted to some extent in the old school at present, as Dr. Ringer tells us. I would also direct attention to the Homœopathicity of *Glonoin* and of *Amyl nitrite* to the cardiac and vascular elements of the disorder. Dr. Edward Blake has communicated to the PRACTITIONER a case in which the subjective symptoms were markedly relieved by minute doses of the latter medicine.

Dr. Lilienthal has made this malady the subject of another of his useful studies of the disease. ✢ He does not seem aware of the observations I have mentioned above; but gives some facts suggesting *Natrum muriaticum* and *Lycopus* as possible remedies. I have myself called attention to the Homœopathicity of *Iodine* to this form also of Goitre; and I notice that Jousset mentions emaciation and Bulimia as occasional elements in the cachexia accompanying it. The higher dilutions of the drug ought to be most serviceable here.

Later experience with this disease has mainly affirmed the recommendations now given —*Belladonna, Iodine* and *Lycopus* being the remedies most frequently used, the two former in the medium dilutions, the latter in the lowest or the mother-tincture. ↓ *Thyroidin* itself (the extract of sheep's thyroid) has been sometimes used with success. The remedy would be one of the isopathic order; but if the dosage be small enough should not on that account be put out of court.

---

* B. J. H., xxv., 187.   ✢ N. A. J. H., xxv., 380.
↓ J. B. H. S., i., 91; iv., 347; vi., 305, 308, 399; vii., 222.

LECTURE XLIV

DISEASES OF THE URINARY ORGANS.

―――o―――

THE KIDNEYS.

―――o―――

BRIGHT'S DISEASE—NEPHRITIS ALBUMINOSA—GRANULAR DEGENERATION—AMYLOID DEGENERATION—FATTY DEGENERATION—ALBUMINURIA.

In the present Lecture I enter upon the DISEASES of the URINARY ORGANS. The affections of the KIDNEYS will first engage our attention ; and of these we shall begin with those morbid renal conditions with which Albuminuria is associated, and which are known under the general name of —

BRIGHT'S DISEASE—Before proceeding to Therapeutics, however, we must agree upon certain points as regards Pathology and Nosology. I was for some time accustomed to use the nomenclature of renal diseases which I learnt from Dr. George Johnson. Now so far as this recognizes the existence of (besides fatty and amyloid change) two distinct forms of Bright's Kidney —the large, white and smooth, and the small, hard and granular, each being of primary and independent origin, and having its own etiology and clinical history,—so far, I say, it is entirely substantiated by all later investigations. The then German doctrine that these two varieties of the disease were but succesive stages of the same process is now rarely held ; it has been rejected by one of the latest and best writers on the subject from that country—Dr. Bartels, in Ziemssen's 'Cyclopædia'. But Dr. Johnson used to call the first of the two maladies a "Chronic Nondesquamative Nephritis," stating that in it the epithelial cells are not found detached after death, nor do they appear in the urine during life ; and that, in fact, the enlargement of the gland consists of a real hypertrophy of its secreting structure. He considered that the disease only occasionally appeared in an acute form, of which, in his book on the subject,* he gives three instances. He does not connect it with the Acute Nephritis of Scarlatina or from cold. The hard contracted kidney he considered the result of a "Chronic Desquamative Nephritis," thinking that the diminution of the size of the organ was produced by the shedding of its epithelial cells.

―――――――――――――――――――――――――――――――

*On Diseases of the Kidney, 1852.

Dr. Dickinson, on the other hand, may be taken as the representative of the present views on the subject when he maintains * that the large white kidney of Bright's Disease is simply the chronic form of the "Acute Desquamative Nephritis" which both authors recognize as the result of cold and of Scarlatina. In the contracted kidney, he considers that the mischief begins in the fibrous matrix, and that the whole process is identical with that which obtains in Cirrhosis of the Liver. He would call the one, accordingly, a "Tubal," the other an "Interstitial" Nephritis. I can have no hesitation in assenting to these doctrines. Dr. Johnson's "Non-desquamative Nephritis" thus dropped out of my Nosology. His acute cases so described, I can without difficulty refer to the category of Renal Congestion, while his chronic ones are mostly, I think, examples of amyloid disease,—when he wrote little understood. And, again, his reference of Granular Degeneration to a Desquamative Nephritis may arise from the fact that the large white kidney (where this process does obtain) may, if its subjects live long enough, undergo what Dr. Bartels aptly calls "Secondary contraction."

Of our Homœopathic writers Jousset is very clear as to the specific distinctness of the two chronic varieties of Bright's Disease (both of which he classes among his "Cachexies"), but hardly as much so in connecting with the former the Acute Nephritis resulting from Scarlatina or from cold. Bahr follows the old German view, and has no distinct idea of the contracted kidney as a clinical entity. The same misconception mars the only Monograph we have on the subject—the "Morbus Brighti" (SIC) of Bunchner, which Dr. Lilienthal has translated for us. Even otherwise I am unable to commend this Treatise, whose thought seems to me as confused as its style; but I shall endeavour to incorporate anything of therapeutical value it may contain. More satisfactory than any of these, both in Pathology and Therapeutics, is the paper "On Bright's Disease, and its Homœopathic Treatment," read by Dr. Kidd before the British Homœopathic Congress of 1855, and printed in the Thirteenth Volume of the BRITISH JOURNAL OF HOMŒOPATHY. The Article on the malady in Marcy and Hunt's 'Treatise' is also of unwonted excellance.

We will speak first, then, of—
NEPHRITIS ALBUMINOSA (which is Rayer's phrase), meaning thereby the "TUBAL NEPHRITIS" of Dickinson, and the "PARENCHYMATOUS NEPHRITIS" of Bartels. In its recent form it is the "ACUTE RENAL DROPSY" or "ACUTE DESQUAMATIVE NEPHRITIS" which results from cold, or occurs after Scarlatina, Diphtheria, Cholera, and some other acute diseases. In its chronic form it

---

*On Albuminuria, 1868.

NEPHRITIS ALBUMINOSA 619

embraces all instances (excluding those of pure Amyloid or Fatty Degeneration) in which the large white kidney is diagnosed or discovered, and among which the Albuminous Nephritis of pregnancy takes a prominent place. I shall best bring its Therapeutics before you by discussing the principal medicines which have been employed.

The drugs whose power of setting up acute hyperæmia and irritation of the kidneys is most obvious, are *Turpentine* and *Cantharides*. It is generally assumed that their action is identiçal, but I think that careful study reveals a considerable difference in the manner in which they respectively affect these organs. You will remember that in the kidneys we have a double circulation, subserving distinct purposes. The arterial blood first passes through the Malpighian tufts, where the urinary water is separated; and then through the capillaries of the cortical portion of the gland, where the epithelium of the convoluted tubes forms from it the urea and other solid constituents of the secretion. Congestion and irritation of the Malpighian tufts will thus show itself in alterations of the quantity of the urine.* and in the presence of such abnormal elements thereof as blood and albumen; while, if the secreting function of the gland be affected, the epithelium will degenerate and be cast off, and the elimination of urea be more or less impaired. Now in studying, in my 'pharmacodynamics', the renal phenomena of poisoning by *Turpentine*, I have shown (upon the data now laid down) that its main influence is extended upon the Malpighian circulation of the kidney; and I have not come since upon any evidence leading me to modify that view. **Terebinthina** is accordingly—as I have pointed out—less suitable in proportion as the Nephritis is Desquamative, and apt to lead to Uræmia, while more so as the presence of blood and albumen, and the diminution of the urinary water, are the leading phenomena. Such indications would determine its choice in any given case.† But, speaking generally, it may be said that they indicate it in Acute Nephritis from cold rather than that which follows Scarlatina, and give it the preference in the Choleraic affection of the kidneys, where the circulation seems primarily at fault, and suppression of urine constitutes the chief peril. They also make it the leading remedy in the ordinary form of the smooth Bright's kidney—the "Chronic Parenchymatous Nephritis" which sometimes remains over from an acute attack, but more commonly develops primarily under the influence of extensive suppurations, exposure to cold and wet, Malaria and such-like causes. Here Uræmia is rare; and the great evils are

---

*Generally in the direction of scantiness, and twice at least with resultant Anasarca (see Goodfellow's "Diseases of the Kidneys", p. 44 and s. 173 of Allen's Pathogenesis).

†They did so with utmost advantage in two cases treated by Dr. Wolston of Edinburgh (ANNALS, viii, 550).

the drain of albumen from the system, and the Dropsy which results from the insufficient excretion of the urinary water. The cases I have cited or referred to from Dr. Kidd, Henderson. Yeldham and Cartier of Lyons will illustrate these positions.*

Cantharis, on the other hand, while not sparing the primary circulation of the kindneys, exerts its main influence upon that which belongs to the secreting function of the glands. In Schroff's experiments with *Cantharidin*, besides blood-corpuscles, pus-globules, and blood, "a quantity of epithelium and fibrinous cylinders" was found in the urinary sediment ; and in a case related by Dr. Dickinson (OP. CIT., p. 50), the administration of twenty-five minim doses of *Tincture of Cantharides* caused pain in the loins and increased desquamation, but no Hæmaturia, and after death there was intense injection of the superficial capillaries—*i. e.*, those belonging to the secreting tubes. Moreover, while the Spanish fly has never caused the œdema characteristic of Bright's Disease, it does produce its head-symptoms—pain, delirium, convulsions and coma ; and as these usually come on some days at least after the ingestion of the poison, they are very probably secondary to the renal mischief it sets up. Accordingly, *Cantharis* is most appropriate in cases of Nephritis where desquamation is considerable, and Uræmia threatens ; and therefore, CÆTERIS PARIBUS, in most cases of Post-scarlatinal Nephritis. I have mentioned Dr. Dickinson's recognition of its similarity and Dr. Ringer's, of its usefulness here. Cornil has since corroborated the one, and Dessan the other.† It has hardly received in the Homœopathic school the attention it deserves, mainly—I think—because the bladder symptoms of *Cantharides*-poisoning are so prominent, that their absence in Nephritis is thought to counter-indicate the drug. I can not see, however, why it should not produce its specific effects upon one part of the urinary tract because another part remains healthy ; and I cordially commend it to my colleagues. It would also be suitable to the Nephritis of Diphtheria.

The only medicine which takes equal rank with *Terebinthina* and *Cantharis* in the present malady is **Arsenicum**. This poison alone produces the œdema of Chronic Bright's Disease ; and Symptomatology and Pathology concur to show that the Arsenical is a Renal Dropsy. I have studied its characters in my lecture on the drug, and have shown its high repute in similar conditions. I have only here to remark upon the occasional production of Hypertrophy of the Heart in the animals whose kidneys were affected by it. I was somewhat puzzled at this as we had been led to connect such cardiac changes exclusively with Granular Degeneration. Dr. Buchner supposes that the renal effects of *Arsenic* are secondary to those it produces in the

---

*See also three good cases of Dr. Pfander's in J. B. H. S., iv., 339
†See M. H. R., xl., 124.

heart. But the condition of the kidneys induced under such circumstances appears to be a venous congestion, resulting in induration ; and altogether different from that which appeared in the experiments to which I refer. The true explanation seems now afforded by Bartel's observation, that when secondary contraction supervenes upon a Nephritis of some standing, the heart at once begins to thicken and the arterial tension to increase. The six cats in whom Quaglio induced Albuminous Nephritis were slowly poisoned in periods of from one to ten months ; and in the four in whom the left ventricle was hypertrophied secondary contraction may well have begun.—The Nephritis of *Arsenic* is not so acute as that of *Cantharis* ; and for this very reason I find it preferable in most cases of Post-scarlatinal Nephritis. In Chronic Bright's Disease it will reinforce *Terebinthina* in many cases, * and would be preferable to it in those of Malarial origin. Its relation to inflammation of the serous membranes gives us another element in its Homœopathicity to the present malady, in which they are so apt to occur ; and indicates its employment, if not previously, at any rate when they show themselves ✝

I must now speak more briefly of some other medicines which appear related to Albuminous Nephritis.

Aconite would obviously be indicated from its general action when recent Nephritis from cold was accompanied by rapidly developed general Anasarca, forming the "Acute Renal Dropsy" of the old authors. But it appears to be actually a specific irritant of the kidneys, as in a poisoning by it the urine was found loaded with albumen and fragments of casts, which speedily disappeared as the patient recovered. ‡

Apis appears, from Therapeutic experience, to act upon the kidneys very much as *Turpentine* and *Cantharides* do, promoting a free flow of urine in congested states of the kidneys, and thus removing œdema. Its Physiological action in the sphere is unknown. It is a favourite remedy with many practitioners in Post-scarlatinal Dropsy, and in the Nephritis of Pregnancy. The presence of great œdema is the main indication for it, as in the following case reported by Dr. Wingfield :

Mrs. W. æt 40, had been ill for five years under "regular" treatment and gradually growing worse, with increasing Anasarca. When first seen the whole body was enormously, œdematous, face so much

---

*Besides the reference in my 'Pharmacodynamics,' see B. J. H., xxxiv., 702 : L. H. H. R., iv., 149 ; and J. B. H. S., i., 187 ; viii., 76. In the last case the *Iodide* was employed.

✝ Dr. Gally Blackley has communicated to the M. H. R., for February, 1894, three cases of Acute Nephritis treated in the London Homœopathic Hospital. All had *Arsenicum* 3x during the acute stage, but two of them required *Plumbum carbonicum* 3x later on. A good recovery was made in every instance.

‡ See UNITED STATES MED. INVESTIGATOR, 1875 ; Vol ii. ; p. 414

swollen that features could not be recognised, abdomen greatly distended with fluid, and legs twice their natural size. Albumen was one-half. She had been delirious on and off for five days, and was given up as hopeless by her friends. As a forlorn hope *Apis* 3_x gtt, ij every two hours was tried. The effect was immediate and astonishing ; large quantities of urine began to pass and Anasarca rapidly decreased. Improvement was steadily maintained. After some weeks *Arsenicum* 3_x was given. Patient rapidly recovered, and all symptoms disappeared, leaving only a trace of albumen in the urine. Patient has now been able to attend to ordinary household duties, and has had no relapse for three years.*

Dr. Goldsborough reports a similar case occuring in a child. This was in a discussion on the subject at the British Homœopathic Society ; and several members concurred in his asignment of a place to *Apis* in the transition from acute to chronic Bright's Disease when there is much œdema present.

Aurum muriaticum cured a severe case of Bright's Disease, with local and general Dropsy, occuring in the Leopoldstadt. Hospital ; ‡ and is recommended by Leidbeck and Buchner. It should be useful where *Arsenicum* was indicated but had failed.

Chelidonium has caused very striking symptoms of Desquamative Nephritis. Besides the general phenomena of renal irritation, examination of the urine in one case showed the presence of cylindrical casts with epithelial cells. The mischief in this case was so considerable that œdematous swelling of the extremities occurred. The relation of *Chelidonium* to Pneumonia here becomes important, because of the frequent occurrence of this inflammation as a complication of Tubal Nephritis in children. Dr. Buchmann gives one case of cure of chronic renal disease by this medicine ; but it was treated at a a distance, and too imperfectly described for identification.

Helleborus niger has much reputation among us as a remedy for Post-scarlatinal Dropsy, and is evidently an irritant to the kidneys. We know not, however, whether its action extends further than this.

Hepar sulphuris is much recommended by Kafka for the same affection, on the Pathological ground of its being a Croupous Nephritis. This, however, I take leave to doubt. The so-called fibrinous casts which appear in the urine are, I believe, simply coagulated albumen ; they vary in number directly with its amount.

Mercurius corrosivus sets up, as by poison, decided Albuminous Nephritis ; and ever since Ludlam first recommended it has been our main-stay in this condition when occuring in Pregnancy.

The case of poisoning by **Phosphorus** which I have related in my lectures indicates its power of causing a decided Nephritis ; and Sorge states that in his experiments "the urine several

---

*M. H. R., xxxix., 17. †J. B. H. S., viii., 109, ‡B. J. H., xvi., 500

times contained a number of epithelial scales and pus and mucous corpuscles, in six cases albumen, in two exudation-casts and in one blood-corpuscles". Putting this together with the profound action of the drug upon the blood and its power of causing Pneumonia, it ought to play an important part in the treatment of Bright's Disease. I agree with Bahr in thinking it specially appropriate to those cases (not Amyloid) which arise in the course of chronic suppurations.

Sabina and Scilla both cause scanty, bloody and albuminous urine and might find places in the treatment of the present malady,—the former when it occurs in pregnancy, the latter when it assumes the form of Acute Renal Dropsy. Solania also —the active principle of *Dulcamara*—produces similar effects ; and the repute of its parent plant in affections resulting from cold and wet might make it serviceable in the early stages of Chronic Albuminous Nephritis so caused.

As regards the occasional incidents of this form of Bright's Disease, I have already mentioned *Arsenicum* as most suitable for the serous inflammations, *Chelidonium* and *Phosphorus* for the Pneumonia. Of Uræmia and its effects I shall speak when I have discussed that other form of the malady to which it more especially belongs.

I have only to add that there is nothing in the specific medication I have recommended to make unsuitable or needless, such adjuvants as the milk-diet advocated by Donkin, or the diaphoretic measures so praised by Bartels. In so grave a disease as this, no aid is to be despised. One may even go further. Dr. Searle, of Brooklyn, who has had large and special experience in Bright's Disease, has summed up the results of this in the HAHNEMANNIAN MONTHLY for February, 1894, and May, 1895. He is "confident that it can frequently be cured — always, when taken in time." He depends chiefly on *Arsenicum*, *Apis* the ("business end" of the bee in trituration) and *Mercurius corrosivus*. But he writes—"In this as well as many other chronic forms of the disease, I have derived inestimable benefit from a combination of the milk, rest and water cures. Indeed, it is amazing to see what can be accomplished by these alone, while, without them, drugs may be set aside as of little use in Chronic Bright's Disease."

Of the other leading form of Bright's Disease I will speak under the name of—

GRANULAR DEGENERATION OF THE KIDNEYS.—This is the genuine primary contracting kidney, the "Chronic Desquamative Nephritis" of Johnson, the "Renal Cirrhosis" of Dickinson and Grainger Stewart, the "Nephrite Interstitielle" of the French Pathologists. It is a very serious matter; and Homœopathy, like traditional medicine, has to acknowledge that its ordinary termination is death. I have always pointed out that our most hopeful outlook is in the direction of Plumbum. The complete Homœopathicity of the drug to the disease, I have fully argued in the 'Pharmacodynamics'; and it corresponds, not only to the renal lesion, but to such coincident features of the malady at the arterial changes, the Amaurosis, the tendency to hæmorrhage, the Cachexia and depression of spirits. I have not however, any more favourable experience to add to that recorded in my former work; and Jousset has to confess his disappointment with it. Dr. Samuel Jones communicated an interesting case of the kind to the Twelfth Volume of the American Homœopathic Observer. The tabular view of the weekly analysis of the urine given by him shows well the progressive diminution of albumen and increase of urea under the influence of the medicine which was given in the 30th trituration. The patient (who was 52 years of age) "exchanged his pasty yellow look for the ruddy hue of health," and regained his ordinary health and vigour. But the improvement was not permanent. The patient passed into the hands of another physician, and died in about a year.*
Dr. Searle thinks he has seen good results from *Mercurius corrosivus*; Bartholow and Hale commend *Aurum muriaticum*; and Dr. Pritchard speaks highly of *Ferrum muriaticum*, in the ordinary tincture, of which he gives 1-5 drops three times a day. "It causes," he writes, "the specific gravity to creep up, the digestion to become better, the pale cheeks to take on colour, the albumen to become less and less, the casts to grow fewer and finally to disappear, until only a few epithelial masses are observed."

While, however, we should give our patients the advantage of the continued use of one of these medicines—which, if beneficial at all, must be radically so—we shall probably help them best by endeavouring to meet the complications of the disease. Of these perhaps the most annoying and injurious is the Dyspepsia with its accompanying vomiting. Dr. Jousset speaks warmly of the value of Nux vomica here;—we have seen under its influence," he writes, the digestion re-established, the vomiting checked, the thirst and Polyuria diminished, the powers returning." He gives the dilutions from the 12th

---

* See J. B. H. S., iii., 112; but also Vol., i., p. 90, where several cures are spoken of.

to the 30th. Dr. Kidd speaks hardly less warmly of **Nitric acid**, in more substantial doses. Perhaps, as much of the stomach disturbance arises from the excretion of urea by the gastric mucous membrane, and as this is speedily converted there into *Carbonate of Ammonia*, the *acid* may have a Chemical action, The cardiac hypertrophy does not ordinarily call for treatment, as it is a compensatory change ; but if it caused trouble through over-action of the heart *Cactus* would be suitable here as elsewhere. The serous inflammations which are apt to occur should be treated as those of Nephritis Albuminosa : for the Bronchitis which is so prevalent in this form of Bright's Disease I should suggest **Kali iodatum**. Of the Amaurosis, I have spoken under the head of Albuminuric Retinitis among the diseases of the eyes.

I have only to add a few words as to the treatment of uræmic symptoms, which manifest themselves with especial frequency in this variety of the malady. Pathology has not yet made up its mind as to the rationale of these phenomena, as may be seen from the balanced conclusion at which Bartels has to arrive after his exhaustive examination of the subject. The views of those who believe the Coma and Convulsions to arise from œdema of the brain are supported by the rapid results which often follow pure Homœopathic medication. Dr. Drury declares *Opium* to be often of striking efficacy ; and Dr. Marcy has seen excellent effect from *Cannabis Indica*. Still more general testimony is borne to **Cuprum**. Dr. Kidd has found the *Acetate* useful in relieving the Cramps of the later stage of the disease ; but Drs. George Schmid and Buchner commend it in Uræmic Eclampsia and Coma. Dr. Goodno prefers it in the form of the *Arsenite*, which he gives in the 2x and 3x trituration. Even when renal disease is advanced, he says and without accessory measures, it is capable of clearing away the Coma, provided Convulsions are present ; and it exerts a favourable action on the subsequent course of the Nephritis.* I would also suggest **Carbolic acid** as strikingly Homœopathic to Uræmic Coma. But, nevertheless, the evidence in favour of the ultimate dependence of such symptoms upon blood contamination of some sort is so strong, that I should advise you not to content yourself with internal medication, but to promote Diaphoresis to the utmost extent in your power : at by hypodermic injection of about gr. $\frac{1}{8}$th of *Pilocarpine*.

---

* North Amer. Journ. Of Pom., June 1896.

626 DISEASES OF THE URINARY ORGANS

AMYLOID DEGENERATION of the kidneys—of old styled WAXY or LARDACEOUS, and by Dr. Dickinson (upon the hypothesis of its etiology) named "DEPURATIVE INFILTRATION"—appears to be in nearly if not quite in all cases the result of chronic ulceration and suppurations. TOLLERE CAUSAM, therefore, whenever practicable, ought to be our chief indication for treatment. But, in seeking for a Homœopathic remedy appropriate for it (we have no experience of the kind on record), I have come upon **Phosphoric acid** as promising most. This remedy has well-known virtues in the hectic of the suppuration from Phthisical lungs and Carious bones; it might also remedy the more remote consequece now before us. Its close relative, *Nitric acid*, has cured the same Degeneration in the liver, and *Phosphoric acid* has an affinity almost equal for the kidney, as we shall see further on. Dr. Dickinson also noted the constant diminution of *Phosphoric acid* in the urine in this disease.

The pulmonary complications of Amyloid Degeneration probably call for the same treatment as those of Tubal Nephritis. The œdema and Diarrhœa ought not to divert our attention from the main current of the treatment; and indeed no more suitable remedy for the latter could be given than the *Acid* I have suggested.

FATTY DEGENERATION is a not uncommon accompaniment of the last-named and indeed of every form of albuminuric disease. Correspondingly, it has been caused and may be cured by **Arsenicum**. But whenever it presents itself, as in the cases described by Dr. George Johnson, as an idiopathic and substantive affection, I would direct your attention to **Phosphorus**. You already know the relation of this medicine to fatty change as such; and I have just called your attention to its specific affinity for the kidneys. In this connexion it is interesting to note that in one of Dr. Johnson's cases the affection (which came on in three weeks' time) appeared to be the immediate result of sexual excess. Moreover, Fatty Degeneration of the kidneys has been observed in connexion with Acute Yellow

Atrophy of the Liver ; and the power that *Phosphorus* has of setting up this morbid state is familiar to you.

Before leaving the subject of the albuminuric diseases of the kidneys, I must say a few word upon.
ALBUMINURIA itself.
That this condition may exist prior to, or even independently of renal disease is unquestionable. You cannot read a better defence of this position than Dr. Meyhoffer's Papers in the MONTHLY HOMŒOPATHIC REVIEW for 1866-7. Claude Bernhards, experiment, by which irritation of the nervous centres induced Albuminuria as well as Glycosuria, suggests the frequent neurotic origin of such cases. Phosphoric acid and Helonias will then claim your attention. One of Dr. Meyhoffer's cases, and another in Hempel SUB VOCE, well illustrate the action of the former ; of that of the latter you will find evidence in the Article on it in Dr. Hale's 'New Remedies'. When, as sometimes happens, a drain of albumen continues after all other symptoms of Nephritis have subsided, *Plumbum* is curiously effective. I have mentioned Lewald's results of this kind in my 'Pharmacodynamics.' Dr. Edward Blake relates * a case of Post-diptheritic Albuminuria, in which the 6th trituration of the *Carbonate* was the curative remedy. He mentions, also, an observation of Dr. Galley Blackley's, in which, while the inmates of a house showed various symptoms of Saturnism from drinking water impregnated with Lead, one of them, the subject of Post-scarlatinal Albuminuria, lost his complaint and steadily improved in health.

---

* M. H. R., xxxiv., 348.

LECTURE XLV

DISEASES OF THE URINARY ORGANS
(concluded)
—o—

THE KIDNEYS (contd.)
—o—

DIABETES MELLITUS—DIABETES INSIPIDUS—CHYLURIA
—AZOTURIA—GRAVEL.

In my last Lecture I spoke of those morbid conditions of the kidneys with which Albuminuria was associated. I shall occupy the present one with those maladies which, though apparently renal, in most if not in all instances lie further back than the organs through which they manifest themselves to our observation. These are DIABETES (in its two forms), CHYLURIA, AZOTURIA and GRAVEL. We will speak first of—

DIABETES MELLITUS.—I do not enter here into the dietetic treatment of this disease. It must always be of high importance. But it is not, in the nature of the case, and by the confession of its advocates, curative. Sometimes indeed under its use Nature, relieved of much of her burden, asserts her recuperative power; and when the patient returns to his usual diet, he finds it unattended by its pristine consequence. But too often the Diabetic regimen proves but a continuous and most irksome palliative; the least abatement of its rigid restrictions is followed by an increase of the malady; and the patient at length succumbs under pulmonary disease, Carbuncle, or simple exhaustion of the powers of life. Until we can do more than cut off the supplies, until we can attack the morbid process itself, we cannot consider ourselves in a position to cure Diabetes.

In a paper on this disease in the Volume of the BRITISH JOURNAL OF HOMŒOPATHY for 1866, I endeavoured to estimate our resources for effecting this end. I found traditional medicine giving us nothing but *Opium* and *Kreosote*, and not attaching more than palliative virtue to the first and very uncertain powers to the second. I should have added the Alkaline waters of Vichy and Karlsbad, which—TAKEN AT THEIR SOURCES—have long enjoyed no mean repute. From Senator's Treatise on the malady,' in Zeimssen's 'Cyclopædia' and Silver's in Quain's 'Dictionary, I find that no addition has been since made to its Drug-therapeutics; and that the prognosis is considered less unfavourable only when a suitable diet can be borne and has a decided effect upon the quantity of sugar eliminated in the urine. We have, accordingly, now as then to look to Homœopathy for anything like curative resources in the treatment of the malady.

In the literature of the new system we found on the one hand report of decided benefit in the Diabetic cases from general and symptomatic treatment ; and on the other certain complete or proximate cures with medicines presumbly Homœopathic to the essential lesion. Of these I would fix your attention here on *Phosphoric acid* and the *Salts of Uranium*.

Acidum phosphoricum stood at that time unquestionably in the highest place among the remedies for Diabetes. The first notice of it I can find, is contained in the Sixteenth Volume of the BRITISH JOURNAL OF HOMŒOPATHY. Three very interesting cases are there recorded by Dr. Walker of Manchester, of which the following is a summary. The first is briefly told. Sugar was present in the urine, with the usual symptoms ; improvement ensued and the disease was for some time kept at bay by *Phosphoric acid* and the saccharated (!) *Carbonate of Iron* (dose not stated) ; but the patient eventually sank under pulmonary disease. Case 2 was equally marked. Its subject was put upon rigid diet, and took three times a day a dessert-spoonful of a solution of 14 grains of anhydrous *Phosphoric acid* in six ounces of water. The sugar and the general symptoms soon disappeared ; and when, six months after, the patient returned to his usual diet, he felt no ill-effects : he was cured. In case 3, the *Phosphoric acid* was given in the same manner, but the diet was unrestricted. The specific gravity of the urine fell in eight days of this treatment from $1035°$ to $1023°$. The ultimate issue of the case is not recorded. In the Ninteenth Volume of the same Journal, Dr. Ransford contributes two cases in which *Phosphoric acid* was the main remedy.—in the first in the 6th dilution, in the second in grain doses of the anhydrous *Acid*. The usual restrictions were put upon the diet. In both, the sugar disappeared from the urine, and the patient got well. Two other cases are cited in my paper in which the disease was kept at bay or nearly cured by the medicine ; and I may add to them those recorded by myself that Thirty-first Volume of the BRITISH JOURNAL (p. 369), and by Dr. Dudgeon in the Thirty-Seventh (p. 371).

As to the rationale of this unquestionable influence of *Phosphoric acid* over Diabetes, I have suggested in my Paper that it is of a Homœopathic nature,— the drug having aggravated the symptoms of the disease in man and actually induced it in animals. Dr. Black, in the valuable study of Diabetes he has contributed to the Thirty-Seventh Volume of the BRITISH JOURNAL, analyses the observations I have referred to with unfavourable results, and I am quite ready to regard the questions an open one. Perhaps the frequent origin of Diabetes in nervous strain or depression is the main reason why *Phos-*

phoric acid should do it good ; and it would be when such antecedents were traceable that we should preferably resort to it. But of this I will say more when I have considered the claims of the other chief remedy we have for the malady.

This is the new and rare metal **Uranium** given in the form of one of its soluble salts (the *Nitrate* or *Muriate*). In my 'Pharmacodynamics' I have adduced, in some detail the evidence for the Homœopathicity and efficacy of this drug. The report of the Committee of British Medical Association upon "The action of Uranium salts in Glycosuria" to which I then looked forward has not yet seen the light ; and I have only to add here, the testimony borne to its value by Dr. Jousset. "This substance" he writes in the Second Edition of his MEDICINE PRACTIQUE", ' which produces an artificial Diabetes in dogs, causes in Diabetes the disappearance of the sugar without any restricted regimen. There are even a certain number of observations in which the malady has been completely cured. The practitioners who have employed the *Nitrate of Uranium* have generally given strong and increasing doses of the first decimal triturations (Curie, Ozanam). However, we have one fine instance of perfect cure with the 6th dilution (Love). Eight years of experience have confirmed to any mind the favourable action of the drug in the treatment of Diabetes. It rarely produces a radical and definitive cure, but nearly always effects a considerable amelioration in the general condition of the partient. The principal indication for it is excessive thirst."

As regards the distinctive indication for the two remedies now named, I feel more and more convinced that the main one is that which I have laid down when lecturing on *Uranium*, that "it is best-suited to cases originating in Dyspepsia or assimilative derangement, while *Phosphoric acid* excels it where the starting-point of the disease was in the nervous system." I am glad to see that Senator recognises these as the two leading forms of the malady ; we have, he says, "a Diabetes proceeding primarily from the nervous system (neurogenic), and a Diabetes proceeding primarily from the intestinal canal or the liver (gastro-enterogenic and hepatogenic)." I was myself led to perceive the existence of these two forms from the action of the drugs which cause and cure them. I am inclined to think that Diabetes is most frequently "neurogenic", and that thus *Phosphoric acid* is more often required in its treatment than *Uranium*. E. G., in the last three cases I have had to treat, the disorder could be traced, in the first, to anxiety connected with failure in business in the second to Hemiplegia, in the third to a long-continued and depressing illness (which had not, however, involved the digestive organs).

This was the state of our knowledge up to 1881. From 1888, however, experimentation on animals with *Uranium salts* was instituted by fresh hands and abundant confirmation as to its power of causing Glycosuria was supplied. In that year, Chittenden tested the drug on rabbits, confirming Blake's results as regards Albuminuria, and showing this to depend upon a Parenchymatous Nephritis ; but adding Glycosuria, which appeared in seven out of the nine animals experimented on. Woroseilski, in 1889, in his trials used mainly a *Tartrate* of *Uranium* and *Sodium* ; and had similar results, including the ulcerations observed by Blake. In 1891, our own Dr. Cartier published his "Glycosuries Toxiques." In his chapter on *Uranium*, he summarises and discusses all foregoing experimentations, and adds further work done by himself on one dog and ten rabbits. Glycosuria, Albuminuria, Phosphaturia, diminution of salts and urea, Oxaluria, Acetonuria—these are the phenomena noted by him as occuring in the urinary sphere. He discusses the rationale of the first ; rejects the hypothesis that the action of the drug on the liver (though undoubted) will account for it ; thinks that of sub-oxidation, impairing the combustion of sugar, insufficient to do so ; and concludes that the drug acts by increasing sugar-formation through the nervous centres.

In 1895, Dr. Samuel West brought before the meeting of the British Medical Association three cases which, he maintained "pointed to the conclusion that we possess in *Uranium*, a drug which has a powerful effect upon Diabetes." Much comment ensued in our journals and in the November number of the MONTHLY HOMŒOPATHIC REVIEW for that year, I published a chronological history of the use of the metal in medicine, —showing that its application to Diabetes was both an obvious inference from the rule SIMILIA SIMILIBUS and one actually made with considerable success for a length of time. The difficulty Dr. West expressed with regard to the dosage seemingly required and actually followed in his cases was seen to disappear on a wider survey of the facts. Very much smaller, even infinitesimal, quantities had often sufficed to produce as good results. I summed up by saying ; "What shall be the exact place of *Uranium* in the treatment of Diabetes, to what forms and varieties will it prove specific, are as yet open questions. As far as we can see at present, it corresponds to the definite symptom—Glycosuria, and thus to all the other symptoms due to the drain of sugar by the kidneys. But Diabetes may be—perhaps we may already say is—a larger thing than mere Glycosuria, just as Bright's Disease is more than Albuminuria ; and forms of it may occur in which the general symptoms are more important, as guides to the selection of the remedy than the changes in the urine. The unquestionable efficacy of *Phosphoric acid* and *Syzygium jambolanum* in its treatment points in this direction ; for with the former there is very slight, with the latter there is no evidence of any power of inducing a Glycosuric condition. We must wait and watch.

and perhaps ere long we shall be able so to differentiate between our Anti-diabetics as we are between our Anti-pneumonics and our Anti-choleraics, that success with them may yet be further enhanced."

We have made no nearer approach to such goal since I wrote ; and the only further experience with *Uranium* appearing in old-school literature has been that of Dr. C. H. Bond in 1896. Reading a paper on "The Relation of Diabetes and Glycosuria to Insanity," before the Medico-Psychological Association, he mentioned that in all the cases in which this complication was observed, by the administration of *Uranium nitrate*, the excretion of sugar in the urine could be entirely stopped. In our own school, perhaps more interest has been aroused in the drug I have just mentioned—the **Syzygium jumbolanum**. This Indian plant is in some native repute ; and Dr. Dudgeon, reading of this, was led to obtain the seeds from that country, and prepare a tincture from them. His experience with it is narrated in the Third Volume of the LONDON HOMŒOPATHIC HOSPITAL REPORTS. In some cases it was without effect ; but in two ladies it so reduced the amount of sugar as to eliminate the Pruritus which is one of its most distressing effects, and in a gentleman of 56 it completely removed the disease. Dr. Dudgeon refers to some favourable experience with the drug in the ordinary medical journals. In our own, Dr. C. H. Viche reports a cure. He appears to have given the tincture, in 8 to 10 drop doses ; but Dr. Moffat found that in such quantity the drug caused much intestinal irritation. He thenceforward attenuated it gradually, and now reports the 12th dilution as giving the best results.*

An interesting experience is that of Dr. Stiegele. He found that *Syzygium* diminished the quantity of sugar in the urine, but had no effect on the general health, whilst *Arsenicum* improved the general health without diminishing the quantity of sugar. He therefore combined *Arsenicum* 6 with *Syzygium* 3x as a double medicine and gave it in six cases without change of diet except deprivation of sweets, with curative results, complete or closely approximate, in every instance. This brings us to **Arsenicum** as an Anti-diabetic. It is obviously indicated when cachexia is present, especially when the alimentary mucous membrane is red and irritable. But it has yet more cogent claims on our notice here. † Yeldham, Grauvogl, Crepel and Dodge each report a cure from it :—Crepel giving it alternately with *Uranium nitricum* and Dodge with *Terebinthina* ‡ Elb relates two cases in which it proved curative single-handed : in one he gave the 30th, in the other the 3x. ↓ To complete the

---

* J. B. H. S., iii., 21i, 330 ; xii., 356.
† See, for old-school experience, IND. MED. RECORD, Aug., 14, 1901.
J. B. H. S., iii., 214, 333, ↓ IBID., ix., 98, 181

evidence of its suitableness to Diabetes, we have a case of Dr. Edward Blake's observation, in which all the classic symptoms of the disease supervened on a long-continued medical use of *Arsenic*, and cleared away rapidly on its suspension.*

But for Dr. Moffat's experience, we might unhesitatingly follow the absence of pathogenetic evidence, and set down *Syzygium* as Antipathic to Glycosuria — reducing it by exerting a Physiological action only. In the case of another substance we have evidence for an opposite conclusion. *Phloridzin*, a glucoside obtained from the bark of several fruit-trees, has a unique power of inducing saccharine urine, more constant than that of *Uranium*, and obtaining in the absence of sugar-forming food, and when the liver is deprived of Glycogen or even extirpated. Our late colleague Dr. Gibbs Blake gave an account of this substance in the Fortieth Volume of the MONTHLY HOMŒOPATHIC REBVIEW; and spoke of having obtained Therapeutic results with it which in some cases were very satisfactory. Another of our practitioners, Dr. Platt, has argued that there is an essentially renal Glycosuria, and that it is this which *Phloridzin* causes; † and Dr. Paillon, adopting the same view, relates three cases treated by the drug, in two of which it showed decided curative action.

In Dr. Paillon's third case, *Phloridzin* failed to influence the malady, and improvement only set in when pancreatic extract was given in its place. This bit of "Opo-therapy" is warranted by the reasoning and experience of Dr. Jousset, PERE ET FILS; the former advocating the origin of the disease in pancreatic inaction rather than hepatic over-action, and both relating cases of cure. ‡ It is especially when the patient is thin that the pancreatic preparations prove effective. They might be reinforced by a medicine like Iris, which in two recorded cases showed considerable Anti-diabetic power. † Also, where the patients are not emaciated, it is possible that the liver is the starting-point of the morbid process; and looking for a suitable medicine in such cases, we should remember that Dr. Sharp has published two cases in which *Chamomilla*, in the first dilution, proved effective, without any great restriction of diet. ‖

Again, we sometimes meet with Diabetes pursuing an extremely rapid course, and threatening life in a few weeks or less (D. ACUTUS and ACUTISSIMUS). Here, I think, we should invoke the aid of those neurotic medicines which experiment on animals has shown to be capable of causing Glycosuria. I speak especially of **Morphia** and **Curare** — our authority for whose properties of this kind is Claude Bernard himself. ✢ I made

---

* M. H. R., xxxiii., 410. † HAHN, MONTHLY, Jan., 1897
‡ L'ART MEDICAL, June and Dec. 1895.
† J.B.H.S., vi., 396; ix., 181. ‖ Essays on Medicine p. 791.
✢ LONDON MEDICAL RECORD, i., 725.

this suggestion in 1878. I do not know whether it has been acted on after this specific manner; but Dr. Burkhard, of Berlin, has lately advocated the use of *Curare* in Diabetes generally. He relates three cases in which sugar disappeared from the urine under the administration of the 4x trituration. In one of these no alteration whatever was made in the diet. *

What, finally, are we to do in those sudden cerebral intoxications which sometimes present themselves in the course of Diabetes, analogous to the Uræmia of Bright's Disease, and—from the poison with which the blood is supposed to be charged—called (provisionally) Acetonæmia ? I should hardly think that any dynamic remedy is likely to avail us here, and that—as in Uræmia—we should do most by setting the skin to work. In addition to this, transfusion with the normal Salt solution might be tried; and I believed that some good results have been obtained from copious draughts of a solution of *Bicarbonate of Soda*.

As a remedy for—
DIABETES INSIPIDUS you will naturally seek medicines of the order "Diuretics." Of these, Scilla deserves your best attention. The first case in which I gave it was an Indian officer, who had for two years been passing an inordinate quantity of pale urine. There were no special symptoms present, but the drain seemed to keep his health and strength below par. *Phosphoric acid*, which I first gave, did no good. He then got *Scilla* 2, three drops in water twice daily. After taking this for three or four weeks, he reported that the urine had fallen to its normal quantity, and that he was feeling quite well. I have since given it in similar cases with equally good results.

Besides the ordinary Diuretics, medicines like *Argentum* and *Murex purpurea* have sometimes proved curative. The remedies for Diabetes Mellitus, *Phosphoric acid* and *Uranium*, are also applicable here: the latter is chiefly indicated when the urine is acrid. Diabetes Insipidus, however, so often depends upon

---

* J. B. H. S., v., 293.

incurable lesions of that part of the brain whose irritation can set it up that its prognosis is rarely favourable.

CHYLURIA is rarely seen in this country, being apparently indigenous to tropical and sub-tropical regions. It is natural to suppose it dependent upon some leakage from the chyle-vessels into the urinary passages, and though it is admitted that no such communication has ever been traced, it is still believed in. Of late, moreover, the presence of the parasite Filaria Sanguinis Hominum Nocturna, which had formerly been reckoned incidental to the disease, has come to be regarded as its essential cause.

If this be so, there is little hope from dynamic medication; and we must think of such parasiticides as *Thymol*. As however, there have been instances of the disease occuring in England,* there is just a possibility of its having a constipational origin, and we may think what drugs would be likely to benefit it. The most promising seems to be **Phosphoric acid.** Dr. Chapman, mentioning the value of the remedy in nutritive derangements of children associated with a milky state of the urine, suggested its use in the Chyluria of the West Indies. † If now you will read in the BRITISH MEDICAL JOURNAL for 1860, p. 772, Dr. Lionel Beale's account of the constitutional symptoms of the disease, as observed by him in several cases, you cannot fail to see the Homœopathicity of the medicine, and to be encouraged to try it. Should you have to look further, I can refer to you two cases, reported by Dr. Partridge, observed in residents at Barbadoes, ⸸ where great benefit was obtained from *Uva ursi* ; and to a statement that a Cuban physician has found *Kali bichromicum* very beneficial in the form of the disease known as "Hæmatochyluria." ‡

AZOTURIA—i. e., excess of urea in the renal secretion—has been either more frequent, or more frequently observed, of

---

* Quain's Dictionary, 2nd Ed. *Sub voce.*   † B. J. H. vii ; 391.
⸸ IBID., iv., 420.   ‡ J. B. H. S , ii., 485.

late years than formerly; but the only reference I can give you to our literature on the subject is to a Paper read by Dr. Gibbs Blake before our Congress of 1888 and the discussion which followed. Dr. Blake, having found excessive passing of urea a not uncommon cause of debility, low spirits, loss of flesh and so forth, collected the observations made as to its causation by drugs, and presented his results at the meeting. *Calcarea muriatica* and *Euonymus* were the members of the group which had served him best in practice—the former mainly in children. In the discussion, Dr. Drysdale reminded us of the increase of the solids of the urine caused by **Senna**, and which had led him to a good cure, as recorded in the Twenty-Fifth Volume of the BRITISH JOURNAL He gave four-drop doses of the tincture twice a day. I mentioned the experience I had had with the affection, leading me to trace it to one of two causes—excessive ingestion or imperfect assimilation of Nitrogenous food on the one hand, nervous exhaustion and waste on the other. In both forms Hygiene and regimen played the chief ameliorative part; but in the latter I could speak well of **Causticum** as a medicine, which I continue to do.

I have, lastly, to speak of the treatment of—

GRAVEL—It is necessary to have clear ideas about the various morbid states included under the term. I will divide them into four groups.

1. There may be actual EXCESS of *Lithic* or *Phosphoric acid* formed in the system, and eliminated by the urine. This is indeed rare, especially as regards *Phosphoric acid.* Excess of Lithic acid is of course characteristic of the Gouty diathesis; and I have already told you what we can do to modify this. The only additional question raised by this manifestation of the diathesis is that of giving Alkalies. I cannot think that we should refuse the temporary aid of these remedies (especially in the form of natural mineral waters) when we have reason to apprehend concretion; but I am quite opposed to their continued use. Excess of Phosphoric acid implies waste of nervous tissue (more rarely disease of bone, as Mollities Ossium). Its best medicine would probably be *Phosphoric acid* itself in the dynamized form.

2. There may be DEPOSIT, without excess, of Lithic acid or Lithates on the one hand, or Phosphates on the other. They arise, as you know, the one from a too Acid, the other from a too Alkaline urine. Again there can be no objection that I can see, to redressing temporarily the balance of an over-acid urine

by Chemical measures. But you will be too wise to expect its radical cure from anything but proper diet and mode of living. In this category you will consider the regulated use of Lemon-juice, of whose value Dr. Kidd has furnished so many striking illustrations.* Deposit of Lithates is generally connected with some temporary derangement of health, and here requires no special treatment. Its occurrence in a permanent form, as one of a group of symptoms pointing to digestive derangement, tells of the liver being involved. I have always found it an indication for Lycopodium ; but the recent re-proving suggests Sepia, as also appropriate in such cases. If, however, the symptoms be rather Neuralgic, the presence of abundant Lithates leads me to Quinine. I give you this as a bit of experience ; but it is amply borne out by Noack's proving. Alkaline urine, when secreted so by the kidney, must depend upon a depressed state of the general especially the nervous system. Phosphoric acid is here again likely to help as a medicine ; and if you like to give it in material doses so as to obtain its Chemical as well as its dynamic effects I at least shall not quarrel with you. But I apprehend that Alkaline urine is most frequently the result of inflammation of some part of the urinary mucous tract, and requires the treatment proper thereto.

3. I suppose that the use of *Nitro-muriatic acid* in OXALURIA is one of the most satisfactory bits of the ordinary practice. What is the rationale of its action ? There is no Alkaline condition here to be chemically neutralised : indeed, the appliances of the Oxalic are rather with the Lithic than the Phosphatic diathesis, as Dr. Bence Jones has demonstrated. I suspect that the *Nitro-muriatic acid* is a TERTIUM QUID different both from the *Nitric* and the *Muriatic* ; and that its action is specific and dynamic, i.e., Homœopathic. When I wrote this in my 'Therapeutics', I could only suspect ; but now I can maintain. When the Homœopathic College was first established in the University of Michigan, a professor from the other side said to one of the Homœopathic students : "According to your Law, *Nitro-muriatic acid*, which is so effective in Oxaluria, ought to produce it in a healthy person." Dr. Samuel Jones, who then filled the Chair of Materia Medica in the Homœopathic College, got this student to prove the *Acid* on his own person. As a result, the presence of Oxalates in the urine was demonstrated on two occasions, to the chagrin of the challenger. Even without this evidence, I should have advised your employment of the remedy ; but I do so now with yet more confidence.

I would add that—upon the analogy of the usefulness of *Phosphoric acid* in the Phosphatic diathesis—I have given *Oxalic acid* itself, in the *12*th dilution to a case of Oxaluria, and with very satisfactory results. I am glad to have my experience

---

*B. J. H., xxi, 43.

confirmed by such good observers as Dr. Bernard Arnulphy *
and Dr. Clifford Mitchell. † Dr. Allen states that Dr. Heermann,
of Paris, has had remarkable success from *Kali sulphuricum*,
considering it almost a specific in this condition ; and he adds
that he has himself "repeatedly verified the generalisation." ‡

4. When, in connexion with any of the causes and varieties
of Gravel, it is formed in particles of such size that their passage
from the kidney excites pain, we are in the presence of another
Therapeutic problem. It might fairly be doubted whether
Homœopathy had anything to say to such a condition (the Renal
or Nephritic Colic of the books), as the difficulty is mechanical,
and the pain inseparable from the presence of the grains or
concretions of solid matter. Certainly, if the pain demanded it,
we should be quite justified here in giving repeated small doses
of *Morphia* or inhalations of *Chloroform*. But the analogy of
the power of *Calcarea* over Biliary Colic suggests that here also
Homœopathically-acting remedies may be found : and they
seem to exist in **Berberis** and **Pareira brava**. The evidence for
the value of the former I have mentioned in my 'Pharmacodynamics' ; I can myself add to it. The latter, long in repute
for urinary troubles, has been tested in this affection by Dr.
Turrel, and found eminently serviceable, in all strengths from
the mother-tincture up to the 12th dilution. § Dr. Jousset confirms
its efficacy from his own experience.

I can since add that *Calcarea carbonica* itself has been found
effective in Nephritic as well as Hepatic Colic ; and in as high
or higher dilution. Such was the testimony borne by Dr. Sands
Mills in an Essay presented to our Paris Congress of 1900, and
substantiated by five illustrative cases, which you may read in
the Transactions or in L'ART MEDICAL for September in that
year. *Sarsa* is an analogue of *Berberis* : its pain is characteristically AFTER urination. *Ocimum canum* is a Brazilian plant
bearing a similar relation to *Pareira brava*. It was introduced
into our Materia Medica by Dr. Mure, upon clinical evidence
solely ; but more recent experience has seemed to show it effective
in the dilutions. ǁ

---

* CLINIQUE, Jan., 1887.   † HAHN. MONTHLY, May, 1898.
‡ N. A. J. H., Feb, 1895, p. 121.

§ See his Paper translated from the BIBLIOTHEQUE HOMŒOPA-
THIQUE for 1875 in the Thirty-third Volume of the BRITISH JOUR-
NAL OF HOMŒOPATHY.

ǁ See J. B. H. S., iii., 208 ; iv., 336. Also iv., 77, compared with
M. H. R., xl., 133.

LECTURE XLVI

DISEASES OF THE URINARY ORGANS.
——o——

KIDNEYS (*concld.*) BLADDER, URETHRA & THE MALE SEXUAL·ORGANS,
——o——

RENAL CONGESTION—SUPPRESSION OF URINE—HÆMATURIA—HÆMOGLOBINURIA—SUPPURATIVE NEPHRITIS—PYELITIS—CYSTITIS—IRRITABLE BLADDER—STRANGURY—PARALYSIS OF THE BLADDER—STONE IN THE BLADDER—CANCER OF THE BLADDER—TUBERCLE OF THE URINARY TRACT—STRICTURE—ORCHITIS—SARCOCELE—IRRITABLE—TESTICLE—NEURALGIA TESTIS—SATYRIASIS—IMPOTENCY—STERILITY—SPERMATORRHŒA—HYDROCELE—VARICOCELE—RETRACTION OF THE TESTICLES—SEMINAL VESICULITIS—CHRONIC ENLARGEMENT OF THE PROSTATE GLAND—PROSTATITS—CHANCROID—BALANITIS—EPITHELIOMA—INFLAMMATION OF THE SCROTUM

I have hitherto been speaking of disorders in which renal mischief is but one element, however important ; but I must now tell what we can do when the KIDNEY itself is primarily and solely affected.

RENAL CONGESTION, of ACTIVE character and RECENT occurrence, is recognized by Bartels simply as a consequence of the elimination by the kidneys of certain irritating substances, as *Turpentine* and *Cantharides*. I think, however, that it is not very uncommon effect of cold. I have met with it several times, and have always found **Terebinthina** (which I have usually given in the third decimal dilution) most effective in its treatment. Should we encounter it as caused by *Cantharis*, as by blistering, **Camphor** seems (from Dr. Reginald Southey's experience *) to be as effective as for the Strangury thus arising.

The CHRONIC and PASSIVE forms of Renal Congestion is nearly always due to the embarrassed circulation of obstructive disease of the heart · and its Therapeutics belong to those of Cardiac Dropsy.

Renal Congestion probably lies at the bottom of most cases of simple—

SUPPRESSION OF URINE ; and **Terebinthina** accordingly occupies the first place among our means of removing this perilous condition. Dr. Yeldham has reported a case cured with the first dilution, in which no urine had been passed for four days. † Suppression of Urine has been also observed in cases of poison-

---

* Ziemssen's Cyclopædia (Engl. Transl,) xv., 196 (note).
(† ANNALs, i., 386.

ing by *Mercurius corrosivus*, *Arsenic*, *Cantharis* and *Kali bichromicum*, so that we have some medicines on which to fall back, should *Turpentine* disappoint us. I have mentioned the usefulness of the last-named in the Ischuria which sometimes follows Asiatic Cholera, and threatens the patient's death if not removed.

HÆMATURIA is often another manifestation of Renal Congestion and accordingly **Terebinthina** takes the first place among its remedies, and old-school experience confirming it. I cannot say whether *Arnica* is of service when bloody urine depends, as it frequently does, upon the mechanical irritation of Renal Calculi or Gravel. Jousset says it is the remedy for such cases ; but Bahr thinks that there is lack of evidence for its efficacy. On the other hand when exposure to cold or rough whether can be ascertained, *Aconite* is of undoubted efficacy *

If Hæmaturia is a part of General Purpura, you will of course treat it on the principles laid down when we were speaking of that disease. But you will every now and then meet with cases which do not seem to come under any of the categories just mentioned, or do not yield to the remedies indicated ; and you will wish to know where you can look for further help. You may find this from *Cantharis,* which is certainly Homœopathically indicated, though it seems to require more than the usual Homœopathic dosage. † You may get it from *Arsenicum hydrogenisatum,* the hæmorrhagic action of which is so well-marked in poisoning by it. Dr. Majumdar relates two cases in which the sixth dilution was promptly curative. They were painless, but much prostration was present. ‡ Or you may dip into the bag of pure empiricism, and try the *Thlaspi bursa pastoris* —the Shepherd's Purse of popular language. This is in all probability the "Angioitico" of Mattei's list of specifics, and it is described as "easily arresting hæmorrhage in general." The *Thlaspi* had this repute of old, as may be seen from Gerarde's "Herball" of 1636 ; and its power as a hæmostatic has been vouched for in our own school by Jousset, Rafinesque and Harper, and also by several old-school (especially Rademacherian) practitioners. § This remedy, like *Cantharis*, has to be given in the mother-tincture.

The endemic Hæmaturia of Egypt, Mauritius and other semi-tropical countries seems to depend upon the presence of a parasite, the "Bilharzia Hæmatobia." Whether under these circumstances our remedies can check the loss of blood must remain a question. If they cannot, there seems no other resources, as all known parsiticides are said to have failed to do so.

---

* See J. B. H. S., ii., 91.   † See M. H. R., xiii., 629.
‡ J. B. H. S., iv., 128.
§ See BULL. DE LA SOC. MED. HOM. DE FRANCE, vi., 721 ; xiv., 160 ; M. H. R., xxxii., 614 ; xxxiv., 735 ; L'ART MEDICAL, July, 1888 ; J. B. H. S., i., 182.

HÆMOGLOBINURIA must be mentioned here, though the seat of the morbid process in it lies behind the kidneys in the blood itself. Its interest to us is enhanced by its having followed upon the introduction into the system of several poisons, among which I may name *Chlorate* and *Bichromate of Potash*, *Arseniuretted Hydrogen* and *Carbolic acid*. We should naturally expect to find among these remedial agents for the malady when occurring idiopathically. We are most likely to do this when it constitutes the "Blackwater Fever" of Malarious countries, or occurs paroxysmally. In the former case certainly, in the latter probably, the **Arsenicum hydrogcnisatum** would be the best of the group to choose; while the others remain in reserve for unusual or obstinate cases. The only case I know of in Homœopathic literature is one of the paroxysmal form furnished by Dr. Galley Blackley to the Second Volume of the LONDON HOMŒOPATHIC HOSPITAL MEDICAL REPORTS. *Chininum arsenicosum* and *Anilin* were the medicines tried; both had some effect in postponing the attacks, but neither could be said to have proved curative.

SUPPURATIVE NEPHRITIS.—The kidneys, like the liver, may be the seat not only of diffuse inflammation of the cirrhotic or liquefactive kind, but also of circumscribed inflammation tending to suppuration. Such a Nephritis is that which results from mechanical violence, or from the irritation of Renal Calculi. *Cannabis sativa* receives a good deal of commendation from the older Homœopathists (as Jahr and Hartmann) in this affection; but I must agree with Bahr in doubting whether its action reaches so far as this. I also follow him in thinking **Mercurius corrosivus** the most Homœopathic and effective medicine for the disease. In cases threatening to be CHRONIC, *Hepar sulphuris* should be considered. *

PERINEPHRITIS has no relation to the kidney proper, and must be treated with the remedies and other means suitable to suppurative inflammation of the cellular tissue. It is otherwise with—

PYELITIS, which demands a section of its own. This inflammation may also arise from injuries received from without or within. More frequently, however, it is secondary to vesical or urethral disease and often manifests its existence mainly by symptoms of distress of the bladder. Sir B. Brodie, in his Lectures on "Diseases of the Urinary Organs," has given a capital account of these cases. He believes that they often arise from "an injudicious use of large doses of *Copaiba* and *Cubebs*, especially

---

*See cases in J. B. H. S., iii., 336. It is headed "Pyelitis," but it is difficult to draw the line between these two affections, especially in the absence of microscopical examination of the urine.

the latter ; and that it is here and not in simple catarrh of the bladder, that *Uva ursi* and *Buchu* exert the influence which has given them repute in urinary disorders." He also recommends the tincture of the *Muriate of Iron*. These hints may be of service to us. I am inclined to think **Uva ursi** on the whole the most effective remedy here. If there is drain of pus from the kidney, you will of course keep your patient up by **China** ; and some Chemical influence seems exerted by the *Peroxide of Hydrogen*, which may be conveniently given in the form of Marchand's "*Glycozone*."

Of Cancer and Tubercle of the Kidney, in their therapeutical aspects, I have nothing to say ; and so we will pass on to the urinary passages, which we have already approached when speaking of Pyelitis.

Let us take first the disease of the BLADDER.

CYSTITIS, in its ACUTE form, is rarely met with. When we have to deal with it—as. in some Gonorrhœic cases—**Cantharis** is confessedly its great remedy ; * and it should not (I think) be given lower than the third dilution. Bahr has seen immediate aggravation from the third decimal trituration. If there be much general erethism or fever, *Aconite* may be given ; but not otherwise. There is a SUB-ACUTE form of Catarrh of the Bladder which is apt to result from local damp and cold, and which is very liable to become chronic : here you will find **Dulcamara** very effective. at least when the deposit is mucous rather than purulent. †

Chronic Cystitis is common enough, though generally secondary to Stricture, stone, diseased prostate, etc. You are not the less to apply to it your specific remedies, while of course you will not neglect the treatment appropriate to the primary affection, or such emptying and washing out of the bladder as may conduce to your patient's comfort. But instead of drenching him with decoctions of *Pareira*, *Buchu* or *Triticum repens* study the symptoms of his case, and give him small doses of the remedy most Homœopathic thereto. This may be *Cantharis*, *Cannabis*, *Lycopodium*, *Terebinthina*, *Copaiba*, *Mercurius* or *Pulsatilla* ; and if no definite indications for either are present, you may ring the changes upon them. Still great favourite of my own is the **Chimaphila umbellata** which I have often used with advantage. It has to be given in the lowest dilutions or the mother-tincture.

The following case so well-illustrates what may be done in these chronic cases, that I give it VERBATIM :—

---

* See J. B. H, S., iii., 442 ; iv., 224. ✢ See IBID., ii., 219.

C., æt. 80, consulted me on September 11th on account of extensive Chronic Catarrh of the Bladder, which he had had for six months. For some time previously he had suffered from difficulty of urinating, and the urine then appeared as a greasy muco-purulent fluid mixed with blood, and was discharged by drops every half-hour or oftener, with great pain in the urethra and glans penis, and much straining—which was often ineffectual. He complained also of painful evacuation of scanty, slimy faeces. The calls to pass urine tormented him also at night, until he fell asleep from exhaustion during which he passed his urine unconsciously, and woke in the morning with his bed soaked. His general health was indifferent, but his strength was fairly maintained. Examination showed Hypertrophy of the Prostate, but it was not particularly painful. I gave *Merc. sol.* 2 every three hours alternately with *Canth.* 3. On October 1st, he came again. A few days after commencing the medicine amendment commenced. He now felt quite well; he had fewer calls to pass urine—only twice in the night; he had no pain, though the bladder was only emptied slowly. No more Enuresis. The urine was nearly clear, with slight slimy sediment. Stool nearly normal; no pain in anus, urethra or glans. The prostate, though still enlarged, was not more so than is common with old men. (Gross, in ALLG. HOM, ZEITUNG, cxxxiii., 178).

IRRITABLE BLADDER, without inflammation, pain, or morbid state of the urine, is often a symptom of Gout, when **Nux vomica** is very helpful for it. It may also arise from disease elsewhere, as in the kidneys, the uterus and the rectum: and here too, though the cause must, if possible, be removed, *Nux* may do much by diminishing reflex irritability. If it seems a simple hyperæsthesia, you will generally get good results from a persevering use of **Belladonna**. I would only make one exception to this recommendation, and that is in cases where the irritability is diurnal only, I advise you here to substitute **Ferrum**. This application of the metal we owe to Dr. Cooper. His cases* are peculiarly instructive. The first was "a light-haired, pale complexioned, delicate little girl," who had been suffering for two weeks from "incontinence of urine, coming on nearly every half-hour, sometimes oftener, but only in the day-time, and invariably ceasing on her retiring to bed at night, and when lying down during the day." She had been taking much Allopathic medicine, chiefly Iron. After *Podophyllum* had been taken for three days without avail, Dr. Cooper suspecting that the Iron had caused the trouble, gave *Arsenicum* as an antidote, and in less than a week no trace remained of her distressing malady. Then the brother of the little girl, two or three months afterwards, was afflicted in a precisely similar manner; and as there was with him no antecedent history of pernicious medication, he got *Ferrum phosphoricum* 1 with speedy and complete success. The next case was of a woman, æt. 65, a teetotaller;

---

* See ANNALS v., 399.

her symptoms were aggravated after drinking Tea. The same medicine and dose cured in a few days; the trouble had lasted six months. The fourth case was after parturition, and the vesical disorder was accompanied with Metrorrhagia and a sense of bearing down and weakness in the hypogastrium. All the symptoms disappeared in a few days under the *Iron*. In these cases the *Phosphate* was given; but in a fifth, the *Acetate* acted equally well, and in the 6th dilution. In the sixth case— a man—the *Phosphate* was again successfully prescribed; it seemed to him as if any fluid he took went right through him ten minutes after. I have myself several times verified this experience. I may also mention *Petroselinum* for this trouble. Dr. Bukk Carleton reports a case of Enuresis in a child of $2\frac{1}{2}$, characterized by sudden irresistible desire to urine both day and night. The 3_x dilution cured in a week this trouble of six months' standing.*

An acute form of Irritable Bladder is described by Bahr as CYSTOSPASMUS, by Jousset as "TENESME VESICAL"; but it is generally known in England as—

STRANGURY.—By this term (of which DYSURIA is a practical equivalent) I mean frequent, difficult, and painful micturition,— a small quantity only being passed at a time. It is, I suppose, an affection of the neck of the bladder, and may be either nervous or inflammatory. When it occurs in an acute form —and I know few seizures more painful—do not care to inquire to which of these categories it belongs, but give your patient repeated dose of **Camphor**, and I promise you that you will earn his grateful thanks. † The same treatment is applicable when absorption of Cantharides from a blister is the cause of the symptoms. In cases of less urgency you will with advantage discriminate between the inflammatory and the nervous variety. In the former, you can hardly do better than give **Cantharis** itself, if your patient be of the male sex. But if the Dysuria occur, as it very often does, in a woman, I commend to you **Copaiba** and the **Eupatorium purpureum**. The cases in which I have seen the former act so well have all been women advanced in life; but I do not know that it has any special suitableness to these. In NERVOUS Dysuria you will find **Belladonna**, in the 1st dilution. a rarely-failing remedy. If you should want another, you may consider **Apis, Capsicum**. ‡ and again *Petroselinum*. ↓

PACE Sir Henry Thompson. I shall still continue to speak of— PARALYSIS OF THE BLADDER.—His term "atony" may

---

* N. A. J. H., Oct. 1896, p. 660. † See Pharmacodynamics, SUB VOICE.
‡ See a striking case in REV. HOM. FRANCAISE, Oct., 1895.
↓ J. B. H. S., viii., 80.

be preferable, but for the present the affection is best-known by the other name. It sometimes occurs idiopathically, as in a case described by Sir B. Brodie. * Here **Opium** ought to be its remedy ; and the same medicine might help the catheter to prevent accumulation of urine in Typhus. More commonly it is a result of over-distension, and **Arnica** is under such circumstances extremely helpful, in addition to the mechanical (and perhaps Electrical) aid you will of course afford. When Paralysis of the Bladder occurs in connexion with disease for injury of the spine, it might be thought that little could be done for it, But I have seen power return, and Ammoniacal urine become healthy, in a case of this kind, under the influence of drop-doses of the tincture of the *Muriate of Iron.*

There are forms of Paralysis of the fundus of the Bladder—the detrusor urinæ ; and constitute the paralytic form of RETENTION of urine. But the same condition may obtain in the sphincter, causing partial or complete INCONTINENCE—Enuresis. Of the nocturnal form of this trouble, so common in children, I shall speak when upon their special maladies. As occuring in adults you will occasionally find **Gelsemium** or **Conium** † useful for it, and still more frequently **Causticum.**

STONE IN THE BLADDER calls for our medicines only to diminish the inflammation it sets up ; and of these I have spoken under Cystitis.

CANCER OF THE BLADDER is hardly likely to be touched by anything you can do for it ; but the hæmorrhage to which it gives rise may be checked by *Hamamelis* or *Thlaspi.* There is a form of morbid growth here, however, hitherto known as "VILLOUS CANCER", but which ought—Sir Henry Thompson says—to be accounted Simple Papilloma. Here the power of *Thuja* over papillary growths generally might be brought into play, and better results still obtained than in Dr. Ord's case related in Lecture XXII. At present, however, we have no reports of its use ; but Dr. Mason, having three or four times seen multiple Papillomata of the surface disappear under the action of *Arsenic*, was led to try it in a case of Papilloma of the Bladder, revealed by the usual hæmorrhage and villous tufts. He gave *Fowler's solution* twice daily, and complete cure resulted. ‡

TUBERCLE OF THE URINARY TRACT is little known ; but I may mention a case of Dr. Hawkes, so designated on good

---

* OP. CIT. (4th Ed). p. 101. † J. B. H. S., ix, 100.
‡ M. H. R., Aug., 1899.

authority, in which entire recovery took place under *Calcarea carbonica* 6, continued for some months. *

Passing now from the bladder to the URETHRA, I have to tell you what Homœopathy can do in the treatment of—

STRICTURE—you may think that I am here presuming upon the province of Surgery ; but it is not so. Let me cite Sir B. Brodie's sketch of the usual history of these cases. "The patient voids his urine in a diminished stream. The diminution gradually increases, being sometimes attended with a slight mucous or muco-purulent discharge. By-and-by there is a complete Retention of Urine. This subsides spontaneously, or is relieved by art. After an interval, which may vary from weeks to months, or even to years, he is overtaken by another attack of Retention. During the whole of this time the stream of urine continues to become smaller ; it is flattened, or otherwise altered in shape, or divided into two. At last the urine never flows in a stream larger than a thread, nor without great effort and striving." Now there are three stages in this melancholy progress in which our medicines will render effectual help.

1. The first is in the attack of Retention, when the Stricture is narrowed by spasm, or inflammation, or both. When pure spasm is present it will generally yield with great rapidity to repeated doses of **Camphor**. When inflammation predominates or complicates, as from Gonorrhœa or irritating injections, you may depend with equal confidence upon **Aconite**. With these medicines, and the warm bath, you will seldom need the catheter ; though you must always be prepared to use it if the distension is great.

2. I think there is no doubt but that the incipient symptoms of organic Stricture of the urethra may be in many cases abolished by the administration of **Clematis**. The testimony to its value is very general, as I have shown in my 'Pharmacodynamics'. There seems no reason why coagulable lymph effused here should not be absorbed, while fresh, as it may be elsewhere.

3. When organic Stricture has become confirmed, so that mechanical dilatation is indispensable, Dr. Yeldham testifies to the great advantage of having such medicines as **Aconite** and **Cantharis** to control all inflammatory and spasmodic tendencies prior to the introduction of instruments. *Aconite*, moreover, administered after their passage has been found to prevent the sometimes perilous rigor which in susceptible persons follows the operation. *Arnica* may be preferable where there has been much mechanical difficulty. †

---

* IBID., June. 1893. † See J. B. H. S., iii., 418.

ORCHITIS

I pass on to the consideration of the maladies affecting the MALE SEXUAL ORGANS, including those of the TESTICLE, the SPERMATIC CORD, the PROSTATE GLAND, and the PENIS and SCROTUM.

Of the diseases of the TESTICLE I shall speak first of— ORCHITIS.—We are most familiar with this disease when occuring secondarily to Gonorrhœa. In these cases it seems to be the epididymis on which the sttess of the mischief falls; while in Orchitis from cold, from sexual excess, or from Mumps, the body of the gland and its investing serous membrane are the parts mainly affected. I do not think that this need cause any difference in the treatment; save that as Parenchymatous Orchitis is generally more painful than Epididymitis, especially if the tunica albuginea is involved, it would require **Hamamelis** in preference to **Pulsatilla**. These are the two great remedies for Orchitis. *Pulsatilla* has hitherto given me every satisfaction; it is the standard remedy for the affection in the Homœopathic school, and Jousset, Yeldham and Jahr express perfect confidence in it. Its reputation has recently leaked out among the ranks of traditional medicine, and numerous testimonies have been borne to its efficiency. But I cannot ignore the warm commendations given by such excellent authorities as Drs. Ludlam and Franklin to *Hamamelis*; and Jousset says that he has found it of much service in the more severe cases. Besides these locally-acting remedies, **Aconite** and **Belladonna** must be held in reserve; the former to be given if there is much fever and arterial tension, the latter (as Dr. Yeldham well says) "when there is great sensitiveness of the nervous system, and intolerance of pain, and where the pain partakes of the character of Neuralgia." I should say that, in citing this author, I am referring to the Third Edition of his excellent "Homœopathy in Venereal Diseases." Jahr, too, I quote mainly from his Treatise on the same subject, which I have mentioned when speaking of Syphilis.

I have not mentioned *Clematis* among the ordinary remedies for Orchitis though it had some repute among the older Homœopathists, and the case Dr. Ransford has communicated to the Twenty-Fifth Volume of the BRITISH JOURNAL OF HOMŒOPATHY (p. 650) shows that it can sometimes act rapidly enough. I know not, however, of any indications which should lead us to prefer it to *Pulsatilla* and *Hamamelis*. Bahr recommends it only in the sub-acute form of the malady which sometimes ensues upon Gleet. The *Mercurius* recommended by this author and others for Gonorrhœal Orchitis, I can hardly think appropriate.

SARCOCELE—This is a term including every variety of solid enlargement of the testis. When the Tumour is Carcinomatous, enchondromatous, cystic or fibro-plastic it hardly comes within the range of medicine; and any interference must be in the way of castration. SIMPLE, STRUMOUS and SYPHILITIC SARCOCELE are the varieties of the disease of whose treatment I shall speak.

1. SIMPLE SARCOCELE means CHRONIC ORCHITIS, with induration. The *Pulsatilla* and *Clematis* I have mentioned in connexion with the acute disease have occasionally proved useful here; but more important remedies are **Spongia**, **Rhododendron**, and especially **Aurum**. The first two seem to act mainly on the tunica vaginalis (of cord and gland); the last—though Dr. Yeldham advises it when neuralgic pains affect chiefly the cord, and when this is palpably enlarged—has a potent influence on the testicle itself. In Dr. Clokey's hands it cured a chronic case of Epididymitis showing an enlargement almost as hard as bone, with pains shooting up the cord. The whole trouble disappeared after six weeks of the 3_x trituration. * In another case a man had a hard enlarged testicle on the right side, painful, particularly to touch. *Clematis* 1_x aggravated. The 6_x dilution of the same drug, and *Iodine* 3_x had no effect; and castration was recommended. *Aurum metallicum*, in the 15th trituration, was now given three times daily: the testicle gradually assumed its normal size and became softer, and in six weeks the patient was discharged cured. † It is probably the most active remedy we have in Simple Sarcocele; and I have had excellent results from it.

2. STRUMOUS SARCOCELE may be either chronic Orchitis in a patient having this diathesis, or actual Tubercular deposit—the latter generally in the epididymis. In the one case **Spongia** would bid fair to be useful. In the other I should have suggested, as heretofore, that a general Anti-scrofulous treatment, medicinal and Hygienic, would probably give the best results. Dr. Wassily, however, has shown that by calling **Tuberculin** to the aid of our *Silica* and *Calcarea* we can do more, than could have otherwise been expected. †

3. Of SYPHILITIC SARCOCELE we have spoken when discussing Anti-syphilitic treatment generally. *Aurum* plays here also a prominent part, though *Mercurius biniodatus* has Yeldham's weighty commendation.

IRRITABLE TESTICLE is so often a symptom of other mischief—as Varicocele, disease of the prostate or prostatic urethra

---

* N. A. J. H., Nov., 1892.   † IBID., April, 1893 (p. 249)
† J. B. H. S., v., 396 : See also a cure with *Teucrium scorodonia* in IBID., iv., 131.

IMPOTENCY. 649

—or a result of improperly-regulated sexual functions, that TOLLERE CAUSAM must be its usual treatment. *Ignatia* might be a helpful medicine.

NEURALGIA TESTIS may be said to exist when, without or besides morbid sensibility of the gland, paroxysms of sharp pain occur in it from time to time. This, too, is frequently caused by self-abuse, so that a causal treatment might be the most effectual. When it cannot be accounted for, you will think of **Aurum**, **Hamamelis** and **Colocynth** for its relief. The first is suggested by Dr. Yeldham's experience with it in Orchitis. To the second we are led by the symptoms elicited in Dr. Burt's proving of the drug on himself.* I have myself seen it of much benefit in a case of neuralgic pain in the testicles, with heat and morbid sensibility. The action of *Colocynth* on the spermatic and ovarian nerves was developed in the Austrian provings; and, though verified principally in women, bids fair to find its application to the male sex also. † A case is related in the CLIN QUE for September, 1899, as cured by *Oxalic acid* 6_x, the indication for the remedy being that the pain returned whenever the patient thought of it.

Passing now to the FUNCTIONAL DISORDERS of the TESTES, we will speak of—

SATYRIASIS—This affection in its higher grades where it constitutes almost a form of Mania, is happily very rare. Should you meet with it, the most helpful medicines would be **Phosphorus** and **Cantharis**,—the latter if any local irritation can be discovered, the former when the derangement seems of nervous origin. In less severe cases, where the patient himself comes to consult you for the sexual excitement with which he is worried, **Picric acid** (fairly high) is the first medicine you should think of. In some cases **Nux vomica** or **Platina** might be useful,—the former in strong adults, addicted to Alcohol and Coffee, the latter in young persons of feminine constitution and temperament. Here, too, *Origanum*, is to be thought of. ‡

IMPOTENCY—In undertaking the treatment of a case of this kind, you will of course begin by ascertaining whether your patient has any discoverable disease of the testis or cord, or of the kidney; whether he is Dyspeptic, or has Oxaluria; and whether it is moral treatment rather than medical which is required. When these causes of Impotency have been eliminated

---

*See Pharmacodynamics, SUB VOCE. † See M. H. R., xii., 733. ‡ See J. B. H. S., v., 95.

there remain three others to which his trouble may be traced, and which require treatment accordingly.

1. The fault in many instances is in the nervous centres. Sometimes the sexual weakness is one element in general Paralysis especially Locomotor Ataxy. Sometimes there is a history of a blow or fall, when you think of *Arnica* or *Hypericum*. You will observe cases of this variety, moreover, in which the loss of power is not in the testicles, but in the ejaculatory, erectile, and intromittent functions. This, which is a true Paralysis, has been caused and may be cured by *Arsenic*. In some cases of conjoined sexual atony and cerebral depression **Kali bromatum** might prove useful ; and **Selenium** is to be considered.

2. Impotency may be the result of over-indulgence of the sexual function, in which event it is usually complicated with Spermatorrhœa (q. v.). Rest to the exhausted organs, and the administration of **Phosphorus** and **Phosphoric acid** according as the symptoms are erethistic or atonic, are the remedies.

3. A premature senility, or a sort of general eunuchism with or without atrophy of the testicles, may be the condition of the patient who consults you for Impotency. **Baryta carbonica** is good here ; and **Conium** is so Homœopathic that it ought to be of service. The same may be said of **Agnus castus**, which Stapf states that he has several times used with success in Importence. Perhaps **Camphur** should be added to the list.

STERILITY in the male subject—i. e., capacity for sexual intercourse but inability to procreate—so generally depends upon organic causes that it rarely comes within the reach of medicine. If it be associated with atrophy of the testicles, the medicines capable of causing this atrophy, viz., **Iodine** and **Conium**, might be tried.

SPERMATORRHŒA—We owe to Lallemand the demonstration of the frequent dependence of this trouble upon chronic inflammation of the prostatic portion of the urethra, with the seminal ducts and vesicles, and the prostate. But we are not, I think, to follow him in the treatment of such cases by the local application of *Nitrate of Silver*,—roughly Homœopathic though it be. * We shall accomplish the same end by our internal medicines, which by elective affinity seek out and influence the affected part. The chief of these are **Cantharis**

---

* A milder local treatment is advocated by Dr. Vaughan-Hughes in a paper on this disease, under the title of "The Irritable Prostate," in Vol. v. of the ANNALS. You will weigh his recommendations in unusually obstinate cases.

† ANNALS, v., 131.—Sir H. Thompson cures such cases by blistering the perineum : is he not using the specific influence of *Cantharis* in so doing ?

and Staphisagria. Dr. Kidd speaks highly of the former; † and I have myself seen great benefit result from the latter.

Excluding the comparatively rare instances in which Spermatorrhœa results from rectal irritation, which must be treated with reference to the latter region ; and from suppressed cutaneous eruptions, where *Sulphur* is required, the only other form of Spermatorrhœa we have to combat is the tonic, from masturbation or sexual excess. Hahnemann and his immediate followers, as Hartmann, consider **China** specific in this condition. It would suit the condition of morbid irritability in which it commences admirably. "The frequent and morbid excitement of the sexual organs, resulting in an involuntary emission of semen, and caused even by slight abdominal irritations, is permanently relieved by *Cinchona* :" so writes Hahnemann. Latter on **Phosphorus** and **Phosphoric acid** became our most suitable medicines, the former (as before) when irritable weakness, the latter when simple debility is present ; and, in alternate use and varying dilutions, will be found very serviceable.

This is my experience ; but other authors speak highly of **Sulpher** and **Nux Vomica**—Jousset saying that he owes a radical cure to the former, in the *12*th and *30*th dilutions. Bhar commends **Digitaline**, in the third decimal trituration, as the most effective remedy we possess against too frequent emissions. I have several times adopted this piece of practice with success. Jahr gives *Phosphoric acid 18* in the passive form of Spermatorrhœa, supplemented (if need be) by *Sulphur*, *Conium*, and *Sepia*; and *Nux vomica 30* when the condition is more erethistic, following it where required with *Phosphorus* and *Calcarea*. Dr. Olive, of Barcelona, relates a series of cases in which *Dioscorea* (from the 3rd upwards) has proved helpful after *China*; and Dr. C. W. Roberts gets good results from substantial doses of the mother-tincture of *Thuja*.*

HYDROCELE, in its common vaginal form, has not unfrequently been cured by Homœopathic remedies. "Acute Hydrocele," i, e., inflammation of the tunica vaginalis independently of the other contents of the scrotum, would probably find its best remedy in **Spongia**. But Chronic Hydrocele is rather a Serous Dropsy, **Pulsatilla**, **Rhododendron** and **Aurum** are again medicines which have done good service to the testicle ; but **Graphites** is to be added. Cases illustrative of the action of *Pulsatilla* and *Graphites* by Dr. Black may be read in the Seventh Volume of the BRITISH JOURNAL OF HOMŒOPATHY (p. 525) ; and there is a case cured by *Rhododendron* by Dr. Hastings in the Eighteenth Volume of the same Journal (p. 351). I have myself seen a Hydrocele disappear under *Aurum*.

---

* J. B. H. S., v., 210, 291

In cases which refuse to yield to this treatment, you will consider the arguments of Dr. Jousset, to which I have already directed attention, * and which go to prove that the **Iodine** injections so successful in Hydrocele cure, not by setting up inflammation, but a specific alterative influence exerted upon the serous walls of the sac. He recommends the injection of *"Eau iodee"* with a capillary trocar. I have seen the fluid become absorbed under the internal and local use of the *Iodide of Potassium*. Dr. Hempel says that in children *Calcarea* is an excellent remedy.

The disorders of the SPERMATIC CORD which come before us for treatment are Varicocele and Retraction of the Testicles.

VARICOCELE is as open to specific treatment as is varix occuring elsewhere in the body, and by the same medicines, viz., **Hamamelis** ⚥ and **Pulsatilla**, whose affinity for the testicles gives them especial power over this local variety of the complaint. You may use a suspender or apply the pressure of a truss as you please ; but I think you will find that the "radical cure", of Varicocele is better obtained by the use, internal and external, of these specifics than by any of the operative procedures now in vogue.

RETRACTION OF THE TESTICLES must imply a spasm of the cremaster muscle. We are familar with it as a symptom of the passage of a Renal Calculus ; and even in apparently idiopathic irritation at the bottom of it. But if none such is discoverable, you will do well to consider the frequent appearance of this symptom among the subjects of Lead-poisoning, and also Teste's statement, that he has employed **Plumbum** with particular success in "an excessively painful Retraction of the Testicles and Penis, which seemed to re-enter the hypogastrium (in consequence of prolonged venereal excesses and repelled Tetters)."

It is only lately that we have been enabled to speak of affections of the SEMINAL VESICLES. Mr. Dudley Wright has made our own the information that has been acquired regarding —

SEMINAL VESICULITIS, and has enriched it from his own experience. ‡ He finds *Oxalic* and *Phosphoric acid* the most useful medicines, according as *Oxalates* or *Phosphates* are observed in the urine ; but attaches most importance to emptying the distended sacs PER RECTUM in a way he fully describes.

When now we come to the PROSTATE, you will naturally think of that CHRONIC ENLARGEMENT of its substance which

---

* Pharmacodynamics, SUB VOCE, Iodium.
†See an illustrative case in J. B. H. S., iv., 141. ‡M. H. R., xliii., 589.

is one of the troubles of old age. I cannot tell you that medicine has any power to reduce this ; but Mr. Dudley Wright has here again helped us, by showing how much may be done by *Ferrum picricum*. in the 2_x and 3_x dilutions, to relieve the symptoms which accompany this enlargement, and even to check its onward progress.*
Contenting myself with a reference to this, I will speak of the treatment of inflammation of the gland.

PROSTATITIS is rarely seen save as a complication of Gonorrhœa or Gleet. When so occuring, as a recent thing, opinion seems divided as to the superior value of **Mercurius** and **Pulsatilla** ; but all authorities agree that these are the two leading remedies. The only exception is Jahr, who would have us rely upon *Nitric acid 30*. If the inflammation tends to linger in a sub-acute form, Dr. Yeldham recommends the administration of grain doses of *Kali iodatum*. CHRONIC PROSTATITIS may be helped by *Pulsatilla*, † or again (according to Jahr) by *Nitric acid* ; but it finds a still more efficient remedy in **Thuja**, on which – in varying dilutions—its subject should be kept for a long time. ‡

A fresh candidate for honour in Chronic Prostatitis has lately appeared in the saw palmetto, **Sabal serrulata**. Dr. E. M. Hale's pamphlet on the drug sets forth its claims to confidence, and a discussion in the BRITISH HOMŒOPATHIC SOCIETY, which you will find in the Eighth Volume of its JOURNAL, shows how these have been received and tested by practitioners in this country. It seems to act much as Mr. Wright has found *Ferrum picricum* to do, relieving symptoms of irritation without altering the fundamental evil.

The treatement of Prostatitis must be somewhat modified if suppuration is probable, or has actually occurred, which often happens in Strumous subjects. Here, whatever other remedies may be given, **Sulphur** becomes of prime importance, Yeldham recommends the tincture in the acute stage to aid *Mercurius* ; and Jahr relies on the 30th dilution, in concert with his *Nitric acid*, in chronic suppurations of the gland.

We have lastly to consider the diseases affecting the PENIS and SCROTUM. We have already discussed Gonorrhœa, but have yet to speak of —

CHANCROID.—Soft Chancre, with its suppurating Bubo, is now generally recognized as a local, though specific and contagious affection. The very reasons which have led me to maintain that **Mercurius** is Antipathic in relation to the Hard Chancre

---

* IBID , xlii., 414, Later, Mr. Wright has had equal or better results from *Picric acid* itself (J. B. H. S., viii., 154.)

† See M. H. R., xxxix., 632   ‡ See B. J. H., xxiv., 499.

show that it is Homœopathic to the Soft ; and you may rely upon it with the utmost confidence, and in quite moderate dosage. It cures, not because of the influence it exerts upon the Syphilitic virus, but in virtue of its power of causing ulceration generally and at this particular spot. **Nitric acid** is here, as in ulcers of the mouth, an effective ally to it ; and the two medicines often come in usefully to reinforce one another's action when it is flagging.

The BUBO which accompanies Chancroid calls for no change in medication when *Mercurius* is being employed, and Yeldham and Bahr concur in recommending persistence with it. **Hepar sulphuris** may be substituted if suppuration appears inevitable. The former was in the habit at one time of opening the abscess early, but he had so frequently seen it disperse without breaking that he latterly gave it a longer chance of doing so. Jahr and Caspari have had corresponding good results from *Carbo animalis.*

BALANITIS is not a very serious matter ; but any one will thank you for telling how promptly it may be subdued by *Mercurius solubilis* or *Cinnabar.** In neglected cases the local use of *Calendula* (as advised by Yeldham) is most helpful.

Elephantiasis of the penis and scrotum, and Prurigo of the latter, belong to cutaneous diseases ; but I must speak of the form of Cancer which affects the parts, and which is nearly always—

EPITHELIOMA—If this could be seen and treated early, good results might be obtained from **Thuja**. Later, **Arsenic** internally and locally- would probably do all that could be expected from medicine.

INFLAMMATION OF THE SCROTUM is either of the diffuse form affecting the abundant cellular tissue ; or one threatening mortification, analogous to the noma pudendi of the other sex. **Apis** for the former, **Arsenicum** for the latter, would be the suitable medicines. In a case of Erysipelas appearing in the abdominal parietes, and involving the scrotum, the latter was found enormously swollen, dark, and superficially ulcerated. Delirium, high fever, rigors and dry blackish tongue were present. *Arsenicum* 3_x arrested the Gangrenous process, and completed the cure in four weeks. †

---

* See J. B. H. S., vi. 299.   † N. A. J. H., Nov., 1892 p. 656.

LECTURE XLVII
DISEASES OF THE FEMALE SEXUAL SYSTEM.
—o—

THE OVARIES, FALLOPIAN TUBES AND MENSTRUATION.
—o—

OVARITIS—OVARIAN NEURALGIA—OVARIAN DROPSY—SALPINGITIS—MENORRHAGIA—AMENORRHŒA—VICARIOUS MENSTRUATION—DYSMENORRHŒA.

The disorders peculiar to the female sex will next engage our attention, and from the frequency with which they come under our notice will demand a careful consideration. For the same reason, I shall have abundant material on which to draw. Besides the sections devoted to this subject in our systematic works, we have several special Treatises on Gynæcological Therapeutics, among which I may specify those of Ludlam, Guernsey, Leadam, Matheson, Jahr, Croserio, Hale and Peters. Dr. Ludlam's "Lectures, Clinical and Didactic, on the Diseases of Women" have deservedly reached their Third Edition. Though "clinical," and therefore occasional, they are so numerous as to embrace nearly the whole range of the subject: they are brimful of practical observation, and are couched in language which makes them most pleasant reading. The 'Obstetrics' * of Dr Henry N. Guernsey (which is also in a third edition) is of a different type. It represents the choice of remedies upon the grounds of minute symptomatology and "key-notes," of which this physician was a leading advocate, and for this purpose may constantly be consulted; but it is hardly to be read continuously. Dr. Leadam published some forty years ago a Volume entitled "The Diseases of Women, Homœopathically treated" and a Second Edition of 1874 embodies the results of his experience since that time. Dr. Matheson has given us some valuable practical material in his four lectures. "On some of the Diseases of Women, their Pathology and Homœopathic Treatment" delivered in 1876 at the London Homœopathic Hospital. "Jahr's "Homœopathic Treatment of Diseases of Females and Infants at the Breast," and Croserio's Homœopathic Manual of Obstetrics," represent an older and more limited Homœopathy; while Dr. Peters has founded on Ruckert's collection of recorded experience several of his useful treatises.

---

* More fully, "The application of the principles and practice of Homoeopathy to Obstetrics and the Disorders peculiar to Women and young Children."

656 DISEASES OF THE FEMALE SEXUAL SYSTEM.

Dr. Hale, in his "Diseases of Women," of which the Second Edition dates from 1880, deals mainly with Dystocia and Sterility. I shall also have to refer you to other contributors on a large scale to uterine Therapeutics, in the pages of our journals, among whom I may specify my industrious friend, Dr. Edward Blake.

I begin with the diseases of the OVARIES. Very little was known at one time of the action of medicines upon these organs ; and we had to rely mainly upon their homology with the testes for the ascertainment of remedies suitable to their corresponding morbid conditions. Experience confirmed indeed the soundness of the interference ; but we have now, from the large amount of USES IN MORBIS on record, and from the many provings instituted by women, a number of well-defined ovarian remedies, and can use them with much precision.

I will first speak of OVARIAN INFLAMMATION—

OVARITIS —There is much difference of opinion among Pathologists as to the frequency of the occurrence of real inflammation of the ovaries, and as to its ever appearing save as secondary to uterine disease. My own judgment goes with Dr. Ludlam (who has devoted two excellent lectures to the subject) in favour of both the frequency and the primariness of Ovaritis, at any rate in a sub-acute form. Sudden suppression of the menstrual flow, as from cold or coitus ; inordinate sexual indulgence or ungratified sexual desire ; mechanical violence or the irritation of emmenagogues these are some of its must common causes, and suggest the form of disease I wish to have in your mind as our object of treatment.

In managing recent Ovarian Inflammation, whether acute or sub-acute, the most important indication for our choice of remedies is the presence or absence of involvement of the investing peritoneum. Should this feature exist — as indicated by the character of the pains—you will do well to make it your first consideration. All our remedies for Peritonitis are available here, and have been found useful, as **Belladonna** by Bahr and Ludlam, **Colocynth** by the latter, **Bryonia** by Jahr and Leadam, **Mercurius corrosivus** by myself. The general indications for these medicines regulate their employment here, and I need not repeat them. When, by one or other of them you have eliminated the peritonitic element of the case, or when it is absent from the first, **Pulsatilla and Hamamelis** are our remedies, as in Orchitis. Here also the former suits the sub-acute, the latter the more intense forms of the malady ; and either may be aided by *Aconite* if required. Of late, **Apis** has received much commendation in Parenchymatous Ovaritis : "stinging pain" is said to be a special indication for it. Dr. Guernsey places *Cantharis* also in the first rank among the remedies for this state.

By these medicines, with suitable general management, you

will generally succeed in preventing Ovarian Inflammation from becoming chronic. Should you find it, however, in this condition, you may undertake its treatment, with good hope of success. The first question must be whether you have induration or abscess to deal with. In the former case **Conium, Platina** * and **Graphites** † are in most repute ; Sterility in the married, tardy and scanty menses in all, are indications for these drugs. Dr. Guernsey adds **Thuja**, when the left ovary is affected, and there is much pain, with great aggravation at the catamenial period. *Palladium* is another medicine which, though little-known as yet, seems to have a true ovarian action, and must not be lost sight of. In Ovarian Abscess, **Lachesis**, first recommended by Dr. Hering, has found several praisers ; but you must not neglect our accredited remedies for suppuration elsewhere, as *Mercurius* when it is threatening, *Hepar sulphuris* and *Silicea* to moderate it when established, and *China* and *Phosphoric acid* to combat the drain on the system.

The foregoing is what I wrote on the subject in 1878. Since then, Dr. Fralich has shown what a bolder use of *Palladium* can do. In a case of Chronic Ovaritis and Salpingitis, of many years' standing, the 3_x trituration effected in three months a nearly complete cure. The mischief was on the right side. ‡ In an equally good case, left-sided, with Leucorrhœa, thick, white and acrid, *Iodine*, given because of some concomitant symptoms, effected complete recovery. The dilution is not stated. ⊕

Sabal serrulata also must be considered in this connexion. Its proving upon women show a marked irritant action on the ovaries ; and Dr. Mullins, who conducted one of them reports much success with it in diseases of the uterus and its appendages. He gives the third and sixth dilutions. ||

OVARIAN NEURALGIA—Of all our authors, Ludlam and Guernsey alone devote a section to this malady. It is true that a large proportion of the cases so called depend on a chronic subinflammatory state of the surface of the organ and of the adjacent peritoneum (Ovarian Folliculitis and Pelvic-Peritonitis). When it is so (as suggested by the presence, in addition to the occasional paroxysms of permanent tenderness and enlargement, and perhaps continuous pain) medicines should be selected suitable to the inflammatory as well as the possible neuralgic element in the case. Such are Hamamelis and Colocynth,—the first being appropriate where the ovary itself,

---

* See B. J. H., xxv., 157. † Sec IBID., xxxi 183.
‡ N. A. J. H. Oct., 1896, p. 660. ⊕ J. B. H. S., iv., 226.
|| IBID., v., 199.

the second where its peritoneal envelope is the part affected; while both reach to Neuralgia of the part. *Apis*, also, may prove a useful alternative here. * But there may unquestionably be a pure neurosis of the ovary, answering to the irritable and neuralgic testicle. When you have sought for and removed any eccentric sources of irritation which may lie at the root of such a malady, you will seek its remedies among our neurotic medicines. Dr. Ludlam speaks, highly of **Atropia**, in the 3rd trituration at the time of attack, and of **Zincum**, in the form of the 3x trituration of the *valerianate*, in the intervals. He also mentions **Naja** as having proved useful; it has become my own favourite medicine for obscure Ovarian Pain, not frankly inflammatory. Dr. Guernsey commends *Staphisagria* where the affection is of mental origin; and the undoubted action on the ovaries of *Sabal serrulata* may be utilised in this place also.

OVARIAN DROPSY—In thinking over the possible curability of this disease, it must be remembered that it corresponds not with Hydrocele, but with cystic disease of the testicle. As the only help for the latter is castration, so it would appear that Ovariotomy is quite in place for the former. Dr. Leadam considers this to be true as regards the multilocular growths, but thinks from his experience that Homœopathic remedies have considerable power over those of unilocular character. He has seen many such "which have been left untouched, either from the patients having been delicate, too feeble, or supposed to have a tinge of Consumption about them, or of Cancer, go on perseveringly with treatment for a long time, and at the last their forms have gradually diminished, and their strength has recovered." He mentions several instances of the kind. Dr. Guernsey extends this favourable prognosis to all kinds of ovarian enlargements. "The profession has come to realise," he says, "that all such growths are of dynamic origin, and that the persistent use of a remedy Homœopathic to the particular case in question will certainly so contract the diseased condition as to make the Tumour disappear." In the HAHNEMANNIAN MONTHLY for December, 1877 he collects a number of cases in which this result seems to have followed upon Homœopathic treatment.

It was only fair to place these hopeful statements before you, though I confess that they go beyond my own experience and expectation. However, as there is no hurry about Ovarian Dropsy, it is worth while allowing them to encourage us to try the effects of treatment before resorting to operative measures,

---

* See J. B. H. S., vi., 312.

The medicines recommended for consultation by Dr. Guernsey are *Apis, Arnica, Arsenicum, Belladonna, China, Conium, Graphites, Iodium, Lachesis, Lycopodium* and *Zincum*. Of these **Apis** and **Iodium**, are the two which seem to have most evidence in their favour. Several cases showing activity on the part of the former have come from America; and a German colleague has communicated one in which a complete cure resulted from the use of the *Iodine*-waters of Hall. Dr. Jousset would bring *Iodine* to bear more directly by injecting "*Eau iodee*" into the sac. Another hopeful medicine is **Kali bromatum**, to which we can credit at least three apparent cures. *

If Ovariotomy is decided upon, our remedies for Peritonitis and vomiting go far to improve the chances of the patient's recovery from the operation.

Since writing the foregoing, a good deal of evidence has accumulated as to the occasional efficacy of remedies—especially of *Apis* and *Kali bromatum* in Ovarian Tumours. The question is such an important one, that I must state the case in favour of it in some detail.

First, as regards *Apis*. Besides the American reports previously mentioned, we have had the following:—

1. Dr. Craig, of Bedford, has given details of two cases in which, after a primary tapping, *Apis* 3 was given thrice daily for a considerable time. In one, an unmarried lady of 24, there was no reaccumulation of fluid for two years, when six quarts of fluid were withdrawn. There was no further recurrence. The second patient was a lady, also single, of 72, with a left Ovarian Tumour. She dies six years after the single tapping, and a post-mortem examination revealed a shrivelled cyst of the size of a walnut attached by a pedicle to the ovary. †

2. Dr. Percy Wilde has recorded two well-marked cases of unilocular ovarian cyst, both of which were rapidly cured by *Apix* 3x. In one four years, in the other, two had elapsed since the recovery, and in neither had there been any re-filling of the cyst. ‡

3. Dr. Hallock reports a case in which what seemed a fibro cystic ovarian growth, consequent on a kick in the region, disappeared under *Apis* 3, though an operation had been recommended. †

4. Dr. Weidner was consulted about a right ovarian cyst, so diagnosed by a specialist, and condemned to operation. It was about the size of an apple and dated from a confinement nine months previously. Soreness and pain were felt on much walking. Patient has lost flesh and become Anæmic. *Apis* 3_x was prescribed, and afterwards *Apisin* 6, with rest and freedom

---

* See Pharmacodynamics, SUB VOCE.   † M. H. R., xxxix., 570.
‡ IBID., xxxiii., 337.   ⁋ N. A. J. H., Dec., 1893, p. 802.

from worry. Improvement began from the first, and in four months she had gained nine pounds in weight, and the Tumour had quite disappeared. *

5. Dr. Bourzutschky reports two cases. The first was preceded by ovarian Dysmenorrhœa dating from the first appearance of the menses; patient was now 18. Gradual abdominal swelling had supervened, beginning on the right side, where were all the physical signs of a Cyst. She got *Apisin*, 5_x trituration, three times a day, with dry food and firm abdominal bandaging. Speedy subsidence set in, and in six months the patient was perfectly well. The second case was that of a woman of 45, who had been operated upon for a right ovarian cyst two years previously. For several months another cyst on the left side had appeared and enlarged rapidly. The same treatment was instituted, and cured in three months. †

And now for *Kali bromatum*. The three cases of cure given in my 'Pharmacodynamics' owed their happy issue to somewhat material doses; and it has been so with the two I have now to add to them,—in the one two grains twice daily, in the other ten grains three times, having been given. You will find these cases in the Third Volume of the JOURNAL OF THE BRITISH HOMŒOPATHIC SOCIETY, and APROPOS of them a discussion initiated by Dr. Burford as to the possibilities of medication in these growths. Dr. Burford himself would encourage such hopes in glandular growths and Parovarian Cysts; but would as strongly discourage them, and advocate early surgical interference, in Dermoid Cysts and Malignant Tumours.

Two cases on record in which *Arsenicum* and *Apocynum* respectively proved curative ‡ might well have been instances of these Parovarian Cysts or cysts of the broad ligament as they are sometimes called. Two cases, so diagnosed by good authority, have in past times been reported as recovering under *Bovista*. †‡

From the ovaries we pass to the FALLOPIAN TUBES, which have of late years become a centre of Pathological interest. This arises from the frequent extension of Endometritis, of Puerperal or Gonorrhœal origin, along the mucous membrane which lines them. We will speak here, then, of—

SALPINGITIS—For a discussion of this disease and its treatment I would refer you to Papers by Dr. Dyce Brown and Dr. Burford in the First Volume of the JOURNAL OF THE BRITISH

---

* J. B. H. S., v., 295. † IBID., vi., 312, See also ix., 175.
‡ IBID., iii. 440 ; iz., 97. †‡ M. H. R., xxv., 474.

Homœopathic Society, and by Dr. Neatby in the Forty-Third Volume of the Monthly Homœopathic Review. Dr. Neatby rightly quotes me as saying that *Arsenicum* is the only drug which has been known to produce Salpingitis (though I should add *Mercurius corrosivus* now). He says that he has used the drug between the attacks of Peritonitis which are apt to occur in chronic cases, and in some instances the attacks have become less frequent and less severe, finally ceasing. "During mild peritonitic attacks,' he writes, "*Colocynth*, answers well ; and Dr. Southwick has found it, when indicated by the pains, actually curative of the Salpingitis itself. * In Pyo-salpinx *Mercurius corrosivus* is Homœopathic, and *Hepar* asserts its usual powers. ✢ Dr. Hawkes commends *Eupion* to our notice ⁝ ‡ and *Sabal serrulata* must not be forgotten. $

I will take next the disorders of MENSTRUATION, which occupy a common ground with diseases of the ovaries and those of the uterus ; and will speak first of —

MENORRHAGIA—I think the best division of the cases in which this trouble occurs to be that of Dr. Guernsey, who classifies Menorrhgia, as Organic, Sympathetic and Functional. Organic Menorrhagia, implies that some local diseases of the womb is present, of which the hæmorrhage—generally intermenstrual as well as menstrual is but a symptom. Sympathetic Menorrhagia is that which appears in Brights' Disease and Tuberculosis, in the inhabitants of Malarious districts, and in the subjects of Lead-poisoning. The persistent treatment of these cases must of course be that of the primary disease. But you must not therefore suppose that you cannot diminish the profuseness of the menstrual flow at the time. What Dr. Kidd has told us may be done with *Sabina, Secale* and *Ferrum* in the Menorrhagia of fibrous tumours ❙ — Dr. Jousset speaking of similar results from *Ledum* and *Platina* in more attenuated forms — is true also of other instances of the Organic and Sympathetic forms of the disease.

While, therefore, I shall be speaking of the remedies for Functional Menorrhagia only, you will understand that the indications given for them are those which should also influence our choice in cases where the affection is secondary.

The remedies for Menorrhagia are, in the first rank, *Crocus, Sabina* and *Ipecacuanha* ; in the second, *Arsenicum, Belladonna, Calcarea, Chamomilla, China, Ferrum, Hamamelis, Nux vomica, Platina,* and *Secale.*

---

* J. B. H. S., viii. 259.   ✢ Ibid,, i., 376.   ‡ M. H. R., xlv., 663.
£ J. B. H S., v., 199.   ❙ See B. J. H., xx, 52.

Crocus is invaluable in Functionl Menorrhagia, when the discharge is blackish, and lumpy or tenacious like pitch. There is no medicine I have given more frequently, or with better effect, than this, when the trouble has occurred in youngish women. I have generally administered it during the period, and *China* in the interval. The dark and clotted condition of the discharge has been my indication for its choice : I have never met with the "sensation as if something were alive in the abdomen," which is said to be so characteristic of it.

Sabina is suitable where the blood is bright red, with which the accompanying symptoms generally correspond to indicate hyperæmia—approaching to inflammation—of the uterus. I find such a condition present in Menorrhagia less frequently than that which calls for *Crocus* or *Ipecacuanha* ; but when it occurs, *Sabina* is very effective in its removal. Dr. Matheson (who has an excellent Lecture on Menorrhagia) esteems it "a remedy which will cure a large number of cases of simple and uncomplicated Menorrhagia and Metrorrhagia than any other medicine in the whole Homœopathic Materia Medica." If Metrorrhagia is included, I agree with him. It should be given both during and between the periods.

Ipecacuanha may be given where neither *Crocus* nor *Sabina*, nor any of the more specially-defined remedies of which I shall speak presently, is indicated. It is particularly called for where much nausea is present. It is most suitable at the time of the period itself.

The other Anti-menorrhagic remedies are called for under the following conditions :—

Arsenicum, in material doses, has proved curative in some obstinate cases, perhaps of Chronic Endometritis. ∗

Belladonna may be given when the menstrual and uterine symptoms are those of *Sabina*, but the cerebral and general condition is that belonging to the polychrest, which is also indicated by the uterine tenesmus characteristic of it.

Calcarea is suitable, during the intervals, in cases where the Menorrhagia is but one element of general mal-nutrition. The patient should be one suitable for the remedy, though she need not have the damp cold feet so much insisted upon by Drs. Guernsey and Skinner. According to Hahnemann, the period should anticipate, as well as be in excess, if *Calcarea* is the remedy.

Chamomilla has undoubted control over hæmorrhage from the womb ; and may be given in Menorrhagia when it has been brought on by disturbing emotions, and where sensibility, local and general, is abnormally exalted. A black and clotted dis-

---

∗ See Hahnemann Mat. Med. Part I., p. 18 (Arsenic). Conversely, Mr. Hunt noticed Menorrhagia, with pelvic tenderness and pressure, occuring in a young woman taking *Arsenic* for *Alopecia*, and ceasing on its discontinuance.

MENORRHAGIA. 663

charge, with pain in the back, indicates it; and also an extreme irritability of temper occuring at every period.

China is of course the best medicine for relieving the debility incident to Menorrhagia. But it is also Homœopathic to the disorder itself, producing a flow like that of *Crocus*; it is accordingly specially useful to reinforce that medicine in the menstrual intervals. It helps, moreover, to restore the periodicity in cases of irregularity.

Ferrum, not too low, is a most Homœopathic and useful remedy in young subjects, of sanguine temperament, and liable to nose-bleeding.

Hamamelis, like *Ipecacuanha*, may be often given with advantage at the time of the flow, when no special indications for other medicines are present.

Nux vomica is a useful adjunct to the Hygienic remedies on which we must mainly depend when Menorrhagia occurs as a consequence of a too stimulating diet, with sedentary habits, in comparatively plethoric subjects.

Platina has long been a favourite Homœopathic remedy for this trouble: it seems best suited for cases due to premature or excessive development of the sexual instincts, and where in older women it is associated with Melancholia. Its Catamenia are too early and long-continued, as well as profuse.

Secale seems, at first sight, suitable only as an Antipathic palliative to give temporary aid in extreme cases. But the evidence of dosage to show that it has a true Homœopathic relationship to uterine hæmorrhage, for it often proves curative in the dilutions from the 6th upwards. * Even in this form it seems best-suited to atonic conditions of the uterus, as in women who have long resided in tropical climates; Dr. Guernsey adds that its appropriate subjects are thin and cachectic.

The foregoing remedies are those to which my own knowledge and experience relate as helpful in Menorrhagia. Several others, however, are indicated by our various authorities, of some of which I must speak; though I cannot do more than refer you to the list of eighty-four characterized by Dr. Guernsey. Bahr mentions *Phosphorus* where the menses are delaying but profuse, and cause much debility and back-ache also when Menorrhagia occurs in nursing women (Dr. Guernsey indicates *Calcarea* and *Silicea* here). He thinks that Menorrhagia often depends upon the stasis of the blood caused by Heart Disease, and that *Digitalis* is here required. Jousset considers Menorrhagia to have frequently the same significance as Bleeding Piles and in such cases gives *Nux vomica* or *Ignatia* — the

---

* See Teste, SUB VOCE.

latter if the menses also anticipate. Otherwise he relies upon *Arsenicum.* * Dr. Leadam gives full and valuable indications for twenty medicines, including most of those above mentioned ; his list may well be consulted in difficult cases. He has had good effects from the constitutional course of treatment recommended by Dr. Patzack, consisting of *Calcarea, Sulphur, China* and *Nux vomica* given in rotation during the intervals. Dr. Matheson's recommendations are much the same as my own ; and so also are those of Dr. Carfrae, in a clinical lecture on Menorrhagia which appears in the Eighth Volume of the ANNALS, save that he makes more use of five-drop doses of the mother-tincture of *Secale* than seems to me consistent with genuine Homœopathic treatment. Dr. Hawkes relates a case cured, after many failures, with *Trillium.* ✢

A fresh accession to our Therapeutic means for Menorrhagia has been furnished of late years in the shape of **Hydrastis** ; and though the medicine is ours, its application to the trouble is of old-school origin. You will find a full account of the matter in the LONDON HOMŒOPATHIC HOSPITAL REPORTS for 1892. Of the two Alkaloids which the golden seal contains, *Berberin* and *Hydrastin*, the latter is found to monopolise the curative virtues of the root. It has itself been split up into two constituents, *Hydrastin* and *Opianic acid* ; and it is this *Hydrastinin*, differing in some points of Physiological action from *Hydrastin*, that has been mainly used in the ranks of traditional medicine. Dr. Burford and his colleagues find that, as regards uterine hæmorrhage, there is little difference between them ; and *Hydrastin* on the whole seems more available for practice—two to five drops of a 1 in 350 Alcoholic solution, representing at the utmost one seventieth of a grain, being a sufficient dose. *Hydrastinin* has to be given in the 1_x dilution during the loss, in the 2_x or 3_x during the intervals. "Given in this way" Dr. Burford writes, "there are few non-parturient uterine hæmorrhages that it will not immediately control, and few contingent uterine conditions that its continued use will not more or less benefit." The rationale of its action is not yet manifest.

This is all I have to say about Menorrhagia, properly so-called ; for other remedies for uterine haemorrhage unconnected with menstruation have yet to come before us, and will do so when we speak of Metrorrhagia.

I have now to direct your attention to the opposite condition—AMENORRHŒA.—I include under this heading all marked

---

* See L'ART MEDICAL., Dec., 1894. ✢ M. H. R., xiv., 674.

AMENORRHŒA

deficiencies of the catamenial flow, whether in quantity or quality, down to its complete absence. I will not now speak of the form of this disorder which comes before us in those entering upon puberty, as I shall have to speak of their troubles under the heading of "Critical Age." I am thinking at present of those in whom the menses are suddenly suppressed, or gradually diminished until they finally disappear.

The menses which a chill or mental emotion has suddenly suppressed may often be restored there and then by the timely administration of **Aconite**, which may sometimes be aided by *Belladonna* or *Glonoine* if the head is much congested. If, however, you are too late for this, and the next period fails to appear, a more directly-acting remedy is required; and this Homœopathy has supplied for the great majority of cases in the shape of **Pulsatilla**. A course of this medicine, continued during one or two intervals, rarely fails to set matters right; it has acted well in different cases alike in the 12th attenuation and in five-drop doses of the mother-tincture. As a rule, I get the best results from the 6th. *Helleborus* (when the system seems overcharged for want of the relief, the head is heavy, and the epigastrium distended), *Cyclamen* and *Senecio* * are alternative remedies of the same kind, and might help us should *Pulsatilla* fail. If Chlorosis has set in, in consequence of the menstrual suppression, it may yield to these remedies; but if it be considerable, you will materially aid the restoration of health by a Chalybeate course. The case I have cited when lecturing upon Anæmia illustrates the advantage of this method.

Cases in which the Catamenia are simply suspended, i.e., fail to occur at the expected time, are generally due to change of climate or mode of life, and rarely cause any derangement of health or require treatment. But the most important variety of Amenorrhœa is that in which the discharge, having diminished in amount for two, three or more periods, or the interval having become longer and longer, has finally ceased. This is generally dependent upon constitutional causes, and the menstrual suppression is but a symptom of the deranged health of the whole system. It is rare that the error is on the side of plethora. Where it is so, **Belladonna** should be given during the intervals, and *Aconite* at the periods; and the obvious Hygienic regulations observed. Far more commonly the general condition is one of malnutrition and debility. If this be simply chlorotic, I would refer you the remarks I have made on the treatment of that malady. If it be (as Dr. Ludlam points out that it frequently is) the incipient stage of the Tubercular cachexia, **Calcarea** — as recommended by him — is an important remedy. When no such definite disorder is present you must treat the patient according to her symptoms with such remedies as *Graphites*,

---

* See J. B. H. S., v., 98.

Sepia, **Sulphur**, *Natrum muriaticum*, **Plumbum** and **Conium**. **Graphites** stands next to *Pulsatilla* in the frequency of its usefulness for defective menstruation. Costiveness and tendency to Eczematous cutaneous eruptions are its special indications; and it is perhaps better when the menses are delayed, scanty and painful, than when they are altogether absent. **Sepia** is most useful when there is much Leucorrhœa, and where the general dyscrasia is considerable; the rectum also may give evidence of the existence of portal or pelvic congestion. **Sulphur** is valuable in Scrofulous or otherwise unhealthy constitutions, with tendency to papular skin eruptions and temporary congestions or flushes of heat. **Natrum muriaticum**, like *Graphites* and *Sepia*, has constipation among its indications, and, with the latter, is most useful in chronic cases with greatly impaired nutrition, as evidenced especially by the appearance of the skin, which is dry, harsh and sallow. The same is to be said of **Plumbum**, which was introduced as a remedy for Chlorosis by Dr. Winter, of Lunenburg. You will find his Paper translated, with some additional remarks by Dr. Drysdale, in the First Volume of the BRITISH JOURNAL OF HOMŒOPATHY. **Conium** is Homœopathic where the Amenorrhœa is part of a general depression of sexual activity; in which case the salts of *Baryta* also might be useful.

VICARIOUS MENSTRUATION is rather an annoyance than a disease of moment. Dr. Leadam recommends *Fcerrum*, and Dr. Dunham *Bryonia*, as ordinarily the most suitable remedies for rediverting the menstrual nisus to its proper seat. *Hamamelis* also has occasionally effected this purpose.

I have last to speak of painful menstruation—
DYSMENORRHŒA—In undertaking the treatment of a case of this kind, you will of course begin by eliminating the purely mechanical variety of "Obstructive Dysmenorrhœa." Whether arising from congenital narrowness of the cervix, or from subsequent flexion of the womb, in either case it seems to require mechanical treatment, though the latter is somewhat (as we shall see) under the influence of medicine.

FUNCTIONAL Dysmenorrhœa implies that the ovaries and uterus (chiefly the latter) cannot perform their periodical duties without pain. This of course may result from their being in a condition of chronic inflammation, in which case nothing is required for the special pain of the period. But even when

DYSMENORRHŒA

they are otherwise sound, they may suffer unduly during the menstrual nisus. Either their natural hyperæmia oversteps the boundary of health, or their nerves are abnormally sensitive ; or the uterine muscular fibres are prone to Spasm or stiffened by Rheumatism. The leading medicines for Dysmenorrhœa will find their place under one or other of these forms.

OBSTRUCTIVE Dysmenorrohœa *i, e.*, where the pain is felt chiefly, if not entirely before the flow is fully established, is (when not mechanical) due to narrowing of the cervical canal by Congestion or Spasm. If from Congestion, limited to the uterus itself, the remedies I shall mention as suitable for the condition— especially *Sabina* or *Sepia* should be given during the intervals, and either **Aconite** or **Pulsatilla** at the time,—the former when the discharge is bright red, and the patient of sanguine constitution, the latter when she is lymphatic, and the blood is dark and clotted. If the Congestion be more general—as shown by Constipation, Hæmorrhoids, hepatic disturbance and so forth— **Collinsonia** is a good medicine both at the periods and between them. For the spasmodic form I find **Gelsemium** (not higher than the 1st decimal dilution) a most excellent remedy ; it is best given, as Dr. Ludlam recommends, in WARM water, even a teaspoonful of cold fluid being apt to bring on the pains in this affection. *Gelsemium,* however, is scarcely more than palliative at the time ; and **Caulophyllum** is the best medicine to be given as curative during the intervals. Its action upon the uterus is like that of *Secale*, but with the difference (so important here) that it influences the cervix as well as the fundus. The **Viburnum opulus** has been much used of late in this form of Dysmenorrhœa, both at the time and prophylactically. Its MODUS OPERANDI is uncertain ; but the lowest dilutions seem required.

Another form of Obstructive Dysmenorrhœa is only secondarily so,—the primary fault being in the uterine mucous membrane. I speak of the affection called "MEMBRANOUS DYSMENORRHŒA," in which the menstrual decidua is so abnormally large and thick as to cause severe pain in its expulsion. This is sometimes the result of chronic uterine inflammation or congestion, as in a case recorded by Dr. Matheson, and cured by him with *Belladonna* and *Mercurius*. * More frequently, I apprehend, ovarian irritation is at the bottom of the morbid exfoliation of the lining membrane of the uterus ; and here we must look for more recondite remedies. The most promising is **Borax**, cures with which have been reported by Dr. H. Bennet from the old school, and Dr. E. M. Hale from our own. ✢

---

* See ANNALS, viii., 252

✢ See B. J. H., xxix., 746.—In a case recorded in the MEDICAL CENTURY of August, 1898, the cure was effected by the 6_x trituration. The fear of downward motion characteristic of the drug was present here.

Material doses were employed; but the drug has unquestionably a specific relation to morbid and painful uterine conditions. Dr. Ludlam has reason to think from observations he has made that this malady is often traceable to repercussion of a cutaneous eruption; and here finds *Sulphur* of service.

Non-OBSTRUCTIVE Dysmenorrhœa, where the pain continues during the flow, means an abnormal sensitiveness of the nerves of the ovaries or uterus, or of the both. It is probably in ovarian Dysmenorrhœa that the virtues of **Hamamelis**, which is praised by many in this disorder, find their scope. It is good also for intermenstrual pain, which is pretty surely ovarian. When it is rather the uterus which suffers Neuralgic pain in the performance of its monthly function, **Chamomilla** and **Coffea** are recommended; and will often (the former especially when the temper is much disturbed by the suffering) give full satisfaction. Should they not succeed, or should the general hyperæsthesia calling for either be absent, I can commend to you the **Xanthoxylum fraxineum** - one of the indigenous American remedies. I am in the habit of giving this medicine in most cases where Dysmenorrhœa co-exists with some degree of Menorrhagia; and can speak of several cures from it. If Dr. Massy's key-note for its—"prolongation of the pain down the crural nerve"—is confirmed, it would seem to correspond to ovarian Dysmenorrhœa also.

There are certain cases of this affection in which the uterus seems to be "Rheumatic," as it might well be in common with other muscles. *Guaiacum* has been, since Dewee's time a favourite remedy for this condition in the old school; in our own **Actæa recemosa** takes its place.

There is little to add as from others. Guernsey and Leadam give their usual long list of possible remedies. Dr. Jousset mentions *Magnesia carbonica* as having often succeeded with him where the periods delay, and especially when the flow is arrested during the pains.

So I wrote in my 'Therapeutics', practically breaking ground on the subject. It has frequently been treated of since, and I must give you an account of how some of our writers have dealt with it.

1. In the MONTHLY HOMŒOPATHIC REVIEW of 1881, Dr. Dyce Brown published a Lecture on Dymenorrhœa, and entirely confirms from his experience what I had written about the place and value in this trouble, of *Gelsemium, Caulophyllum, Actæa* and *Xanthoxylum*. He adds **Cocculus**, when general abdominal disturbance co-exists. All these are for the paroxysm. During the intervals he would give *Sulphur, Sepia, Pulsatilla* or *Platina*, according to their indications; and here, too, he thinks with me, comes in the place of *Collinsonia*.

2. Eighteen years later, Dr. Neatby brought the subject before the BRITISH HOMŒOPATHIC SOCIETY, as you may read in

the Seventh Volume of its JOURNAL. He, too, lays most stress on prescribing for the patients during the intervals ; but at the time gets good results from *Secale* in the Spasmodic, *Sabina* in the Congestive form —both given in medium potencies. In the discussion which followed Drs. Burford and Madden regarded *Gelsemium, Viburnum* and *Xanihoxylum* as palliatives only, but attached real curative virtues in the Spasmodic form to *Caulophyllum* -3_x in the intervals, 1_x in the attack.

3. *Xanthoxylum* has in other hands approved itself of more permanent value than these colleagues will allow. Dr. Barrow has recorded a striking instance of its efficacy. A lady of 27 had for years suffered so much at the period that life had become almost unbearable. She had all kinds of treatment, including dilatation of the cervix, without result. Two years after the operation, worn to a skeleton with suffering, she came under Dr. Barrow's care. He prescribed *Xanthoxylin* 1x three times a day for a fortnight before the menstrual period. At the next recurrence of the period there was very little pain. The remedy was continued for some time, and when left off the patient was completely cured, and had remained so for three years when the report was made. * An Indian colleague, Dr. Ghose, writes : "I have treated nearly ninety cases of Dysmenorrhœa with complete success, and the majority of these yielded to the almost magical influence of *Xanthoxylum*. He relates several cases. The drug was used, he says, "Indiscriminately," but the majority had the discharge profuse. The pain was excruciating, and felt down the thighs anteriorly. The remedy acted most promptly on women of spare habit, nervous temperment, and delicate organization. ✣

4. *Viburnum* is another medicine which has come much to the front of late. Its proving on the female subject has shown it to be Homœopathic to spasmodic uterine pain, and it is perhaps more frequently used now-a-days in such Dysmenorrhœa than any other remedy. ‡ Dr. Jousset is warm in its praise. He gives the mother-tincture in about half-drop doses.

---

* M. H. R., xl., 751.   ✣ N. A. J. H , Dec., 1899.
‡ See N. ENGL. MED. GAZETTE, April, 1900 (p. 199).

LECTURE XLVIII

DISEASES OF THE FEMALE SEXUAL SYSTEM.
—o—
THE UTERUS.
—o—

CHRONIC METRITIS—HYSTERALGIA—ENDO-METRITIS-CERVICO-METRITIS—LEUCORRHŒA—DISPLACEMENTS OF THE UTERUS—UTERINE FIBROIDS—UTERINE POLYPI—UTERINE CANCER.

I now come to the morbid states of the UTERUS itself. Taking the organ first as a whole, we have to consider its hyperæmic conditions. Of these Acute Metritis is rare, save after parturition, where it will receive subsequent attention. Chronic hyperæmia of the uterus—as from sub-involution and the various causes of determination or stasis of blood in the organ—is common enough, and the only questions is whether we shall call it congestion or inflammation. The general CONSENSUS of recent writers is in favour of the latter view, so I will speak here of—

CHRONIC METRITIS—I think nevertheless that a difference must be made in our treatment according as the phenomena are more purely congestive or present (at times at least) frank signs of inflammation. The former class of cases are those most apt to rise from excessive or abnormal sexual excitement and from Obstructive Dysmenorrhœa on the one hand, from venous stasis, owing to portal or pelvic congestion on the other ; the latter are chiefly those consecutive upon Acute Metritis or Subinvolution. We thus have three forms of uterine hyperæmia which we may roughly designate as ARTERIAL CONGESTION, VENOUS ENGORGEMENT, and PARENCHYMATOUS INFLAMMATION respectively ; and to these three forms we may adapt our remedies.

For ARTERIAL CONGESTION of the womb your choice will generally lie between **Sabina, Belladonna** and **Lilium tigrinum.** The first should be chosen in preference where there is much tendency to hæmorrhage, and consentaneous rectal or vesical irritation, or both ; the second where there is the characteristic sensation of pressure downwards, as if the contents of the pelvis would be forced out, which I have described as tenesmus of the cervix ; the third where there is much general nervous depression or irritability and local pain and sensibility, with tendency to Diarrhœa.

For VENOUS CONGESTION the highest place is taken by *Sepia*, which controls the whole range of the malady, and rarely fails to benefit it. An alternative remedy is **Murex purpurea**, which is preferable where the Catamenia are free—those of *Sepia* being rather scanty. Where the liver is much at fault, **Magnesia muriatica** often relieves both that and the accompanying uterine troubles; while, when the rectum is the starting-point of the affection, **Belladonna**, may be of the utmost service.

In genuine INFLAMMATORY conditions, Dr. Matheson (one of whose Lectures is on Metritis) would have us rely almost exclusively upon **Collinsonia** of whose efficacy (in the lowest dilutions) he speaks in the warmest terms. In cases of old-standing, where induration has supervened, several practitioners have obtained excellent results from **Aurum**. Dr. Leadam advises that, whatever other medicines are given, a frequent resort should be made to intercurrent courses of **Sulphur** as an "Antipsoric," and Dr. Jousset also lays much stress on the constitutional origin of Metritis.

HYSTERALGIA.—By this name I would describe the "IRRITABLE UTERUS," which is sometimes a congested one, and still oftener a flexed one, and requires treatment accordingly. But when all such cases have been eliminated, there remain behind some to which the description of Gooch and Ferguson applies, in which the uterus, without any recognisable lesion, is a constant source of trouble in itself and to the whole system. None of the old remedies are so good for this complaint as the **Actæa racemosa**. The frequent presence of a Rheumatic tendency in the patients strengthens the indications for it. I recommend you to continue its use in varying dilutions, for a considerable length of time. The *Lilium tigrinum*, also, may possibly be found useful here.

I need hardly point out the importance of the general management of such cases. It is fully sketched by Dr. Ludlam, who has a most excellent Clinical Lecture on the malady.

ENDO-METRITIS.—I use this term to designate inflammation of the mucous membrane lining the body of the uterus. It is rarely met with save in its chronic form, when it constitutes one of the forms of Leucorrhœa. When you feel sure of its existence, I would advise you to rely upon **Arsenicum** in its treatment. This medicine is especially useful when Menorrhagia is a prominent symptom of the disease.

I come now to the important and difficult subject of the treatment of the INFLAMMATIONS, INDURATIONS and ULCERATIONS of the OS and CERVIX UTERI. Some of these belong to Metritis and some to Endo-metritis ; but they occupy so special a place of their own that I prefer to discuss them separately, which I will do under the heading of—

CERVICO-METRITIS—The tendency of all inflammations of this part being to form ulcers, their treatment has, in the old school, mainly consisted in the employment of the *Caustics* which are so liberally used in similar breaches of the surface in other parts. To the Homoepathists, however, no such inference is possible. There seems to him no reason, A PRIORI, why ulcerations of this part should not be as curable by internal remedies and healing applications as those which occur elsewhere. Yet the prejudice in favour of local *Caustics* is so strong, and the temporary relief they afford is so obvious, that their relinquishment is one of the most difficult tasks, the convert to Homœopathy has to perform. I am persuaded that he must perform it, if he wishes to be thorough in his new system, and not a mere eclectic. In this view, I am supported by nearly all those in our ranks who have cultivated Gynæcology. Dr. Madden's published experience is especially instructive upon this point. Having devoted a good deal of attention to uterine diseases, and feeling far from satisfied with the results of internal medication in Ulceration of the Cervix, he proposed and for some time practised the local application of *Caustics*. You will find an elaborate Paper from him to this effect in the BRITISH JOURNAL OF HOMŒOPATHY, Vol. ix., p. 11. But before many years had passed over, we find him candidly avowing that he had found the practice ultimately injurious, leading to the development of diseases in other parts. For this see Vol. xi of the same Journal, p. 638. He finally told us * that he never used any stronger application to the uterus than a weak *Calendula* lotion. Dr. Ludlam represents a similar view, saying, ✝—"That the general profession will one day and very soon, concede and decide that the cauterisation of the neck of the womb for ulceration is quite as indefensible and harmful as the cauterisation of the throat and larynx in Diphtheria, I have no doubt." Dr. Jousset and Matheson both think *Caustic* applications rarely required ; while the more strictly Hahnemannian school, as represented by Drs. Guernsey and Skinner ‡ and (to some extent) Lcadam, tells us that internal remedies are all-sufficient without any local treatment whatever. The only really dissentient voices I have heard from our ranks are those of Dr. Moore, of Liverpool, who—from thirty years'

---

* ANNALS, v., 129.
✝ In his paper on Uterine Therapeutics, read at the British Homœopathic Congress of 1875 (see M. H. R., xix., 673).
‡ See B. J. H., xxxvi., 194.

experience—concluded that though simple ulcers of the womb can be healed without local applications, Granular Ulcers, deep-seated Scrofulous and Syphilitic Ulcers, required *Caustics* for their cure ; and Dr. Edward Blake, who appears to find the whole Gynæcological apparatus of the old school necessary for the treatment of the diseases of women.

If, however, we are to dispense with these potent measures we must all the more carefully select our specific remedies. The main distinction I apprehend to be between true Cervical Metritis, which is a Parenchymatous Inflammation, and what we may call ENDO-CERVICITIS, or Catarrh of the mucous lining of the canal. Correspondingly, we may have ulceration within or without the cervix ;—the surface affected in the former case being that of a freely-secreting glandular organ, covered with columnar epithelium,—in the latter that of an ordinary mucous membrane with squamous epithelium, covering a fibro-muscular structure. Now Endo-cervicitis and ulceration within the cervix always come before us clinically in the form of Leucorrhœa, and under that heading I will immediately speak of them. Cervical Metritis sometimes occurs in an acute form, as in a case well-described by Dr. Ludlam. More frequently we meet with it as a chronic affection, and generally in connexion with a similar condition involving the body of the womb. In all these cases **Belladonna** is the great medicine, and should be persevered with until all tenderness and engorgement have disappeared, or until its action seems exhausted. Dr. Matheson has the utmost confidence in it ; and Dr. Moore states that its influence in hyperæmic states of the os uteri is "most marvellous." If you need an ally to it, you may find it in **Tartar emetic**, which Dr. Ludlam has lately praised in this condition, which he calls "Chronic Corporeal Cervicitis." Should ulceration have occurred, but be superficial only, **Mercurius solubilis** (as recommended by Dr. Matheson) or **Arsenicum** (the latter if the pain is burning, the patient weak, and the discharge thin) should be given internally, and injections of *Calendula* (one part to eight, or weaker) employed. If it be more deeply excavated, and the visible portion of the os and cervix be swollen and indurated, **Mercurius corrosivus** is my favourite medicine ; and, as this condition nearly always exists in chronic cases, I always begin with it in them, using *Calendula* or *Hydrastis* as an injection. Besides these medicines, Jahr recommends *Nitric acid* and Leadam *Lycopodium*, in Ulceration of the Os,—the later giving a long list of possible remedies for it, with their indications, which you may consult in difficult cases.

You will of course look carefully after Syphilis in your patient, and treat its local manifestations as you would do if they appeared elsewhere.

The foregoing, about inflammation of the Uterus and its Cervix, I have brought before you in the words of my 'Therapeutics of 1878. It represents the Pathology of that time, while anticipating a revulsion from the strong measures then adopted for coercing the cervix to health, and healing the "ulcers" to which it was supposed to be so unaccountably subject. The Article on diseases of the womb in Quain's 'Dictionary' of 1894, written by Dr. Playfair, shows that this revulsion has occurred ; but unfortunately it has been made on Pathological rather than Therapeutical grounds. The "red, strawberry-like abrasions round the os, which, under the name of ulceration, have formed so fruitful a subject of controversy in uterine disease in no sense of the word constitute an ulceration, since the epithelium is the only structure destroyed. Their detection is of much importance from a diagnostic point of view, but chiefly as leading to a knowledge of the more deep-seated changes which have produced it as a secondary result, which are themselves beyond the sphere of observation, but which are truly at the root of the evil." This is good, and shows that in dealing with the condition so revealed by internal remedies and nothing but soothing applications we have been on the right track. But the Therapeutic violence which I so earnestly deprecated when it assailed the cervix has only transferred itself to the lining membrane of the uterine body. The mildest agents of intra-uterine medication are strong solutions of *Carbolic acid* and *Iodine* ; then comes *Nitrate of Silver* in similar form or in the solid stick ; and barbarity is carried to its utmost in the applications (recommended by the Dublin Physicians) of fuming *Nitric acid*, the cervix having been first dilated with tents. I cannot protest too strongly against thus breaking into the house of life Is the uterine mucous membrane so different from that which lines other tracts that it should be assaulted in this rude manner ?

Homœopathy shows us a more excellent way. By observation and experiment it finds what drugs can, when taken otherwise into the system, inflame the lining of the womb ; and it administers these by similar channels when Endo metritis is already set up, knowing that they will by elective affinity seek out the irritated surface, and gently, harmlessly, peaceably exert upon it the alterative influence desired. Are we not, in so acting, already in the van as regards endo-uterine Therapeutics, as we were when I formerly wrote in respect of Cervical Ulceration ?

Let us now see what advance or modification the progress of years has brought in the recommendations I have already made.

1. To what I have said on the treatment of Chronic Metritis I have little to add, save to emphasize the recommendation of *Aurum*. If you will read the section "5exual Organs" of Dr. Washington Epps's excellent Monograph on "Aurum, its

LEUCORRHŒA 675

Pathogenesy and Therapeutics" in the transactions of the International Homœopathic Congress of 1896, you will find abundant evidence of its virtues in this sphere. You will notice also, that it seems to act best here in one of the double *Salts* it forms either with *Sodium* or *Potassium*.

2. I have mentioned *Arsenicum* alone among remedies for Endo-metritis where the body of the uterus is the seat of the catarrh ; and you will rarely require anything else. Dr. Deschere, however, contributes an alternative which may be useful when the kind of Leucorrhœa he mentions is present. *"Carbolic acid,"* he writes,* "has proved serviceable in several cases of displacement of the womb, with a co-existing catarrh of the utero-vaginal mucous membrane. Discharge from this, if present, is always offensive. The symptoms first relieved are the agonizing Backache across the lions, with dragging sensation down the buttocks and into thighs. The improvement of the local symptoms, except the displacement, follows gradually but surely." He uses the *30*th dilution.

3. The question of dynamic medication as against *Caustics* in the so called *"Ulceration"* of the cervix you will find threshed out in the papers presented and the discussions on them held at the International Homœopathic Congress of 1881. My sympathies were with Drs. Dyce Brown and Matheson against their opponents, and I think that the trend of later experience has been in their direction. Dr. Brown gives very full and clearly-marked indications for our chief medicines suitable to this condition, which you cannot do better than consult when you have it to treat.

I have now to speak of—

LEUCORRHŒA—This is indeed a symptom rather than a disease, and it may be associated with many of the uterine maladies we have already considered or shall yet have to consider. But there are several varieties of Leucorrhœa which come before us for treatment as such ; and the remedies for these I shall now consider.

First, we have Leucorrhœa occuring in connexion with general debility—as from residence in tropical climates, over-

---

* N. A. J. H., Sept., 1896, p. 596.

lactation, &c., implying an atonic state of the uterus, but nothing more. In addition to the general measures you will here adopt for strengthening the system, you will remember the special virtues of **Helonias** as a uterine roborant. If, nevertheless, the Leucorrhœa persists, you will find **Pulsatilla** here as elsewhere the specific remedy for the morbid activity of the glands of the cervix.

A still more common form of Leucorrhœa is that which comes before us in those who have had severe abortions, or who have borne children too frequently. Here, I apprehend, besides debility, there is arterial or venous congestion of the womb. Accordingly, **Sabina** and **Sepia** are our chief remedies; and with the aid of general and local bracing will do great things for our patients.

When Leucorrhœa from either cause, but especially from the latter, has lasted for some time, irritation going on to inflammation and ulceration of the glands of the cervix is set up, as has been shown by Tyler Smith. Accordingly when the remedies I have already mentioned have been fairly tried, but without success, or when from the symptoms or a specular examinatian you diagnose Endo cervicitis, you must resort to more deeply-acting medicines. If the discharge is white and milky, but profuse, **Calcarea** carbonica is generally remedial. Sometime a trituration of roasted egg-shells was recommended in America for this trouble, in place of the preparation of oyster-shells we ordinarily employ ; and, as Constantine Hering used to call the latter *Calcarea ostrearum*, the former might be named *Calcarea ovorum*.* I have frequently verified the suggestion giving the second and third triturations. When the discharge degenerates into an acrid and offensive fluid, **Kreasote**, from the 2nd to the 6th, is an excellent remedy. ✝ In cases having no special features, you may bethink yourselves of the experience of an old-school physician, which is cited in the Third Volume of the JOURNAL OF BRITISH HOMŒOPATHIC SOCIETY. He commends the persistent use of *Cantharis in this trouble occuring in young unmarried women, where local examination is undesirable. His dose is very small, and no strangury or other unpleasant symptoms are produced. "The action of the drug," he says, "has been uniformly satisfactory."

Dr. Southwick, who is well-known as a Gynæcologist, has lately written on the Therapeutics of Leucorrhœa. His remedies are much the same as those already mentioned, viz., *Calcarea phosphorica*, *Helonin*, *Kreosote*, *Sepia*. He also commends *Stannum* for profuse discharge of yellowish or white mucus, with great debility and aching in the back.

---

* It was introduced as *"Ova testa"* evidently a misprint for *"Ova tosta"* but the error has been perpetuated ever since.

✝ See J. B. H. S., v., p. 106.

Of Vaginal Leucorrhœa I shall speak when I come to the affections of that canal. I will only mention here that it is in this form of the flux that *Borax* exerts its really great powers.

As to vaginal injections in Leucorrhœa, my own experience is decidedly in their favour. Free irrigation of the os and cervix daily with cold water is of unquestionable service; and something is to be said for the injection of a solution of the medicine which is being given internally, or of **Hydrastis** or **Calendula**. The use of medicinal astringents, however, still more of *Caustics*, I do not recommend. In Endo-cervicitis there is no advantage in injections, as they hardly reach the interior of the cervical canal; but Dr. Ludlam finds the occasional insertion of a tampon saturated with Glycerine to be of much assistance.

DISPLACEMENTS OF THE UTERUS—including Ante and Retroversion and Prolapsus—will next engage our attention. It may be thought that medicines can have little to say to these mechanical disorders. ·But remember how often the flexions of the womb depend upon congestion of the organ or the presence of fibrous tumours in its walls, aud how Prolapsus generally implies weakness of the uterine supports; and the place of medicines as remedial agents is evident. What they can sometimes do may be illustrated by the following case.*

In 1858, I was called to see an unmarried woman of thirty who had been ill for three years, and had never got much relief from any medical advice she had received. I found her general health much impaired, with constant pain in the back and pelvic region, with extremely painful menstrution, her spirit depressed, and herself convinced that no one had understood her case, and feeling that there could be no cure for her. In my examination of the case, I learned from her that, three years previously, while assisting her father to lift some heavy article, she had felt something given way, and had become sick immediately; had kept her bed for some time after; had got little help from any medicine, and had slowly recovered so as partially to resume her labours, but had never been well since, nor ceased to suffer in the back and lower part of the abdomen.

On making the necessary examination, I found the uterus retroverted, the os pressed high up against the pubes, the fundus low down in the hollow of the sacrum. The slightest attempt to replace the organ gave such severe pain as to make me desist immediately: and after two futile attempts, I decided to try *Sepia* 30, and see her again in a few days. I then found her feeling better, but she said that each repetition of the medicine gave pain from the inguinal region to the pubes, "a kind of drawing pain." I ordered a continuance of the *Sepia*, and saw her again about a week after my first examination. To my great joy I found the cervix uteri had descended an inch or more, and the fundus correspondingly ascended. I can hardly express the delight felt at this discovery, believing from

---

* Amer. Hom. Review, v., 321.

that moment that the idea so long cherished would be fully realised, and that my patient would be really cured when the uterus had regained its normal position, and I did not doubt that the means which had so well begun the work would complete it.

I need only add that the first menstruation after the treatment commenced was accomplished with comparatively little suffering and that as the cure progressed the suffering ceased. The cure wet steadily on, and at the third examination the position was norman; and, although the patient was obliged to rise several times each nigl t to wait on an aged grandmother, and did not relax from her usuhl duties about the house, she had no relapse. Some two years afteraI went to ascertain if she still remained well, and found that she ha d steadily gained in health, and had no return of the disease.

This case is reported by the late Dr. Mercy Jackson, of Boston ; and by a reference to the Article on *Sepia* in my 'Pharmacodynamics' you will see that to the end of her career she continued to get similar results from the medicine.

I may also refer you to a Paper by Dr. Liedbeck, of Stockholm, in the Twentieth Volume of BRITISH JOURNAL, in which he relates some experiences with *Belladonna* as a uterine remedy. Two of the cases cured by it were of Retroversion. He prefers using it in the form of an ointment, which is to be rubbed into the hypogastrium and thighs. There are also some cases of Prolapsus on record cured by *Secale* ; * and Dr. Preston communicates † experience with *Ferrum iodatum* in Uterine Displacements in general, which seems to have been very satisfactory.

You will thus see that we have no inconsiderable evidence as to the power of Homœopathic remedies over the various forms of Uterine Displacements. Dr. Guernsey goes so far as to say that there is no case of the disease in which, replacement having once been effected, and rest in a suitable posture being secured, complete recovery may not ensue under the administration of the suitable medicines. It is true that the case he instances, in which a fallen womb of ten years' standing, being restored to its position, returned no more after the administration of *Conium* does not prove much. It is no uncommon thing for such a proceeding to be followed by a cure without *Conium*, or any other medicine,—adhesions forming between the (generally) ulcerated cervix and the vagina, which prevent the return of Prolapse. But his vast experience can hardly deceive him when he speaks of the general curability of these displacements by medicinal means, without the use of pessaries or uterine supporters of any kind ; and I think I am justified in advising you in all save the most purely mechanical cases to begin (at least after reposition) with medicinal treatment alone. The remedies already mentioned—**Belladonna, Ferrum, Secale** and **Sepia**—are those which seem most frequently service-

---

*See B. J. H., i., 407.   † See IBID., xxv., 49.

able; and I may add to them **Stannum**, which in Prolapsus has really great power; **Lappa major** and **Helonias** of which—in atonic cases—the same may be said; *and **Lilium tigrinum** † Dr. Guernsey gives indications for some fifty drugs, which you may consult if you have a troublesome case to manage.

Even if after a fair trial of remedies, mechanical support seems indispensable, do not therefore discontinue them, as they may hasten the time when a radical cure shall have been accomplished, and pessaries be no longer needed.

I have now to speak of the medicinal treatment of the MORBID GROWTHS of the uterus. And first, of —

UTERINE FIBROIDS—The main use of remedies in the management of this disease has hithrto been to check the hæmorrhages which accompany it, at any rate in its interstitial and sub-mucous forms. Of these I shall speak under the head of Metrorrhagia. Whether we can depend upon specific medication to reduce the size of the growths, or favour their diminution or expulsion, has been uncertain. There is a Paper on the subject by Dr. Kidd in the Twentieth Volume of the BRITISH JOURNAL. He bears testimony to the value of *Mercury* in discussing these Tumours, recommending the *bichloride* where profuse muco-purulent excoriating Leucorrhœa exists, and the *biniodide* in cases characterized by a stony hardness of the Tumour without much excoriation. Both are to be given in low potency. The cases he relates, however, hardly bear out his suggestions, as in one of the four only was any impression made upon the Tumour. Here, moreover, *Mercurius corrosivus* was the remedy, although no Leucorrhœa was present. Dr. Helmuth, who has contributed a paper on the subject to the Twenty-Third Volume of the same Journal (p. 538), is less sanguine as to the results of Homœopathic medication; and Dr. Jousset expresses himself to the same effect. He writes, however,—"I have just obtained the complete disappearance of a Fibrous Tumour which had reached the size of a fœtus at term. The patient was treated principally with *Platina*, administered for the hæmorrhages symptomatic of her malady." He does not mention whether this occurred at the Menopause, or after childbirth—periods well-known to be favourable to the sponta-

---

*See J. B. H. S., i., 280; viii., 253.   † IBID., vii., 336.

neous decay of these Tumours, and of which we may avail ourselves in endeavouring to make an impression upon them.

Since these writers handled the subject, however, some solid contributions have been made to the medicinal treatment of Fibroids.

1. The late Dr. Alfred Beebe, of Chicago, has from time to time communicated favourable results obtained from **Calcarea iodata**. A Paper in the MEDICAL ERA of February, 1892, summarises his experience and gives references to his previous deliverances on the subject. He gave about gr. $\frac{1}{60}$th for a dose, repeating two, three or four times a day. He never failed, he said, to control the hæmorrhage by this means, and often accomplished a notable reduction in the size of these Tumours. I have had a similar experience in a well-marked case. Dr. E. A. Sears relates one, * where the Menorrhagia had made the patient quite Anæmic. Ten grains were dissolved in a pint of water, and a teaspoonful taken after each meal. When last seen she had lost all Anæmic look, had gained flesh, and was bright and cheerful. The periods had become quite natural, though the tumour had not perceptibly diminished in size. In two cases, one interstitial, one sub-serous, great reduction in size was observed by Dr. Sarah J. Millsop under the use of the 2_x dilution. † Dr. Neatby, who in the LONDON HOMŒOPATHIC HOSPITAL REPORTS for 1894 and 1895 relates the history of thirty-four cases which had come under his notice up to that time, in 1898 brought the subject before the British Homœopathic Society, ‡ and summed up the Therapeutics by saying that his sheet-anchor for reducing both hæmorrhage and size, had become the *Iodide of Lime*. "I give," he writes, "the American preparation which contains 12·5 per cent. of free *Iodine*, about one-fifth of a grain for a dose four times a day."

2. There is thus good prospect of help in this direction; and another in which we may look is towards the curious virtues of *Thyroidin*. In a deeply interesting Paper, embodying a large experience in the extra surgical treatment of Fibroids, Dr. E. S. Bailey relates nine cases in full and refers to others. Among them are contained several showing good effects—sometimes of a striking character—from *Thyroidin*. He finds it act well, if not even best, in the triturations up to the 3x, so that it is not its Physiological action which is exerted. Dr. Bailey's Communication appears in the CLINIQUE for January, 1898. In the same Journal for February 1899, you may see the results of a large testing of the remedy on the part of his colleagues. They show an undoubted power on the part of this substance (usually in the 1x trituration) to relieve the symptoms and often to reduce the size of these growths.

---

* J. B. H. S., ii., 94.   † IBID., i., 375.   ‡ IBID., vi., 30.

3. Baumann has been able to extract the active principle of the thyroid gland, and finds it to be an organic compound of **Iodine**. That this drug is the pre-potent element in the *Calcarea iodata* has already sufficiently appeared; and Dr. Gaudy has reported some cases of Fibroid, where in the form of *Kali iodatum* as weak as the 3_x dilution, it has produced remarkable effects. Large doses had generally been given first, but had been without influence save for evil.

It is thus to *Iodic* preparations that we must look for control over Uterine Fibroids.

UTERINE POLYPI—There are several instances recorded in Homœopathic literature in which Polypi have been expelled from the uterus apparently under the action of Homœopathic remedies. Dr. Petroz, considering them to be a manifestation of the "Sycotic" diathesis, treated them with *Thuja*, and relates † a case in which under its influence a large one came away which had caused distress for a long time. In the Twenty-Sixth Volume of the BRITISH JOURNAL OF HOMŒOPATHY are recorded two cases, in one of which five Fibrous Polypi were expelled from the interior of the uterus under the use of *Conium*, and in the other one from the vagina under *Thuja* and *Calcarea*. I confess I am more inclined to view these occurrences as spontaneous than as effects of medication. The analogy of Nasal Polypi, in which our medicines are so often helpful, hardly holds good here; as uterine growths of this kind are either Fibroids which have become united to their original site by a pedicle only, or mucous follicles which have enlarged and protruded the mucous membrane that covers them. Dr. Guernsey, who is generally so satisfied with internal medication, recommends surgical measures here; and Leadam is in favour of removal at first and subsequent Homœopathic medication to obviate recurrence.

UTERINE CANCER—There are three main forms under which this terrible disease may present itself, and in which we have to consider what Homœopathic medication can do for it.

1. The first, and most common, is SCIRRHUS OF THE OS and CERVIX. If you can catch this morbid condition in its incipi-

---

* JOURNAL BELGE—D' HOMŒOPATHHIE, March—April, 1899.

† MEMOIRE SUR LA SYCOSE, in Cretin's Edition of his collected writings.

ence (which is unfortunately rare), I think that something may be done for it by **Arsenicum iodatum**, in the lower triturations. Our experience is not decisive enough for me to say more at present, but I commend this to you as a promising piece of practice. I cannot say whether it or any other medicine is of use when ulceration has set in.

2. We next have the 'CAULIFLOWER EXCRESCENCE' OF THE Os, which—when malignant, is an Epithelioma. I say, when malignant, for there seems no doubt that papillary growths of perfectly benign character may occur from Gonorrhœa or from local irritations. **Thuja** would unquestionably be curative of these, but it is uncertain whether it can modify malignant Papillomata. In the case so diagnosed recorded by Dr. Quin in the First Volume of the ANNALS, it seemed of striking service, but Jahr says that he has never derived the least benefit from it. An old-school physician—Dr. Welsch, of Augsburg—has lately written of the drug: "Very good results have been observed from its application in erosions and ulcerations of the vaginal portion of the womb. I have seen better and more rapid cures of cases suspiciously like Cancer from *Thuja* than from any other remedy."* Jahr, with Wahle and Kurtz, has much confidence in **Kreosote** in these cases; and it certainly bears some Homœopathic relationship to them. Dr. Daudet reports a case in which digital examination, together with the constitutional state and appearance of the patient, led him to the diagnosis of Epithelioma of the cervix. He prescribed *Hydrastis 12*, a dose three times a day. Two days later, a copious, fœtid, blackish, hæmorrhage set in; and in three or four days more the morbid growth came away in blackish masses having a sickening odour. All local symptoms disappeared, and the patient became quite well. †

3. The third form of Uterine Cancer of which I would speak is SARCOMA. I have hitherto suggested *Silicea* for this growth; ‡ but Dr. Helmuth's experience would point to *Thuja* here also, and the persistent brownish Leucorrhœa which characterizes it to *Kreosote*. We have no experience of its treatment on record.

This is all I can tell or suggest as to curative treatment of Uterine Cancer; and it would seem to leave the knife a surer resort. Where, however, from any cause this is not employed, though we may not be able to cure we can do much by way of palliation, prescribing according to the symptoms. Your patients with Uterine Cancer may be thus led in comparative case down the path of decline till death closes the scene.

---

* J. B. H. S., i., 284.   † REVUE HOM. FRANCAISE, July, 1893, p. 291.
‡ See Therapeutics, p. 309.

LECTURE XLIX

DISEASES OF THE FEMALE SEXUAL SYSTEM

—o—

UTERUS (*concluded*)—THE PERI-UTERUS, VAGINA, VULVA, MAMMAE, AND COCCYX.

—o—

METRORRHAGIA—HYDROMETRA—PHYSOMETRA—PERIMETRITIS—PELVIC HÆMATOCELE—PELVIC CELLULITIS—PELVIC ABSCESS—VAGINITIS—VAGINISMUS—PROLAPSUS VAGINÆ—VULVITIS—ACUTE LABIAL ABSCESS—CANCER PUDENDI—NYMPHOMANIA—VASCULR TUMOUR OF THE URETHRA—STERILITY—INFLAMMATION OF THE MAMMÆ—MAMMARY SCIRRHUS—COCCYGODYNIA.

An accident which may occur in connexion with any of the uterine affections hitherto mentioned, but which requires its own special treatment, is—

METRORRHAGIA—For arresting an existing uterine hæmorrhage we have excellent remedies in *Ipecacuanha, Sabina, Secale* and *Hamamelis*. Ipecacuanha is suitable where no very distinctive features are present. Jahr says that he always begins with it, unless any other medicine is plainly indicated and often finds it sufficient. Sabina is of the utmost value where the hæmorrhage is connected with uterine congestion or inflammation, and when the patient is robust and florid, and the flow bright-coloured. Secale takes its place when the constitutional and local state is of an opposite character. But unless forcing pains are present, I hardly think the medicine Homœopathic; and am in the habit of relying upon **Hamamelis** where the flow is dark, passive and painless.

For obviating the tendency to Metrorrhagia the remedies suitable to the disease on which it depends are generally the most effective. But where this symptom calls for treatment of its own, medicines like *Ferrum, Plumbum* and above all **Arsenicum**, are indicated. Dr. Ludlam has communicated some valuable experience with **Nitric acid** in those passive but prolonged Metrorrhagias which sometimes follow abortion, and which he connects with an injured state of the mucous lining of the uterus. Drs. Claude and Amermann endorse his experience. *

The medicines I have mentioned under Menorrhagia may

---

* J. B. H. S., i. 85.

684 DISEASES OF THE FEMALE SEXUAL SYSTEM

also come into play here. As regards particular forms of the trouble, I can only say that Jousset has found *Ledum*, *Platina* and *Argentum* of most value in that which accompanies Uterine Fibroids. The writer also signalises an empirical remedy, the *Thlaspi bursa pastoris*, as one that has frequently rendered him good service in obstinate cases. He gives the mother-tincture.

Since I wrote the foregoing in my 'Therapeutics,' several fresh contributions have been made to our knowledge of the therapeutics of Metrorrhagia.

1. As a hæmostatic at the time, Dr. Ludlam has had good results from *Cocaine*. He puts about gr. $\frac{1}{12}$th in half a tumblerful of water, and gives a teaspoonful frequently till the flow diminishes. * Mr. R. K. Ghosh sends a similar experience from India, saying that the remedy often acts like a charm. †

2. When Metrorrhagia is fœtid, *Kreosote* is as effective as when a similar condition obtains in Leucorrhœa. Dr. Aldrich and Sybel concur in testifying to its efficacy here. ‡

3. The Shepherd's Purse, (*Thlaspi*) which I mentioned as recommended by Dr. Jousset in Metrorrhagia, has come quite to the front of late as an anti-hæmorrhagic, as I have told you when speaking of Hæmaturia. Dr. Julia Button relates a curious experience with the drug. She gave it in a Climacteric case—fifteen drops of the tincture to half a glass of water, a teaspoonful every hour. It controlled the hæmorrhage, but caused a severe constrictive Headache; the patient said it seemed as though her skull would crack if she did not move her head with great care. *Glonoine* relieved this, but the hæmorrhage returned. Finally the 1_x dilution was substituted. This controlled the bleeding without producing Headache; and the trouble had not returned for six months when the report was made. $ Dr. Mason records a case following on a miscarriage, in which, after not medicines only but operative procedures had failed, *Thlaspi* cured. The drug was given in infusion, and its too long continuance seemed to cause a recurrence of the hæmorrhage, for the latter quickly ceased on suspending it. ‖

4. I would add to the remedies I have already mentioned two others. One is a rarely-used herb—the Lesser Periwinkle, **Vinca-minor**. I have found it, acting on the suggestion of Dr. Henry Madden, excellent for checking hæmorrhage recurring some years after the Climacteric, and making one fear that malignant disease was impending. The other is Trillium. Drs. Burford and Neatby concur in esteeming this drug the most effective hæmostatic we have where Fibroid growths cause the

---

* J. B. H. S., iii., 336. † IBID., iv., 132. ‡ IBID., iii., 215.
$ IBID., 379, i. ‖ IBID., iii., 105.

loss ; * and Dr. Hawkes has lately told us of a cure with it of Menorrhagia degenarating into Metrorrhagia in a young subject. †

HYDROMETRA and PHYSOMETRA. In case you should ever encounter these rare affections in that idiopathic form for which alone remedies are useful. The first has subsided under *Sepia*. ‡ For the second, Dr. Guernsey recommends *Bromine*, *Phosphoric acid* and *Lycopodium* ; but Dr. Ludlam relates a case brought on by worry and fatigue after Parturition, where *Belladonna* proved curative.

Before leaving the uterus, I must speak of some affections which belong to its surroundings and connections. These are PERIMETRITIS and PELVIC HÆMATOCELE ; PELVIC CELLULITIS and ABSCESS.

By —
PERIMETRITIS I mean to designate the Pelvic-Peritonitis of Bernutz and Goupil, which is, as its name imports an inflammation of that portion of the peritoneum which dips down into the pelvis, and constitutes the broad ligaments of the uterus. I thus exclude the "Parametritis" of the Germans, the "PELVIC CELLULITIS" of our English Nomenclature, which will be considered in its proper place.

The only one of our authors who mentions Perimetritis is Jousset, who in his LECONS relates two cases, and discusses the Pathology and Therapeutics of the malady. The medicines he recommends are **Aconite** (in pretty strong doses), and **Colocynth**, and (from the analogy of its action on the Pleura) *Cantharis*. I can hardly advise more suitable remedies than the two first-named, unless *Mercurius corrosivus* should be found as useful here as it is in inflammations of the abdominal peritoneum.

PELVIC HÆMATOCELE—We owe to Dr. Jousset a lecture on this accident also ; and his remarks, with a paper communicated by Dr. Dyce Brown to the BRITISH HOMŒOPATHIC SOCIETY, § constitute the only Homœopathic literature of the subject with which I am acquainted.

There are three occasions in the clinical history of pelvic Hæmatocele at which our medicines may interpose with advantage. The first is where the primary hæmorrhage is still going on. Here **Hamamelis** would suit both the nature of the trouble

---

* Dr. Royal reports a case in which, not only did the Menorrhagia abate, but the Fibroid withered (M. H. R., xxxviii., 688).
† M. H. R., xlv., 674. ‡ NORTH AM. JOURN. HOM., iii., 89.
§ See B. J. H. xxxiv.. 99.

and the source whence it proceeded. The second when the effusion is intra-peritoneal, and has set up inflammation. The medicines already recommended for Pelvi-peritonitis would now come to our aid. Lastly, when all was quiescent, the re-absorption of the effusion might be aided by **Arnica** and **Sulphur**. Dr. Brown's case did very well under such treatment,—*Aconite, Belladonna, Mercurius corrosivus* and *Arnica* being the medicines successively given.

PELVIC CELLULITIS most frequently occurs in the Puerperal state, and we shall discuss its treatment there under the head of Puerperal Fever. As it does supervene, however, upon other traumatic incitements, a word must be given to it here.

Apis and **Rhus** are the main remedies for areolar inflammation, and the former would be most appropriate to the Non-puerperal, the latter to the Puerperal form of Pelvic Cellulitis. If fever runs high, there is reason to think that **Veratrum viride** will do more for it than *Aconite* or *Belladonna*. Should suppuration occur, the case resolves itself into one of—

PELVIC ABSCESS, which may of course arise from other morbid processes, as Tubercle and Hæmatocele. However it originates, **Hepar sulphuris** and **Silicea** are its main remedies, and under these—especially the former, quite extensive collections of pus have been known to undergo absorption. If the effusion have not yet undergone a purulent transformation we may bethink ourselves of *Palladium*. In a case of Dr. von der Goltz's as a sequel of pelvic inflammation following an Abortion three years previously, the uterus was retroflected, painfully sensitive and immovable; and both parametria were a compact mass, filling out the lower pelvis. After two courses of three doses each of *Palladium* 30, at three week's interval, the patient returned to report herself pregnant. On examination, nearly all inflammation was found to have subsided.*

The less important morbid states of the VAGINA and VULVA must next come under our notice.

VAGINITIS may come before us either as ACUTE or as CHRONIC.

1. ACUTE VAGINITIS is generally the main element of Gonorrhœa in the female. When it is so, and *Aconite* and *Cantharis* have been given if required, instead of the *Cannabis* we should administer to the other sex, I recommended **Sepia**. In simple Acute Vaginitis, as from cold, *Aconite* may be followed by **Mercurius**, as advised by Bahr. In Diphtheritic Vaginitis, as occasionally observed in the course of the toxæmic diseases, local antiseptic measure seems the best aid we can give to the remedies for the general affection.

---

* J. B. H. S., v., 289.

2. CHRONIC VAGINAL CATARRH is the basis of vaginal as distinguished from uterine Leucorrhœa. *Mercurius* and *Sepia* are here also principal remedies (Dr. Jousset recommends the latter in the *I*st and *2*nd triturations) ; but *Calcarea* is good in scrofulous subjects, *Pulsatilla* in those that are chlorotic, and *Kreosote* where the discharge is of bad character and acrid quality. Of late years I have always begun the treatment of Vaginal Leucorrhœa with **Borax** in the 2_x or I_x trituration, and have rarely found it to fail. When ulceration has occurred, *Nitric acid* might be useful. *

VAGINISMUS—In undertaking the treatment of a case of this distressing malady, the first necessity is to ascertain if the husband is at fault. Scanzoni has usefully directed us to this element of the trouble, † and we may with advantage adopt his hints as to the general management of the patient. But cases will often occur in which such measures are insufficient, and you then have a substantive malady to treat – a reflex hyperæsthesia of the nerves of the part. Dr. Skinner ‡ tells us that Sir James Simpson, who saw multitudes of instances of the affection from all parts of the world, admitted that in a great many of them it was a pure Neurosis, only to be reached by long-continued courses of Anti-neuralgic medicine like *Iron* and *Arsenic* ; and that, in spite of these remedies and surgical measures, failure to cure was the rule in his hands. Dr. Skinner himself records two cases of apparent cure. In the first, *Silicea*—given because of the concomitant head symptoms—removed these and the Vaginismus in a fortnight ; and, as the patient had not applied to him for two years since, he fairly counts her recovery to have been permanent. In the second case, a temporary removal of the trouble (which had lasted two years) twice occurred—the first time under **Nux vomica**, the second under **Ignatia**, A few weeks after the change wrought by the latter, her husband was drowned, so it is impossible to say whether the trouble might not have returned. Dr. Villers also has recorded a case which recovered under the **Belladonna.** ||

These remedies seem excellently suited to the Pathology as well as the Symptomatology of the disease, and should be considered in any case which may come under our notice. I may mention that Vaginismus has been observed as one of the effects of Lead-poisoning, which gives us *Plumbum* as a possible remedy for it.

PROLAPSUS VAGINÆ, after reposition, and with the aid of recumbency, may be materially benefited by **Stannum**.

---

* See J. B. H. S., viii., 75. † See PRACTITIONER, i., 381.
‡ THE ORGANON, i., 76. || J. B. H. S., ii., 93.

VULVITIS, as occuring in children, will be considered hereafter. In adults, Acute Vulvitis rarely occurs save in connexion with Vaginitis, of which it forms a part and in whose treatment it shares. When it does appear independently, there being no drug which has so intense an action upon the external genitals as *Arsenicum*, I should be disposed to rely upon it in preference to any other medicine. Chronic Vulvitis is either Eczematous under our notice in connexion with the diseases of the skin. For the latter, *Mercurius*, *Thuja*, and *Sepia* have been recommended.

ACUTE LABIAL ABSCESS (I speak of the circumscribed variety, generally, if not always, an inflammation of the vulvo-vaginal glands) requires different remedies from those of Vulvitis in which the surface is the part mainly affected. There is a case in the Twenty-Fourth Volume of the BRITISH JOURNAL OF HOMŒOPATHY in which **Apis** seems to have arrested the progress of the inflammation. Jahr says that "an inflammatory swelling of the labia major, if not very intense, generally yields to a single dose of *Sepia* 30, and if acute, and threatening to suppurate, to a single dose of *Mercurius*."

CANCER PUDENDI is, like that of the external generative organs of the other sex, usually of the epithelial variety, and is somewhat amenable to treatment. **Conium**, **Arsenicum** and **Thuja** are the medicines likely to help. In a case which I had the opportunity of treating for a short time I saw marked relief from the lancinating pains afforded by the higher dilutions of the two former medicines.

NYMPHOMANIA is generally associated with some irritation of the external parts, and I accordingly mention it here. It is happily rare in the present day ; but our older Homœopaths seem to have had some experience in its treatment. Hahnemann himself has recorded a case, * in which **Hyoscyamus** was the principal remedy. **Platina** also is generally recommended ; it would be especially serviceable when ovarian irritation lay at the root of the symptoms. *Gratiola* is said to have caused, and *Origanum* to have both caused and cured this form of Mania. † Mr. R. K Ghosh tells a remarkable story of Nymphomania occuring in a young Hindoo bride, to the distress of her husband, who found himself quite unequal to the tasks imposed upon him. *Ptatina* caused only temporary relief, but *Coca*, in the I_x dilution and mother-tincture, effected a steady and fairly rapid cure. ‡

---

* See B. J. H., vii., 494.   † See N. A. J. H., xv., 62.
‡ J. B. H. S., iv., 139.

INFLAMMATIONS OF THE MAMMÆ 689

The treatment of the affection of the urinary organs in the female, does not differ from that of the similar disorders occurring in the male subject. But one of these is peculiar to the former sex, and deserves special mention. I mean –
VASCULAR TUMOUR OF THE URETHRA.—Before resorting to surgical measures for this trouble, it might be well to try the administration of **Thuja**, to which medicine its nature and origin strongly point ; or of the **Eucalyptus globulus**, with which a very competent observer, the late Dr. Woodbury, of Boston, U.S.A., professed to have obtained several cures.

Before leaving the female organs of generation I must say something about—
STERILITY.—Many of the ovarian, uterine and vaginal diseases already enumerated are associated with Sterility, and the treatment of the latter will accordingly be that appropriate to the former. But if none of these exist, and no mechanical impediment to the ingress of the Spermatozoa be present, and there be no fault on the husband's side, then a course of Homœopathic medication may be tried with fair hope of success. The constitution of the patient, and any symptoms of ill health she may have, must be taken into account in your prescription. Apart from these, **Borax** and **Conium** are the medicines most in repute ; the former is said to be indicated by the co-existence of an acrid Leucorrhœa, the latter is suitable to depressed ovarian activity. I have twice verified the recommendation of *Borax*.

The diseases of MAMMÆ, of most frequent occurrence and practical importance, are those which occur during Lactation. These will be considered among the disorders incident to the Puerperal state. But I must speak here of the INFLAMMATIONS and the TUMOURS which occur during the dormant intervals of the breast's existence.
1. There are TWO inflammatory states to which the mammæ are liable. The FIRST is rather HYPERÆSTHETIC CONGESTION ; it is that which in some women occurs at every menstrual period. The SECOND is what is used to be called 'IRRITABLE MAMMARY TUMOUR' ; and which I have hitherto described under that name, likening it to Ovarian Neuralgia and Irritable Testicle. Mr. Birkett, in Quain's 'Dictionary', adduces good reason for believing it to be a CHRONIC LABOUR MASTITIS.
Now for these inflammatory conditions we have three prime remedies in **Conium, Belladonna** and **Phytolacca**. It is difficult to distinguish between them ; but *Conium* (of which in "Irritable Mammary Tumour," Sir Astley Cooper had so high an estimate) had seemed to me most useful when painful glandular enlarge-

ments have followed blows upon the breast. It is, however, effective enough in the catamenial form. * *Belladonna* would be the better-indicated, the more obvious was the inflammatory condition; Dr. Wingfield gives a case in the Thiry-Ninth Volume of the MONTHLY HOMŒOPATHIC REVIEW (p. 143) where a Tumour of six months' standing, suspiciousiy like Cancer, disappeared in a fortnight under the 1_x dilution. *Phytolacca* has been used successfully by Dr. E. M. Hale for the tendency of the breasts to grow tender and painful at the monthly period. † Jousset praises *Murex* for the pains of these cases calling it nearly infallible; and Jahr speaks of dispersing the Tumour with *Calcarea, Chamomilla, Belladonna, Lycopodium* and *Phosphorus*. More recently, two of the American indigenous remedies have acquired high repute in the treatment of Mammary Tumours. These are **Phytolacca and Hydrastis**. The action of *Phytolacca* upon the breasts is well-illustrated by Dr. E. M. Hale in an Article upon it in the Twenty-First Volume of the BRITISH JOURNAL OF HOMŒOPATHY. He states that he has treated several cases of Irritable Mammary Tumour successfully with *Phytolacca* in the lowest dilutions. *Hydrastis* has a still more general reputation. I shall have to speak directly of its claims as a remedy for Mammary Scirrhus. But if you will read Dr. Bayes's Paper on the subject in the ANNALS (Vol iii, p. 489). and the discussion following, you will find that even those who doubted its efficacy in the Malignant, spoke highly of its power over the Simple Tumours of the Breast. It may be used externally as well as internally with advantage.

MAMMARY SCIRRHUS.—I speak only of this form of Cancer of the Breast, as there is no doubt that the encephaloid variety ought to be removed by operation as soon as detected. But as we have some prospect of being able to curc, or at any rate to retard the progress of Scirrhus in this situation, the question between submission to immediate surgical measures and a trial of Homœopathic medication may fairly be raised.

In speaking of the power we have over MAMMARY SCIRRHUS, I am not referring to anything which our ordinary medicines can do,—not even including **Conium**. Dr. von Viettinghoff speaks of this medicine as "specific in Cancerous induration of the mammæ attended with lancinating pains" But his cases do not bear out his assertion, That it will to some extent relieve the pains themselves I do not doubt, but I think it has yet to be proved that it has power of checking the progress of the disease. The remedy whose introduction has given us new hope is the **Hydrastis Canadensis**. You will remember the facts and cases I brought forward when lecturing upon this

---

* J. B. H. S., iii., 207.   † B. J. H., xxi, 205,

drug. * Should a patient come before you affected with this disease, you will do well to look over the observations to which I have there referred. If the case be one of those in which benefit may, upon those data, reasonably be expected from *Hydrastis*, viz., "Scirrhus in an early stage occurring in well-developed breasts," you will do well to give it a fair trial. Administer it internally, in varying dilutions, and apply it externally in not too strong a lotion (20 drops of the tincture or strong infusion to a pint of water for continuous use, 3j to 3jj to relieve the pain.) When the medicine acts, the improvement is speedy ; so that if after a month or two there is no change for the better there is no longer hope from this source to stand in the way of an operation, if that be otherwise admissible. If, moreover, after temporary improvement from *Hydrastls* a relapse occur, there is little use persisting in it. Dr. Dudgeon records a case where *Hydrastis* aggravated, but *Curdurango* cured an apparently Malignant Mammary Tumour. †

Should operation be inevitable, you will consider the evidence adduced by Drs. Marston and MacLimont in favour of enucleation by *Chloride of Zinc* in preference to excision by the knife. Their papers on the subject are in the Twenty-First and Twenty-Third Volumes of the BRITISH JOURNAL. Dr. Edward Madden, of Birmingham, has taken up their practice, and tells me he gets excellent results therefrom.

Silica in substance, and *Arsenicum* in the higher dilutions, have been found palliative of the pains of Scirrhus while unbroken ; *Chlorate of Potash* and *Citric acid* locally when ulceration has occurred.

The COCCYX is so intimately related with the female sexual organs, that I may speak here of the only malady of which it is the seat—

COCCYGODYNIA.—A full account of this not unfrequent affection is given by Dr. Guernsey, with indications for a number of medicines. I can confirm his view as to "traumatism" being the most frequent cause of the pain—the injury is often, I think, received during childbirth ; and also as to the value of **Arnica** under such circumstances, though I have not found a "very high potency" necessary. In other cases owing the same origin, **Rhus** or **Ruta** may be useful ; and where the pain is not traceable to injury, **Phosphorus** or **Lachesis**. The last medicine is specially indicated (Dr. Guernsey says) when all the suffering is experienced on rising from a sitting posture.

---

*See a striking case by Dr. Kidd, in his 'LAWS OF THERAPEUTICS' (p. 230). † H. W., xxiv., 543.

LECTURE L

DISEASES OF THE FEMALE SEXUAL SYSTEM

—— 0 ——

PREGNANCY, PARTURITION, THE PUERPERAL STATE AND LACTATION,

—— 0 ——

DISORDERS OF PREGNANCY— MISCARRIAGE—DISORDERS OF PARTURITION—POST-PARTUM HAEMORRHAGE—PUERPERAL CONVULSIONS—DISORDERS OF THE PUERPERAL STATE-PUERPERAL INSANITY—DISORDERS OF LACTATION—MASTITIS—PHLEGMASIA ALBA DOLENS.

I have now to consider the maladies—hitherto purposely omitted—from which the woman is liable to suffer in discharging her great function of maternity. We will take first the DISORDERS of PREGNANCY. The treatment of these is very fully discussed in the Treatises of Leadam and Peters ; and I shall make much use of their recommendations. I shall draw also upon an excellent little manual by Dr. Pope, entitled, 'A MEDICAL HANDBOOK FOR MOTHERS'.

There are two primary facts about every pregnant woman—that her blood is super-fibrinated' and her nervous system hyperæsthetic. The former lies at the bottom of the subfebrile condition which is sometimes met with in the early, but more frequently in the latter months of pregnancy. This is greatly under the control of **Aconite**. The excess of fibrin, is a Physiological, not a Pathological change ; and it has overstepped the boundary of health when fever is induced by it. The Hyperæsthesia, also, need not be morbid. It does not take much, however, to fret it into irritability of temper, sleeplessness, and other mental disturbances. It is probably also the cause of the readiness with which other organs sympathize with the uterus,— reflex excitability being increased. Hence also the Cramps and Spasms and "Fidgets," and the "False Pains," which are observed in these subjects. The remedies for each of these will be given as we go on. I mention the general condition chiefly to suggest that it indicates the higher dilutions of our medicines as most suitable for the Disorders of Pregnancy,—an indication which experience has generally confirmed.

I will take the ailments of the pregnant woman in the same order as that in which I have been considering the maladies of the human species in general. Accordingly, having already spoken of the fever which is her special blood-disease, I will

PREGNANCY 693

pass on to the disorders of her brain, spine, and nervous system in general.

MENTAL DIORDER—in fully developed Mania or Melancholia—attacks not so much the pregnant as the puerperal woman. But there is a condition of mind met with in the former, which is unquestionably morbid. It is characterized by irritability of temper, readiness to shed tears on slight provocation, undue fear of the approaching confinement, and so on. A good many medicines are mentioned by Peter and Guernsey as suitable to special shades of this state of mind. I myself have found **Actæa racemosa** so beneficial for it, that I have rarely had to resort to any other remedy. If I needed such, I should expect to find it in **Pulsatilla**, which Dr. Leadam commends highly. When crossness is the most evident symptom, **Chamomilla** is useful; and when the dread of death in the approaching confinement amounts to Monomania, **Aconite**.

The HEADACHE of pregnant women is not, to my knowledge, different from that which they have at other times, and whose treatment we have already discussed. In the early months it is usually Nervous, in the later months Congestive. You will remember of course, that it is sometimes one of the warning signals of the supervention of Albuminous Nephritis *

SLEEPLESSNESS in these subjects often arises from a febrile state of system, and will be removed by **Aconite**. When this cause is not operative, you will find **Coffea** or **Pulsatilla** useful, when the patient cannot get to sleep for a long time after retiring; **Nux vomica** or **Sulphur** when she sleeps at first, but wakes early in the morning and cannot get off again. In the latter months sleep is often hindered by Cramps in the Calves, or a sense of painful restlessness in the lower extremities, which they call "Fidgets." Here I have found **Chamomilla** very beneficial. Dr. Leadam speaks highly of **Veratrum** for Cramps.

The digestive organs sympathise with the gravid uterus more, perhaps, than any other part of the body. Toothache, Salivation, Vomiting, Heartburn, Constipatton—are well-known troubles of Pregnancy. Let me give you some hints as to their treatment.

The TOOTHACHE of Pregnancy may either be a sympathetic Neuralgia, or may arise from Caries of the Teeth produced or furthered by the patient's condition. In the latter case **Kreosote** (and, as some say, **Staphisagria**) will act as well as in other circumstances. But in the former the ordinary medicines—

---

* In a case where it occurred during a POTS-PARTUM Albuminuria, *Picric acid* 12 proved curative both of cause and of consequence. J. B. H. S., i.. 74.

Aconite, Belladonna, Coffea and *Chamomilla* – will rarely give more than temporary relief ; while uterine medicines like **Sepia** and **Magnesia carbonica** are curative, **Calcarea**, also, is recommended, perhaps best in the form of its compound with *Fluorine*.

SALIVATION is one of the most obstinate of this class of affections. *Mercury* and *Iodine* are Homœopathic enough ; I wish I could say they were curative. The newer medicine, **Jaborandi** may prove more effective. I have myself hardly found it so ; but others have reported more favourably of it.* Dr. Leadam recommends *Sulphur,* followed by *Natrum muriaticum* (when there is much gastric and buccal disorder) or *Arsenicum* in obstinate cases.

The VOMITING of Pregnancy must generally be treated otherwise than as an affection of the stomach. **Nux vomica,** which is perhaps its most important remedy, probably acts by diminishing the reflex excitability which enables the uterus to disturb the stomach. **Kreosote,** whose sphere is "Sympathetic Vomiting," is a remedy of the same kind. Again **Sepia** is reputed to be one of our best medicines for this trouble ; and here we must suppose that the action is upon the uterus itself, the starting-point of the morbid circuit. It is especially useful when the uterus has previously been unhealthy. It is only when the stomach has become irritable, and most of the food is ejected as soon as taken, that **Ipecacuanha** is suitable ; and even here it is in my experience best alternated with *Nux vomica. Apomorphia* should be considered in obstinate cases ; also *Cuprum aceticum* and *Arsenicum.* †

HEARTBURN is often a great trouble with these patients. It is not necessarily associated with Acidity ; if the latter be present to any extent you may give **Calcarea**, and let our patient take freely of the sub-acid fruits, which are always grateful to her. If the Heartburn stands alone, **Pulsatilla** and **Capsicum** are the most useful medicines.

Respecting the strange TASTES and LONGINGS which pregnant women not uncommonly display, I think it well to gratify them unless the substance desired be injurious, as chalk or cinders, or the digestive organs be obviously disordered. In the latter case, treat these upon the usual principles. The longing for chalk often implies Acidity, and that for cinders Flatulence, so that **Calcarea** and **Carbo vegetabilis** may remove the symptoms. Other medicines are recommended for the various morbid

---

* See J. B. H. S., ii., 99.   † IBID., i,, 177 ; viii,, 155,

cravings by Leadam, Guernsey and Peters; but I know not on what grounds.

CONSTIPATION is no uncommon accompaniment of Pregnancy especially in the early months, when I suppose it to depend upon a sort of congestive inertia of the lower bowel. Better than all the ordinary remedies of this trouble (which, however, must be used if especially indicated) I find the **Collinsonia Canadensis**, which I recommend to be given in the 1st, 2nd or 3rd dilution. It is no less useful for HÆMORRHOIDS, when these occur in connexion with Constipation.

DIARRHŒA is far less common than Constipation. **Pulsatilla** is generally its remedy, the characteristic indication being often present that the stools occur mainly at night. Secale and Phosphorus or Phosphoric acid, are sometimes, preferable,—the latter especially when there is prostration and loss of flesh. In obstinate cases, Leadam and Jahr concur in recommending **Sulphur**.

An abdominal trouble connected—in the mind, at any rate—with Pregnancy is its simulacrum, PSEUDO-CYESIS. When it is the movements of the child that are simulated, *Crocus* may be, as it has been,* effective to remove the sensations.

The only symptoms of the respiratory organs with which I am acquainted in connexion with Pregnancy are COUGH and DYSPNŒA. The Cough is either from vascular fulness of the chest, when **Aconite** will relieve; or is a spasmodic one, from reflex excitation. **Belladonna**, in the first decimal dilution has been my favourite medicine in the latter case. But should any of the indications, now familiar to you, for *Ipecacuanha*, *Hyoscyamus*, *Corallium*, *Drosera* or *Conium* be prominent, you will do well to give these medicines as though no Pregnancy were present. The Dyspnœa and oppression often complained of in the latter months is gastric rather than pulmonary; and I can quite believe Dr. Leadum that **Nux vomica** is its best remedy, though. *Lycopodium* and and *Apocynum* must be remembered.

The BLADDER, from its proximity to the uterus, is even more liable to be affected than the rectum in Pregnancy. In the early months it is usually a sympathetic tenesums of the neck which is present. I have found **Belladonna** here again very useful, in the 1st decimal dilution; but Jahr says that **Pulsatilla** will hardly ever fail to relieve. *Nux vomica*, *Ferrum* and *Cantharis* are possible alternatives, and smelling at *Camphor*

---

* J. B. H. S., i., 176

will often give temporary relief. Once, in an obstinate case, *Staphisagria 6*, proved curative in my hands. Towards the end of the time, the frequent calls to pass water are, I think, of mechanical origin,—the capacity of the viscus being diminished by the pressure of the womb.

A much more important affection of the urinary organs induced by Pregnancy is ALBUMINURIA, with its accompanying Anasarca. This is an indication (as you know) of the supervention of a form of Bright's Disease in the kidneys. I had thought it a Venous Congestion, of mechanical origin, liable to go on (like that of cardiac disease) to induration and atrophy ; and had supposed *Colchicum* to be its most Homœopathic remedy. Later observation, however, has shown it to be a true Tubular Nephritis ; and we thus explained the repute which **Arsenicum** and **Apis** have gained in its treatment. Dr. Ludlam speaks still more decisively in favour of **Mercurius corrosivus**. With one or more of these remedies you should ply your patient, so that she may not incur the risk of Eclampsia involved in her reaching the time of Parturition with albumen still passing in her urine.

Dr. Burford has shown * that simple renal inadequacy, without inflammation, may be the condition induced by Pregnancy ; but hitherto no remedies have restored the lacking function.

And now of the troubles which the GRAVID UTERUS causes to itself, and to other parts of the female sexual system —

Sometimes the commencing ENLARGEMENT OF THE WOMB is attended with much distress. Here Leadam recommends **Nux vomica, Pulsatilla** or **Belladonna** —according to the symptoms, or the patient's constitution.

In others the natural ENLARGEMENT OF THE BREASTS at this period causes undue pain and tension. **Conium** and **Pulsatilla** are suitable here when Neuralgia predominates, **Bryonia** and **Belladonna** when the symptoms are rather inflammatory.

PRURITUS PUDENDI is a very troublesome accompaniment of early Pregnancy. **Collinsonia, Caladium** and **Ambra** are its best internal remedies ; but local palliatives are required. You must not forget that Follicular Vulvitis (Q v.) is sometimes present as the cause of this trouble ; in which case you will think of **Borax**.

As the uterus increases in weight, it often causes a very distressing dragging PAIN IN THE LUMBER REGION. I mention this pain because it has often been relieved by a curious medicine for it, **Kali carbonicum**. Leadam mentions *Nux-vomica, Rhus* and *Arnica* as occasionally required.

---

* J. B. H. S., viii., 128.

MISCARRIAGE

Sometimes the uterus itself is the seat of pain, and resents pressure and the movements of the child. This is described by Cazeaux as RHEUMATISM OF THE WOMB. Actæa racemosa, with or without Aconite, ought to benefit it. Two cases are mentioned in the NORTH AMERICAN JOURNAL OF HOMŒOPATHY for February, 1896, in which this symptom was removed by *Opium*—not given as a narcotic but in the sixth dilution.

The "FALSE PAINS" of later Pregnancy have generally been checked by **Chamomilla** in my hands ; but Drs. Drury and Leadam both recommend the higher potencies (*12*th or *30* th) of **Pulsatilla**. Sometimes, when they seem truly uterine, and recur regularly as if Parturition were beginning, I have seen them rapidly banished by giving after each a drop of the mother-tincture of Secale. Caulophyllum also is suitable here.

MISCARRIAGE—The treatment of this accident is prophylactic as well as curative. The fault which causes the tendency to its occurrence may lie with the ovum, with the placenta, or with the uterus itself. If the ovum be the cause, it is usually that it is Syphilitic. If the mother also manifest symptoms of this taint, by treating her accordingly, you may remedy the infant's condition. But if she be free, I think it well to try whether the administration of occasional doses of a high dilution of **Mercurius** may favourably modify the nutrition of the fœtus. This plan has proved successful in the case of Scrofulous offspring—*Sulphur* and *Calcarea* being the medicines given.*

The error of the placenta which leads to Abortion is usually Fatty Degeneration. It should be worth while trying the administration of **Phosphorus** in cases where this change was deemed likely to supervene. When the womb itself, without extraneous reason, is given to casting untimely fruit, medicine can do much in the way of prevention. Ascertain first whether its irritation is secondary to that of the ovaries ; and if so, treat the latter organs,—as with **Apis** which Dr. Guernsey recommeds, and which has caused Abortion when given to pregnant women. If not, remember that the muscularity of the uterus is small during the earlier, greater during the later months of Pregnancy. In Abortion occurrring during the earlier months accordingly, **Sabina** would be more suitable than **Secale**, and VICE VERSA if the contrary obtained. These are the medicines most in repute for the prevention of the habit of Abortion.

When hæmorrhage and pains indicate that Miscarriage is imminent, we have some remedies which will materially aid perfect rest in adverting the accident. First, you will ascertain the cause ; and if this be mechanical, will give **Arnica**, if

---

* See M. H. R., xxxiv., 603.

emotional—as from fright or other nervous agitation **Chamomilla**, or **Aconite** if the fear continues. If neither of these causes is in operation, and the symptoms have occurred spontaneously, the **Sabina** or **Secale** already recommended as preventives will be no less useful as curatives. * If pains are present, it is best to give a dose after each ; but if there is hæmorrhage the doses must be frequently repeated.

Should Abortion prove inevitable, you must take the proper measures for promoting the complete emptying of the womb, and the subsequent recovery of the patient. Medicines do not play an important part here ; but Dr. Guernsey has found **China** of great help when "the membranes of an early ovum remain for weeks, keeping up a more or less constant hæmorrhage." It is, he says, not only of value as remedying the results of the loss of blood, but as "serving in a remarkable manner to arouse the expulsive action of the uterus."

I come now to the DISORDERS incident upon PARTURITION. This, like Pregnancy, ought to be a Physiological process ; but too often in our day and society it presents Pathological features. These we are often enabled by Homœopathic medication so to modify that they give place to the normal phenomena of the process. Many of them, of course, are beyond the reach of such means ; and you will understand that in those dystocic conditions I have left unmentioned, you must do your best upon the common principles of the Obstetrical Art. Perhaps we have fields here yet to conquer ; for indeed this is a department which has not been assiduously cultivated by Homœopathic practitioners. The position in which most of us are placed in this country at least, makes it impossible for us to attend confinements. The result is that we have little practical experience of the application of our remedies to the accident of Labour ; and I shall therefore rely mainly, in addition to my own limited experience, upon the recommendations of those few who have devoted themselves to this branch of practice. They were few when I wrote thus in 1878. But the Homœopathic Journal of Obstetrics, Gynæcology and Pedology, now in the twenty-fourth year of its existence, shows that America at least has not failed to attend to this department of our art ; and the Papers read by Mr. Rean before the British Homœopathic Society, † by Dr. Robertson Day before the Congress of 1891, ‡ and by Dr. S. P. Alexander before the Western Counties Therapeutical Society, ○ show, both in themselves and in the discussions they evoked, warm interest in the subject.

---

* See IBID, xlii., 323 and J. B. H. S., vi., 397, for confirmation from both schools as to *Secale.*
† ANNALS, x., 413. ‡ M. H. R., xxxv., 578. ○ IBID., xxxvii., 76,

There is an ante-partum opportunity for medicine here. Can we do anything to approximate the labours of civilised women to those of their Indian sisters, who will drop out of a march to produce their babies in a convenient wood, and rejoin the column ere it has gone too far? Mr. Rean says we can with **Arnica**, and Dr. Day reports like results (which many have had before him *) with **Actæa** and **Caulophyllum**—all in the 1_x dilution. Dr. Alexander confirms the experience of the two last medicines, but suggests that they should be chosen not in a routine manner, but on the strength of the symptoms present at the time of administration, or dreaded thereafter.

The earliest object for which you may have to administer medicines to an actually parturient women is to rectify a MAL-PRESENTATION. It seems at first unlikely that such an effect can be looked for from drugs. But we have a sure basis on which to act, viz., the occasional occurrence, and therefore the possibility, of spontaneous version. If the uterus can effect this change to the norm, there is no reason why it should not be aided towards it by specific remedies. **Pulsatilla** (generally given in high dilutions) is the medicine credited with the power of furthering natural version. In a Paper on "Homœopathic Tocology," by Dr. Fincke, in the Sixth Volume of the AMERICAN HOMŒOPATHIC REVIEW, you will find a collection of the cases in which under Homœopathic treatment a mal-presentation has been rectified; and further experience of the same kind is recorded by the late Dr. Mercy Jackson, in the Transactions of the American Institute of Homœopathy for 1875. They may of course have been coincidences; but you cannot do wrong, should you encounter a case of this kind, to give a dose of *Pulsatilla 6 to 30*, and wait a while for a chance of a favourable change. Dr. J. S. Ayres has reported two cases in which the 6th dilution seems quite unmistakable to have effected such purpose. †

The next CONTRETEMPS which may need help is a RIGID and UNDILATABLE CONDITION OF THE OS UTERI, hindering progress. Dr. Leadam tells us that results of magical rapidity may almost always be obtained here from the *30th* dilution of **Belladonna**. ‡ EXPERTO CREDE is all I can say. Dr E. M. Hale reports a case of this kind in which, after the failure of *Belladonna*, *Pulsatilla* and *Aconite*, **Caulophyllin**, in half-grain doses every fifteen minutes, effected Dilatation in an hour. Dr. Guernsey gives indications for (besides these remedies) *Aconite*, *Chamomilla*, *Actæa*, *Gelsemium* and *Lobelia*. I should have thought that the last two could only have acted antipathically. Mr. Rean has verified Dr. Hale's experience, but not Dr. Leadam's and of Dr. Guernsey's medicines can only speak well of *Aconite*. Dr.

---

* See J. B. H. S., ii., 481; iii., 200, 324; iv., 414; vi., 218.
† J. B. H. S., ii., 99   ‡ M. H. R., xii., 657.

Higbee commends *Belladonna* when the os is really rigid, *Gelsemium* when it is simply inapt to dilate. The uterus may seem to contract the wrong way. ‡

We wlli suppose that now the os is properly dilated, but the PAINS are too feeble to bring the child into the world without assistance. Dr. Leadam tells us that we have two excellent medicines for this condition, **Pulsatilla** and **Secale**, both in the 30th dilution. As far as I can make out the distinctive spheres of the two, according to his experience and that of Croserio, it is that *Pulsatilla* is most suitable when the pains are from the first irregular and unsatisfactory, *Secale* when they are weak from general or uterine exhaustion. I can confirm the praises of *Pulsatilla*, though in the lower dilution ; but confess that this action of *Secale* in infinitesimal doses is at present a mystery to me. But it is well vouched for, and the following case from Croserio seems to show what it can do.

"In the case of a woman, 26 years of age, in her first labour, in whom the sacro-pubic diameter of the superior strait did not offer more than two inches aud a half, I had the patience to wait for seventy-two hours the natural efforts of labour. The head being in the first position, at the end of the second day it began to engage in the superior strait. At the end of the third day, the pains slackened very much ; the woman became very feeble, was pale, exhausted, and had lost all hope. I put *Secal. cor, 30*, into a glass of water. and gave her a teaspoonful at 11 o'clock in the evening. Some minutes after she fell asleep, and slept very quietly for three-quarters of an hour, when, awakened by a violent pain, she made a curageous effort ; and two hours after gave birth to a child, pale and in a state of Asphyxla, but which was recalled to life by proper care. The recovery of the mother proceeded in a regular manner."+

Coffea or **Chamomilla** may be useful if the pains are hindered by being excessively felt or by the general nervous susceptibility of the patient. Where there is entire inertia, the patient making no effort, Dr. M. E. Douglas speaks highly of *Causticum*. † Should the inertia arise from the fœtus being already dead, Dr. Leadam states that a dose of *China 18* before *Pulsatilla* or *Secale* is very serviceable. The same medicine should be of service if loss of blood is the cause of the deficient pains.

And now with or without these aids, the infant is born- but the PLACENTA has not been extruded from the vagina. Can we aid its detachment by medicine ? It seems that we can. A dose of **Arnica** may in all cases be given as soon as the child is separated. If this is insufficient, *Pulsatilla* or *Secale* may be given as for deficiency of uterine contractions during the previous stage. "But in some nervous subjects" writes Dr Leadam, "where tremors supervene during this stage, an

---

* J. B. H. S., 337. ✢ To anticipate an obvious criticism, let me say that such a case should properly have been one for the forceps. ‡ J. B. H. S., ix., 177,

equally or in cases more especialy where there is a tendency to hæmorrhage, even a more singularly effective remedy, is **Ignatia** 3." It is said that the tendency to adherent placenta may be combated by *Hydrastis*.

Once again a dose of *Arnica* may be given before the patient is left, as a prophylactic against AFTER-PAINS. Of these more anon; but I must not leave the subject of parturition without noticing its two most formidable accidents HÆMORRHAGE and CONVULSIONS.

Of—
POST-PARTUM HÆMORRHAGE, Dr. Leadam writes,— "Its treatment by Homœopathic remedies offers to the patient an immunity from danger—not unfrequently the difference between life and death—compared with which Allopathic practice in the most experienced hands is a perfect nullity." Dr. Guernsey speaks still more strongly of the efficacy of our medicines in this perilous accident. But you will say, "Surely the one thing we have to do in Post-Partum Hæmorrhage is to obtain contraction of the uterus. We accomplish this most effectually by cold and pressure. We hardly care even to give *Ergot*, so little time have we for waiting for medicinal action. The administration of infinitesimals seems too supererogatory here to be thought of." I must confess that I should sympathize with you in this objection, so far as the primary importance of such measures as the application of cold (or strong heat) and pressure is concerned. I cannot think that our attention shouid be diverted from these potent means of inducing uterine contraction by any question of medicines. Nevertheless, our old-school teachers have been wont to tell us that *Ergot* has its place in the prevention, at any rate, of Post-partum Hæmorrhage. To give, when this is apprehended, one or two doses of the drug during the last pains, or before the extraction of the placenta, is always reckoned good parctice. Here then, our medicines have their sphere in lieu of *Ergot*, as before in undue protraction of labour. "The circumstances," writes Tyler Smith, "which interfere with efficient uterine contraction after delivery, or produce intertia, are many of them the same as those which lead to powerless labour. Amongst these circumstances are, a general relaxed habit of body, weakness of the abdominal muscles, and Umbilical Hernia. Such conditions are frequently found in the greatest degree in woman who have resided in tropical climates. They occur also in woman who have borne large families." Here **Secale** is indicated; and if the efficacy of the 30th dilution be substantiated, it will be better than the crude drug. "The uterus often flags when Labour has been long delyed from any cause, whether the womb be simply inert, or worn out by prolonged

---

* IBID., v., 91,

action." **Pulsatilla** would be called for by inertia, **Arnica** by fatigue of the organ. "The same result may sometimes, but far less frequently, spring from exactly opposite causes. After a very rapid Labour, or after the extraction of the body immediately after the birth of the head, the uterus may suddenly fail." Here **Ignatia** would be suitable.

For administration during Hæmorrhage itself, Dr. Leadam recommends *Ipecacuanha, Sabina, Crocus, Chamomilla, Belladonna, Hyoscyamus, Ferrum* or *China,* according to the well-known indications for each, such as I have mentioned when speaking of Menorrhagia and Metrorrhagia. D. Guernsey gives indications for many more drugs. He is so confident of the efficacy of the suitable remedy, that he puts aside all the measures ordinarily employed as needless, and relies upon medicines alone. "The most prompt and most efficient measure in such cases," he writes "according to my experience and that of a very large number of able Homœopathic practitioners, is to apply that remedy which is Homœopathic to the totality of the case. This can be done as quickly as any other procedure, and will be found efficient even in those cases where the blood flows PLENO RIVO and threatens almost immediate dissolution." I must confess that my own faith has not been hitherto robust enogh to dispense with the pressure and cold by which I had learnt in student-days to check Post-partum Hæmorrhage, and which I have always found effectual. I do not doubt, however, that the medicine most appropriate to the Metrorrhagia present may be of service ; and the power of **China** to relieve exhaustion, and of *Ferrum* to remove the quasi-congestive head symptoms resulting from this cause, is beyond dispute.

PUERPERAL CONVULSIONS must be discussed here ; as they more frequently complicate Labour, present or imminent than the Puerperal state proper. In treating a case of this kind you must fiirst ascertain if Albuminuria is present, and the Convulsions are uræmic. Should it be so, you may give the remedies whose indications I shall mention presently ; but your main duty is to relieve the pressure on the kidneys by emptying the uterus as speedily as possible.

Abnormal reflex excitability is at the bottom of Non albuminuric Puerperal Convulsion. For this **Ignatia** and **Hyoscyamus** —the latter especially—are most valuable remedies ; and one or other should be administered whenever you see reason to dread Convulsion. **Chamomilla** and **Coffea** are less frequenty indicated :—if the pains, or the sense of the pains, be excessive, they might be suitable. If the patient is actually in a convulsion, or the fits are recurring rapidly, **Belladonna**, is the classical remedy. But I would suggest **Hydrocyanic acid** as a possible alternative, especially in uræmic cases. Mrs. Rean finds it far superior. While you are giving frequent doses of the proper medicine, you will see that no eccentric irritation – gastric, rectal, vesical—which you can remedy exists or remains. But I would not advise you to interfere with the uterus.

I think that by these means you will be able to dispense with the once universal blood letting in Puerperal Convulsions. **Aconite** may sometimes be given with advantage, when of old the lancet would have seemed demanded by the symptoms. The *Chloroform* inhalations of modern practice are not open to the same objection; and in the uræmic form at least I should have no hesitation in using them as temporary expedient till I could effect delivery, should Homœopathic medicines seem insufficient for the purpose.

A dose or two of **Opium** is often very useful for relieving the condition of brain left behind after Puerperal Convulsions; and should Uræmia in parturient women take rather the form of Coma, I should prescribe it in preference to any other medicine.

Some cases by Dr. Wielobycki illustrating the action of several of these medicines may be read in the Fifth Volume of the BRITISH JOURNAL OF HOMŒOPATHY. I may to encourage you conclude with what Dr. Leadam says of the treatement of Puerperal Convulsions : "This is one of those diseases in which the superior efficacy of Homœopathic remedies is beyond doubt. The extreme severity of the attack, the imminent danger, and the fearful consequences would daunt the moral courage of a man who had not perfect confidence in his remedial results; and the contrast between the action of the VIS MEDICATRIX NATURE, which must be slow, and the rapid effects which follow the application of the Homœopathic remedy is sufficient here, at any rate, to determine to what influence recovery is due."

The DISORDERS of the PURPERAL STATE will next engage our attention.

When the patient is a multipara, your first thought must be to diminish the severity of her AFTER-PAINS. For this purpose the dose of **Arnica** I have recommended you to give, before you leave your patient will do much. But if at your next visit you find that the pains are distressing, you must prescribe specially for them. **Gelsemium**, in the *1*st decimal dilution, is the medicine on which I am accustomed to rely; and Dr. Leadam confirms my recommendation. *Chamomilla* or *Coffea*, and sometimes *Ignatia* or *Pulsatilla*, may be required,—the two former by the excessive sensibility of the patient. When the pains are intestinal rather than uterine, **Cocculus** is the most suitable medicine; and when they press upon the rectum or bladder, **Nux vomica**.

IF THE PERINÆM IS TORN, but not badly enough to require stitching up, you will find the local application of **Calendula** of the utmost service to promote healing and union.

The BLADDER may at this time require assistance. If no urine has been passed within twelve hours of the labour, you will do well to give a dose of **Aconite**—Say the 3rd decimal – every fifteen minutes, and wait to see the effect. If this should not succeed in an hour, give **Belladonna** (in a higher dilution) after the same manner. * You will rarely need the catheter. Should the tendency to retention persist, try **Eqisetum** 1_x. ✝ I know nothing of "Incontinence of Urine" after Labour (the dribbling from an over-distended bladder must not receive that name); Dr. Leadam recommends *Arnica* and *Belladonna* for it.

Very painful HÆMORRHOIDS are sometimes developed after Labour. Dr. Leadam recommends **Pulsatilla** 30 for this trouble, and relates a striking instance of its efficacy. In a case I once saw, very repaid relief was given by *Aconite* and *Belladonna*, *Hamamelis* locally, in the form of *Pond's Extract*, is a useful adjunct.

Morbid conditions of the LOCHIA occasionally require attention. If the sanguineous character continue too long, **Sabina** should be given. If the discharge becomes offensive, without uterine mischief or neglect of cleanliness to account for it, *Sepia*, *Secale*, *Carbo animalis* and *vegitabilis* have been recommended; but the most general consent is in favour of *Kreosote*, which I have myself seen act very satisfactorily. Suppression of the Lochia nearly always indicates supervening fever or inflammation, and is the signal for **Aconite**. If the Lochia continue too long, but of natural quantity and quality, Dr. Leadam speaks highly of **Calcarea**, 30. This is generally a symptom of Sub-involution of the Uterus, and Dr. Lawrence Newton esteems *Calcarea* the best of remedies to promote the restoration of the organ to its norm. ‡ **Caulophyllum** 3 has also been given with success; and Dr. Ludlam has found good effect from *Secale* of the same strength. In Sub-involution itself, following Parturition, Dr. Burford has been led to *Potassium*, especially in the form of the *Bromide*, as the most helpful medicine in recent cases, and to *Aurum* in those more advanced. He has had a double *Bromide of Gold* and *Potassium* prepared, from which he gets excellent results. $ (You will remember the the value of the double

---

* See B. J. H., xxvii., 390.   ✝ M. H. R, xii., 286.
‡ B. J. H., xxviii., 241. $ M. H. R., xi., 94.

Chloride of Gold and *Sodium* in uterine enlargements otherwise occurring.

A few words upon the MANAGEMENT OF THE BOWELS after Labour. I need hardly say that Homœopathy, always repugnat to purgatives, repudiates them here with especial abhorrence. We regard them us unnecessary, and often injurious. Tyler Smith says that "left to themselves, the bowels would probably pass a week or ten days in a state of inactivity." The real fact is that spontaneous evacuation generally takes place about the fourth or fifth day. If it be delayed beyond the sixth you may with advantage treat the patient as for Constipation, premising a simple enema to remove accumulations. The rectum is generally at fault, and Collinsonia is the most applicable remedy; but Dr. Leadam speaks highly of *Veratrum* and *Zincum*. If the torpor seem to be in the colon, *Bryonia*, *Opium* and *Nux* are more suitable, according to the usual indications.

DIARRHŒA is not common: when it occurs, **Hyoscyamus** or **Pulsatilla** will be the remedy,—the latter when the evacuations are most frequent at night.

The DISORDERS OF LACTATION play an important part among puerperal maladies; but of these I will speak separately further on. I have now to discuss the treatment of the great Phlogoses and Neuroses which attack the lying-in woman. This I shall do under the heading respectively of PUERPERAL FEVER and PUERPERAL INSANITY.

PUERPERAL FEVER.—The pathological questions raised by this disease are of the utmost interest. Are the various inflammations—Metritis, Peritonitis, Pelvic Cellulitis, Uterine Phlebitis—of the puerperal state only local manifestations of a febrile blood-poison? Is this latter anything PER SE, or is it only an altered form of the Erysipelas with much—if not with other Toxæmiæ —it is interchangeable? What are its laws as to spontaneous origination, epidemic influence, and spread by contagion?— These are some of the points which obstetricians are actively discussing. I have hitherto thought that for therapeutical purposes we need not go beyond the conclusions arrived at by Gooch. * There are two leading forms of the disease. In the first, the inflammation, wherever it is seated, is primary, and the fever is sympathetic therewith. In the other the symptoms of an adynamic fever are present from the commencement, and local affections may or may not be developed. I still think that such a classification stands good. But there must be subdivision under the second head, according as the infection,

---

* See his Essay on Puerperal Fever in the New Sydenham Society's Edition of his works.

which seems always its cause, travels by the lymph-channels or by the veins, according therefore as we have Puerperal Septicæmica or Puerperal Pyæmia to deal with. Let us consider its treatment under these heading.

1. When a chill, followed by the development of pain and tenderness, indicates the supervention of inflammation, you would naturally put your patient upon *Aconite*; or you might do worse. Evidence has been accumulating of late, however, in favour of **Veratrum viride** as more suitable in the premonitory stage of these inflammations, which are always somewhat Erysipelatous in nature. Thus, Dr. Ludlam writes :—"It appears to be especially adapted to the relief and removal of puerperal inflammation. For many years I have been in the habit of prescribing it whenever, in a lying-in woman, the first symptoms of the pelvic or peritoneal congestion show themselves and when my directions have been faithfully followed, the result has been most happy. It restores the milk and lochia when these have been suddenly suppressed, quiets the nervous perturbation. relieves the Tympanites and the tenesmus, whether vesical or rectal, and frequently cuts short the attack. When called in season, I have seldom failed to set aside a threatened Cellulitis by the same means. My custom is to give it in the second or third decimal dilution."

Should, however, the symptoms gain ground, you must substitute or alternate a more locally-acting medicine. When the uterus itself is inflamed, so as to present Puerperal Metritis, I can confirm Hartmann's recommendation of **Nux vomica**, in the higher dilutions. I have been astonished at the rapidity of its action. When the inflammation attacks the peritoneum, and we have Puerperal Peritonitis, **Belladonna** is most frequeutly required, though *Bryonia* and *Mercurius corrosivus* must not be forgotten. **Colocynth**, which is quite Homœopathic to Peritonitis is recommended where Tympanities is excessive. Should the areolar tissue be the seat of the mischief, and Pelvic Cellulitis is before us, **Rhus** is the medicine most likely to avert suppuration ; if this is inevitable, *Hepar sulphuris* should be administered to favour the completion of the process. I have spoken more in detail of this inflammation in my last Lecture.

2. In the most virulent form of Puerperal Fever proper, which kills in a day or two, the only hint I can give for treatment is Tyler Smith's statement that "the blood in these cases resembles that of persons killed by lightning or **Hydrocyanic acid.**" In less FOUDROYANT cases you will give, besides free support and stimulus, either **Rhus** or **Lachesis**; and to these, general consent gives **Hyoscyamus** as a valuable auxiliary. Dr. Custis regards *Rhus* as the main remedy here. "I never saw a case," he says, "where it was not called for sooner or later. So constant has been this experience, that I anticipate the condition by giving it in the absence of other directly indicated remedies, or when

the temperature remains stationary, not improving under the medicines previously prescribed.

So far I have been speaking of Puerperal Septicæmia. Should the mischief begin by uterine Phlebitis or present itself from the first under the pyæmic form, the remedies for that condition indicated in Lecture XLIII. must be brought into play.

PUERPERAL INSANITY may take the form either of Mania or of Melancholia. **Stramonium, Hyoscyamus** or **Cannabis Indica** ought to help Puerperal Mania. The distinctive indications for the two former I have already given when speaking of Simple Mania. The Indian Hemp would be especially called for when the mental delusions were of an exalted character. For Puerperal Melancholia *Platina, Pulsatilla, Aurum* and *Agnus castus* are suitable ; but I have most confidence in *Actæa racemosa*.

The DISORDERS of LACTATION are greatly under the control of our medicines.

At the first coming in of the milk, **Aconite** will hasten the resolution of the fever, and **Bryonia** will relieve undue engorgement of the threatening inflammation.

If the milk is late in appearing, or becomes afterwards diminished in quantity, **Agnus castus** and **Asafoetida** * are the medicines recommended. Sometimes a single dose of *Calcarea* will effect the improvement.

Sulphur, Calcarea, Silicea or **Mercurius** may be given according to the constitutional symptoms when the quality of the milk seems to be at fault, and the child rejects it.

SORE NIPPLES require local applications, among which *Calendula* is important. **Phellandrium,** or in the event of its failure, **Sabal serrulata,** is said to remove the pain felt in these, after each application of the child. Where this pain is of a Neuralgic character, and shoots from the point of the nipple through to the scapula, Dr. Guernsey speaks in high terms of the value of **Croton.**

In WEANING, **Bryónia** will prevent engorgement of the breasts, and **Pulsatilla** or **Calcarea** is recommended to diminish the flow of milk.

---

* See B. J. H., ii., 417, and J. B. H. S., vii., 83.

708 DISEASES OF THE FEMALE SEXUAL SYSTEM

China is, as might he supposed, of the utmost value against the effects of OVER-LACTATION.

And now of the treatment of Acute—

MASTITIS—the much-dreaded "MILK-ABSCESS." I can nearly always promise you an arrest of this inflammation if taken sufficiently early. Bryonia is the great medicine for the purpose, in the 6th or 12th dilution. I have often seen it act most rapidly. **Belladonna** is much praised by Dr. Jousset, and is said to be preferable "when the tumid breast exhibits a surface with Erysipelatous redness, and is glossy ;" but I have never had occasion to use it internally, though before I became aquainted with Homœopathy the external application of the ointment was a favourite practice of mine. Guernsey speaks highly of *Graphites* in cases where there are so many Cicatrices from former suppurations that the milk can s arcely flow. **Phosphorus** is recommended when it is too late to prevent suppuration, to relieve pain, hasten the termination of the disease, and promote the healing of the Abscess. It has several times cured a fistulous condition of the breast left behind after Milk-Abscess. These recommendations as to *Bryonia, Belladonna* and *Phosphorus* I owe to a Paper on the subject from the pen of Dr. Mery Jackson in the Twenty-Fourth Volume of the BRITISH JOURNAL OF HOMŒOPATHY. When the "Caking" of the breast, whether Acute or Chronic is very great, **Phytolacca** is recommended to us by Dr. E. M. Hale ; and from what I have seen of its action I am disposed to confirm his good opinion of it. *

The Last Puerperal Disorder of which I shall speak is the "White Leg" or—

PHLEGMASIA ALBA DOLENS.—When the symptoms of this disease depend upon a Phlebitis extending from the uterine into the crural veins, **Pulsatilla** or **Hamamelis** will pretty speedily effect their removal. But I imagine that the lymphatic vessels (for which we have no such medicines) are often as much to blame as the veins ; and that the latter are as frequently obstructed by coagula from a distance as primarily inflamed. I have certainly found it an obstinate affection ; and Dr. Leadam's indications for remedies read as if hypothetical rather than the result of successful experience. The present view seems in favour for its being a Cellulitis, starting from the parametrium, in which case *Apis* or *Rhus* should be the best medicines for it.

---

* See M. H., xl., 440.

LECTURE LI

DISEASES OF THE SKIN.

—o—

EXANTHEMATA, PAPULAE, VESICULAE, PUSTULAE & SQUAMAE.

—o—

ERYTHEMA—URTICARIA—LICHEN—PRURIGO—ECZEMA—
HERPES—PEMPHIGUS—IMPETIGO—ECTHYMA—
PITYRIASIS—PSORIASIS—ICTHYOSIS.

I have now to speak of the Homœopathic treatment of Cutaneous Diseases. We had not much special literature on the subject till 1877, when Dr. Lilienthal gave us his "Treatises on Diseases of the skin"—a compilation, it is true, but a very useful presentation of our knowledge of cutaneous Therapeutics. We could, however, claim mainly for Homœopathy in the essential meaning of the term, a book that was once a classic in the old school—Mr. Hunt's "Guide to the Treatment of Diseases of the Skin"; * at least that portion of it, quite seveneights of the whole, which deals with the use of *Arsenic*. As such a claim may cause surprise, and as *Arsenic* is now employed (if at all) in cutaneous therapeutics simply as "nerve-tonic," I must make my assertion good before we go further.

Mr. Hunt undoubtedly belonged to the traditional school of medicine; but Homœopathy resides not in the name so much as in the thing. When a medical practitioner publishes a work containing the results of a vast experience in the treatment of the diseases of a particular organ by a single drug specifically related to that organ, we hail it at once as a contribution towards the development of that essential truth of which system called "Homœopathy" is the embodiment. Homœopathic treatment involves an electic affinity of the drug for the part affected; its capacity for affcting such part in a manner resembling the disease; its power, if given in too large dosage, of aggravating the morbid condition; and its superior efficacy when administered singly. Well, Mr. Hunt, maintaining that *Arsenic* is an almost unfailing remedy in cutaneous diseases not Syphilitic or Tuberculous in nature, regards this remedical power as dependent on a specific action of the drug upon the skin (p. 160), and mentions the supervention of mild forms of Pityriasis and Lichen under its medicinal use (pp. 34, 25). He advocates its administration in doses too small to disturb the system generally (p. 17), in one case giving as little as $\frac{1}{480}$th of

---

* My reference are to the Fifth Edition, dated 1861.

DISEASES OF THE SKIN.

a grain of *Arsenious acid* (p. 73); and states that large doses often aggravate cutaneous diseases, which will nevertheless yield to smaller ones. He further urges that *Arsenic* should always be administered singly, and says that "if there be any medicine more dangerous and unmanageable than another, it is the villainous compound of *Arsenic, Iodine* and *Mercury* known by the name of "Donnovan's Solution" (p. 28). By his own testimony, then, the *Arsenic,* Mr. hunt has employed so successfully in skin disease, is a Homœopathic remedy. He admits this explicitly in reference to the irritation of the gastro-intestinal mucous membrane which not unfrequently complicates the disorder of the skin. "It is not generally known," he says, "that *Arsenic,* which in large doses irritates the bowels, in small doses soothes them, and is of eminent utility in checking the Chronic Diarrhœa and gastric irritation" of cutaneous cases (p. 22). Fortunately, this fact is generally known among Homœopathic practitioners, and was proclaimed by them many years before Mr. Hunt's First Edition appeared. His words, in a note appended to his statement, might fairly proceed from the mouth of every contributor to Homœopathic literature, :—"this assertion has been treated with ridicule, but I venture, after twelve year's further observation, to repeat it."

But some of my hearers, who have imbibed the prevalent "nerve-tonic" theory of the cutaneous action of *Arsenic* may ask for further evidence than Mr. Hunt's, of its specific action on the skin. I would ask such to read the section devoted to the subject in my 'Pharmacodynamics,' and $ 24-44 of the posisonings by the drug presented in the 'Cyclopædia of Drug Pathogenesy.' You will there find examples of well-nigh every form of altered nutrition, of inflammation, and of Neurosis from which the skin suffers idiopathically to have been eaused by it as a toxic agent; and we are thus entitled to ciaim from the method of Hahnemann whatever good has resulted from it in this sphere as a remedy. We who avowedly practise according to such method may resemble the present dermatologists rather than Mr. Hunt as to the frequency with which we use it, but this is only because we have other remedies which seem to us more appropriate. When we do use it, we know and acknowledge that we are Homœopathizing.

There is another point in which Mr. Hunt's cutaneous therapeutics is essentially that of Homœopathy, viz., that it seeks to cure skin diseases from within, by internal medication, rather than to suppress them by local measures, as it is now the fashion to do. However untenable Hahnemann's Psora-doctrine is as regards the definite malady, Scabies, with which he connected it, it is—I believe—entirely true in respect of skin-disease in general. It is very rare that this is primiarily parasitic or purely local. It nearly always has its root in the system at large,—at any rate in the recesses of the part at which it appears; and we

ERYTHEMA.

hold it bad practice, and fraught with injury, to be content with abolishing its superficial manifestations. It is much easier to do this, and quicker in the doing, than to cure the morbid state on which the cutaneous malady depends; and the Homœopathic treatment of these affections is often slow in comparison with that of the specialists of the old school. But I think that if you could trace the subsequent medical history of a dozen patients treated on one of the other plan respectevely, you would be satisfied of the superiority or internal medication in regard to the interest of the patient as a whole. Dr. Burnett has devoted one of his little books * to working out this thesis and has done is very effectively.

My classification of skin diseases will present little that is novel. It will be substantially that which has prevailed in the English school since the days of Willan; but I shall fill in the outlines from Mr. Malcolm Morris's excellent Manual.

In the order EXANTHEMATA we shall have to consider (Erysipelas having already come before us as a general disease) ERYTHEMA and URTICARIA.

ERYTHEMA occurs under two forms.

In the FIRST the blush is continuous, and the skin smooth. It is that which arises from local irritation, from frequent suffusion of the skin (as in the face from Alcoholic drinks or Dyspepsia), and from insolation. The cause having been removed, **Belladonna** will be found an excellent remedy for Erythema of the face or the upper part of the body, and **Mezereum** for that of the legs (where it often occurs in oldish people from obstructed circulation, and is called Erysipelas).

Of the SECOND form the Erythema Nodosum is the type. This eruption approximates to the true Exanthemata, being preceded and accompanied by pyrexia, with articular pains. It is supposed by some to be a rheumatic affection—it is called by Hardy, "Rheumatic Purpura." It differs anatomically from Simple Erythema in that some localised effusion has occurred. The benefit obtained from **Quinine** in old-school practice is so great, and its power of causing an Exanthem (mostly Erythematous) has now received so many illustrations, that I am much inclined to suppose it to exert a specific influence here, especially as (according to Jousset) its relation to Acute Rheumatism is of the Homœopathic kind. **Rhus** is indicated on like grounds. Dr. Hansen reports a case in which the patient a woman of 42— had for eighteen years never been free from it save for the three summer months. There were shooting pains in the legs having the modalities of *Rhus*, and causing much restlessness. The *Venenata* variety was given, 5 drops of the 3_x three times a

---

* "Diseases of the Skin from the Organismic Standpoint." London. 1886. "Diseases of the Skin," 3rd Ed., 1894.

DISEASES OF THE SKIN.

day and a complete cure was effected. *Apis* and *Arnica* also may have to be considerded.

Several kinds of Erythema—formerly distingushed as Papulatum, Tuberculatum, Annulare, Circinatum, Marginatum, and so forth according to the shape of the patches—are now classed together as "Erythema Multiforme." They follow the "Nodosum" variety ln being ordinarily associated with pyrexia, and *Quinine* and *Rhus* would be indicated for these as for that. The latter would be preferable in "Erythema Iris", on account of its tendency to form vesicles and bullæ. The **Copaiba** rash a'so frequently simulates Erythema Multiforme. Of Lupus Erythematosus I shall speak when I come to Lupus itself, and of Rosacea under Acne.

And now of—

URTICARIA.—In this disorder—the familiar "Nettle-rash"—the most obvious Homœopathic remedy would be the **Urtica urens**, the *stinging-nettle*, whose effects the malady so much resembles, and which has caused the characteristic wheals when taken internally by its provers. I believed that it is esteemed by some practitioners, and Bahr counts it the principal remedy. I have myself always treated the acute affection (which I have twice had in my own person) with **Apis**, which is no less true a simile to the exanthem, and corresponds better to the nervous and circulatory disturbance often present. Under its use I find the symptoms disappear within three days, while Erasmus Wilson states their natural duration to be seven. *Apis*, I may add, is the better-indicated as the Urticaria approaches the œdematous from ; and the preparation of the sting of the wasp—*Vespa*, it might be called—would be as well if not better-indicated.

In Chronic Urticaria—where any unusual article of diet or change of temperature will bring out the rash—these remedies will rarely be sufficient, and resort must be had to others of a profounder and longer action. *Anacardium, Antimonium crudum, Arsenicum, Chloral, Copaiba,* and *Dulcamara,* have all been found capable of producing the eruption, and may find place in its treatment. **Antimonium crudum** is most suitable, with regulation of the diet, when the exciting cause is gastric ; **Dulcamara** when it is atmospheric ; **Anacardium** when it is emotional (this medicine corresponds especially to the form known as U. TUBEROSA). Mr. Hunt gets excellent results from Arsenic in obstinate cases : and Drs. Dyce Brown, Burnett and Clifton have shown the virtues of *Chloral,* in about grain doses. I used to treat these cases, when without special indicatains, with *Arsenicum* and *Apis* in alternation ; but of late have found

PRURIGO

Chloral (in the 1_x trituration) a single and sufficient substitute. In one case which bids it defiance, I succeeded with *Antipyrin*.

One species of the order PAPULÆ—STROPHULUS—belongs to the maladies of children. The other two are LICHEN and PRURIGO.

For the simple form of—
LICHEN we have no better medicine than **Sulphur**, whose eruption is characteristically papular. For LICHEN URTICATUS, Apis is preferable, and the "PRICKLY HEAT" of the tropics seems to belong to this category. In the LICHEN AGRIUS of the old writers (and also in the LICHEN RUBER of Hebra) **Arsenic** is indispensable.

LICHEN has been almost analysed away by Mr. Morris. According to him, the "Simplex" and the "Agrius" varieties are forms of Eczema ; the "Urticatus" is one of Urticaria itself, and "Prickly Heat" is Miliaria in a tropical degree. Nothing is left but Hebra's "Ruber"—Erasmus Wilson's "Planus"—and while *Arsenic* is a specific for it, such large and long-continued doses are necessary that the practitioner has to be warned against medical poisoning. We must see if we can show a more excellent way, and perhaps we may do it by giving our *Arsenic* in the form of the *Iodide*. Dr. Mackechnic narrates a case of a month's standing, which went on increasing for ten weeks under *Sulphur, Apis* and *Graphites*, but yielded in three or four weeks when *Arsenicum iodatum*, in the 3_x trituration was substituted. *

PRURIGO, when occurring in its "Mitis" form, will generally yield to **Sulphur**, and if you like to apply this substance locally also in the form of baths there is little fear of "throwing in" the eruption. Prurigo Ferox is a tenacious and distressing affection. Here, too, you need not debar your patient from any relief which bran-baths, or those of alkaline, borated and sulphurated nature, may afford ; but you will not be limited to such resources, as the old-school dermatologists of the present

---

* M. H. R., xlii., 51.

day appear to be. They have given up *Arsenic*, which in Mr. Hunt's hands had, with perseverance, done marvels; and have nothing to supply its place. We should not follow them in such neglect, and should use **Arsenicum** as the fundamental medicine, whatever vegetable drugs we may alternate or intercalate with it. Of these we have hitherto depended mainly on the *Rhuses—Rhus toxicodendron* and *venenata*. Some striking cures by these plants, given from the 3rd to the 6th dilution, are recorded in the NEW ENGLAND MEDICAL GAZETTE for March, 1875, by Dr. Conrad Wesselhœft. I have myself mainly depended in these cases on **Mezereum**, of whose action on the skin I have spoken fully in my 'Pharmacodynamics.' *Morphia* and *Chloral* cause great itching of the skin; and Dr. Burkhard commends the former, in the 3rd dilution, alternated with *Terebinthina*, in recent Prurigo. A new candidate for our favour has lately appeared in the Cowhage—*Mucuna*, or, as Linnæus names it, **Dolichos pruriens**. The adjective indicates its power, like the nettle, of irritating the skin by local contact; and though we have not, as in the other plant provings, evidence of the power of doing the same by elective affinity when introduced into the system, clinical experience points in that direction. It was first tested by Dr. Mifflin, of Brooklyn, and Dr. Jean de We'e, of Brussels, in the itching which is apt to accompany Jaundice. Dr. Cartier then employed it in other forms of Pruritus, and with excellent effect. † "It almost always relieves," he say, "even in the most rebellious cases. The dose," he adds, "is a matter of experiment. I now begin with two drops of the mother-tincture a day, and increase the dose by one drop every other day. I have seen the itching stop with two, five and ten drops a day, and have again as much as fifty drops in an extremely difficult case of Senile Prurigo." This is the general experience as to dose; but Dr. de We'e in one of his cases found the 3_x dilution sufficient.

It is right to say that "Prurigo Senilis" is not at the present day recognized as a true instance of the papular eruption, but a generalised Pruritus only. The genuine disease, it is maintained, always begins, if not congenital, in childhood. I would call attention, moreover, to Mr. Hunt's experience of the frequent necessity of Antiphlogistic means in the course of Prurigo. In his day, they often included blood-letting; in ours, the fact may give us a hint as to the possible need of **Aconite**, with a cooling diet and regimen, in addition to our armamentarium hitherto described.

---

* J. B. H. S., i., 177, 278.
† IBID., ii, 219; N. A. J. H., May, 1896, and Sept., 1899.

ECZEMA

I now pass to the order VESICULÆ, which is headed by one of the most frequent and important of skin affections—

ECZEMA—In simple recent Eczema you will very rarely have occasion to use any medicine but **Rhus**. It is exquisitely Homœopathic, and rapidly curative. Its only rival is **Croton**, with which I often precede it when the itching is unusually severe. *Rhus* is Jousset's and *Croton* is Bahr's principal remedy for Eczema Simplex ; so I have good support for my recommendations.

In Eczema Rubrum, **Mercurius** ought to be the specific remedy, as this is pathologically identical with the Eczema Mercuriale. I have found it, especially in the form of the *Corrosive sublimate*, of much value. Jousset recommends, *Cantharis* in the early inflammatory stage ; and here also *Mezereum* must not be forgotten.

In Eczema Impetiginodes, I am inclined to think **Antimonium crudum** the most suitable remedy. I do not follow the latest pathologists in including under this heading all the forms of Impetigo. which is—at any rate clinically—a distinct cutaneous affection.

In Chronic Eczema—when the original vesicles have become transformed into Crusts, Rhagades and Thickenings—**Arsenic** is again an excellent remedy ; but Homœopathy has discovered another in **Graphites**, with which, as a rule, you will do well to commence the treatment. 'Quite recently," writes Bahr, "we have cured an Eczema of seventeen years' standing with *Graphites*, the patient being otherwise in perfect health. She had to continue the remedy for over six months in the fourth to sixth (decimal) trituration, but even the excessively hypertrophied ears finally resumed their normal shape." The oozing of a glutinous moisture is considered by Dr. Guernsey a special indication for this drug.

Some local forms of Eczema deserve special mention. On the hands it appears, when affecting the dorsum, as "Bakers," and "Grocers' Itch," when **Bovista** is recommended ; in the palms it is "Psoriasis Palmaris" and here, besides *Graphites*, **Hepar sulphuris** is excellent. Dr. Cooper commends *Calcarea carbonica*, in low trituration, * and Drs. Royal and Bourjutschky *Petroleum*—the latter having caused the affection in the healthy subject †. When occurring behind the ears, Eczema is a very troublesome disorder, and often needs local measures. *Oleander* however. has cured it. ‡ Eczema Pudendi is especially amenable to *Croton* § ; and when occurring on the face, to *Carbolic acid*. ‖ **Sulphur** and its *Iodide* may be thought of in obstinate cases. ⁕

---

* J. B. H. S., i., 189.   † IBID., ii., 361.   ‡ IBID., iv., 133.
§ B. J. H., xvi., 420.   ‖ J. B. H. S., ii., 102 ; iii,' 322
⁕ IBID., ii., 330, iv., 134.

HERPES, when occurring on the face, should it need treatment at all, would probably get it best from *Natrum muriaticum*, which has caused it. In its Preputial form, *Mercurius solubilis* is equally Homœopathic and curative. But the three most common and important forms of Herpes are SHINGLES, HERPES CIRCINATUS, and DERMATITIS HERPETIFORMIS.

1. SHINGLES (from CINGULUM, in allusion to its generally girdling the waist)—HERPES ZOSTER, ZONA—is a common and interesting disease. It has been treated Homœopathically by many remedies,* but I hardly think we need go far afield. When occurring in young or middle-aged persons, I have always given **Rhus**; and my experience has been that of Dr. Russell, ‡ that this medicine is of itself sufficient to relieve pain and itching to shorten the duration of the eruption, and to prevent SEQUELÆ. In old people, however, the latter were apt to occur in the the shape of both Pruritus and neuralgic pain, until (at Bahr's recommendation) I began to substitute **Mezereum** for these subjects, with which I have been thoroughly satisfied. *Ranunculus*, *Cistus* and **Arsenic** are other drugs which have caused the phenomena of Herpes Zoster, and the latter is forcibly suggested by the vesicular eruption, burning pain and Neuralgia which constitute the affection. Bazin and Trousseau recommend it as well as Imbert-Gourbeyer.

The Neuralgic pains which remain behind after Shingles are sometimes very obstinate; but all remedies above mentioned have been found useful for them, as also the *Dolichos pruriens*, which would cover the Pruritus also.

Two interesting records of experience with Shingles were communicated to the BRITISH JOURNAL OF HOMŒOPATHY for 1877,—the one by Dr. Ker, the other by Dr. Clifton. The former speaks well of *Mezereum* for the remaining pains, and in one case had good results from *Dolichos*, The latter shows how often Neuralgic pains precede by some length of time the eruption, and relates instances in which *Staphisagria* and *Causticum* proved best for these and *Apis* for the eruption. Dr. Garth Wilkinson speaks highly of *Cantharis* lotion locally.

2. HERPES CIRCINATUS (which must of course not be confounded with Tinea Circinata) has in my hands, since the proving of **Tellurium** produced so similar an eruption, always been treated by this remedy; and I have never failed to cure it speedily there with.

3. DERMATITIS HERPETIFORMIS has now been adopted as a generic title under which various vesicular inflammations of the skin, accompanied with great Pruritus, may be classed. Papers upon it have recently appeared from two of our London colleagues, Drs. Washington Epps and Goldsbrough, which

---

* See B. J. H. xx., 492. ‡ IBID., x., 605,

give the clinical history of the malady, besides exhibiting in full detail two histories of cases. * In one *Antimonium tartaricum* in other *Aresenicum* and *Sulphur*, seem to have been the curative medicines. We want more experience here.

We pass on now to the third great member of the order VESICULÆ—

PEMPHIGUS,—"No specific remedy," say the writers of the Article on the disease in Quain's 'Dictionary,' "for Pemphigus yet been discovered; the nearest approach to one is **Arsenic**, which in some cases of relapsing Pemphigus, especially in early life, exerts a marvellous action on the disease, not only removing all traces of it for the time, but restraining its further invasion during long periods." This statement is made on the authority of Mr. Jonathan Hutchinson. If you wish to know on what principle *Arsenic* acts in exerting this curative power, I may refer you to case 33, of the poisonings by the drug collected in the 'Cyclopædia of Drug Pathogenesy,' where you will find a general pemphigoid state, involving also the mucous membranes, set up by it. I should prefer **Rhus** in the rare Pemphigus Acutus, of which I have had a case exhibiting its virtues; and in the Pemphigus Foliaceus should feel disposed to rely rather on **Mercurius**. Dr. Hansen has reported a case of the ordinary kind in a man of 37, in which *Arsenic* did nothing but relieve the accompanying pain. As he complained of night-sweats, and expectorated much mucus, *Mercurius solubilis 1* was given, and a Mercurial-salve applied to ulcers that had formed. In a month he was well. He denied Syphilis. †

The order PUSTULÆ to which we should next come, has since Willan's day been well-nigh refined from the face of the earth. Rupia may indeed be relegated to the class of cutaneous Syphilides, and Porrigo Capitis, with Crusta Lactea and Serpiginosa, are doubtless primarily Eczematous. I do not, however, feel disposed to give up Impetigo as a distinct clicical entity, or Ecthyma as an important variety of it.

---

* See J, B. H., ii,, 242, and M. H. R., xxxviii., 324.
† HAHN. MONTHLY, May, 1895. Cases are referred to in which *Ranunculus bulbosus* proved curative and *Arum triphyllum* where the fluid is acrid (IBID., Oct., 1901).

IMPETIGO is chiefly interesting now-a-days in its contagious form, where it seems to be caused by inoculation of pus cocci. Parasiticide applications are in order here, especially of a Mercurial kind; the white precipitate ointment is the most innocuous. Duhring and Kaposi, however, describe non-contagious forms of Impetigo, and from my own experience I believe them to be right. *Antimony* is here the leading remedy, because of the truest simile, as *Arsenic* is in other cutaneous inflammations. The 'Cyclopædia of Drug Pathogenesy' displays this also especially in Nos. 15-22 of its poisonings by *Tartar emetic*; and herein, I may remark, shows that pustulation of the skin may proceed from internal causes, and is not a mere local irritation as Dr. Liveing maintains.

Impetigo comes before us not unfrequently as a disfiguring eruption on the face. *Tartar emetic* has removed this *; but the best *Antimonial* preparation for it seems to be the *Golden sulphide* (*Antimonium sulphuratum aureum*). The *Black sulphide Antimonium crudum*, answers best—as a rule—for Impetigo of the general surface, † *Kali bichromicum* is a possible alternative to *Antimony* here and *Viola tricolor* in recent Impetigo of the face.

ECTHYMA—"The pustules," says Erasmus Wilson, "following the irritation of **Tartar emetic** are Ecthymatous;" and in the simple form of the disease no remedy should be more effectual. In Ecthyma Cachecticum, deeper-acting medicines are required; and these we may find in **Arsenicum** or **Lachesis** if the pustules appear on the arms, **Secale** if they invade the legs.

And now of the SQUAMÆ which are Pityriasis, Psoriasis and Icthyosis.

PITYRIASIS is, in its simple form, the most frequent among the cutaneous changes induced by **Arsenic**, and Pityriasis Rubra has been observed as an effect of the drug. I can hardly recommend any other medicine, and in this I am supported by Jousset and Bahr. Sometimes the *Iodide* will be found more effective than the *Oxide*. ‡

---

* See J. B. H. S., xxiv., 311 ; xxix., 402.
† Ibid., xxiv., 312., xxxii., 241
‡ See J. B. H. S., vii., 223, 324.

PSORIASIS

PSORIASIS, also, has found in **Arsenic** so specific a remedy, that, as it has also been caused by it, we need hardly look further for its help. It is Jousset's chief medicine for it. *Sepia* is another drug which has been commended ; it would be specially suitable to women with uterine ill-health. I have myself had very good results with *Mercurius solubilis* in recent cases. *Carbolic acid* and *Manganum* have found favourers in France.

So I wrote in 1878. adding that the affection formerly called "Lepra," seemed now to be recognized as merely a Circinate form of Psoriasis ; and that where, in a case I once treated, the constitutional symptoms led me, after *Mercurius,* to *Iodtne*, a speedy and permanent cure rewarded my choice. The whole subject, however, in the light of later observation, need considering afresh.

1. I am not so clear as I was about the Homœopathicity of *Arsenic* to Psoriasis as such. When I said that it had been caused by the drug, I was basing my statement on a case cited by Stille, in his "Therapeutics and Materia Medica". * Reading it again now, it seems to me rather referable to Pityriasis Rubra (in that severe form which has been called "Dermatitis Exfoliativa") than to Psoriasis. I had noted in my 'Pharmacodynamics' that in Dr. Imbert-Gourbeyre's exhaustive list of cutaneous phenomena induced by *Arsenic*, squamous eruptions were not found. That Pityriasis is simulated by it, there is abundant evidence ; can it produce the dry insensitive scale patches of true Psoriasis ?

Therapeutic experience lends more countenance to the belief in the Homœopathicity of the drug, but it is not decisive, I have mentioned Mr. Hunt's curative experience with gr. $\frac{1}{180}$th doses ; and Dr. C. E. Wheeler has had similar results from the 6th dilution. † Both these were cases of Psoriasis Guttata ; but in Psoriasis generally Dr. Wheeler says he has done much better with the 6th dilution than with the 3_x trituration or *Fowler's Solution*. Dr. C. H. Evans relates a case where a patch on the leg had lasted for seventeen years, during which the patient had suffered many things of diverse physicians. The one subjective symptom was that the spot burned night and day, and on the strength of this *Arsenicum* 6 was given, four doses daily. By the end of the third week the heat was reduced by one-half, by that of the fourth it had gone. A week later the scales began to fall off, and a perfect cure soon followed. After seven years there had been no recurrence of the affection.‡ Dr. Arcularius reports two cases actually cured by the 30th dilution. On the other hand, the testimony of old-school Dermatologists is unanimous as to the ordinary necessity of large and long-continued doses. From three to ten minims of

---

* Page 823 of Vol. ii., (4th Ed.),
† M. H. R., xli,, 352.   ‡ CLINIQUE, April, 1893.

Fowler's Solution or one to ten or twelve of the *Pilulæ Asiaticæ*, are to be given three times daily for months. There is general agreement in deprecating its use in acute forms of the disease, where hyperæmia is marked, and in alleging that its first effect is to render the skin redder and more inflamed. "It is of no value" also (so writes Mr. Morris) in the prevention of recurrence.

The facts now brought before you bring me to the same negative conclusion, as that arrived at by Dr. Galley Blackley, in a Paper which you may read in the Thirty-Fourth Volume of the BRITISH JOURNAL OF HOMŒOPATHY. Any scaly appearances observed as the effect of *Arsenic* are secondary to inflammation, not—as in true Psoriasis—Primary; and in old-school Therapeutics it acts simply as an irritant. I have been unable to verify his positive hypothesis, that it is where the output of urea is notably reduced that *Arsenic* acts beneficially in Psoriasis; and would rather rely on symptomatic indications. It is where the surface is hyperæmic and irritable, where burning or itching is much felt—in the very instances, that is, in which traditional medicine forbids its use, that Homœopathy directs it.

2. The recent use of **Borax** internally for Epilepsy has revealed an elective affinity on its part for the skin, and Sir William Gowers has three times observed it cause Psoriasis. * Dr. Mc Clatchey reported most fovourably of its use in the idiopathic disease; †and I have many times verified his experience. I give the 2_x trituration, in three-grain doses.

3. *Carbolic acid* (as I have mentioned), *Cuprum, Kali sulphuricum* and *Thuja* have all recived favourable mention from writers of our school. ‡ But the most promising candidate for honours in this field lately arisen is **Thyroidin.** Noting the "intense desquamation of the skin" occuring in Myxœdematous patients under treatment with thyroid extract, Dr. Byrom Bramwell drew the curiously Homœopathic inference that the remedy might be suitable for Psoriasis, and found it so, to a high degree. He gave it in ordinary small doses. Dr. Halbert, however, reports equally good results from the dilution from the 3_x upwards—"the proportion of cures being," he writes, "beyond my most sanguine expectations." †Dr. C. D. Collins also cured a Psoriasis Diffusa with the 2_x trituration in six weeks. ‖

---

* LANCET, Sept. 24, 1881.   † HAHN. MONTHLY, Feb, 1883
‡ J. B. H. S., ii, 368 ; iii., 455 ; v., 108 ; vii., 328 ; B.J.H., xxxv., 380
†CLINIQUE, Feb., 1897.   ‖ IBID., July, 1899.

ICTHYOSIS

This last experience may be useful in the third of the Squamæ.

ICTHYOSIS—Of this happily rare disease, generally congenital or at any rate inherited, I have hitherto said that it seems little amenable to treatment, even with *Arsenic*; and have contended myself with suggesting *Hydrocotyle* as a possible remedy for it. Thyroidin now bids fair to do more for it than could have been expected. Dr. Swift, in communicating (from Australia) his experience with this drug in cutaneous disease, writes that the class of cases that has derived the greatest amount of benefit has been that of Icthyosis and the allied conditions of Xerodermia and Sclerodermia. He has had twelve cases of Icthyosis and two of Xerodermia under his care, and in only one instance (Xerodermia) has the treatment failed to produce a most beneficial effect on the skin, all the harsh, dry and withered scales being removed, and the skin beneath rendered soft, supple and elastic. He generally begins by giving one-five-grain tabloid twice a day to adults, and gradually increases the dose. In young children he commences with half-a-tabloid PER DIEM. When recovery is well-advanced it is wise to lessen the dose gradually, and give only sufficient to keep up the effect. *

In view of the one exception noted here, I may mention that Dr. Burkhardt, of Berlin, has cured in a girl of 17, a case of Icthyosis dating from birth with *Sulphur* and *Graphites*.

I have now discussed the recognized "orders" of Cutaneous Diseases, and must reserve its remaining varieties for another lecture.

LECTURE LII

DISEASES OF THE SKIN (*concluded*)

—o—

PAPILLAE, GLANDULAR APPARATUS, HAIR-FOLLICLES, GENERAL, LOCAL AND SPECIAL AFFECTIONS OF THE SKIN, NAILS & PARASITIC AFFECTIONS.

—o—

VERRUCA—SEBORRHŒA—MOLLUSCUM—ACNE—HYPERIDROSIS—BROMIDROSIS—MENTAGRA—ALOPECIA—LUPUS—RODENT ULCER—LEPROSY—FURUNCLE—CARBUNCLE—DISEASES OF THE NAILS—ULCERS—TINEA—SCABIES—ELEPHANTIASIS—ACTINO-MYCOSIS—PRURITUS.

I will now speak of the affections of the SEVERAL CONSTITUENTS OF THE SKIN.

The only disease of the PAPILLÆ which can come before us is—

VERRUCA, the WART, including under this name CORNS, CALLOSITIES and HORNS. When a single Wart presents itself for treatment, it is usually cauterised with *Acetic acid* or *Caustic potash*. You may, however, cause its withering away more painlessly, if less rapidly, by touching it daily with the mother-tincture of **Thuja**. It is, however, when crops of Warts appear that this medicine shows its specific power over them; but it is then administered internally. The medium dilutions have generally been employed; but Dr. Orrin Smith gives a case, and refers to another and to his general experience, as showing that it acts well in drop doses of the tincture.* Should it not be entirely successful, follow it up with **Calcarea carbonica**.† This, which is my own experience, is substantiated by most of our Therapeutic writers; though Jahr adds *Natrum carbonicum* and *Causticum* as remedies frequently effective; and the first of the two has several times proved curative in the hands of Dr. Turrel.‡

A recent case which defied both *Thuja* and *Calcarea* led me to look further afield, and my search was rewarded by seeing the excrescences disappear under small doses of *Liquor arsenicalis* as recommended by Erasmus Wilson. Dr. Cooper finds *Ferrum picricum* very effectual. He seems to use the 3_x dilution; but three cases are reported in the HOMŒOPATHIC RECORDER for August, 1898, in which the action of the 6th was all that could be desired.

---

* J. B. H. S., vii., 225. † IBID, vi., 314; vii., 321.
‡ BIBLIOTHÈQUE HOM., Nov., 1876.

It is more especially in "CORNS" that this last medicine has won repute. You may smile at treating such formations by internal remedies, deeming them the mere effects of ill-distributed pressure ; but, like Warts, they too often occur in crops, and are too idiosyncratic altogether in their behaviour to be so considered. Dr. Cooper related a case in the HOMŒO-PATHIC WORLD of June, 1887, in which quite a bevy of these indurations disappeared rapidly under a 2 per cent. solution of the Salt. Referring to this case at our International Congress of 1896,* he adduced two others exhibiting the same result. When the thickening of the skin of the soles is so extensive as to be called a "Callosity" rather than a Corn, you will do well to consider the facts, Pathogenetic, and curative, I have brought forward in my 'Pharmacodynamics' when speaking of **Antimonium crudum**. ✝ The subject of cutaneous "Horns" was brought before us at the same gathering I have just mentioned by Dr. Samuel van den Berghe. The case he alleged, in which the excrescence came away while the patient was taking *Causticum* 30, was not very convincing ; but the discussion tended to show that when such growths were real papillary hypertrophies, and not mere accumulations at the mouth of a sebaceous gland, they might disappear under **Thuja** as Warts do.

I came now to the glandular apparatus of the skin. The affections of the SEBACEOUS GLANDS are SEBORRHŒA MOLLUSCUM and ACNE.

SEBORRHŒA, I place provisionally here, though I am aware of Unna's argument in favour of referring it rather to the sweat-glands. There is an excellent Article upon it by Dr. Washington Epps in the Fourth Volume of the LONDON HOMŒO-PATHIC HOSPITAL REPORTS. While, however, it encourages us in the result of treatment, it does not throw much light on what remedies are likely to be most effective. In the six cases related, as many medicines were given, with two to the last. They were *Graphites, Sepia, Hepar sulphuris, Sulphur* and its *iodide, Thuja* and *Staphisagria.* General Hygiene and mild local Antiseptics played a large part in the treatment.

The form in which Seborrhœa most frequently comes before us in ordinary practice is that in which it effects the scalp, causing DANDRUFF. Kafka is the only one of our authorities who mentions it ; he recommends various medicines, especially *Natrum muriaticum.* I would suggest *Iodine* as of promise. The improvement in the beauty of the hair and the cleanness of the scalp which I have mentioned as following its use in

---

* See its Transactions, iii., 224.   ✝ See also J. B. H. S., iv., 235 (palms and soles).

Scrofulous subjects probably depends upon an influence of the sebaceous glands of the part. An obstinate Dandruff cured by a *Sulphur*-lotion may be read of in the Third Volume of the JOURNAL OF THE BRITISH HOMŒOPATHIC SOCIETY (p. 452).

The sole fact about the treatment of—
MOLLUSCUM which I can find in Homœopathic literature is a case mentioned by Dr. Dudgeon in Part I. of the "Hahnemann Materia Medica." * In this, he states, the Tumours were disappearing under the influence mainly of *Silicea* and *Lycopodium*. As I suppose, however that Wen is simple Molluscum, it seems to the point when I refer you to a case of Dr. Belcher's, in the Twenty-Seventh Volume of the BRITISH JOURNAL OF HOMŒOPATHY, in which a crop of these excrescences on the scalp disappeared under the action of **Kali iodatum**. In connexion with this, it is interesting to note what Mr. Morris writes of Iodic eruptions—"From the elementary lesions various more complex forms of eruption—Ecthymatous, Condylomatoid, Molluscoid, &c.—may arise."

The simple form of—
ACNE, as it occurs in young people, may, if recent, be often cured by **Belladonna** if the patients are full blooded, by **Pulsatilla** if they are pale and slender. The connexion of the affection with sexual evolution probably explains the value of these remedies. In more chronic cases, which yet are Acne Simplex, **Sulphur** is indispensable, ✝ or **Hepar sulphuris**, if suppuration has occurred ; and local application of one or the other is helpful and harmless. I have no experience of the *Lycopodium* (15) so warmly commended by Dr. C. D. Collins. ‡ When Acne Indurata is present, or when Acne Vulgaris resists Sulphureous medication, **Kali bromatum** is indicated by its well-known Pathogenetic effects. It must be given low "One of the prettiest, and at the same time most striking illustrations of the Homœopathic Law," writes Dr. Deschere, "is the curative action of certain *bromides* in various forms of Acne. *Potassium bromide* rarely fails me in Simple Acne of the face and upper part of the body. The *1*st or *2*nd decimal dilution, or one grain of the crude Salt, given three times daily for a week, will remove every trace of the eruption, especially in nervous hyperæsthetic females, without reference to puberty." Dr.

---

* Page 50 of the Article on *Kali bichromicum*.
✝ See J. B. H. S., iv., 230 ; viii., 157. ‡ CLINIQUE, March, 1899.

Cushing speaks as warmly of the *Arsenicum bromatum*, which he gives as high as the $4x$.*

Acne Rosacea is now accounted as a form of Erythema, and classified under its second name—the adjective being made into a substantive. Its treatment, however, moves upon the lines of Acne. *Sulphur* and *Arsenic* (best in their *iodides* or the *bromide* of the latter) and *Carbo animalis* have done most in its medical treatment. Dr. Salzer recommends **Hydrocotyle** and from my own experience I should be disposed to endorse his choise. Bahr, both here and in Acne Simplex, thinks most of *Sulphur* locally,—as by a wash of two drachms of *Sulphur lotum* to two ounces of water.

A word further as to the recommendations of our other authors in Acne. Jousset advises *Kali iodatum* and *Tartar emetic*. Kafka praises *Phosphorus* in obstinate cases, and *Hepar sulphuris* when the diseases assumes a pustular form. Dr. Arcularius, in the latter case, has most confidence in *Cicuta*. Dr. Washington Epps, in an interesting post-graduate lecture on the disease,† expresses his conviction that an excess of both Sugar and Common Salt in the diet will aggravate Acne if it will not actually cause the acneiform condition, and places *Natrum muriaticum* at the head of its medicinal remedies.

Coming now to the SWEAT GLANDS, we have to consider excessive and morbid perspiration.

HYPERIDROSIS, as a general affection, comes before us chiefly as a concomitant of exhausting diseases like Phthisis. Of the sweats of this malady, I have spoken when upon it. I will only add here, to the *Iodine, Stannum, Phosphoric acid* and *Jaborandi* there specified, **Silicea**. Dr. Snader has recently called our attention to this remedy. Of 62 cases in which sweating was a predominant feature in pulmonary affections treated by him in the Hahnemann Hospital of Philadelphia, in 43 the perspirations were stopped, and in 13 they were lessened. The dilutions used were from the 3rd to the 30th, and Dr. Snader thinks that the higher potencies as a rule acted best. ‡

Another malady in which sweat is apt to be excessive is ACUTE RHEUMATISM. Its presence, especially when mal-odorous, always conducts us to **Mercurius**, and this generally suffices for the syndrome as well as the whole morbid state. Dr. Frohling, however, reports a case in which the perspiration persisted and had continued for weeks when **Jaborandi**, in the 4th trituration, was administered. This acted quickly; after the first few doses the sweats ceased entirely, and the patient made a rapid recovery. *

I find *Jaborandi* also very useful, when the flushings of the Menopause are accompanied with undue perspiration. When this last is brought on too readily by exertion, *Phosphoric acid* is very effectual.

So much for general sweating, though its occurrence as a symptom of *Opium*-poisoning must not be forgotten, and Dr. F. H. Pritchard's statement that his experience with checking, exhausting and colliquative perspiration was unsatisfactory until he was led to give *Opium* for it. † *Sambucus*, however, must be remembered—especially in the sweats of child-bed. Local Hyperidrosis, as in the axilla, perinæum and feet, is mostly Bromidrosis, and will be considered under that heading. In an inoffensive way, however, it is apt to occur in the hands, where *Fluoric acid* has chased it from the palms and *Phosphorus* from the fingers. ‡ Unilateral sweating has been checked, in Dr. Ringer's hands, by small doses of *Pilocarpin*. ɔ

BROMIDROSIS is most frequently met with, and here in connexion with Hyperidrosis, in the feet. The usual treatment for this trouble—especially common, in my experience, among domestic servants consists of repressive local applications. Dr. Gallavardin has shown, by copious evidence, that such practice is injurious ; his cases also exhibit **Silicea** as invaluable in first restoring the suppressed secretion, and then bringing it to normal quantity and quality from within. It may also cure in the first instance. ‖ I early had a hint from Dr. Henry Madden that **Petroleum** 2 or 3 would cure this malady, and I have often verified the recommendation. *Thuja* and *Nitric acid* have also proved curative. ⴲ When the odour comes from the axilla ("Sudor Hystericus"), *Sepia* is said to be curative. When it seems to emanate from the entire body, including the secretions, we might be driven to that very dubious and unsavoury medicament "*Psorinum*," ** but a case recorded by Dr. George F. Dunham shows that we may have an alternative in *Nitric acid*. The patient had been troubled by foul-smelling sweat for five years ; stool and urine also being extremely offensive. Ten drops of the 3_x dilution were mixed with four ounces of water, and a teaspoonful taken four times a day. Two prescriptions completed a cure. No external applications were used. ††

---

* J. B. H. S., v., 92 † HAHN MONTHLY, Feb., 1896.
‡ N. A. J. H., April, 1898. ɔ See PRACTITIONER, Dec., 1876.
‖ See J. B. H. S., v., 204. ⴲ IBID., iii., 451 ; iv., 492.
** See IBID., ii., 223. †† N. A. J. H., Sept., 1896, p, 595.

LUPUS

Under the head of affections of the HAIR-FOLLICLES, I have to speak of MENTAGRA and ALOPECIA.

MENTAGRA is more commonly called "SYCOSIS MENTI," but I have used the term Sycosis for another purpose. It is essentially a chronic inflammation of the hair-follicles of the beard. **Tartar emetic** and **Cicuta** have cured it ; and Bahr has had excellent results from **Graphites** (4th and 6th decimal triturations). Jahr says that he has cured a number of cases with *Calcarea* 30, in rare doses. Dr. Stens relates a case cured by *Fowler's Solution*, after *Arsenicum* in the potencies has had little effect.*

ALOPECIA includes as its simplest form the "FALLING OF THE HAIR" which results from local or general debility. **Phosphoric acid** is often very serviceable in these cases. If the BALDNESS be complete, whether general or in patches, you will of course first inquire after a Syphilitic history ; and if the taint be detected, you will, I think, find **Fluoric acid**, the specific medicine for this local manifestation of it. In Non syphilitic cases, Mr. Hunt leads us to expect great things from **Arsenic** ; and, as this drug has caused Alopecia, even in the "Areata" form, † you will feel encouraged to follow his guidance. *Vinca minor* has cured a case where there was great itching of the scalp ; ‡ and *Thallium* must be borne in mind. ††

I will now treat of a number of miscellaneous affections of the skin and the subcutaneous cellular tissue, which I will take as I find them in our official Nomenclature.

Among GENERAL DISEASES are ranked LUPUS, RODENT ULCER and true LEPROSY.

LUPUS occurs in two forms, the "ERYTHEMATOSUS" and the "VULGARIS"—these fairly corresponding with what used to be called the "non-exedens" and "exedens" variety respectively. Though these affections are specifically distinct, they have been so mixed up in time past that much confusion has been caused as to the results of treatment. The Article in my own 'Therapeutics' is vitiated thereby, and I must cancel it in favour of what I shall now say.

1. LUPUS ERYTHEMATOSUS is named by Mr. Morris "ERYTHEMA ATROPHICANS"—a term that well expresses its characters. Unlike its fellow, it is non-tubercular and does not ulcerate.—the only point of contact being that its favourite habitat is the face,

---

* J. B. H. S., ii., 352. † See Cyclo. of Drug Path , ii., 42
‡ J. B. H. S , i., 62 †† IBID., x., 116.

where, spreading over the nose from either cheek, it forms the well-known "BAT's-WING" patch. Of all the cases of Lupus I can find in our literature, two only seem to me to belong to this category. They were reported by Dr. Wingfield in the Forty-First Volume of the MONTHLY HOMŒOPATHIC REVIEW (p. 30). In the first, a solution of *Hydrocotyle* in Glycerine was used as a paint, and *Kali bichromicum* 3_x given internally. Complete cure resulted in a month, though the disease had lasted for eleven years. In the second case the same local application was made, but the *Hydrocotyle* was also given internally in the l_x dilution. Great improvement resulted in a fortnight, when the patient had to leave the city, and passed from observation. In addition to these medicines *Phosphorus* has been commended,* and I would suggest *Thyroidin* for consideration.

2. In regard of LUPUS VULGARIS, our old school authorities are diametrically opposed about treatment. "In healthy subjects," writes Mr. Hunt, "*Arsenic* internally administered is a specific. No local treatment is required." On the other hand, Mr. Morris declares that "*Arsenic*, the administration of which is a kind of ceremonial observance which some practitioners consider indispensable in all cases of skin disease, is useless"; and his Therapeutics of the disease consists in a series of destructive local proceedings, which are as painful as they are formidable. I need not say on which side our sympathies lie, and our own recorded experience corroborates that of Mr. Hunt. "*Arsenic*," writes one of our Belgian colleagues from large dispensary experience, "does not act on Lupus Erythematosus only. It seems to be nearly specific in Lupus of the face, and especially when this is Tuberculous. The lower triturations (2_x to 3_x) have given me the best results, producing primary aggravation with rapid formation of an ulcer. This soon heals after the discontinuance of the medicine or its administration in higher dilutions." † Dr. George Clifton exhibited lately on "Consultation-day" at the London Homœopathic Hospital a case cured, though with many a scar, by *Arsenicum iodotum* 3x to 6x with a weak *Arsenical* paste locally. ‡ But we are not limited in our treatment to *Arsenical* preparations. The *Hydrocotyle* and *Kali-bichromicum* we have already mentioned as benefiting the Erythematous form are useful also here. Dr. Andouit, the introducer of the former into European practice, reports a case of Lupus Exedens cured by it, $ and Dr. James Jones has contributed another.‖ Of the power of the latter Dr. Edward Blake has recorded two instructive cases; he found the 5x dilution more effective then the 3x. ⁕ Dr. Hansen finds it necessary in most cases to supplement *Arsenic* with *Kali iodatum*, in what he calls its "original dilution," but tells of a case cured by this

---

* IBID., iii., 329.   ⁕ JOURN. BELGE D'HOM., Mar.—Apr. 1900.
‡ M. H. R., xli., 35. $ B. J. H., xi., 585.
‖ M. H. R., xx., 509.   ⁕ B. J. H. xxxii., 643.

LEPROSY

medicine alone in the first centesimal. * Bahr commends *Aurum muriaticum*, whose elective affinity for the nose would operate favourably here; and Jousset *Hydrastis*. With this drug, he writes, internally and externally used, he has achieved several cures in cases very far advanced. Dr. Veit Meyer long ago communicated in the Second Volume of the ANNALS OF THE BRITISH HOMŒOPATHIC SOCIETY a case in which the disease, commencing in the left lower eyelid, completely disappeared thence under *Apis 4.* but showed its virulence by recurring in the ala nasi of the same side.

At this point Dr. Meyer's narrative stops; and we are reminded that Lupus is unquestionably a Tuberculosis of the skin, and, whether treated topically or by medicines acting in virtue of local affinities, tends to recur. In view of this, we are led to enquire whether *Tuberculin* will do something for us here. On its introduction into general practice, one of its chief applications was to Lupus; and at first it was thought to be a specific. The hopes awakened soon died down; but Mr. Morris is satisfied that while it does not of itself cure, it prevents recurrence when the disease has been destroyed by other means. This is significant; and perhaps here, as in Pulmonary Tuberculosis, our infinitesimal doses may enable us to give it with results unattainable by the ordinary fractional ones, even though administered PER OS like other medicines.

RODENT ULCER seems to be a deep-seated or at least deep-burrowing—Epithelioma of the face. We have Homœopathic experience in its treatment; but this would be a suitable case in which to try Dr. Mitchell's plan of using **Arsenicum** in trituration internally and locally.

LEPROSY is of course no disease of the skin merely, but it is in this tissue that the ravages of one form of it—the LEPRA TUBERCULATA—are mainly displayed. This terrible scourge of the past, seems to be exhibiting signs of recrudescence in our day, and we ought to be equipped for dealing with it, should it come under our notice. You may be questioning in your mind whether any medicinal treatment can avail here; but indeed there is more evidence in its favor than might be expected. Dr. Nureing, who has treated 40 cases, can speak of two complete recoveries, and of apparent benefit in the majority, from two tropical plants, the *Gynocardia odorata* and the

---

* HOM. WORLD, xxvi., 801.

Dipterocarpus turbinatus. The *"Chaulmoogra"* and *"Gurjun" oils* derived from these respectively have in his hands and those of others been the main instruments of these benefits, and small doses only seem required. We are thus encouraged to believe what has appeared in our own literature about **Hydrocotyle** and **Anacardium**. Of these drugs I have told the story in my 'Pharmacodynamics.' The usefulness of *Hydrocotyle* in Lupus tells in its favour; and the hyperæsthesia of the *Trigeminus* displayed in its provings suggests the first stage of Lepra Anæsthetica. *Ancardium,* also, has a double action on the nervous system and the skin, and the tradition as to its Leprosy-producing power in those who handle it is not to be hastily rejected.

"Arsenic," too, "is sometimes of marked use, especially in the skin variety." So writes Mr. Morris; and the cutaneous condition induced by the over-use of the drug shows sufficient Homœopathicity to what we have in Lepra Tuberculata. Further, as Lepra Anæsthetica is essentially a Neuritis, there is no reason why *Arsenic,* which is pre-eminent of the poisons that induce these inflammations, should not benefit it here.

Lastly, Dr. Jousset says that he has obtained a brilliant success in a Leper of 16, in the ulcerative period of the disease, from *Hydrastis,* given internally in the mother-tincture, and the same applied locally to the sores, diluted to one-tenth or one fifth with water.

I hope that those of our faith who practise in India and other tropical climates will give us their experience in the disease. The only contribution of the kind known to me is a Brochure issued by Dr. S. C. Durand, of Harda, Centrae Provinces, India, who says he has had considerable experience with Leprosy. He finds that *Secale cornutum,* one part of the tincture to two of Alcohol and three of water, a teaspoonful once daily, will make some very marked cures. It is certain that some features of Ergotism strongly resemble especially the anæsthetic form of Leprosy, and there is no reason why *Secale* should not play a prominent part in the treatment of the idiopathic disease.

And now of some more LOLAL, or at any rate LOCALISED affections of the skin.

FURUNCLE—ANGLICE, BOIL—is a trouble with which you will be glad to know our means of dealing, as it is very common and very painful. I can recommend the following bits of treatment to you with much confidence. If you can catch a Boil in the stage of inflammatory engorgement, before matter has formed,—the "BLIND BOIL" of popular language,—it may almost always be blighted by repeated doses of the first dilution of Belladonna. Whether this will act better than the local application of the same drug, or that of *Tincture of Iodine*—as advised by Mr. Morris, or than the *Arnica* compresses of Dr. Clotar Muller or the Lime-water of Dr. Wyld, I cannot say. They present alternatives for your consideration. Even later, I learnt from Dr. Madden that progress may be arrested by the third trituration of **Silicea**. Further, when Boils, like sorrows,

"Come not single apiece
But in battalions"

—if they recur again and again, the tendency may nearly always be checked by a course of **Sulphur** 12.

CARBUNCLE is often nothing more than a large MULTIPLE BOIL, and requires treatment accordingly. Dr. von Grauvogl says that it may be dispersed by repeated doses of **Arnica** internally and similar success has been obtained with *Iodine*, Lime-water and *Camphor* locally applied. Dr. Salzer advises both for Boil and simple Carbuncle the administration throughout of *Apis*.* But when from the outset the inflammation is of a low type, and accompanied with fever and prostration, special measures must be adopted. Both Jousset and Bahr recommend **Arsenicum** to be given, and no better remedy could be chosen for the general symptoms; but they do not claim for it any modifying influence over the progress of the Carbuncle itself. Jahr says that, finding it (with several other remedies) inoperative towards forwarding the suppuration and dispersion of the phlegmon, he at last hit upon **Bryonia**, which "hastened the process of suppuration, sometimes reducing the period to five or six days," instead of two or three weeks. 'In two cases," he writes, "where I was called at the commencement, I was even enabled to effect the dispersion of the swelling." †

The later medicinal treatment of Carbuncle consists in giving **Silicea** to check excessive suppuration, with **China** or **Lachesis** if there is evidence of exhaustion or blood-poisoning.

I confess that none of these medicines has seemed to me to exert any real control over the progress of Carbuncle; and I hailed the American recommendation of **Tarantula cubensis**—the bite of this spider setting up a localised phlegmonous inflammation very like that of our present disease. I have been able

---

* See J. B. H. S., vi., 9'. † Dr. Lippincott writes to corroborate this experience of Jahr's, but gets his results from the tincture instead of his predecessor's 30th (J. B. H. S., iii., 324).

repeatedly to verify the experience, and this remedy has become my first and last one in the treatment of Carbuncle. To control the suppuration I rely upon *Calendula* locally. Dr. S. G. A. Brown has lately related a case that well illustrates its powers. After operation by crucial incision the mischief went on spreading till a solution of the *Succus, 1* in *6,* was applied. "The effect was marvellous. Pus began to disappear rapidly, the inflammatory extension ceased instantly, and temperature dropped." *

For checking the recurrence of Carbuncular inflammation the place of *Sulphur* is taken by *Arsenic,* which I think acts best in drop-doses of *Fowler's Solution.*

The NAILS, as appendages of the skin, must come in here; and there are three of their affections which need therapeutical consideration.

MAL-NUTRITION of the nails may show itself in hypertrophy, when Dr. Hirsch's successful use of *Graphites* locally ✝ may be followed; in Softening, in which case von Grauvogl's *Thuja* or Dr. Babault's *Plumbum* may cure ‡; or in dryness and brittleness, for which at present we have no known remedy, though *Mercury* and *Arsenic* are worth consideration.

2. ONYCHIA is happily very rare, for here also we have no clinical experience and are without even pathogenetic suggestion. The sprinkling with powdered *Nitrate* of *Lead,* mentioned by Dr. Helmuth in his "Surgery," appears to be helpful. Dr. McLachlan commends *Fluoric acid.* $

3. PARONYCHIA, "WHITLOW," is much more common, and is well under the control of our remedies. *Silicea* and *Fluoric acid* have been hitherto our main remedies for it. Dr. McLachlan says that the latter is indicated when there is relief from cold and aggravation from heat, while with the former it is the other way. If we needed any confirmation of the influence of *Silicea* we might obtain it from the excellent case of the late Dr. Kafka's, which you may read in the Fifth Volume of the BRITISH HOMŒOPATHIC SOCIETY'S JOURNAL (p. 110). Here the trouble had

---

* HAHN. MONTHLY, March, 1898.   ✝ B. J. H., xxiii., 300.
‡ J. B. H. S., i., 187. $ HAHN. MONTHLY, Oct., 1898, p. 668.

lasted three months, and removal of the nail had been advised; but I have found the drug no less effective in blighting cases in their incipience. Of late, much commendation has been given to the *Myristica sebifera*, of Brazil (which must not be confounded with the *Myrica cerifera*), in this malady.* Dr. Lippincott finds his Bryonia 0 as useful here as in Carbuncle. †

I will speak next of—

ULCERS—These, of course, are not diseases of the skin; but I cannot well range them under any other category. All, except sometimes the "weak" and "indolent," require and repay constitutional treatment; but all, save the "Scrofulous" need local applications also. These last will often heal spontaneously as the general health improves under such medicines as **Sulphur** and **Calcarea**. When they are slow to fill up, the *Phosphate* may be advantageously substituted for the *Carbonate of Lime*. according to Dr. Beneke's suggestions. ‡ "WEAK" and "INDOLENT" ulcers should be treated by the local application of **Calendula**, in the proportion of a drachm of the tincture of *Succus* to an ounce of water. You should see that the lint soaked in the solution fits accurately to the ulcerated surface, and does not overlap the surrounding skin. If *Calendula* fails to heal, apply **Kali bichromicum**, a grain to eight or twelve ounces of water, in the same manner. These applications are tolerably efficacious even by themselves: but they are much aided by the well-understood management which includes rest and support.

The remaining forms of Ulcer require both constitutional and local treatment. For the "INFLAMED" Ulcer, if it is the raw surface itself that is red and hot, **Arsenicum** will be most suitable with water-dressing; if the surrounding skin is the seat of chronic inflammation, give **Belladonna** and apply *Calendula* or *Hydrastis* in the manner practised in Dr. Yeldham's time at the London Homœopathic Hospital. ‖ The "Irritable" Ulcer is rather intractable. I think **Lachesis** a good medicine for it; but find it usually necessary to seal it up, so as entirely to exclude the contact of air. *Lachesis* is no less useful for "PHAGEDÆNIC" and "SLOUGHING" Ulcer, as also is *Arsenicum*: the best local applications for these are a lotion of **Hydrastis** or **Kreasote**. For the "VARICOSE" Ulcer, when threatening, I can again recommend *Lachesis*, which will often arrest the mischief. When established, its treatment is that of the Varicosis itself; and if *Hamamelis* be the drug selected, it can with advantage be applied locally. Dr. Windelband recommends *Carduus marianus* for this Ulcer, and Dr. Jousset *Clematis vitalba*. ‖

---

* J. B. H. S., iii., 208; iv., 335; vii., 86.
† IBID., iii., 324. ‡ B. J. H., xvii
‖ See ANNALS, v., 356; and M. H. R., xi., 520. ❙ J. B. H. S., i., 286.

To these hints, derived mainly from my own experience, I may add some observation from others. Jahr speaks warmly of the advantage of commencing the treatment of all chronic Ulcerations with **Sulphur** 30, * and Dr. Clotar Muller praises the same drug in the tinctura fortissima. † Next to it, he ranks **Mercurius** ; and the power of this poison to induce ulceration of the skin ought certainly to be turned to more use than it has yet received. A list of medicines suitable to ULCERS, with their respective indications, is given by Dr. Franklin in his "Surgery", and by Dr. James Jones in the Twentieth Volume of the MONTHLY HOMŒOPATHIC REVIEW. I would remind you, so, of what I have said in my 'Pharmacodynamics' of *Asterias* and of *Pœonia*. *Mezereum* is recommended by Dr. Dunham for Mercurial and Mercurio-syphilitic Ulcers of the lower extremities.

I have now to say a few words upon the PARASITIC DISEASES of the skin - RINGWORM, SCABIES, FAVUS, and the rest. Of all of them I would say two things. First, it is simply foolish to neglect local applications in these affections. If a patient came to you complaining of itching at any part of the surface, and you found lice to be present, you would of course adopt measures for killing the vermin, and would not think of prescribing medicines Homœopathic to the sensations caused by them. So is it with Scabies and its fellows. But, secondly, you should not fail to treat with the suitable remedy any derangement of health which may co-exist ; and you may not uncommonly in this way obtain a spontaneous disappearance of local disorder—the parasite seeming to be starved out, as it were, by the alteration in the quality of its soil.

And now of the SPECIAL DISORDERS—Reserving Ringworm for the Diseases of Childhood, I shall speak here of the other forms of TINEA and of SCABIES.

TINEA is a generic name, applicable to all parasitic affections, whether they be of animal or of vegetable origin. The "TINEA TONSURANS" is the Ringworm of the scalp, whose consideration I have deferred. "TINEA FAVOSA" is now commonly called "FAVUS." Teste curiously enough says that the treatment of this disease is one of the triumphs of Homœopathy, recommending *Sulphur, Dulcamara, Viola tricolor, Oleander,* and *Hepar sulphuris* according to the symptoms. I must follow Bahr, Jousset and Kafka in recommending epilation and parasiticidal

---

* IRJD., iv., 241   † B. J. H., xxxii., 237

applications. "TINEA CIRCINATA," or RINGWORM OF THE SURFACE (which must not be confounded with Herpes Circinatus, which is a constitutional affection), must be similarly" treated (without epilation), as also "TINEA" or "PITYRIASIS VERSICOLOR." * *Sulphurous acid* makes an excellent lotion for these affections.

SCABIES—It was a long time before the followers of Hahnemann, influenced by his mistake in connecting chronic diseases with the Itch-eruption, could bring themselves to believe that Scabies was a purely local disorder, produced by the presence of an acarus. Bahr, in maintaining this view in 1863, speaks apologetically of differing herein from the majority of his colleagues. Now, however, I apprehend that there is no diversity of opinion on the subject. Jahr, who fairly represents the older Homœopathists, is as convinced as Bahr that Scabies cannot be cured by internal remedies alone, and that those who profess to have effected such cures must have been mistaken in their diagnosis.

Most of us use *Sulphur*-ointment to destroy the acarus ; but Jahr recommends a more agreeable substitute in the form of the *Oil of Lavender*, which he finds very effectual. Internal remedies are only needed when scratching or the violent local applications have induced great irritation of the skin. **Sulphur** itself is quite applicable here ; as also are **Croton** and (where Ecthymatous pustules have been developed) **Sepia.**

Recent Pathology has added two other diseases, phenomenally CUTANEOUS, to the category of parasitic infections. These are ELEPHANTIASIS and ACTINO-MYCOSIS.

ELEPHANTIASIS is surnamed "ARABUM" by Mr. Morris,—I suppose to distinguish it from Elephantiasis Græca, which is true Leprosy. "It is characterized," he writes, "by chronic hypertrophy of the skin and subcutaneous tissue, giving rise to enormous enlargement of a particular part of the body, generally one, and in rare cases both, of the lower limbs ; sometimes it is the scrotum or one of the labia that is affected. The face is occasionally the seat of the disease. It is often ushered in by febrile disturbance ('ELEPHANTOID FEVER')." In the tropical climates in which it is ordinarily seen, it is found to be due to obstruction of the lymph-stream by the Filaria. Sanguinis Heminis ; but it is admitted that simple inflammation of the lymphatic ducts may cause it. In such cases our remedies may

---

* I have called this ' Chloasma" in my 'Therapeutics.' That name however, had better been reserved for the non-parasitic "liver-spots" not unfrequently met with, and generally disappearing under *Sepia* or *Caulophyllum.*

do something for it and it is worth-mentioning that in a case of "BARBADOS LEG," acquired in the Island so-named, I obtained great benefit from *Hydrocotyle.*

Under the title "ELEPHANTIASIS NOSTRAS" Dr. Burkhardt has described a chronic œdema and hypertrophy of the leg, a sequel of Phlebitis and Varicosis ; and finds *Carduus marianus* and *Hamamelis* its remedial agents.

ACTINO-MYCOSIS is an infection from a fungus chiefly haunting straw and hay. I mention it mainly because Mr. Morris, who in the Edition of his Treatise dated 1894 relegated its treatment entirely to Surgery, in 1896 declared that *Iodide of Potassium* was "almost as certain a specific here as in Tertiary Syphilis." * The interesting thing is that the *Iodide* produces when over-used, just such "Tumours and Nodosities" of the skin as are displayed in Actino-Mycosis, and of which it "causes rapid subsidence." I have had an interesting case presenting all the features of this malady, though the Actino-myces could never be found. No medicine did good but *Kali iodatum*, and on raising this from the 1_x dilution to two-grain doses a final cure was effected.

I have last to speak of—

PRURITUS —This malady is so often dependent on Phthiriasis, that inquiry must first of all be made as to the presence of Pediculi, and, if they are found, treatment be instituted accordingly. Idiopathic Pruritus, in its general form, his happily not common. If you have a case to treat, try first what can be done by attending to the general health, and improving the condition of the skin by baths, frictions, &c. If it does not thus yield, consider the exact nature of the itching, and the circumstances under which it is aggravated or relieved, and look out for these symptoms in a good Repertory. In this way, you will possibly find in *Opium, Nux vomica, Mercurius, Sulphur,* or some less-known medicine (such as the *Dolichos* I have mentioned when speaking of Prurigo) the remedy of which you are in search.

The local varieties of Pruritus—all haunting the intracrural region—are generally symptomatic, and demand a careful inquiry into their causes. *Sulphur, Lycopodium* and *Petroleum* are sometimes useful for Pruritus Ani, and *Caladium, Ambra, Carbo vegetabilis* and *Collinsonia* (Jousset and Bahr add *Lycopodium* and *Conium*) for Pruritus Pudendi. But local Pruritus is very rebellious against internal remedies ; and you will generally have to resort to external applications, among which *Borax, Carbolic acid* and *Murcury* in various forms are the most effective. Sometimes a lotion of *Hamamelis* is of much service.

---

* LANCET, June 6.   † See J. B. H. S., ix., 76.

LECTURE LIII

DISEASES OF THE LOCOMOTIVE ORGANS·— CASUALTIES

—o—

MUSCLES, BONES & JOINTS—ACCIDENTS

—o—

MYOSITIS—MYALGIA—LUMBAGO—STIFF-NECK—OMODYNIA—PERIOSTITIS—NODES—OSTEITIS—CARIES—NECROSIS—EXOSTOSIS—MOLLITIES OSSIUM—ACROMEGALY—ENCHONDROMA—SYNOVITIS—WHITE SWELLING—ARTHRALGIA—BURSITIS—GANGLION—WOUNDS—CONTUSIONS—STRAINS—BURNS—SCALDS—CHILBLAIN—STINGS—FRACTURES—SUNSTROKE—SHOCK—EMOTIONAL DISTURBANCES.

As I am now entering the surgical sphere (though on its medical side), it will be well that I should mention our sources of information as to what Homœopathy can accomplish here. They come principally from America, where alone until lately our practitioners have been sufficiently numerous to allow of their cultivating Surgery as a speciality. I would name Dr Franklin's "Science and Art of Surgery," Dr. Helmuth's "System of Surgery," and Dr. Gilchrist's "Homœopathy in Surgical Diseases," as especially worthy of your attention. I have not seen the "Cyclopædia of Surgery," edited by Dr. C. E. Fisher, but doubt not that it is thoroughly worthy of consultation.

As the ORGANS OF LOCOMOTION I shall class the MUSCLES, BONES, and JOINTS; and on the present occasion will bring forward what I have to say upon the treatment of their morbid conditions.

And first, of the MUSCLES. As there is no reason why these organs should not be attacked by inflammation, I will speak of—

MYOSITIS, though I confess I know nothing practically about it. Should you encounter it, you will remember what I have said when lecturing upon **Bryonia**, that both the symptoms of the provers and the post-mortem appearances make it probable that this medicine is a specific irritant to muscular fibre. Bahr gives some instructions as to the treatment of "Psoitis," with *Belladonna*, *Mercurius* and *Hepar sulphuris* according to the stage of the inflammation. Chronic indurating Myositis is generally of Syphilitic origin, and I have nothing to suggest for it in preference to *Iodide of Potassium*.

738 DISEASES OF THE LOCOMOTIVE ORGANS

A far more frequent affection of the MUSCLES is—

MYALGIA—I need not tell you how much we are indebted to the late Dr. Inman, of Liverpool, for the identification of Myalgia as a pathological entity. But we owe to Dr. Henry Madden its naturalisation—so to speak—in Homœopathic regions, and the establishment upon a firm basis of its chief remedies. You will find the Paper of his to which I refer in the Twenty-Fifth Volume of the BRITISH JOURNAL OF HOMŒOPATHY, and I feel sure that you will derive many a valuable hint from its perusal. **Arnica** is the grand remedy for Myalgia in all its forms, especially when it results from fatigue or injury of the muscle. Even the heart, when its muscular walls have been strained by over-exertion, as from rowing, may have its integrity restored by this medicine, of which Dr. Bayes has furnished some valuable cases in point.* Another useful medicine for Myalgia is **Actæa racemosa**, which is of special service in women and other nervous subjects. **Gelsemium**, also, is of decided usefulness, as recommended by Dr. E. M. Hale, for Acute General Myalgia, with feverishness, as from unwonted or undue bodily fatigue ; and **Bellis**, the Daisy, has played a large part in Dr. Burnett's hand for more chronic cases of this kind.

I have now to speak of the so-called MUSCULAR RHEUMATISMS, including PLEURODYNIA, LUMBAGO and TORTICOLLIS. I know that there is much question now raised as to the really Rheumatic character of these affections—Jousset and Bahr amongst ourselves denying it as strongly as Garrod in the other school. I am myself inclined to think that each has its "Rheumatic" form, though Lumbago and Torticollis may—as I have said with regard to Pleurodynia—occur under other pathological conditions. I will speak of these two affections, accordingly, as separate maladies.

LUMBAGO—I agree with Jahr that the chief remedy for this affection is **Rhus**. It suits equally well that form which originates in a sudden exertion and that which results from exposure to cold and damp ; though in the former case it may be reinforced by **Arnica**, and in the latter may be preceded by **Aconite**, especially if the lumbar muscles seem chiefly involved. *Rhus* acts mainly, I think, on the Fascia.

Bahr prefers **Tartar emetic** even to *Rhus* and *Arnica* in Lumbago. He gives the second or third decimal trituration. Jousset agrees with his late colleague Dr. Cretin in esteeming

---

* "Applied Homœopathy," SUB VOCE.

Nux vomica very highly. I have found it of much service when the pains have been remittent, and have suggested Spasm of the Muscles as being present. In lingering cases you may think of *Æsculus*. *

Of Torticollis, or—
STIFF-NECK, I have only to say that, in my experience, it has yielded rapidly to **Aconite** when resulting from a draught of cold, dry air, to **Dulcamara** when the cause has been exposure to damp. Of the spasmodic form, I spoke in my Twenty-Eighth Lecture. I see that Dr. Jousset has obtained frequent success from the *Belladonna* I there suggested, giving it in low attenuation or mother-tincture.

Another frequent seat of MUSCULAR RHEUMATISM is the deltoid, where it constitutes—
OMODYNIA—Of ordinary Rheumatic medicines, perhaps *Phytolacca* suits this best. ✝ It has more frequently yielded however, to *Ferrum*. ‡

Of the BONES—
PERIOSTITIS—Of the Syphilitic and Mercurial forms of this disease, which are usually circumscribed, I will speak immediately under the head of "Nodes." The diffuse form is either acute, from cold or injury ; or chronic, from Rheumatism or Scrofula. The specific tissue-irritants of the periosteum which we possess are **Mezereum, Phytolacca, Mercurius, Silicea, Kali bichromicum,** and perhaps **Guaiacum.** In Acute Periostitis, I recommend (in common with Bahr and Franklin) the first of these ; but when suppuration threatens, *Mercurius* should be given, and, if it has taken place, *Silicea* is indicated, and should be preserved with until all symptoms have subsided. The propriety of incision, whether subcutaneous or direct, is a surgical question which I must leave to your discretion. "Periosteal Rheumatism" is hardly an inflammation ; I have already spoken of its treatment under Rheumatism. Chronic Periostitis in strumous subjects will commonly yield in the general diathetic measures you will adopt ; but one or other of the medicines above mentioned may help in its removal. *Ruta* and *Asafœtida* are spoken of as periosteal remedies ; I have no knowledge of them in this capacity. The first is recommended especially in Periostitis from mechanical injury.

---

* J. B. H. S., ii., 216.   ✝ J. B. H. S,. i., 88.   ‡ IBID., ii., 357.

NODES are either "SOFT" or "HARD" **Silicea** which is good for either, is especially suitable to the former. When Soft Nodes form on the scalp, **Kali bichromicum** is perhaps its superior in efficacy. For the genuine hard Syphilitic Node, with its nocturnal pain, we may try **Aurum**, which is Homœopathic enough; but must be prepared to fall back upon the *Iodide of Potassium*, with the action of which in such cases I think that Homœopathy has little to do. I will again refer you to the discussion of the rationale of its influence by Dr. Henry Madden in the Twenty-Sixth volume of the BRITISH JOURNAL OF HOMŒOPATHY. You will see that, if he is right, there is no reason for expecting its virtues to be displayed in infinitesimal doses.

I do not know that *Calcarea carbonica* has found any employment in Homœopathic practice for Periostitis. It is worth noting, however, that "Mother-of-Pearl" workers are subject to a very painful swelling of the bones of the extremities, accompanied by fever, continuing for weeks and even months, but rarely leading to suppuration. The substance in question, the dust of which they are constantly breathing, consists of 95 per cent, of Carbonate of Lime and 5 per cent of an organic substance called Concholine. *

It will be understood that in thus speaking of Periostitis, whether diffuse or circumscribed, I have in view its simple form, and not the acute infective inflammation which Dr. Charles Hayward brought before the BRITISH HOMŒOPATHIC SOCIETY in 1895. † This is what we used to call ACUTE NECROSIS; and from my experience with that inflammation – of which I have treated two well-marked cases – I can support his Thesis that Surgery must here come to the aid of Medicine. Treated with the latter only, one of my patients nearly died; and in neither could I trace any decided benefit to the medicines employed.

OSTEITIS, in the acute form, is secondary either to Periostitis or to Osteo Myelitis Chronic inflammation of bone, whether primary, or extending from the periosteum, is Syphilitic, Mercurial, or Scrofulous. If Syphilitic, the first question is whether the patient has been Mercurialised. If not **Mercurius** suggests itself as in every way a most Homœopathic and suitable remedy. **Aurum** is its important ally; and the two medicines may reinforce and replace one another until the cure is complete. Too often, however, the osseous disease owes its origin to the improper use of Mercury; and here our primary aim must be to antidote the poison. **Nitric acid** is the most important agent we Homœopaths have for this purpose; and then comes *Aurum*

---

* See M. H. R., xlii., 242.   † See J. B. H. S., iii.,379

again, and **Staphisagria**. These medicines are likely to suffice when the Mercurialization has been extreme. But if the patient is in the latter unlucky case, or if the Syphilitic diathesis is very pronounced. I cannot but think the oridinary prescription of *Iodide of Potassium* still more satisfactory.

There is a chronic inflammation of the bone described by Sir James Paget as "OSTEITIS DEFORMANS" and said to be unamenable to any treatment. Dr. Savall, of Barcelona, has reported a case occurring in a boy of 10 (which is unusual), where entire recovery occurred under *Calcarea phosphorica* 3_x, with *Staphisagria* for the pains. *

Chronic Scrofulous Osteitis is nearly, if not quite always, Caries ; of which I shall now speak.

CARIES is reputed to be incurable under ordinary treatment and is relegated to the knife. We have better auguries. Let me cite the following case ;—it is given by Dr. Laurie in his 'ELEMENTS.'

"A boy became affected, after Scarlet Fever, with Caries of the temporal bone, which, during a period of five or six years, periodically broke out afresh, discharged an offensive pus, and then healed again. The entire left side of the cranium was arrested in its growths, and consequently rendered much smaller than the other side : the left eye also appeared strikingly smaller than the right one. The intellect of the boy was, nevertheless, not in any way affected. Several remedies improved, but failed in curing the Caries. After the employment of **Fluoric acid** the attack came on earlier, and in a more aggravated form than usual, but never returned. From that time onward the lesser half of the craninm commenced to grow and the previous inequality of size between the two sides of the head became gradually less, and finally imperceptible."

I can refer you also to two cases of Dr. Cooper's condemned to operation, but recovering under *Calcarea carbonica* and *Silicea* ; ✤ to two of Dr. Kesserling's of Mulheim having the same happy end under *Silicea* and *Calcarea fluorata* (which last, I may mention, is the main remedy for bone-trouble in Schussler's Therapeia) ; ‡ and to quite a series from Dr. James Love, in which *Aurun 30* was curative. $ *Phosphorus* and *Phosphoric acid*, also, are not to be forgotten,—the latter especially when there is much purulent discharge and hectic is present. Jahr advises that in Scrofulous subjects treatment should always be commenced with *Sulphur*, after which, he says, we shall get much better results from *Silicea* ‖ and the other special remedies. If the Caries be Syphilitic or Mercurial, the treatment I have indicated for Osteitis arising from these causes is required.

* IBID., v., 209.   ✤ H. W. Feb., 1894.
‡ J. B. H. S. iv., 232. $ REX. HOM. FRANCAISE, June 1896.
‖ Dr. Windelband's remarkable series of cases cured by *Silicea 3* include several of Caries (ZEITSCHR DES BERLINER VEREINS HOM. AERZTE, xii., 1).

OF—

NECROSIS in its acute form I have already spoken. When supervening on such an acute attack, or primarily chronic, we have to treat a Necrosis already accomplished, and the dead bone awaiting detachment as in Caries the question of surgical interference will arise ; but, as in Caries, I would advise you to refrain. Give Silicea as your basic remedy, with Symphytum to aid in the detachment of the sequestrum ; and you will have more thorough extrusion of the necrosed matter, while your patient's general health will actually improve under the process. A case of Dr. Villers, which you will find in the Second Volume of the JOURNAL OF THE BRITISH HOMŒOPATHIC SOCIETY, will illustrate this.*

For Osteo-Myelitis I have nothing to suggest ; and for—
EXOSTOSIS can only note that it is among the affections which in Dr. Windelband's hands have yielded to *Silicea 3* and that Dr. Majumdar has seen one of the antrum disappear under *Calcarea flourata*.

I must say a few words, however upon—
MOLLITIES OSSIUM.—I was wrong, it seems, in speaking of this as a fatty degeneration and suggesting *Phosphorus* for it. Our only experience in its treatment is that which D. Arnold of Heidelberg has left us. He found *Calcarea carbonicum* 2_x and *Iodine* 2_x to 4_x, in weekly alternation, distinctly remedial. † I do not know whether you have noticed the curious facts which seem to show that the induction of anæsthesia by *Chloroform* (not Ether) has given this disease a turn in the right direction ‡ which may go on to complete recovery. They ought to be turned to systematic Therapeutic account.

For the curious ENLARGEMENTS OF THE BONES, especially those of the hands and feet now known as—
ACROMEGALY we have nothing to suggest which promises better than the "Opotherapeutic" plan of giving an extract of the pituitary body, as that of the thyroid is given in Myxœdema. Excellent results have already been reported from this practice. $

For—
ENCHONDROMA we are better-equipped. I have told in my 'Pharmacodynamics' how von Grauvogl, anticipating Schussler, treated this morbid growth with Silicea on the ground that

---

*H. W., March., 1895.   † See B. J. H. xviii., 155
‡ See J. B. H. S., ii., 105. $ IBID., iv., 343 ; v., 201.

the only chemical differences between cartilage and bone is that flint is present in the latter but not in the former; and got curative results. One of our lady-practitioners in America reports equally good results in a Tumour of like nature on the frontal bone of an infant. Similar growths had occurred in every male child born in the family for several generations, and *Silicea*, disappeared in 48 days. *

I have now to speak of the diseases of the JOINTS, and shall begin with—

SYNOVITIS—This inflammation, in its acute form, is readily manageable by Homœopathic remedies, without the need of the leeches the blisters. or even the continuous cold to which you have been accustomed. If it has been excited by injury, you will do well to keep the joint covered by a weak **Arnica**-lotion. Otherwise simple water-dressing in the only local application necessary. You will of course keep the joint at rest, and, if practicable, elevated. Then, for internal medicine,—**Aconite**, if there is fever or intensity of local action, but alternated with the more specific remedies, **Bryonia** or **Pulsatilla**: the former when, as often happens, the patient is Rheumatic, although the Synovitis be simple; the latter in children, delicate women, and indeed in the majority of the cases in which Synovitis occurs. In some cases, where there is much effusion but little pain (Acute Hydrarthrosis), **Apis** is preferable to either. ✝ The support of strapping or a bandage is all that is afterwards required to cause absorption of the effusion,—the medicines being continued. If suppuration has taken place, you should give **Hepar sulphuris**, and apply a solution of it externally; but I cannot promise you that the matter will be absorbed without evacuation. ‡ Should this latter have taken place, and matter be discharging, **Silicea**, also locally as well as internally, seems preferable to *Hepar*: $

For the simple form of Chronic Synovitis I recommend,—if it be Syphilitic or Mercurial, **Kali iodatum**; if it be Rheumatic, **Mercuris**. But in either or any case the predominance of serous effusion over inflammatory thickening ("Hydrops Articuli") leads to **Iodine** or its compound with *Potash* as the most suitable remedy. Here again Homœopathy occupies common ground with the old school.

Chronic Scrofulous Synovitis, with or without the actual

---

*IBID., iii, 215.

✝ *Cantharis* is an alternative here, according to Dr. Jousset (Rev, Hom. Francaise, June, 1896).

‡ Dr. Cartier relates two cases in this condition which yielded with marvellous rapidity to *Myristica sebifera*, in the 3rd dilution (IBID., Nov., 1898), $ J. B. H. S., i., 378.

deposit of Tubercle, constitutes the joint-disease which I shall call by the old and popular but useful name of—

WHITE SWELLING—This disease may begin, as you know, either in the synovial membrane, the cartilage, or the cancellous structure of the ends of the bones of a joint. The diagnosis of these different origins is important, as, in addition to the general Anti-scrofulous medicines you will prescribe, those influencing the tissue primarily affected with often be serviceable, My counsel, however, will be that you rely mainly on the constitutional remedies of which **Sulphur** and the **Calcareas**, with **Silicea**, stand pre-eminent. From Dr. Wassily we have three cases which show *Sulphur* curative here single-handed ; * to Dr. W. L. Morgan six, in which *Calcarea carbonica* and *phosphorica* played. the leading part ; † and Dr. Windelband includes Tuberculous joints among his victories gained by *Silicea*. If you have to look further, however, then, if Synovitis has been the primary mischief *Pulsatilla* or *Apis will* help ; if inflammation of the cartilages, *Mercurius corrosivus* while if the disease has begun in the bones, *Mercurius* itself, or perhaps *Symphytum* would best follow, though you could hardly do better than persevere with *Silicea* throughout.

These remarks are of course applicabe to DISEASE OF THE HIP —"MORBUS COXÆ"—as of other joints. But here you will find *Colocynth* also a very useful medicine, relieving as it does much of the pain accompanying the disease, from irritation of the neighbouring nerves. You must also bear in mind the domestic reputation of *Cistus Canadensis* in this affection, and Dr. Bradshaw's success with it in a White Swelling of the knee.

ARTHRALGIA is a convenient term, including as it does both the "HYSTERICAL JOINT' and Neuralgia (often sympathetic) haunting the articulations. Hysterical Joints, like Hysterical sufferings generally, are obstinate things to deal with ; and I have no special suggestions to offer beyond what I have said regarding Hysteria generally, save that **Argentum** has sometimes proved curative in Arthralgia seemingly of this nature. Nor do I think that Neuralgia of joints is ever primary, so as to require a special medicine. Should it be so, however, *Plumbum and Zincum* should be thought of.

As closely connected with the joints, I must speak of BURSITIS and of GANGLION. first, of—

BURSITIS—In acute inflammation of these of sacs, *Aconite* and

---

* IBID., iii., 284. † IBID., i., 378

WOUNDS

Belladonna have been efficacious in my hands; but *Sticta* has lately been also commended, and I have found it very effective. In the Chronic form, of which the HOUSEMAID'S KNEE is a well-known instance, **Rhus** internally and externally, and also **Silicea** have proved curative; but you may have to fall back upon the similar use of *Iodide of Potassium*. **Ruta** is sometimes good for BUNION.

GANGLION, also, has disappeared in my hands under **Ruta**: but I cannot tell you that it will always succeed. **Benzoic acid**, rubbed in as an ointment, will often disperse these swellings; and Dr. Turrel has obtained corresponding effects from the internal administration of the drug, in pretty high dilution.*

Before leaving the subject of BONE and JOINT Diseases, let me direct your attention to an excellent Paper on the subject presented to our Congress of 1894 by Mr. Gerard Smith, and printed in the MONTHLY HOMŒOPATHIC REVIEW of that year (p. 456). His experience is much the same as that I have brought before you; but I may briefly state some of his points as those of a very capable observer. For INJURIES of JOINTS he commends *Arnica* 1_x, internally as well as locally, at first; *Ruta* or *Bryonia* if inflammation should supervene; *Rhus* if recovery should linger. If Acute Synovitis inclines to be chronic, he finds *Kali iodatum* 1x very effective. *Mezereum*, he thinks, relieves the pain of Periostitis rather than reducing the inflammation. *Nitric acid* and *Aurum* seem to him to act better in Chronic Osteitis than does *Mercurius*; he has also had considerable encouragement in the use of *Calcarea fluorata*.

I shall now devote a few minutes to the subject of CASUALTIES,—mentioning under that heading what part our medicines play in the treatment of WOUNDS, CONTUSIONS, SPRAINS, BURNS, CHILBLAINS, STINGS, FRACTURES. SUNSTROKE, SHOCK and EMOTIONAL DISTURBANCES.

The division of—

WOUNDS into INCISED, PUNCTURED, CONTUSED and LACERATED is familiar as regards their surgical management; but it bears no less upon their medicinal treatment.

In INCISED wounds your one object is to secure union by first intention. Besides the mechanical measures you will adopt for this purpose, **Calendula** comes in as the most potent "vulnerary" that has ever been discovered. It is not a germicide; that has been ascertainded: † but its influence is entirely inimical to

---

* See BIBLIOTHEQUE HOMŒOPATHIQUE., Nov., 1876.
† N. A. J. H., March., 1893.

suppuration, and, having itself no irritating properties, it may be freely applied to the cut surface and edges. The strength may be from the pure *Succus* * (prepared by Gould & Son) to a mixture of one part of the tincture to seven of water or Glycerine.

PUNCTURED wounds may be aided in their healing by *Calendula*. They often give, however, an amount of local and general trouble out of all proportion to their size ; and Teste appears borne out in his assertion that their specific remedy (even when the sequelæ are severe and distant in time ✝) is **Ledum**, which may be used both externally and internally. If he is right, too, a potency not of the lowest should be selected for both purposes.

In CONTUSED wounds it is generally admitted that the element Contusion is of more moment than the element wound. Hence **Arnica** should be given internally, and used locally (not stronger than one part in fifty) in preference to *Calendula*. The latter may come in afterwards to promote healing, if required.

It was in LACERATED wounds that *Calendula* first gained its reputation ; and if the promotion of healing by first intention were all that was needful, we should not have to look further. But Lacerated are like Punctured wounds in the distress they cause,— both in the part and in the system at large ; and this is especially of "nervous" character. Accordingly, Dr. Franklin has been led to treat them with **Hypericum**, and reports the best possible results from its use. He makes the lotion with one part of the tincture to twenty of warm water. Dr. Gilchrist finds a similar application so soothing to operation-wounds that it quite supersedes the necessity of an *Opiate*.

I will now speak of—

CONTUSIONS.—You know already the repute of **Arnica** for Bruises ; and certainly the manner in which it removes the pain and discoloration is very gratifying, and quite of a specific character. Here it may be used in stronger solution than in Contused Wounds ; but the liability of some persons to an *Arnica*-erysipelas must be remembered, and caution observed.

The only Contusions to which *Arnica* is less applicable are those which involve glandular parts—as the female breast, and the periosteum—as the tibia in kicks on the skin. **Conium** in the former case, **Ruta** and **Symphytum** ‡ in the latter, are its substitutes.

---

* An "Aqua *Calendula*," which is a strong infusion, was used in the earliest experiments made with the plant.
✝ See B. J. H., xxxiv., 337.   ‡ See J. B. H.S., iii., 105.

BURNS & SCALDS

STRAINS are supposed to be more benefited by **Rhus** than by *Arnica* ; and some cases which you will find in the Twenty-Fifth Volume of BRITISH JOURNAL OF HOMŒOPATHY (p. 662) bear out the opinion of its efficacy. It is said to be especially suitable in Strains of ligamentous parts, as tendons and fasciæ, occurring in robust persons, and having the *Rhus* characteristic that the pain is felt most when the parts are first moved, and becomes easier as the motion continues. But **Arnica** is a capital medicine for Strains as well as Bruises, and, when the muscular fibre itself is the seat of the mischief, is superior to *Rhus* or anything else.

BURNS and SCALDS require different medicinal treatment according to their intensity and to the constitutional symptoms which accompany them.

Burns of the first degree—*i.e.*, where Erythema only, or but slight general raising of the cuticle obtains—are best treated internally with **Aconite**, locally with **Urtica urens**, in the proportion of one part of the tincture to twenty of water. Do not remove the rags when once applied, but keep them wet with the lotion.

For Burns of the second degree—*i.e.*, where there is considerable vesication—**Cantharis** takes the place of *Urtica* as the external application. It may even prevent the supervention of the bullæ. In the HAHNEMANNIAN MONTHLY for January, 1897, Dr. Howard Crutcher illustrates the rapid and thorough effect of the application of a third aqueous dilution to a Burn produced by the explosion of burning Alcohol on his own person. "Within five minutes," he says, "my pain was gone entirely, and it never returned. From the severity of the Burn I had expected a crop of ugly Blisters. Within six hours not a trace of discoloration was visible." Dr. Helmuth, also, bears witness to the efficacy of such medication. "As soon as the wound is cleaned," he writes, "it is washed thoroughly with a stream of *Cantharides* water, and then dressed with *Calendula cerate*. This, after long experience, I am convinced is better than the Carbolic acid, Eucalyptol, Icthyol, and others of the newer methods of treatment." * If you are too late for such abortive measures, and have raw surfaces to treat, try *Calendula* dressings till all suppuration has ceased and then, if necessary, call in the aid of **Hamamelis**. Dr. H. H. Chase relates a very satisfactory experience with the fluid extract of Witch-hazel. Pledgets of cotton dipped in it were applied. "There appeared," he writes, "to be sufficient astringency to do away with the fungosities, and some portions of the *Hamamelis* dried into the

---

* N. A. J. H., June., 1895.

surface of the ulcer; whenever this occurred, normal granulations immediately formed underneath, and as these became firm and substantial the *Hamamelis* came off, leaving a good, firm, new skin which rapidly grew in area and thickness.
In the course of ten days I succeeded thus in completely covering the entire dorsum of a hand burnt in a recent fire." *

Of the efficacy of these four remedies—*Urtica, Cantharis, Calendula* and *Hamamelis*—there is no question, and they are in general acceptance amongst us. But we have no such accredited medicine for Burns of the third degree, where the cutis vera is involved and the tissues are carbonised. *Kreasote* and *Causticum* have been thought useful, and I should use the former (a drachm to a pint) with some hope of benefit. But the constitutional treatment is here of more importance than the local, as the eschar must separate, and if it needs aid, may receive it from the ordinary means of Surgery.

The internal treatment in cases of Burn or Scald depends upon the symptoms present. In Burns of the first and second degree the uneasiness of the part affected is the thing chiefly complained of, and **Rhus** will then aid the topical applications in giving relief. But when these are extensive, and in Burns of the third degree, the general symptoms are considerable. For the primary shock, if accompanied with coldness **Camphor** should be given. If with the reaction, fever should set in, after a few doses of *Aconite*, **Arsenicum** should be steadily administered. We must also be on the look-out for the duodenal mischief which Mr. Curling showed to be frequent after severe Burns:—I have already mentioned the value here of *Kali bichromicum*.

Before leaving the local effects of Excessive Heat, I would mention those of undue Cold. Frost-bite is out of the range of medicine, but I may give some suggestions in aid of the treatment of a minor form of this evil—

CHILBLAIN—Painting these enemies to comfort with the mother-tincture of *Aconite* or *Agaricus*—the former if they are inflamed, the latter if simply irritable—gives great relief. Internally, **Pulsatilla** may be administered; and is often useful to moderate or extinguish the proclivity to this complaint with which some persons afflicted. Dr. Balzer has found *Hepar sulphuris* effective for the latter purpose. †

* J. B. H. S., iii., 327. † J. B. H. S., ii., 365.

And now of—

STINGS—Teste speaks in the strongest terms of the rapid relief given in MOSQUITO-BITES by the application or even internal administration of **Ledum**, as high as the *15*th dilution. I suppose that the same treatment would be applicable to the Stings of BEES, WASPS and other VENOMOUS CREATURES. An old popular remedy for BEE and WASP Stings, the application of moist earth is generally quite successful in speedily removing the pain and swelling. For SNAKE BITES the use of *Arsenic* in the form of the Tanjore Pills is sufficiently specific and even Homœopathic for us; and so also is that of *Cedron* just lately received. * I should not, however, with our present knowledge allow these to supersede the usual *Ammonia* and stimulants in such cases.

You will hardly think that Homœopathy finds any place in—

FRACTURES—Besides, however, the use of *Aconite* and *Arnica* for Shock, Fever, and Startings in the broken limb, we have not uncommonly to deal with cases where the bones seem disinclined to unite. Cogswell has shown what medicinal treatment can do here by his use of Iodine in Scrofulous subjects—a recommendation I have verified. Should no such cause be traceable, you may rely upon **Symphytum**. The claims which this plant makes by its very name to efficacy here, which popular tradition asserts, and which Jahr and others strongly confirm, may well lead us to give it in every case of Fracture, especially in those of the patella and the neck of the femur, where the disinclination in question is strongly marked. † As alternatives, I may mention Dr. Henrique's successful use of *Ruta*, suggested by its action on the periosteum, or Hering's and Grauvogl's stimulation of osseous production by *Calcarea phosphorica*. Particulars of these experiences will be found under the heads of the respective medicines in my 'Pharmacodynamics.

SUNSTROKE finds a most Homœopathic and effective remedy in **Glonoin**. Many cases are on record of its speedy efficacy in removing the acute symptoms; and I have found it no less useful in some of the after-effects which linger with the patient. It is only when these are of a continuously hyperæmic type that they call preferably for **Belladonna**.

---

* M. H. R., xiv., 684. † See M. H. R., xi., 601.

I have advisedly said "Sunstroke" and not "Heat-stroke" here. That there is a Heat-stroke, producing phenomena far more general than those which occur from the COUP DE SOLEIL, I fully recognize. Aconite would probably do all that medicine can do for it but abstraction of heat by the cold douche or pack is so obvious and so well-accredited a remedy that I hesitate to advise in this condition any dependence on internal medication.

SHOCK may take two forms—the Torpid and the Erethistic. Dr. Howard Crutcher, of Chicago,—one of the American Homœopathists who have so distinguished themselves in Surgery of late, writes—"For Shock, *Camphor*, *Veratrum album* and *Carbo vegetabilis* are pre-eminent. Coldness is the main feature of *Camphor*; blueness calls for *Carbo*; and the well-known cold sweat on the forehead and over the body points to *Veratrum*. I have repeatedly witnessed the efficacy of these remedies in Surgical Shock." His fellow-citizen, Dr. J. S. Mitchell, says of one of them, *Veratrum*, that it is one of the best heat stimulants we have; and that he "can get as prompt results from it, in the 3_x dilution, as he can from a hypodermic of *Strychnia*." Dr. Helmuth adds his testimony to the same effect. In the Erethistic form *Arsenicum*, in a pretty high dilution, would be preferable.

EMOTIONAL DISTURBANCES have received especial study from Homœopathic Therapeutics; and the following are the main conclusions at which they have arrived.

The immediate effects of FRIGHT are best controlled by a dose—some say of *Opium*, others of *Aconite*. I should prefer the latter. But when Fright has given rise to genuine Neurosis, as Chorea or Epilepsy, **Ignatia** is more suitable than any other medicine.

For the effect of GRIEF also *Ignatia* bears away the palm, especially when the emotion is suppressed. If it be longcontinued and wearing, **Phosphoric acid** is preferable.

When ANGER has been the disturbing emotion, **Chamomilla** removes its effects, even when these reach as far as Jaundice.

Beyond these well-tested recommendations, a good deal that is very hypothetical has been written about the remedies for the effects of emotion. The fun that was made out of this material by the first Lord Lytton in "My Novel" was fully provoked. The subject, however, is not the least worthy of further and more experimental study.

LECTURE LIV

DISEASES OF CHILDREN

—o—

GENERAL DISEASES OF THE NERVOUS SYSTEM

—o—

INFANTILE REMITTENT FEVER—RICKETS—INFANTILE SYPHILIS—TUBERCULAR MENINGITIS—HYDROCEPHALOID—HYDROCEPHALUS—CONVULSIONS—INFANTILE PARALYSIS.

I have finally, in the next two lectures, to bring before you what we can do for the special diseases which wait upon CHILDHOOD. You may call this an arbitrary division, and may perhaps be disposed to criticize it as unfitting to a scientific classification. Perhaps it is, yet I cannot doubt that it is practically useful to present under one view the distinctive maladies in question, and the modifications of ordinary disease which there subjects show. The "jucunde" element in Homœopathic treatment naturally makes it sought to for children, * so that we have large experience in the treatment of their disorders. The results of such experience I think it well to put before you in a connected form: and I do not think that you will find the arrangement otherwise than convenient.

I will begin by passing down to classes of diseases already identified, and noting the treatment of such of them as are peculiar to children, or offer special characters in early life. In addition to what I shall myself bring forward, you may consult the special Treatises on Diseases of Children by Hartmann Hartlaub and Teste,—all of which have been translated into English; and the remarks on the treatment of infantile disorders appended by Drs. Leadam and Guernsey to their Gynæcological Manuals already mentioned. I may refer you also to the Monographs on the subject lately issued by Drs. C. E. Fisher and Sigmund Raue; to a "Digest of Ten Years' Work at the Children's Sanatorium, Southport," by Dr. Storrar, published in the Sixth Volume of the JOURNAL OF THE BRITISH HOMŒOPATHIC SOCIETY; to a Paper by Dr. Robertson Day, entitled "A Year's Work in the Children's Department of the Hospital" in the Sixth Volume of the LONDON HOMŒOPATHIC HOSPITAL REPORTS; and to a Lecture on "Homœopathy and the Diseases of Children," by Dr. James Love, of Paris, reported in the Thirty-Ninth Volume of the MONTHLY HOMŒOPATHIC REVIEW.

Among the GENERAL DISEASES we have to treat of a fever—the INFANTILE REMITTENT, and a disorder of nutrition—

---

* See M. H. R., xxxix, 86

DISEASES OF CHILDREN.

RICKETS : we have also to speak of the form which Syphilis takes in the first few months of life.

I know it is a question at the present day whether—
INFANTILE REMITTENT FEVER is a distinct Pathological entity. The question may now, indeed, be regarded as settled in the negative. Nonetheless, however, has it a clinical existence, and presents itself as a true primary fever, independent of local inflammation. An excellent account of it is given, evidently from the life, by Dr. Guernsey. Its antipyretic is **Gelsemium**, as first indicated by Dr. Ludlam ; and I recommend you to give this medicine in all obscure febrile disorders of infancy in which remittency is marked. It will generally need an ally to remove the gastric symptoms, and this I have always found in **Pulsatilla**; though you must not forget *Antimonium crudum*. Should the head symptoms be prominent, the most suitable medicine is *Hyoscyamus*.

Sometimes a condition like that of Remittent Fever proves very lingering and here Helminthiasis is often present—the "WORM-FEVER" of domestic medicine. Whether, however, Worms are actually in existence or not, you cannot do better in such cases than follow Dr. Chepmell's prescription of *Cina*. * If you want further help, you may consider Stille's prescription of *Spigelia*, which I have quoted when lecturing on that drug.

We are learning more and more, since Sir William Jenner broke ground on the subject, to regard—
RICKETS not as a malady seated in the bones only, but as a true constitutional diathesis ranking with Scrofula and Syphilis —though not like these hereditary. "If a child cuts his teeth late, if it does not walk so early as other children, if the fontanelles are late in closing, the probability is that it is the subject of Rickets.' So wrote Dr. Hillier. † He further defined it as "a general disease of nutrition chiefly affecting the infants, characterized at first by unhealthy alvine secretions, pains in the limbs, perspirations about the head, and subsequently by great muscular weakness and retarded ossification and dentition, with abnormal growth of cartilage, causing various deformities in the head, trunk and limbs. In the spleen, lymphatic glands and liver, there is degeneration with enlargement, sometimes also in the cerebrum."

---

* See his "Hints for the Practical Study of Homœopathic Method," p. 35.   † "Clinical Treatises on Diseases of Children." 1868.

Knowing these facts about Rickets, it would seem probable that regulation of defective diet and Hygiene, and administration of COD-LIVER OIL and suitable medicines for the digestive derangements present, would be all that was required for treatment. That this is not so, however, appears from the avidity with which our old-school colleagues have seized upon the use of Phosphorus as a medical remedy for the disease. They were led to it by the experiments of Wegner, which I have fully related in the Article on the drug in my 'Pharmacodynamics.' These showed a power on its part of exciting osteogenetic activity, and so of counter-acting a supposed depression of this function which obtains in the disease we are considering. I had already pointed out, however that such excitement was pathogenetic rather than physiological; and what Wegner himself had found that (to quote his own words) "under the simultaneous influence of feeding with *Phosphorus*, and of the deprivation of the organic substances, especially of Lime, the mode of growth of bones is altered so as exactly to correspond to what we are accustomed to call Rachitis," This has been substantiated since, by the experiments and arguments of Kassowitz. * What really obtains in Rickets is a morbid activity of the osteogenetic function, producing cartilage instead of bone, because of the lack of the mineral pabulum it needs for the latter. *Phosphorus* is thus truly Homœopathic to the condition present, as Kassowitz himself acknowledges ; and this is further shown by the minuteness of the dosage required and the general influence of the remedy. Kassowitz's maximum dose is half a milligramme, *i.e.*, about gr. $\frac{1}{130}$; and that this may be far too strong is shown by a case extracted in the AMERICAN HOMŒOPATHIST of December, 1899, where gr. $\frac{1}{300}$ when taken three times a day for a fortnight caused Fever and Diarrhœa, with enlargement of the lymph-notes behind the sterno-mastoid ; and later, Eczema on the scalp and petechial eruptions on the extremeties, going on to Purpura Hæmorrhagica, so that the child died of exhaustion. † Conversely, the extensive literature quoted by Kassowitz shows that the Convulsions, Laryngo-spasm, Insomnia and restlessness which prevail in Rickets are more benefited by this than by any other drug.

I do not know whether the Homœopathic treatment of Rickets has undergone much modification from these new views as to the Pathology of the disease or these experiences with *Phosphorus* in its therapeutics. Writing ere they had well-risen above the horizon, I professed myself unable to expect much from the *Ruta. Staphisagria, Mezereum, Lycopodium* and *Pinus sylvestris* suggested by Hartmann ; still less from the *Mercurius*

---

* See M. H. R., xxviii, 402 ; N. A. J. H., Nov., 1897.

† The ready way in which this hæmorrhagic condition was set up by the drug corresponds to what Dr. Eustace Smith notes, that "in the child Scurvy is rarely seen apart from Rickets."

solubilis, Colchicum and *Sulphur* which are Teste's eccentric recommendations. "Nor can *Calcarea*," I wrote, be regarded as a specific remedy for the Rachitic diathesis ; though there can be no doubt of its occasional usefulness, * especially (as Bahr says) when a sour-smelling Diarrhœa is present. There is something more here, even in the bone, than deficiency of Lime-salts. To Phosphoric acid, on the other hand, I can follow Hartmann in ascribing great powers for good ; and to it I will add Silicea. The former corresponds to the Diarrhœa and the pains in the limbs, and perhaps to the bone-disease and the albuminoid degeneration. The latter covers the perspirations about the head, the sensitiveness of the surface, and the tendency to increased growth of cartilage. With these medicines, and especially with the latter, I can encourage you to expect great things in the treatment of Rickets. Two cases, one of Hydrocephalus, one of Ascites, in Rachitic children, have lately recovered in a marvellous manner under, its influence in my hands—the potencies from *12* to *30* being those employed.

For—

INFANTILE SYPHILIS, in its full constitutional manifestation, I have nothing better to propose than the small doses of Mercury which form its classic treatment. They may, however, be very small. Infantile Syphilis is a condition in which we may safely follow Hahnemann's directions and give our specific in high attenuation. I have long been in the habit of treating my dispensary patients manifesting this taint with the *30*th potency of the *solubilis*, and they do very well. I tried at one time the *Kreasote* so warmly commended by Teste, but found it effective only against the cutaneous manifestations of the disease. If Condylomata appear, *Nitric acid* must be given ; and if the cachexia is considerable you may with advantage fall back upon *Aurum*.

I pass now to the DISORDERS OF THE NERVOUS SYSTEM as they occur in childhood. I need not tell you how excitable their little brains are, and how readily they can be fretted into morbidity. Besides the judicious general management so important in these cases, you will find the utmost benefit from some of our medicines. On the one side stand those suitable for nervous

---

Dr. Dayesteems it highly. giving the 6th trituration,

erethism simply, which are *Chamomilla, Coffea, Cypripedium, Ignatia, Hyoscyamus, Scutallaria* and *Stramonium* ; on the other, those which reach to inflammatory mischief, of which *Belladonna* is FACILE PRINCEPS. I have told you what great things this medicine, by virtue of its Homœopathicity, can accomplish. But there is one inflammatory state of the brain in which you will not find it curative, and that is Acute Hydrocephalus, as we used to call it, or, as it is more correctly styled nowadays—

TUBERCULAR MENINGITIS—This is partly, perhaps, because it is a Meningitis ; and the brain MEMBRANES are hardly within the sphere of the medicine. Yet it is not only that ; for others that, like *Bryonia*, ordinarily influence them potently have little efficacy here. It is chiefly because it is Tubercular ; because the inflammation is lighted up by no intangible and passing agency, but by these persistent virulent presences—of bacterial or cellular origin it matters not—by Tubercles.

I devoted several pages of my 'Therapeutics' to the treatment of this disease. I told of all medicines that have been recommended, all that have seemed to do good ; but the upshot of the whole story is that we, like our brethren of the old school have found the malady practically incurable. There are few of us, probably, who have not seen an isolated case recover ; but the medicines which appeared effective here have failed utterly next time and henceforward and we doubt if the case that recovered was not simple Meningitis after all. I concluded that, on the whole, the most hopeful outlook was in the direction indicated by Jahr—to give up treating these cases as inflammations and effusions, and medicate them with constitutional drugs like *Calcarea* and *Sulphur.*

I have seen (I know not why) but little of Tubercular Meningitis since then, and have not had opportunity of working in this direction. Occasional cases of recovery from these and other remedies have been reported in our Journals. Dr. Kroner sends one, in which *Sulphur* 6 and *Apis* 3 were the remedies,—improvement coming to a standstill when the 30th dilution was substituted. * Dr. Gutteridge contributes another recovering under *Belladonna* and *Stramonium,* † and an Indian practitioner a third in which *Apis* 30 followed by *Stramonium,* 30 seemed curative. ‡ Dr. Molson has had a successful result from *Zincum phosphoratum* 3_x . Dr. Victor Arnulphy can boast of three cures,—the first with *Sulphur 12*, the two last with *Helleborus* 6 and *12*. In the first and second, improvement or convalescence was accompanied by the appearance of small multiple abscesses on the surface. ∥ Dr. Damon records a case simulating acute general Tuberculosis, with secondary Meningitis, where yet recovery took place. A critical eruption here also accompanied

---

* J. B. H. S., ii., 103.   † IBID., p. 104.   ‡ IBID., p. 496.
$ IBID., iv., 171.   IBID., p. 350.

the first signs of improvement, in the form of Bullæ going on to Ulcers, Abscesses and Boils. The treatment during the cerebral stage was *Belladonna* 2_x alternately with *Calcarea phosphorica* every hour. * Dr. Douglas Smith, of Liverpool, had a recovery under *Bryonia, Hellebore* and *Sulphur.* † A case of what seemed to be this disease, in a boy of 12, delirium being very marked, presented to Dr. Crossbie's eye so strong a resemblance to poisoning by Cocaine that he put two drops of a 2 percent, solution into half a tumblerful of water, and gave a teaspoonful every two hours. Delirium soon abated, and convalescence set in and proceeded uninterruptedly. ‡

But besides these, two avenues of possible help have opened, to which I would draw your special attention.

1. *Iodine* is one of the medicines which have sometimes seemed curative in this disease. Stille cites several reports as to its efficacy, when given in combination with *Potassium* ; and Dr. Jousset thinks he has seen the disease arrested by the administration of a mixture of one drop of its tincture in 200 grammes of water. In the shape of **Iodoform**, however, a more decided efficacy has been ascribed to it. By rubbing well into the shaven scalp an ointment made with a drachm of this substance to an ounce of lard, four out of five successive cases were cured. This was reported some ten years ago, and I am unable to give you the reference ; but it deserved the attention it evoked. The effect of the inunction could not be a derivative one, *Iodoform* having no irritative influence ; it must have resulted from absorption of the drug and how limited this must be through the unbroken surface needs no demonstration. But when it is freely absorbed, as when applied to a wound, what are its effects on the brain ? Do they throw any light on its remedial action when introduced in smaller quantities ? I think that no one can read the cases of poisoning from this cause collected in the 'Cyclopædia' of Drug Pathogenesy without seeing a striking resemblance between Iodoformic intoxication and the malady we are now considering. There is high fever, rapid pulse, and disturbance of the cerebral functions which may, Schede says, "take the form of Acute Meningitis . . . and tend to a fatal termination." The conclusion can hardly be resisted that *Iodoform* is Homœopathic to Acute Hydrodephalus and that any control it exerts over the idiopathic disease must be due to this relationship.

The first to turn such interference to account was Dr. W. S. Miller. He brought before the Homœopathic Medical Society of the country of New York in 1815, a case, diagnosed as Tuberculous by several physicians of repute, and given up by them, which recovered under the inunction ; and in the discussion which followed Dr. O'Connor, pointing out the Homœo-

---

* J. B. H. S., V., 107. † Ibid., p. 277. ‡ Ibid. i., 183.

pathicity of the practice said that he had used the 2_x and 3_x triturations internally with such marked result that he was led to look upon *Iodoform* as almost a specific for any form of Meningitis.* Dr. J. W. Martin of Pittsburg, then reported two cases of the Tubercular form making complete recovery under the 2_x trituration. † Dr. Wheeler brought before the British Homœopathic Society in 1897, a case in which cerebral symptoms like those of Meningitis supervened in the course of Pulmonary Tuberculosis, and cleared away completely under the same potency. ‡ In the discussion, Dr. Neatby spoke of having had a recovery from the use of the 3_x. Lastly, a case having all the appearanc of the disease was rescued from imminent death by its administration (the patient was breathing only from two to four times a minute, and the pulse varied from 84 to 120) at the hands of Drs. Butler and Clapp. $

2. An outlook perhaps yet more hopeful is in the direction of **Tuberculinum.** If Dr. Arnulphy could get such fine results from dilutions of this substance when the Tuberculous process attacked, in an acute manner, the lungs, why should not a similar process be modified by it when occurring in the brain ? The localisation of action noted in its pathogenetic effects is present here also. I will not lay too much stress on the Headache mentioned in Koch's own experiments on the healthy, as that may have been a part of the fever which was in so slight degree induced. But Drs. Burnett and Clarke in this country, and Dr. Boocock in America, have proved *"Bacillinum"* on their own persons, ‖ and concur in speaking of the severe Headache—"deep in the brain"—which it sets up, without any fever to account for the pain. The first of these, moreover, has had some experience in the therapeutic use of the substance. In a paper read before the American Institute of Homœopathy in 1894 ✝ it was said— "Dr. J. Crompton Burnett, in his work on Tuberculosis reports many cases of genuine Tubercular Meningitis cured with his *Tuberculinum.*" I need not say that our late colleague, with all his enthusiasm, made no such extravagant claims. From his own practice he relates four cases bearing on the subject. Two (cases 2 and 3) were acute feverish attacks occurring in brothers of a family where "numerous near relations had died of Consumption at different periods, and one young cousin had died of Tuberculosis of the brain coverings." Both had cerebral symptoms, and both resisted the ordinary Homœopathic remedies ; whereas a single dose of *Bacillinum* turned the tide, and initiated recovery. The two other head-cases he reports (cases I and 24) were rather of the chronic type ; though in the

---

* J. B. H. S. ix., 226. † IBID., V., 196.
‡ IBID., p. 299. $ IBID., viii., 157.
‖ See pp. 4. 233, 263 of the 3rd Ed. of Dr. Burnett's 'Cure of Consumption by *Bacillinum*'. ✝ See p. 845 of the Transactions.

first actual Hydrocephalus existed, with cerebral disturbance and pyrexia, and in both another child of the parents had previously died from the acute disease. In the third edition of his book, Dr. Burnett cites a case from Dr. Chas. W. Roberts of Scranton, Par., U.S.A., which—though too loosely described—certainly reads like Tubercular Meningitis, and which was rapidly worsening under other remedies, while *Bacillinum* brought about a cure.

This is all the experience we have at present; but it is sufficient, I think, to incite to further trials.

Besides Simple Meningitis, there is another affection which may simulate ACUTE HYDROCEPHALUS, and confuse the inferences from treatment.

This is—

HYDROCEPHALOID—Since the time of Marshall Hall and Gooch this disorder has been well-established as liable to occur in children suffering from any exhausting disease, especially Diarrhœa, *China* has not proved of the advantage which might have been expected, but the **Phosphorus** and **Zincum** praised by Jahr received general commendation from our authors. The latter is that most frequently prescribed. *

HYDROCEPHALUS, in its chronic form is as Watson says, a Dropsy, while Acute Hydrocephalus is an inflammation. It is also as a rule, a symptom of some more general cachexia—as a Scrofula or Rickets—rather than an independent local disorder, We can understand therefore Jahr's experience with it—"What **Sulphur** and **Calcarea** 30 are capable of accomplishing in this not very unfrequent disease is almost incredible." I have lately cured a well-marked case with these remedies given (as he advises) in rare doses with long intervals between. Dr. von Grauvogl maintained the effusion in chronic cases to be due to imperfect ossification of the cranial bones, and its best treatment to be the promotion of this process by *Calcarea phosphorica*. *Arsenicum* is commended alike by Jahr Bahr, and Jousset, but by the first two only as an adjunct to *Calcarea*; and *Helleborus* must not be neglected as an intercurrent remedy.

---

* See J. B. H. S., ii., 102; iii, 136,

CONVULSIONS 759

It may even be the primary one (as in a case which you will find in the second volume of the JOURNAL OF THE BRITISH HOMŒOPATHIC SOCIETY, p. 357) when the effusion has resulted from the causes of Hydrocephaloid.

CONVULSIONS, in children, are so frequently a symptom of an eccentric cause that I need hardly indicate our first duty to be the search for this, and, if possible, its removal. But there will remain to classes of cases in which special treatment will be required. The first is where a morbid condition has been set up in the brain by some such irritation, but does not disappear although you have acted on the maxim TOLLE CAUSAM. *Belladonna, Hydrocyanic acid, Ignatia, Cicuta* and *Oenanthe* are here the most important remedies; the first when the patient is full-blooded, the second when he is of the opposite constitution, the last three when the Convulsions seem rather spinal than cerebral, *Belladonna* is most frequently required; and Bahr and Jahr agree that, when indicated, it will nearly always prevent the recurrence of the fits. Then again we frequently encounter Convulsions as a symptom of idiopathic brain disorder, or of the disturbance of that organ incidental to other disease—as the Exanthemata. The main indication for distinctive choise of remedies is, as well-expounded by the late Mr. Hitchman, the presence of excitement or depression of the brain, as indicated by the elevated or depressed fontanelle. The former requires *Belladonna*, and sometimes *Aconite*; if it come on suddenly, *Glonoin* may be preferable. The latter is best help by *Zincum* —the lowest trituration of the metal or its *Sulphate* being most in favour.

Whatever medicine you select, you will best give it in the intervals between the attacks, as for instance a dose after each fit. During the paroxysm itself, you may let the child smell at *Camphor*, which, Dr. Leadam says, will often calm a powerful Convulsion instantly.

I should add that Teste, after recommending *Kreasote* (24) for the Convulsion of Dentition (of which I will speak hereafter) and *Stannum* (30) for those resulting from Worms, states that when Convulsions in nursing children seem to be idiopathic, the only medicine to oppose to them is *Helleborus*. Also, I would say for myself that when Convulsion take the form of carpopedal contractions, they are best met,—if tonic, by *Cuprum*. if clonic, by *Ignatia*.

Finally, there is a form of Paralysis so peculiar to childhood that it is known as—

INFANTILE PARALYSIS—I do not mean by this the Hemiplegia which is not uncommon in children which is of cerebral origin, and dates nearly always from a Convulsion if it be not a symptom of organic disease. The "ESSENTIAL PARALYSIS" of infancy is spinal; usually ushered in by a feverish attack; more or less general at first, but afterwards, if it do not altogether disappear, limited to a group of muscles, and accompanied with atrophy of the latter organs. I think that all evidence is in favour of inflammation being the starting-point and of hyperæmic softening and atrophy of the grey matter of the antoro-lateral-columns lying at the bottom of the confirmed cases. I have accordingly recommended *Belladonna* in the early period, to favour the natural tendency to recovery; and *Secale* and *Plumbum* later on. I am bound to say, however, that what good has been actually effected in this disease has rather resulted from *Gelsemium* and *Calcarea*.

APPENDIX TO LECTURE LIV.

For the sake of completeness, I give here the counsels and experiences summarised in the foregoing Lectures from my 'Therapeutics' of 1878.

"Hartmann groups together the Tubercular and Non-Tubercular forms of Meningitis, and hence his estimate of our power over the disease seems too flattering. He recommends *Bryonia*, *Pulsatilla* or *Zincum*, according to the symptoms, for the stage of incubation; *Belladonna* and sometimes *Bryonia* in that of inflammatory excitement; and *Helleborus* and *Sulphur* when exudation has set in. Teste admits that Tubercular Meningitis is incurable; but speaks warmly of *Belladonna* and *Bryonia* in the simple variety. His translator into English. Dr. Pulte, confirms the value of *Bryonia* when effusion is impending; but recommends its alternation with *Helleborus*. Leadam and Laurie appear to speak theoretically only, and Guernsey admits the unfavourableness of the prognosis in spite of the remedies whose indication he gives. Dr. Bayes relates * a fatal case; but states that he has generally been successful with *Pulsatilla* in insidious

---

* B. J. H., xxi., 22.

APPENDIX TO LECTURE LIV

forms of the disease, and with *Belladonna* and *Aconite* in those of acuter types. Dr. Whale, in an Article on the disease in the Second Volume of the BRITISH JOURNAL (p. 285) commends *Bryonia*, *Helleborus* and *Sulphur*; Dr. Elb considers *Zincum* effectual against Paralysis of the Brain in the last stage; and Dr. Rummel regards *Sulphur* as the fundamental remedy throughout. Dr. Russell relates * a case, apparently of the Tubercular form, recovering after effusion had set in under *Aconite* and *Arsenicum*; and Dr. Watzke had a similar result from the persevering use of *Digitalis* and *Veratrum*. ✝ *Digitalis* proved curative in Dr. Battman's hands also. ‡ More recently, America has given us *Veratrum viride* for the inflammation, and *Apocynum* for the effusion. Lastly, in a German prize essay on the subject, $ *Glonoin* and *Apis* are regarded as specific in the two stages respectively. The first of these is also praised by Kafka and the second by Wolf.

"I think that the general agreement as to the value of certain medicines—notably *Belladonna*, *Bryonia*, *Helleborus* and *Sulphur*——points to a true power exerted by our remedies over Meningitis as such, though there is no proof that they have cured a case where Tubercle was the exciting cause. The possibility of the presence of the latter, however, in a given instance may affect the prognosis rather than the treatment, and in the chance of its absence 'nil desperandum' must be our motto. The following may be sketched as a general accepted system of Homœopathic Therapeutics for the disease :—

"In the premonitory stage, where digestive derangement is the prominent feature, you must remember the commendations given to *Pulsatilla* (in the medium dilutions), which, indeed, corresponds well with the symptoms present and the usual temperament of the patients. The presence of copious deposit of Urate of Ammonia in the urine I have found (with Dr. Bayes) an especial indication for it. But do not continue it too long especially after vomiting has set in. Then go at once to Belladonna, which is now your sheet-anchor. Some say, the higher dilutions are the best, but I have more confidence in the lowest: I have often seen the permonitory symptoms of cerebral mischief in children clear away under the 1_x dilution, alternated with *Aconite* if the fever is active. Dr. E. H. M. Hale consider *Veratrum viride* to unite the virtues of both the drugs :—I have no experience with it. *Belladonna* continues to be the proper medicine as long as effusion keeps off, unless you see good to substitute or interpose Sulphur, which you may wisely do if the symptoms do not abate ; or you may go on to Bryonia. In the brain, as elsewhere, impending effusion is the indication for this medicine, as completed effusion is for

---

* ANNALS, i., 12.   ✝ B. J. H. vi., 170.   ‡ IBID. xii, 496.
$ Translated in UNITED STATES MED. AND SURG. JOURNAL, i., 237.

Helleborus or *Digitalis*. In doubtful cases, *Belladonna* and *Bryonia*, or *Bryonia* and *Helleborus*, may be alternated, as recommended by Teste and Pulte. Here, again, *Sulphur* may be resorted to if the usual medicines fail. Beyond these I feel leaving firm ground : and can say nothing definite about the other remedies proposed.

"It is with much interest that we turn to the sections on the disease in Bahr and Jousset, feeling sure that they will at least be pathologically sound, and that if they can speak with any confidence as to treatment we can depend on their discernment. The former thinks that even when questionable cases have been eliminated, a sufficient number remain to substantiate the fact that Tubercular Meningitis can be cured with Homœopathic remedies. He advises *Bryonia*, *Arnica* and *Veratrum album* in the incipient stage, *Digitalis* when effusion has set in, *Cuprum* when Convulsions occur. Jousset regards Acute Hydrocephalus distinctively a BACILLAR Meningitis, and not necessarily Tuberculous. He thinks he has seen it arrested by *Iodine* in the incipient stage ; but considers *Helleborus*, *Digitalis* and *Secale* its most suitable remedies.

"I will add Jahr's experience. "The only remedies which can do essential good in this disease (provided anything at all can be accomplished by treatment) are *Calc. carb.* and *Phosph*. Having lost in the first years of my practice two young patients whom I had treated for Tubercular Meningitis with *Bellad.* and *Bry.*, I later treated a similar case with *Calc. carb.* 30, three globules in water, a teaspoonful every three hours uptil health seemed restored ; and in another case I wound up the cure with the *Phosph.*, which I gave for the remaining pains. If the disease is not correctly diagnosed at the commencement, and the inflammation is allowed time to reach the climax of its development. *Calc.* will no longer afford any help, nor will any other remedy. I must say that I think our best hope of controlling this disease lies in the direction indicated by Jahr. I followed his plan in an incipient case the nature of which I could not doubt at the time, as another child of the same family had died of the disease ; and any diagnosis was sadly confirmed by the death of the little patient himself, with the same symptoms, on a later occasion and under other (old-school) treatment, This time, however, all signs of illness cleared away under *Calcarea* 30, and health and colour returned."

LECTURE LV

DISEASES OF CHILDREN (*concluded*)

—o—

AFFECTIONS OF THE EYES, EARS, DIGESTIVE ORGANS, RESPIRATORY ORGANS, CIRCULATORY ORGANS, URINARY ORGANS & GENITAL ORGANS, CUTANEOUS DISEASES, MISCELLANEOUS AFFECTIONS.

—o—

OPHTHALMIA NEONATORUM—STOMATITIS—THRUSH— CANCRUM ORIS—STAMMERING—MORBID DENTITION—DIARRHŒA—CHOLERA INFANTUM—COLIC—CONSTIPATION—PROLAPSUS AN —TUBERCULAR PERITONITIS—LARYNGISMUS STRIDULUS—PERTUSSIS— CROUP—BRONCHO-PNEUMONIA—LYMPH-ADENITIS—TABES MESENTERICA—ENURESIS NOCTURNA –NOMA PUDENDI - INTERTRIGO—CRUSTA LACTEA—PORRIGO CAPITIS —STROPHULUS – RINGWORM—CEPHALHÆMATOMA—NÆVUS—HERNIA—MASTITIS NEONATORUM—ICTERUS NEONATORUM—SCLERODERMA NEONATORUM—TRISMUS NEONATORUM.

I resume my consideration of the DISEASES of CHILDREN.

The only affection of their EYES or EARS which requires special notice is—

OPHTHALMIA NEONATORUM—All that I have said when upon Purulent Conjunctivitis applies to this malady, especially as regards the internal use of *Agrentum nitricum*, on which, with careful cleansing of the eye, I entirely depend in its treatment. Leadam and Jahr, however, speak so warmly of Aconite 30, in the early stage of the disorder that you can hardly do wrong in at least initiating your treatment with this medicir

I come now to the diseases of the DIGESTIVE ORGANS occurring in children, and take first the affections of the mouth. I have already, in my Thirty-Third Lecture, studied with you the drugs which act on the buccal mucous membrane, and favourably influence its morbid states. I have simply now to apportion them in the field we are at present traversing.

STOMATITIS may be SIMPLE, APHTHOUS, or MALIGNANT. I will speak of the two latter under the titles of THRUSH AND CANORUM ORIS respectively, SIMPLE STOMATITIS, which is an exudative inflammation of the mucous surface, has no better medicine than Kali chloricum, which we have seen to be confessedly Homœopathic to the morbid condition. I have treated a good many cases in children by the I_x trituration with very satisfactory success.

In the treatment of—

THRUSH, also, we occupy common ground with the old school but maintain the Homœopathic specificity of the Borax we give, as well as they. It will cure when internally administered only, and in almost any dilution; but there seems no reason why its local application should not be conjoined. I give the I_x trituration, and allow it to melt in the mouth. Hartmann commends also *Sulphuric acid* and Teste *Muriatic acid*,—both advising the local as well as the internal use of the medicines. These same remedies are esteemed by Leadam and Bahr; but the latter thinks with me that *Borax* is specific and always to be prescribed first.

CANCRUM ORIS is the "NOMA" of the old writers. The well-known tendency of *Mercury* to cause this serious disease would justify us in opposing one of its preparations to at least the primary manifestations of the malady. The only case I have seen occurred subsequently to Measles, and yielded fairly to *Mercurius solubilis* and *Muriatic acid*. But you should always hold *Arsenicum* in reserve, as the medicine (of all others) best-fitted to cope with the disorganizing process we are now considering. In an epidemic of Cancrum Oris occurring in Germany, Arnold found this medicine, in the 3rd and 4th decimal triturations, the only curative. * It cured a case resulting from *Calomel* in Dr. Banerjee's hands; but in one, supervening on Malarious Fever Dr. Sircar preferred to use *Lachesis* (6) which saved the child (as he expresses it) from the very jaws of death. † You must also bear in mind the facts about *Kali chloricum* which I mentioned in my Thirty-Third Lecture.

As a CHILD's AFFECTION of the TONGUE—though it is more than that—I will speak of—

STAMMERING—Great good may often be obtained in this affection by the persevering use of *Stramonium*. This is Teste's recommendation; and it is sustained by some cases which you will find in the Eighteenth Volume of the BRITISH JOURNAL OF HOMŒOPATHY. The medium dilutions seems most suitable.

---

* See B. J. H., xi., 147.
† CALCUTTA JOURN. OF MED., March and April, 1894.

DENTITION

Coming to the TEETH, we are brought to the large subject of—

MORBID DENTITION—I am unable to agree with those who set down to teething almost all the troubles to which the yearling is subject. The cutting of teeth is as truly a Physiological process as is the growth of the bones; and in healthy children should and does pass off with hardly more disturbance. Without doubt, however, when there is predisposition to blood disease or to nervous disorder, the increased activity of the whole system during the process of Dentition will tend to throw out these morbid proclivities, as in the shape of cutaneous eruptions or of Convulsions. Again, if a child be or become cachectic, especially if he acquire Rachitic tendencies. Dentition, like every other nutritive process, will be badly and so painfully performed. And then, if once the teeth come to be cut pathologically instead of Physiologically, the mouth becomes indeed the starting-point of other evils.

If you can assent to these views, you will follow me in a much more sparing use of the gum lancet than is fashionable around us: and will egerly inquire into the medicinal resources at our command for restoring Dentition to its normal quietue.

There is a general agreement that **Calcarea** (**carbonica** or **phosphorica**), in the higher dilutions, is a most valuable medicine when the teeth are cut slowly and painfully, and the bowels are much disordered in sympathy with the mouth. But we are indebted to Teste for pointing out that there is not unfrequent form of Morbid Dentition in which **Kreasote** is a superior remedy. The latter shows itself in thin, irritable, or cachectic children; it is characterized by extreme agitation and wakefulness while the teeth are being cut, and they often seem to decay as soon as they appear; the neighbouring parts are much inflamed, and the bowels tend to Constipation. I can add my testimony to the great value of *Kreasote*, 12 to 24, in such a condition. It may be continued both in the intervals, and while the teeth are coming through. But if you are giving *Calcarea* as the contitutional remedy, you will require **Aconite** or **Chamomilla** at the time of cutting. The former is preferable when fever is present, the latter when nervous symptoms predominate; and either in its place will give most grateful relief. *Coffea* acts like *Chamomilla*, and might be preferable if sleeplessness was the predominant symptom.

The Convulsions of Teething are best averted by the persevering use of the remedies for Morbid Dentition, but if they seem to be threatening, go at once to **Belladonna**, which exactly meets that state of the nervous centres of which Eclampsia is the outcome.

DIARRHŒA in young children is always a serious disorder, and you will find it a great comfort to yourselves and to the anxious mothers of your patients if you can treat it successfully.

Let me try to indicate the most suitable remedies for its many varieties.

1. The EARLIEST DIARRHŒA of human life is that which affects children who are brought up by hand, and whose intestines reject the unnatural diet. No amount of approximation to mother's milk will render artificial feeding tolerable by these children; and if medicine will not help them the only alternative lies between a wet-nurse and death. I have found two medicines of great service in this condition, *Nux vomica* and *Lycopodium*. *Nux*, in the 1st dilution, I give in non inflammatory cases; *Lycopodium* in the 30th, where Muco-Enteritis has evidently been set up. This last piece of practice I owe to Teste.

2. An ACUTE INFLAMMATORY DIARRHŒA is much more common in infants and young children than in adults. It would run on, suppose, if not checked, to Dysentery, its seat seems to be the colon. *Mercurius corrosivus*, generally alternated with *Aconite*, is the medicine on which I have depended, and with every reason to be satisfied. Sometimes, especially when the inflammation is in the rectum, *Podophyllin* is a capital medicine. The following is a case in point.

Sept. 15, 1866—About 3 o'clock this afternoon I saw a little boy between two and three years old who had been taken ill at noon. From that time till now he had been seized every quarter of an hour with severe pain in the abdomen, followed by passing of a small quantity of mucus and blood. There was no vomiting or fever. I should nearly always have given *Podophyllin* in such cases, but have looked upon the occurrence of prolapse of the rectum at each stool as pathognomic of the remedy. The absence of this symptom in the present instance, and the prominence of the colic, led me in preference to *Colocynth*, of which I gave a drop of the second dilution every two hours.

6th. 11. 30 a.m.—No improvement whatever; the pain and purging have continued every quarter-of-an-hour or so during the night, and the poor child looks much exhausted. I now fell back on the tried remedy, and gave half-a-grain of the 3rd trituration of *Podophyllin* every two hours.

7th.—The little boy came walking into the room to see me to-day, looking quite himself again. The mother informed me that after the third dose of new medicine (*i e.*, in four hours after beginning its administration) the pain and purging had both caused and had not returned since.

3. One of the most frequent causes of Diarrhœa in Children is DENTITION. If moderate, it is hardly well to interfere with it; not improbably it acts as a safety-valve. But if you do treat it, remember its origin: and whatever medicine you give for the bowels, alternate it with one that acts on the nervous circuit

CHOLERA INFANTUM

along which the irritation has travelled. Such are pre-eminently *Chamomilla* and *Belladonna*. They will, especially the former, sometimes cure alone; but it is generally well to reinforce them by a medicine acting more specifically on the intestinal mucous membrane. **Mercurius** is most frequently required; it is the better-indicated, the more wide is the departure from the natural colour of the motions, and the more slimy they are. *Calomel* ("*Mercurius dulcis*") is often its best form. **Rheum** and **Magnesia carbonica** are not unfrequently useful (some of us can remember with sorrow the "*Rhubarb* and *Magnesia*" of our childhood),—the former when the motions have a very sour smell, and there is a good deal of colic; the latter when the stools consists mainly of green mucus. Other Anti-diarrhœic medicines may be required; you will find their characteristic indications excellently epitomized by Dr. Guernsey at p. 786 of his Treatise.

4. There is then the Diarrhœa which sooner or later accompanies all the "WASTING DISEASES" of children. **Phosphoric acid** and **Phosphorus**, **Arsenicum** and **Calcarea** are its medicines when it requires special treatment. An indication for the first given by Dr. Guernsey is that "the Diarrhœa does not seem to debilitate much, although of long-continuance; and the mother wonders that the child remains so strong with it all." With *Arsenicum* in the 3_x trituration, I have many times arrested such a Diarrhœa in cases seemingly desperate. *Calcarea* is highly esteemed by Jahr; and a striking case cured by a single dose of it has been put on record by Dr. Dunham. *

5. Another form of the Chronic Diarrhœa of childhood is the so-called "LIENTERIA," in which the food passes away by stool little, if at all, digested. *Ferrum* has some claim to be considered specific here. Teste recommends *Arsenicum*, *Oleander* and *China*. I have only seen two cases of the disorder; both got well under the last-named medicine.

6. Children are as liable as others to the Diarrhœa set up by hot weather, and the same medicines are applicable to them as to adults. But they have a form of SUMMER-COMPLAINT quite peculiar to themselves, of which I must speak separately by its American name of—

CHOLERA INFANTUM—Profuse vomiting and purging

---

* 'Homœopathy, the Science of Therapeutics,' p. 470.

(generally serous), characterize it; and it is a highly dangerous disease. I cannot feel that we have any very effective medicines for it, and a "Symposium" on the subject contained in the MEDICAL CENTURY of August 15th, 1894, seems to show a similar conviction on the part of American practitioners. *Veratrum album*, which appears indicated, and which Jousset esteems as its principal remedy, has always failed in my hands; *Arsenicum* has only been one degree better. *Iris*, of which I had great hopes at one time, will check the vomiting speedily but leaves the bowels untouched. I gave *Tartar emetic* a fair trial one summer, but it was very uncertain; and from *Elaterium* I got no results whatever. Dr. Madden's Australian experience, * combined with Dr. Hempel's reiterated recommendations, makes it probable that *Aconite* should be the first medicine given in these cases. After this, *Croton* deserves a trial; it is said to be especially indicated when the stools are ejected with great force. *Podophyllum* also may prove of service; profuse, offensive stools, most frequent in the early morning, call for it, The *Euphorbia corollata* has been much used of late for this disorder in America, and it is quite Homœopathic to the morbid condition. In spite, too, of the apparent demonstration of the inertness of *Æthusa cynapium*. Dr. Deschere continues to esteem it as the best remedy we have where the deep lines from the alæ nasi to the corners of the mouth express the collapse and anguish of the little patient. ✝

Sometimes CHOLERA INFANTUM, after beginning more or less acutely, subsides into a chronic form, and threatens to carry off the child by MARASMUS. The mucous membrane of the intestines is then profoundly altered, and the condition called Gastro-and Entero-malacia is present. *Calcarea acetica* and *Arsenicum*, in low potencies, have done most in my hand here; but it is a not uncommonly fatal disease. Jousset adds *Phosphoric acid* to its possible remedies.

COLIC is the name often applied to all the abdominal pains of sucking infants; but I think it inadvisable. There are many cases in which there is no disorder of the bowels, and the gripings are evidently caused by the child having sucked in atmospheric air with its food, and distension or irregular contraction of the intestines being produced thereby. There is no disease present and *Chamomilla* and *Colocynth* will make no impression. But give the baby a few drops of *Chloric Ether* in a teaspoonful of some aromatic water, and the "carminative" will indeed charm

---

* See ANNALS, v., 37. ✝ HAHN. MONTHLY, June, 1895.

the pain away with the Flatulence. Another so-called Colic in infants consists in the gripings which accompany Diarrhœa or disordered motions. Their presence will rather help you to the right remedy for the primary malady than induce you to select a special remedy for themselves; but if they are very severe, a dose of **Colocynth** *6* or *12* will relieve them. It is said to be an indication for this medicine that each onset of pain is heralded by sudden anger and by the throwing away of whatever happens to be in the child's hands. If moreover, the child is being brought up by hand, you will always do well to let it, under these circumstances, take Lime-water instead of aqua pura with its milk.

True COLIC occurring in children is amenable to the same treatment as that for adults. But an additional remedy is recommended by Teste, in the shape of **Cina** *6* to *12*, a dose every quarter-of-an-hour. "The child tries," he says, "but in vain, to go to stool. At the most, he succeeds in the expulsion of gas, and incomplete stools, which give him no relief. The principal seat of the pain is a fixed point above the umbilicus. The pulse is normal, sometimes a little frequent; but the face is pale and pinched."

For the—
CONSTIPATION of infants and young children my chief reliance is on **Bryonia** *30*. Where it is associated with Colic, *Plumbum* may be preferable; and where it evidently depends on inertia of the lower bowel, *Alumina* is often effective.

PROLAPSUS ANI is a not uncommon complaint in these subjects. I mention it more especially because I have, following Dr. Madden, found *Podophyllum 12* so excellent in its treatment. Dr. Schmey, having observed that children so affected generally showed signs of Rickets, has been led to treat them with small doses of *Phosphorus*, and has in all cases obtained therefrom a definite cure * It has generally been when the anus seems paralysed and unable to close that this medicine has availed in Homœopathic practice. Dr Spalding has found *Aloes* 3_x almost a specific for Prolapsus Recti. †

---

*N. A. J. H., Dec., 1900. † See L'ART MÉDICAL, Sep., 1897, p. 230.

TUBERCULAR PERITONITIS has to be mentioned here, as among the troubles of the abdomen. In one case in which I had every reason to suppose this condition to be present, recovery took place under the steady use of Arsenicum and Calcarea. *China* is recommended by both Hartmann and Teste. Jousset says that he owes a grand success in a case of this kind to *Carbo vegetabilis*.

The DISORDERS of the RESPIRATORY ORGANS constitute a most important group of the maladies of childhood. They include LARYNGISMUS STRIDULUS, WHOOPING-COUGH, CROUP and BRONCHO-PNEUMONIA.

I notice Coryza in these subjects only to say that if *Nux vomica* fails to relieve the "stuffy" condition of the nostrils which so seriously interferes with sucking, *Sambucus* will often succeed.

LARYNGISMUS STRIDULUS, the "ASTHMA MILLIARI" of the old nosologists, has often been confounded with Croup, as I need hardly tell you. It is itself a Neurosis; but long ago it was pointed out how frequently it depended upon the strumous enlargement of the bronchial glands, and now we are learning to regard it as very commonly a symptom of Rickets. In the former case, it is a Paralysis of the Glottis, caused by pressure on the recurrent nerves; there is a constant wheezing present, and inspiration is often seriously impeded. In the latter it is a pure Spasm; inspiration is easy enough, and the expiration is the difficulty. An excellent Paper on the characters and remedies of these two forms of the malady, by Dr. Searle, may be read in the Ninth Volume of the Transactions of the New York State Homœopathic Medical Society; and further experience with the Chlorine recommended by him and Dr. Dunham in the spasmodic variety is contained in the "Homœopathy, the Science of Therapeutics" of the latter. * It is given in a solution of the gas in water, of strength equal to our third dilution. There is some confusion about its appropriateness. In two cases of poisoning by inhalation of the gas, Dr. Dunham observed that while inspiration was easy enough, at most accompanied by a crowing noise, expiration became impossible and asphyxic symptoms appeared. He assumes that this holds good in true Laryngismus Stridulus, and he initiated the successful employment of the drug accordingly. All the writers, however, speak of inspiration as impeded by the spasm, and ascribe the crowing which caused the appellation "Stridulus" to the sudden and forcible restoration of the ingress of air. This is a point which needs clearing up.

Sambucus is another medicine much in repute for the Spas-

---

* See also J. B. H. S., iii., 453.

modic form of the complaint. It is where children wake suddenly at night with Laryngismus—especially, Dr. Searle says, if having been previously in a dry heat, they now break out into profuse perspiration—that it is indicated. Corallium rubrum is lauded by Teste, and may from its calcareous nature be suitable to the diathetic condition present as well as to the laryngeal Spasm. For the paralytic variety, *Ignatia* seems the remedy most Homœopathic to the paroxysms, but deeper-acting medicines must be given if the cause is to be reached. The chief of these is Iodine from which Dunham reports one cure and Bahr five. *

My own experience has led me to believe smelling of Moschus to be the best means of relief during the paroxysms of Laryngismus. If they recur frequently, and are accompanied by carpopedal contractions, and where there is arterial excitement and cerebral Congestion, *Belladonna* must be given; but otherwise I rely upon *Cuprum*. There is no medicine like this for pure muscular Spasm; and when Laryngismus occurs either as a primary affection or in connexion with the paroxysms of Whooping-Cough, threatening Asphyxia or Convulsions, as soon as the child recovers from the paroxysm I put him on *Cuprum aceticum* 3_x, and await the result with assurance. The cold sponging of the chest, recommended by Dr. Ringer, has seemed a helpful adjunct.

I have now to speak of WHOOPING-COUGH,—

PERTUSSIS—I shall begin by sketching to you the treatment of this malady which in the great majority of cases has seemed to me amply satisfactory; and shall then give you the suggestions and results of others, and the most suitable remedies for its complications.

I regard WHOOPING COUGH (with Trousseau) as a specific Catarrh, the Spasm being its differentia, but the Catarrh being no less of its essence. I accordingly begin the treatment with Aconite 3_x and Ipecacuanha 2_+ in alternation. Sometimes no other medicines are required; but if the spasmodic stage be well-marked, Drosera had better be substituted. Whether given according to Hahnemann's plan—a single dose being allowed to act for several days; or as recommended by Dr. Bayes, who administered a fractional dose of the mother-tincture after each fit of coughing; or in the ordinary way, this medicine is of undoubted efficacy. When the Spasm has quite disappeared, it may be discontinued; and should the patient take cold during convalescence, and the cough return, *Aconite* and *Ipecacuanha*

---

* The case cured by it in J. B. H. S., vi., 229, is described as "Spasmus Glottidis," but may have been dependent on enlarged bronchial glands.

should be resumed as at first. Under this plan of treatment I have seldom known uncomplicated Whooping-Cough to last, in its pronounced manifestations longer than a month.

And now for other writers. Hartmann gives indications for many remedies but they seem mainly theoretical. Teste's treatment is altogether a singular one. He begins with *Corallium rubrum* 30, which is taken for four or five days, and then followed up by *Chelidonium* 6 until the Cough has become merely catarrhal, when *Pulsatilla* is given to finish off the case. I once treated a family of children on this plan, and they certainly all had the disease very mildly. Corallium has won commendation in Whooping-Cough from several physicians; and I find it, in the *12*th dilution, a helpful adjunct to *Drosera* when the paroxysms are troublesome at night. Bhar considers *Belladonna* the medicine for the Catarrhal and *Cuprum metallicum* (*3*) for the Spasmodic stage; and Jousset makes considerable use of *Cina* and *Coccus cacti* in the latter. The *Coccus cacti* — the common Cochineal—has become a favourite medicine with me of late years when the Cough attacks adults and where in children there is profuse expectoration and vomiting of mucus.

The only novelty which later years have brought into the Therapeutics of Whooping-Cough has been the introduction of Naphthalin among its remedies. Drs. Hardman and Weaver have written in its praise, both giving it in the 1_x trituration.* The former gives at its chief characteristic "long and continued paroxysms of coughing, with inability to get an inspiration, so that the child is almost suffocated." Dr. Murrell, in 1880, made a beginning of the introduction of *Drosera* into British old-school practice (in France it had commenced two years earlier). † Giving a 1_x dilution, he found five-drop doses cause aggravation, while half-drops cured. ‡ This was very pretty Homœopathy; but it does not seem to have ben followed up. In Homœopathic hands the tendency has been to revert to Hahnemann's usage, whose simple doses were of the 30th. Dr. Day uses the same potency; and Dr. Love, who says that Homœopathy is quite reputed in Paris for its treatment of Whooping-Cough, relies mainly on *Drosera* 12.

Complications occur either on the side of the lungs or on that of the brain. The attack often sets in with acute symptoms of Pulmonary Congestion; and these yield rapidly to *Aconite* and *Phosphorus*. I should trust to the same medicines in the event of Bronchitis or Broncho-Pneumonia supervening in the course of the malady; though Jousset relies here, as elsewhere on *Ipecacuanha* and *Bryonia*. Lobar Pneumonia is rare; but here, if ever, Teste's *Chelidonium* should be of service. Convulsions are a serious matter. When they are attended with symp-

---

* J. B. H. S., v., 28 ; vi., 313 † See 'Pharmacodynamics',
SUB VOCE. ‡ See 'Pharmacodynamics', SUB VOCE.

toms of Cerebral Congestion, the brain never properly recovering itself between the frequent paroxysms, *Belladonna* should be given. But if the Convulsions seem just an extension of the essential spasm, and the symptoms approximate to those of Laryngismus Stridulus, *Hydrocyanic acid* or *Cuprum* (Jousset says the latter has always succeeded with him and from my latter experience I can bear a similar testimony) is the best medicine. Convulsions, however, are, more easily prevented than cured ; and their best prophylactic is the medicine which is most effective in diminishing the violence and frequency of the spasmodic cough.

CROUP is one of the most important of children's disease, from its often FAUDROYANT accession, its violent symptoms, and its strong tendency to end in death. You will be pleased to know, therefore, that Homœopathy has remedies capable of coping with it in all its forms ; and indeed counts its treatment one of her chief Therapeutic triumphs. Besides the full and satisfactory account given of its treatment by Hartmann, you will find a study of the several Croup medicines in the Fifth Volume of the BRITISH JOURNAL OF HOMŒOPATHY, an elaborate Article upon it, in the Tenth Volume by Dr. Elb, senior, and cases by Professor Henderson in the Eighth.

You will perceive from all these sources of information (to which I may add one of our own, Hale's "Lectures on Diseases of the Chest") that the two leading remedies for Croup are *Aconite* and *Spongia* ; and in the so-called "CATARRHAL CROUP" you may leave these medicines to be taken in alternation every hour or two, and be tolerably certain of finding your patient improved at your next visit. It is possible that many a case of true Croup has been arrested in its incipience by this treatment ; but when membranous exudation is patent or plainly to be inferred, you should look for yet more potent remedies. I am not disparaging the great service to Therapeutics rendered by Hahnemann in indicating *Spongia* as the leading remedy for Croup when I give my preference to the **Iodine** itself which is its most important constituent. * To Drs. Koch and Elb we owe the establishment of the value of this medicine here. Its volatility, moreover, enables its inhalation to be added to its internal administration, —a practice which has many times been followed with the utmost advantage. The very similarly-acting **Bromine** has often been used with success, as you will see by the references I have

---

* J. B. H. S.' vii., 85

given when lecturing upon that drug. It is probably best suited to the asthenic forms of the disease, such as occur in unhealthy neighbourhoods. **Kali bichromicum**—of all medicines most Homœopathic to Membranous Croup—has frequently cured it. A perusal of the cases given in the Appendix to Dr. Drysdale's schema of the drug in the "Materia Medica, Physiological and Applied," and of those furnished by Dr. Paul Belcher to the Fifth Volume of the old NORTH AMERICAN JOURNAL OF HOMŒOPATHY, and by Dr. Wright to the Fourteenth Volume of the same Journal, will satisfy you on this head. I have never used it; but it is a medicine in which I have the utmost confidence in all the morbid states to which its proving points and in which I have tested its powers.

Whatever medicine you choose, I recommend you to alternate it with *Aconite*. Croup is a Neurophlogosis, and the spasmodic paroxysms need help as well as the continuous inflammation. *Aconite* will give this, and will do sometime for the inflammation itself. It is often well to begin the treatment of a case of Croup by administering it alone, giving (say) the 3_x every half-hour or so until the symptoms abate. It will sometimes dispel the whole attack single-handed; and will at any rate prepare the way for what is to follow. When active disease has subsided, you will find *Spongia* or **Hepar sulphuris** useful in restoring the laryngeal membrane to its normal condition, the former when the cough is hard and dry, the latter when it is hoarsely mucous.

I must not leave the subject of Croup without referring to the exceptional plan of treatment advised and warmly commended to us by M. Teste. "*Ipecacuanha* and *Bryonia*," he writes (but given concurrently for both would be inert alone) are in all cases, whatever be the form of the attack or intensity of the disease, the great modifiers of Croupal Angina." He recommends the dilutions from *6* to *12*; and frequent repetition of the dose. This was long before Curie had demonstrated by experiment the power *Bryonia* has of producing false membranes in the air-passages. As *Ipecacuanha* unquestionably corresponds with the neurotic element in Croup, the prescription is soundly based; and there are not wanting testimonies to its efficacy. Its comparative merits, further experience must decide.

You will see that I have been speaking of Croup as a distinctive and primary disease, standing quite apart from Laryngeal Diphtheria. I do this on clinical grounds, without prejudging the pathological question. I thus agree with Bahr, who assumes the German doctrine, but differ from Jousset, who follows the French Pathologists in holding Croup and Diphtheria to be identical. Bahr's treatment is much the same as that which I have sketched above; but he (as also Jahr) recommends

BRONCHO-PNEUMONIA. 775

Phosphorus when the progress of exudation has caused symptoms of Asphyxia to supervene.

I have now to speak of BRONCHITIS and PNEUMONIA as they occur in children. They are more commonly met with conjointly than separately, and the mixed disease may fairly be called—

BRONCHO-PNEUMONIA—This is practically equivalent to the "CAPILLARY BRONCHITIS" and "LOBULAR PNEUMONIA" of authors as the one rarely occurs without the other preceding or following. Let me repeat what I have said upon the Bronchitis of children, in the Paper referred to before upon that disease.

"The characteristic of Bronchitis, as I observed it in children is the extreme rapidity with which the inflammation runs down the mucous membrane, and, involving the ultimate air-cells of the lungs, becomes true Pneumonia. Broncho-Pneumonia, except in this subjects, I take to be very rare—rarer than Pleuro-Pneumonia, and still rarer than Pneumonia Simplex; and it comes fraught with double danger, the narrowing of the air-passages being superadded to the spoiling of the lung itself. When death results, it is from Aponœa, with its blue lips, lived complexion, and cold extremities. I have very rarely seen a case go thus far under Homœopathic treatment; and I have only known one that did so recover.

"Aconite is as valuable in the Bronchitis of children as it is in that of the adults, if it is given soon enough. It will break up the catarrh, and leave nothing but a loose cough, which will be helped by **Ipecacuanha** if it is spasmodic, by **Pulsatilla** if otherwise. But very often we are summoned too late for the success of this abortive treatment. The dyspnœa, the crepitation and the dulness on percussion tell us that we have Broncho-Pneumonia to deal with. Now I do not affirm that *Aconite* does no good here. I only say that it cannot be depended on to cure, however much it may relieve the general distress. For myself, I generally abandon it altogether in favour of the great remedy for this form of the disease—**Phosphorus**."

I am disposed from later experience to modify the recommendation involved in the last paragraph, viz, the discontinuance of *Aconite* on commencing the administration of *Phosphorus*. I am disposed to think that the action of the former on the vasomotor nerves aids the latter in modifying the tissue irritation, and that without it the *Phosphorus* is even liable to cause aggravation; but I continue to rely upon the latter medicines as the main curative.

What are we to do when, in these cases, Asphyxia threatens? Chiefly, I think to ascertain whether it is caused by the intensity of the inflammation, or by the profuseness of the mucus of resolution, or by impending "Paralysis of the Lungs." In the first alternative, we should push on with our *Aconite* and *Phosphorus*. In the second and third, our most potent allies should be **Tartar emetic** and **Solania**, as recommended for Capillary Bronchitis in the aged.

Belladonna is mentioned by several writers as of value in the Pneumonia of children; and in the class of cases described by Dr. Hillier "in which cerebral, symptoms prevail to such an extent as to mask the pulmonary symptoms, and often to mislead the practitioner," it ought to be quite in place. But it is primary "Lobar Pneumonia" in which this complication occurs. In its absence, *Phosphorus* is the medicine to be given; I am not sure whether *Aconite* helps in here or not. But for both Lobular and Lobar Pneumonia in children we must weigh the claims of **Chelidonium**. This again is a medicine recommended, in an apparently arbitrary manner by Teste; but which subsequent experimentation has proved to bear a true Pathological, relationship to the disease. I refer you to Dr. Buchmann's proving of *Chelidonium*, translated in the BRITISH JOURNAL OF HOMŒOPATHY (Vols. xxiii.—xxv.), and especially to his remarks and observations regarding its use in Pneumonia at p. 64 of Vol. xxv. The cases given confirm Teste's recommendation of the remedy, even to its special value when the right side is affected. His mode of administration, however, was not followed which is to give a dose of the 6th or *12*th dilution every quarter of an hour for four or six doses. "This done," he says "we shall in an immense majority of cases observe a marked, sometimes an astonishing, remission of all the local as well as the general symptoms." After this, other medicines may be given. Dr. Pulte appends a note to the American Edition stating that this treatment has been found very efficacious in considerably shortening the attack. and that the administration of the *Chelidonium* in this way is generally followed by the peculiar greenish discharge characteristic of liver affection.

Since I wrote the foregoing in 1878, a good deal of fresh observation as regards acute chest-affection in childhood has appeared.

1. Dr. Watkins has recorded the entire series of cases of Broncho-Pneumonia in children treated by him during his residence in the London Homœopathic Hospital.* They were 14 in number, and all recovered. As the usual old-school mortality ranges from 33 to 48 percent, this is a brilliant record. **Antimonium tartaricum** and **Arsenicum iodatum**, both in the 3_x, trituration, were the main remedies. The latter was especially

---

* J. B. H. S., vi, 231.

relied on when the Pulmonary Catarrh supervened upon Influenza.

2. One of the truly Homœopathic uses of **Tuberculinum** is its application to Broncho-Pneumonia. Dr. Mersch's Pathogenesis of this substance, translated by Dr. Arnulphy in the CLINIQUE of February, 1896, shows this; and both physicians, as also the late Dr. Herber Smith, have found marked results from it. * The latter used it as low as the 3_x trituration.

3. Apropos of a case of infantile Broncho-Pneumonia, in which the breathing was nearly as rapid as the pulse, Dr. Ludlam states that in former days he had never found any remedy so satisfactory in such conditions as *Chelidonium*, and Dr. McCracken states that the same thing held good with him at the present day. †

4. In the MEDICAL CENTURY for February, 1898, and the NORTH AMERICAN JOURNAL OF HOMŒOPATHY for July, 1899, Drs. Deschere and W. T. Laird discoursed on the treatment of Broncho-Pneumonia and Capillary Bronchitis respectively. Their indications for remedies may often repay consultation.

As I have discussed the lymphatic and lacteal system as part of the CIRCULATORY ORGANS this will be the place for considering the affections of the lymphatic and lacteal glands so common in Scrofulous children. I shall do this under the two heads of LYMPH-ADENITIS and TABES MESENTERICA.

LYMPH-ADENITIS—The medicines which meet with most general commendation in the treatment of enlarged lymphatic glands are *Sulphur, Calcarea* and *Silicea* in one class; *Rhus, Dulcamara, Mercurius, Baryta* and *Conium* in another. The first three are considered most suitable when the Scrofulous diathesis is well-marked; the latter when a local affinity for the glands is chiefly desired in the remedy. *Rhus* is highly commended by Hartmann when an inflamed gland is of a stony hardness. He would give one dose of a high dilution, and allow it to act for some time. Teste exalts *Rhus* into the primary medicine for all cases of Scrofulous glands, but gives repeated doses of the second potency. He follows it up by *Mercurius* and *Sulphur*, stating that the latter medicine, if given first instead of last, will only start but not complete a cure. *Dulcamara* is Hartmann's remedy when damp, *Conium* when

---

* IBID., iv., 342; vi., † CLINIQUE, June, 1896.

contusion is the exciting cause,—conditions, I may add, to which the disease is very rarely traceable. He also suggests, on theoretical grounds, *Cistus Canadensis.* Jousset praises *Conium,* and Bahr *Baryta,* which Jahr also extols when induration is present. In the Leopoldstadt Hospital at Vienna, *Clematis* seems to have been the favourite remedy for enlarged lymphatic glands.

I have made pretty full trial of most of these medicines, but have found little satisfaction from any of them. I follow my brethren of the old school in accounting **Iodine** and its compounds the most important medicines for diseases of the absorbent glands. Its specific action upon them I have already argued at some length. *Iodine,* itself, the *iodide* and especially the *Biniodide of Mercury,* the *Iodide of Potassium* (with which I have seen Dr. Belcher obtained very good results at the Brighton Dispensary), and the *Iodides of Barium* and *Calcium*—all are valuable in the treatment of Lymph-Adenitis. As to external applications here, I apprehend that we should use them only to obtain with greater rapidity the specific effects of the medicines. With the external use of *Iodine* as a vesicant we can have no sympathy.

I have given you the foregoing as I wrote it in my 'Therapeutics' of 1878. Since then Surgery has invaded a region hitherto sacred to Medicine ; and the question about enlarged cervical glands is not so much, what remedies we should prescribe for them, as how soon we should extirpate them. You will find it thoroughly discussed in a Paper by Dr. Macnish, read before the BRITISH HOMŒOPATHIC SOCIETY in 1894, and in the discussion which followed. * The conclusions expressed by most of the speakers were that a majority of cases of Adenitis were Tubercular, were incapable of dispersal by medicine, and required the knife ; but that there was a minority which if taken before suppuration had occurred, might yield to suitable remedies. Silicea seems most in favour : Mr. Dudley Wright mentioned a striking cure from it, given in the soluble form, and others have been reported. The Barium waters of Llangammarch have been found effective in some cases, confirming thus the results Dr. E. M. Hale and others have obtained from *Baryta iodata.* Schussler's *Calcarea flourata,* moreover, has achieved some striking success, especially when the glands have indurated rather than softened. † It was really known to us before Schussler wrote as the *"Lapis albus"* of Grauvogl, which is a *Silico flouride of Calcium,* and from which Dr. Dewey has lately reported very favourable experience in these enlargements.

Closely allied to Lymph-Adenitis is the morbid process which results in Adenoid Growths at the back of the pharynx. I

---

* See J. B. H. S., iii., 146. † J. B. H. S., p. 212

mention them to say how often the symptoms of their presence may be caused to subside by the use of the lower triturations of **Calcarea phosphorica.**

TABES MESENTERICA is nothing more than Strumous disease of the glands of the mesentary, and its general symptoms are due to the disturbance of the important part they play in nutrition. There is no reason, therefore, why we should depart from our **Iodine** in the treatment of this malady ; and with it indeed I have made some of the most beautiful cures I ever saw in medical practice. The ensemble of symptoms unmistakably calls for it,—wasting, hectic especially marked by night-sweats, appetite alternately ravenous and deficient, dry laryngeal cough, and Diarrhœa. When the last is severe, **Arsenicum** (not higher, I think, than the 3_x) is of great temporary service ; but it has no curative power over the entire disease.

It is only right, however, that I should say that *Iodine* holds by no means this foremost place in the recommendations of others for mesenteric disease. *Calcarea* is with most the favourite medicine ; there is a case on record cured by it in the Seventh Volume of the MONTHLY HOMŒOPATHY REVIEW (p. 27). Dr. Lidd recommends *Mercurius corrosivus* where there is evident inflammation of the glands, previous to the development of Tabes, and I have followed his suggestion with decided benefit. Teste's prescription is among his most curious singularities, viz , *Sarsaparilla 18*, *Aloes 6*, *Colchicum 12*, in succession, each for a week or more, three or four times a day. From this medication he states that he has "obtained for several years past the most surprising results."

Later experience has shown a renewed esteem of *Iodine* and its preparations. Dr. Wingfield has reported two cases making complete recovery under the 3_x dilution. * Dr. Day read a paper on "Tuberculosis of the Abdomen in Children, at our Congress of 1897 ; and it was interesting to hear both from himself and those who took part in the discussion which followed how, either in its pure form, or in its combination with *Arsenic* or *Lime*, *Iodine* stood FACILE PRINCEPS among medicinal remedies for Tabes Mesenterica. †

---

* M. H. R. xli., 30.   † M. H. R., p. 549.

The chief URINARY difficulty with the children is —

ENURESIS NOCTURNA, which is often a very obstinate affection. Whenever you can trace it to worms, you may give **Cina** or **Santonine** with good hope of success; the former is said to be specially indicated when the urine grows milky on standing.* When Enuresis is accompanied by a high coloured and strong-smelling urine, **Benzoic acid** will generally both render the urine normal and prevent its escape. But in the numerous cases which present neither of these indications you will have to decide between a large number of medicines; and here as elsewhere a multitude of remedies means small success with any. *Belladonna,* in ordinary doses, has not proved effective in my hands; and the best results I had hitherto obtained had been from **Causticum.** Since reading Jahr's recommendation, however, to begin the treatment of every case with **Sulphur** 30, I have often done so with success. He advises, if it fails to cure, *Sepia, Belladonna* and *Pulsatilla* in young girls, *Causticum* for little boys, *Calcarea* if the children are small and fat. Jousset also has had good results from the **Pulsatilla** here mentioned; he thinks it indicated when during the day there are vesical tenesmus and sudden and irresistible desire to urinate.

Having spoken thus in my Therapeutics, I went on to mention *Verbascum* and the *Equisetum hyemale* as having obtained high commendation in Enuresis from American practitioners (I might have added the *Rhus aromatica*); and to refer to cases in which *Plantago* † and *Thuja* ‡ had proven curative. I also suggested *Gelsemium* as an alternative to *Causticum*; and *Opium* when the trouble seemed connected with too heavy sleep. Looking through our literature since that time, I find no confirmation of these recommendations, so far as *Verbascum, Plantago, Thuja* and *Opium* are concerned. As to the others, Dr. Halbert contributes £ two interesting cases of the affection in boyhood. In the first, simple weakness of the sphincters, following Diphtheria, seemed to have been the initial cause, though some catarrh had become engrafted. Here *Equisetum* cured, acting (he thought) better in the 30th than the 3rd. Conversely, Dr. Bickley has had better results with 5 10 drop doses of the tincture. || In the second, irritation of the detrusor muscle was thought to be present, from the tenesmus which followed micturition; and *Gelsemium,* in varying potency, proved remedial, *Rhus aromatica* comes to us from the eclectics, and has ordinarily been given in their doses of about ten drops of the mother-tincture. Dr. Choudhury, however, finds globules saturated with this preparation sufficient. ☧

---

* See HAHN. MONTHLY, Sept., 1898, p. 605.
† B. J. H , xxv. 319. ‡ IBID., xxvi., 491
£ CLINIQUF, April, 1896. || J. B. H. S., iii., 179 ; iv., 494.
☧ HAHN. MONTHLY, June, 1901, p. 412. Comp. J. B. H. S., iii., 108; v., 105.

As regards the older remedies, *Sulphur, Pulsatilla, Causticum* and *China* fairly maintain their repute. Dr. T. P. Cobbe would give *Pulsatilla* where I have indicated *Benzoic acid*, when the loaded urine can be traced to digestive disturbance. * *Atropine* has been introduced in the place of *Belladonna*, and seems effective in minute doses. Dr. T. G. Dunham dissolves a grain of the *sulphate* in an ounce of distilled water, and of this gives a drop for each year of the child's up to 7. Dr. Lambert has seen very great benefit in a chronic case from the 6th dilution, and here *Belladonna* has been previously given without success. † The last-named medicine continues to be in favour in the old-school. Sir Henry Thompson's Article on the disorder in Quain's 'Dictionary' supplies both an appreciation and an explanation of its action, which appears to be purely antipathic. Another practitioner of traditional medicines writes to extol *Lycopodium*. He gives 20 drops of a tincture three times daily, increasing the dose to a drachm, and gets no ill effects. ‡ Perhaps smaller doses would answer, were the more effective Homœopathie preparations used. In our practice it is considered indicated when Uric Acid (red sand) is deposited from the urine.

In **STRANGURY**, which in a slight form is not uncommon in children, as from cold or damp, **Aconite** or **Dulcamara** is serviceable. But unless one or other of these causes be distinctly traceable, you will be safer in prescribing **Belladonna**.

The **GENITAL ORGANS** of male children are rarely the seat of disease; and when such occurs it is surgical rather than medical. The female child, however, is sometimes troubled with a kind of—

LEUCORRHŒA, which not unnaturally causes much trouble in the mind of the mother. It is readily curable by **Calcarea** and cleanliness, or, if caused by Ascarides, by the treatment suitable for these.

A more important disease of these subjects is—
NOMA PUDENDI—This affection appears to be precisely analogous to Cancrum Oris; and here there can be no question between *Mercurius* and **Arsenicum**, the local affinity of the latter being so much the greater.

---

* IBID., iii., 108,   † H. W., Jan., 1897.   ‡ J. B. H. S., vi., 225.

And now of the CUTANEOUS DISEASES of childhood, several of which are very characteristic of this period of life.

INTERTRIGO, besides the obvious local management, is often greatly helped by Homœopathic remedies. **Chamomilla** is good in simple cases ; **Lycopodium** where the chafing obstinately recurs, and seems constitutional : **Mercurius** where the parts affected are raw and very painful.

Impetigo (or shall we say Eczema ?) has two local varieties very common in children, CRUSTA LACTEA and PORRIGO CAPITIS.

CRUSTA LACTEA is an ECZEMA IMPETIGINODES of the face. I have every reason to be satisfied with the **Viola tricolor** recommended by Hartmann for this disease ; but in obstinate cases you may with advantage remember Teste's commendation of **Sepia**.

PORRIGO CAPITIS (SCALLED HEAD) is more difficult to cure. **Calcarea muriaticum** in the first dilution, is my favourite medicine ; but **Sulphur** must often be interposed. **Silicea** is good where there is abundant suppuration, and **Viola tricolor** where itching is distressing. I believe it also to be important not to remove the crusts until there is reason to believe that the tendency to return of the disease is checked.

A papular eruption peculiar to children is "RED GUM"—

STROPHULUS—**Chamomilla** is generally its specific remedy ; but where the digestive organs are at fault *Pulsatilla* or *Antimonium crudum* may be required.

Lastly, I would speak of—

RINGWORM, or, as it is now called. "TINEA TRICOPHYTINA TONSURANS." I have formerly argued, from the occasional disappearance of this disease, when recent, under internal remedies alone, that the theory of its primarily parasitic origin was baseless. I was able to cite the authority of Mr. Jabez Hogg for my contention ; and since then Dr. Burnett has come forward with a vigorous defence of the view of its "constitutional nature and origin." He does not deny the existence of the tricophyton fungus, but maintains that it cannot grow and thrive save on an unhealthy soil.

I know that in suggesting such doctrine I am going counter to the present mind of the proffession, and I have no desire to provoke controversy by doing so in a pugnacious way. The question need not be a practical one. I do not deprecate the use of parasiticides to the invaded spots ; all I care for is that some constitutional remedy suitable to the patient's general condition should be simultaneously administered. As this is generally of a Scrofulous kind, Dr. Burnett is consistent in treating Ringworm with his *"Bacillinum."* In cases which evidence no such derangement of health, **Sepia** may be preferable ; it is generally given in about the 6th dilution.

There are a few MISCELLANEOUS AFFECTIONS of children on whose treatment I shall remark before leaving the subject of their diseases.

CEPHALHÆMATOMA may disappear under the occasional application of a weak **Arnica** lotion ; but should it linger, Dr. Guernsey states that a high dilution of **Calcarea** will always disperse it.

NÆVUS I have seen disappear under **Thuja** 12, *Calcarea, Lycopodium* and *Phosphorus* must also be remembered here.

HERNIA in infants is said to be sometimes curable by internal medicines, especially by *Nux vomica, Calcarea* and *Sulphur.* There can be no harm in trying.

MASTITIS NEONATORUM is generally produced by foolish endeavours on the part of nurses to squeeze out milk from the breasts. **Bryonia** is its specific remedy.

ICTERUS NEONATORUM should be treated by **Chamomilla** followed, if it should be required by **Mercurius**.

SCLERODERMA NEONATORUM you are hardly likely to see, unless you should become attached to a foundling hospital. Should you ever meet with it, I recommend you to try **Bryonia**, which has caused and cured a similar affection (Haningkrankheit) in oxen. * Two cases of Scleroderma greatly benefited by **Thyroidin** may be read in L'ART MEDICAL for November, 1896.

Of—

TRISMUS NEONATORUM I have already said something when speaking of local spasms in general. When arising (as it usually does) from inflammation of the umbilicus, it seems best-treated by **Belladonna**, † whatever else may be given. When

---

* See B. J. H., xxv., 25.   † See J. B. H. S., iii., 456.

resulting from the influence of the mother's emotions through the milk, Ignatia is most suitable.

A word from Hartmann in conclusion. "Small or highly attenuated doses at long intervals are best for a sick child ; provided the remedy has been correctly chosen, which we may easily know from the fact that the child will fall into a sweet slumber after the first dose, and will awake refreshed and in better spirits." He is speaking, of course, of acute diseases.

I have now ended my task. We have surveyed together the whole field of disease, with a view to ascertaining what Homœopathy has done or may yet do towards its conquest. I think you will feel with me that the result of our survey is eminently satisfactory. During the eighty years or so which have elapsed since the establishment of SIMILIA SIMILIBUS CURANTUR as the guide to specific medication, at least eight-tenths of the ills to which flesh is heir have been brought within its range of action. Of the two-tenths which remain, one consists of mechanical disorders requiring mechanical assistance ; and the other may be only awaiting fresh knowledge on our part of diseases and drug for its annexation. It is true that in the territory already won many patches remain whose cultivation is far from perfect, many diseases and varieties of disease for which we crave more perfect remedies. But the number of these is yearly decreasing. Such work as has been done in my present lectures may have, on any who hear them, the influence which Becon's 'DE AUGMENTS SCIENTIARUM' was designed to exert as regards knowledge in general, and by noting deficiencies encourage the labour which shall make them disappear. For here, too, we have an ORGANON of discovery, whose capacities are inexhaustible. We are not only enriched with a treasure of golden eggs, but we have the bird that lays them, and are under no temptation to kill it. The method which Hahnemann has wrought out and bequeathed to us remains in our hands ; and we have but to emulate his faith and zeal and toil in working it to obtain new triumphs every year.

And now I have only to bid you God-speed and farewell. In becoming practitioners of Homœopathy you will have accepted a position which is as onerous as it is advantageous. Use your vantage ground for the promotion of the advance of Medicine as well as for your own success in practice, that there may be a bearing of its ONERA, and not merely a receiving of its MUNERA. I shall not regret then that I have for a long time past spent most of my leisure in putting together the materials for your work.

APPENDIX.

(The subjoined remarks on the MENOPAUSE which were evidently intended to come at the end of Lecture XLIX, were by some accident omitted by Dr. Hughes from the copy furnished to the printer. I am consequently compelled to insert them here.—R. E. D.)

THE MENOPAUSE OR CRITICAL AGE—There are few women to whom the Menopause is not a time of considerable distress. They cannot call themselves, or be treated, as invalids; yet they rarely feel at ease. One of the most common of their troubles they call "flushes." They "come over" as they express it, in sudden heats, sometimes dry, more commonly accompanied with perspiration, but rarely if ever preceded by chill. The attacks last but for a few minutes but recur frequently and cause indescribable discomfort. The Pathological condition appears to be an ataxia of the vaso-motor nerves, analogous to that of the cerebro-spinal system which obtains in Hysteria. There is no arterial tension and *Aconite* does not help. But we have a valuable remedy for it in **Lachesis**. Administered in the 6th or 12th dilution, it will rarely fail to reduce the trouble to a minimum and to gain for us the grateful thanks of our patients. I owe the original suggestion of this medicine to Dr. Madden. Dr. Gray and others have found **Sanguinaria** and Drs. Ringer and Edward Blake **Amyl Nitrite**, useful for these flushes; so that you have something to fall back upon should *Lachesis* fail you. *Jaborandi* promises to be useful when the flushes take the form of sudden perspirations.

There are two forms of distress in the head complained of by menopausic patients. The one appears to be a special local manifestation of that general hyper-mobility of the vascular nerves which I have already described. There is little or no pain; but the patients complain of great GIDDINESS, with rush of blood, throbbing, beating, and roaring, sometimes with noises in the ears. *Lachesis* helps this, but not very decidedly. On the other hand, it finds in **Glonoin** a most efficient remedy. I believe that Dr. Kidd was the first to suggest this medicine for the malady in question; although the Pathogenetic indications for it are so strong as to make it wonderful, no one had pointed out its applicability before. I have always used it as recommended by Dr. Kidd, in the 3rd decimal dilution. *Amyl Nitrite*, also should be useful,

The other head affection of this period of life is a true ache, a burning pressure upon the vertex. Sometimes it is here, as elsewhere, a symptom of debility from loss of fluids ; as when the shifting menses occasionally stream forth profusely. In these cases the patient often complains of a feeling as if the head were opening and shutting. The medicines are obviously **China** and **Ferrum**. Quite as often, however, there is no such cause present to account for it, and the distress is purely sympathetic. In this case I have already failed to relieve with *Lachesis* ; and **Cactus** may supply its place when needed.

The third climacteric affection I have to mention is "SINKING AT THE STOMACH," and is very common. I have reason to suppose that the solar plexus with its ganglia is the seat of this distressing sensation, which is by no means confined to menopausic subjects. In idiopathic cases unconnected with this change in the system, I found **Hydrocyanic acid** an invaluable medicine. But in the sufferers under consideration its place seems to be taken by the **Actæa Racemosa**, "Faintness at the epigastrium" is a symptom of frequent recurrence in its Pathogenesis ; and its relation to the uteru smakes it specially suitable. I give it in the 2nd and 3rd decimal dilutions, and rarely find it fail to relieve.

When speaking of **Aconite** as inapplicable to the flushings of the Menopause, I did not mean to exclude it generally from the treatment of climacteric sufferings. "Of all medicines" says Dr. Leadam, "Aconite is the most soothing at the climacteric period, especially when the individual is robust and plethoric, or if there be any evidence of local or general increased action ;" and Dr. Ludlam writes—"The wonderful influence of *Aconite* over most of the derangements of the circulation at the climacteric has long been known. It is an invaluable and almost indispensable remedy." It acts best, I think, as Dr. Leadam says, at a medium or higher attenuation.

INDEX

A

Abortion, 697.
Abscess of liver, 516; of lung, 559; pelvic, 686; acute labial, 688; milk, 708
Acidity, 484.
Acne, 724.
Acromegaly, 742.
Actino-mycosis, 288, 736.
Acute Alcoholism, 355.
Acute Infectious Disorders, 193, 205, 220, 231, 242, 262.
Acute labial Abscess, 688.
Addison's disease, 612.
Adipositas Cordis, 589.
After-pains, 701, 703.
Ague, 259.
Albuminuria, 627.
Alopecia, 727.
Alternation of medicines, 108.
Amblyopia, 436.
Amenorrhœa, 664.
Amyloid degeneration of kidneys 626.
Anæmia, 311; pernicious, 317.
Aneurysm, 605.
Angina faucium, 467; ludovici, 467; pectoris, 595.
Animals, experiments on, 56.
Antipathic method, the, 75.
Anus, fissure of, 509; prolapsus of, 509, 769; fistula, 510; paresis of, 511.
Aphonia, 541.
Apoplexy, 344.
Appendicitis, 491.
Arbori-vital medication, 114.
Arsenic in Skin Diseases, Hunt's use of, 709.
Arterial degeneration, 606.
Arteries, diseases of, 604.
Arteritis, 604.
Arthralgia, 744.
Arthritis deformans, 298.
Ascarides, 510.
Ascites, 513.

Asthenopia, 441.
Asthma, 548; Milliari, 770.
Astigmatism, 443.
Ataxy, locomotor, 371.
Atheroma, 606.
Atrophy, progressive muscular, 373; of liver, 517.
Aural Vertigo, 458.
Azoturia, 635.

B

Bacteriology, 78.
Bakers' Itch, 715.
Baldness, 727.
Balanitis, 654.
Bilious Remittent Fever, 258.
Bladder, irritable, 643; paralysis of, 644; stone in, 645; cancer of, 645.
Blepharitis, 412.
Blepharospasm, 413.
Boils, 730.
Bowels, ulceration of, 492; haemorrhage from, 492.
Brachialgia, 397.
Brain, disease, of, 337. 346.
Brain, softening of, 343; concussion of, 364.
Bright's disease, 617.
Bromidrosis, 726.
Bronchiectasis, 547.
Bronchitis. 542; acute, 542; capillary, 543; toxæmic, 543; chronic, 544.
Bronchocele, 613.
Broncho-Pneumonia, 775.
Burns 747.
Bursitis, 744.

C

Callosities, 722.
Cancer, 303; of tongue, 465; of stomach, 478; intestinal, 492; of the liver, 520; pulmonary, 573; of bladder, 645; uteri, 681; pudendi, 688.

INDEX

Cancrum oris, 764.
Carbuncle, 731.
Cardiac Dropsy, 593 ; Digitalis treatment of, 597.
Caries, 741.
Casualties, 745.
Catalepsy, 391.
Cataract, 437.
Catarrhus æstivus, 534.
Cellulitis, orbital, 443; pelvic, 686.
Cephalhæmatoma, 783.
Cerebral congestion, 337.
Cerebral tumours, 343.
Cerebritis, 341.
Cerebro-spinal Fever, 247.
Cervico-metritis, 672.
Chalazion, 413.
Chancre, 322 ; soft, 332.
Chancroid, 653.
Characteristics, 101.
Chicken-pox, 221.
Chilblain, 748.
Children, diseases of, 751, 763.
Chlorosis, 312.
Cholera, Asiatica, 262 ; infantum, 767 ; nostras, 495.
Chorea, 386.
Choroidal congestion, 427.
Choroiditis, 428.
Chyluria, 635.
Circulatory System, Diseases of, 580, 604.
Cirrhosis of the liver, 517.
Clergyman's Sore-throat, 470.
Coccygodynia, 691.
Colic 4)2 ; of children, 768 ; lead, 593.
Concussion of brain, 364.
Condyloma, 333.
Congestion of lung, 560 ; kidneys, 639.
Conjunctivitis, simplex, 415 ; purulent, 417 ; phlyctenular, 421 ; membranosa, 422 ; trachomatosa, 422.
Constipation, 499 ; of children, 769 ; chronic, 502.
Continued Fevers, 231, 242.
Contusions, 746.

Convulsions, 759.
Corneal opacities, 425.
Corns, 723.
Coryza, 530.
Cow-pox, 220.
Cramp of calves, 406 ; writer's 408.
Critical age, 785.
Croup, 773.
Crusta lactea, 782.
Cure, theories of, 148.
Curentur, how altered to Curantur, 9.
Cypher Repertory, 100.
Cystitis, 642.

D

Dacryo-cystitis, 413.
Dandruff, 723.
Deafness, 455 ; throat, 451.
Delirium tremens, 354.
Dementia, 352.
Dengue, 228.
Dentition, morbid, 765.
Derbyshire neck, 613.
Dermatitis herpetiformis, 716.
Diabetes mellitus, 628 ; insipidus, 634.
Diaphragmatitis, 577.
Diaphragm, diseases of, 577.
Diarrhoea, acute, 494 ; chronic, 495 ; inflammatory, 495 ; from improper food, 495 ; from noxious efluvia, 495 ; of children, 765.
Digestive Organs, diseases of the, 460, 472, 489, 499, 512, 763.
Dilatatio Cordis, 587.
Dilutions, 127.
Diphtheria, 268.
Disease, the knowledge of, 38.
Dose, the, 122, 144.
Dropsy, cardiac, 593 ; acute renal, 618 ; ovarian, 658.
Duodenitis, 490.
Dynamisation theory, 34.
Dysentery, 496 ; scorbutic, 498 ; typhoid, 498 ; intermittent, 498 ; chronic, 498.

INDEX

Dysmenorrhoea, 666.
Dyspepsia, acute, 481 ; chronic, 482.

E

Ear, diseases of the, 444 ; erysipelas of, 448 ; eczema of, 448 ; polypus of, 450 ; exostosis of, 450.
Ear-ache, 453.
Ecthyma, 718.
Eczema, 715 ; rubrum, 715 ; impetiginodes, 715 ; chronic, 715 ; of ear, 448, 715 ; pudendi, 715.
Elephantiasis 735.
Emotional disturbances, 750.
Emphysema pulmonum, 547.
Enchondroma, 742.
Endo-carditis, 591.
Endo-metritis, 671
Enteralgia, 492.
Enteric Fever, 233
Enteritis, 489 ; true, 490.
Enterodynia, 492
Enuresis nocturna, 780.
Ephemera, 242.
Epilepsy, 380.
Epistaxis, 536.
Epithelioma of penis, 654
Equinia, 283
Erysipelas, 280 ; aurium, 448
Erythema, 711
Eustachian Tube, 451
Exanthemata, the, 205, 220, 711
Exophthalmic Goitre, 615
Exostosis, 742 ; of the ear, 451
External remedies, 114
Eye, diseases of the, 410, 423, 436

F

Facial palsy, 409
Failure of vision, 435
Fallopian tubes, diseases of, 660
Fatty degeneration of kidneys, 626
Fatty liver, 519 ; heart, 589
Febricula, 242
Female Sexual System, diseases of, 655, 670, 688, 692
Fever, Infantitle Remittent, 752

Fever, 46 ; continued, 231, 242 ; Typhus, 231 ; Typoid or Enteric, 233 ; Febricula or Ephemera, 242 ; Simple continued, 243 ; Relapsing, 244 ; Yellow, 245 ; Cerebro spinal, 247 ; Mediterranean, 248 ; plague, 249 ; Intermittent or Ague, 250 ; Malarial, 250 ; Remittent, 258 ; Bilious Remittent, 258 ; Puerperal, 705 ; Infantile Remittent, 752
Fibroids, uterine, 679
Fissure of anus, 509
Fistula in ano, 510
Fistula lachrymalis, 414
Flatulence, 486
Foctor oris, 463
Food, pain after. 484
Fractures, 749
Functional derangements of stomach, 472 ; of liver, 523 ; of, heart, 580
Furuncle, 730

G

Gall-stones, 522
Ganglion, 745
Gangrene of lung, 559
Gastralgia, 479
Gastritis, 475
General Diseases, 193, 205, 220, 231, 242, 252, 280, 301, 319
General paresis, 352
Genito-urinary organs, diseases of, 639
Glanders, 283
Glaucoma, 428
Gleet, 331
Glossitis, 463
Goitre, 613 ; exophthalmic, 615
Gonorrhoea, 330
Gonorrhoeal Ophthalmia, 417
Gonorrhoeal Rheumatism 298
Gout, 288
Granular degeneration of kidneys 624
Gravel, 636
Grocer's Itch, 715
Gumboil, 466

H

Hæmatemesis, 488
Hæmatocele pelvic, 685
Hæmaturia, 640
Hæmoglobinuria, 641
Haemoptysis, 562
Haemorrhage from bowels, 492
Haemorrhage, post-partum, 701
Haemorrhoids, 505
Hahnemannians, the, 64
Hay-fever, 534
Headache, 355; nervous, 356; congestive, 358; sick, 358, 400
Heart, diseases of, 580; remedies, 581; hypertrophy of, 587; dilatation of, 587; palpitation, 586; fatty, 589; valvular disease of, 592; Dropsy, 593
Heartburn, 485
Hemicrania, 400
Hemiopia, 437
Hepatic congestion, 515
Hepatitis, 516
Hernia, 502; in infants, 783
Herpes, 716; zoster, 716: circinatus, 716
Hiccup, 577
High potencies, 124
Hoarseness, 541
Homœopathic method, 74; practice, 136
Homœpathy, its nature and origin, 1; philosophy of, 148; politics of, 179
Homœopathy, history of, 164; in Germany, 194; in Austria-Hungary, 166; in Italy, 167; in France, 168; in England, 169; in India, 171; in Spain, 172; in Spanish America, 173; in Portugal, 174; in Russia, 174; in Scandinavia, 175; in Belgium, 176; in Holland, 175; in Switzerland, 176, in United States, 177

Hordeolum, 412
Horns, 722
Hydrocele, 651
Hydrocephaloid, 758
Hydrocephalus, 758
Hydrometra, 685
Hydrophobia, 375
Hydrothorax, 576
Hyperchlorhydria, 485
Hyperidrosis, 7 5
Hypertrophia c rdis, 587
Hypochondriasis, 353
Hysteralgia, 671
Hysteria, 390

I

Icterus neonatorum, 783
Icthyosis, 721
Ileus, 500
Impetigo, 715; 782
Impotency, 649
Indigestion, acute, 481; chronic, 482
Individualization, 97
Inflammations, the, 47
Influenza, 272
Insanity 349
Intermittent Fever, 250
Intertrigo, 782
Intestinal Cancer, 492
Intestinal obstruction, 500
Intestines diseases of 499
Iritis, 425
Irritable bladder, 643
Irritable testicles, 648
Itch, 735

J

Jaundice, 520; of infants, 783

K

Keratitis, 424
Kidneys, diseases of, 617, 628, 639; granular degeneration of, 624, amyloid degenaration of, 626; fatty degeneration of, 626; congestion of, 639

L

Labial abscess, acute, 688
Labio-glosso laryngeal Paralysis, 370
Labrynthine Vertigo, 458
Lachrymal fistula, 414
Lachrymation, 414

INDEX

Lactation, disorders of, 707
Laryngismus stridulus, 770.
Laryngitis, 538
Leprosy, 729
Leucaemia, 611
Leucocythaemia, 318, 611
Leucorrhœa, 675 ; 781
Lichen, 713
Lienteria, 767
Lips, 463
Liver, abscess of, 516 ; acute atrophy, 517 ; cirrhosis of, 517 ; fatty, 519 ; cancer of, 520 ; pigmentary degeneration of, 520 ; waxy, 520 ; functional derangements of, 523
Local spasms, 406
Lochia, morbid states, 704.
Locomotive organs, disases of, 737
Locomotor ataxy, 371
Lumbago, 738
Lumbrici, 511
Lung, diseases of, 552, 563 ; abscess of, 559 ; gangrene of, 559 ; congestion of, 560 ; œdema of, 560
Lupus, 727
Lymphadenitis, 777
Lymphadenoma, 609
Lymphangeitis, 608
Lymphatics, diseases of, 608

M

Malarial Fevers, 250
Malignant pustule, 283
Mammae, diseases of, 689 ; inflammation of, 689, 708 ; scirrhus of, 690
Mania, 349
Mastitis acute, 708 ; neonatorum, 783
Measles, 221
Medicines, the knowledge of, 53
Mediterranean Fever, 248
Megrim, 400
Melancholia, 350
Meniere's Disease, 458
Membrana Tympani, 451
Meningitis, 338 ; spinal, 367 ; tubercular, 755, 760.

Menopause, 785
Menorrhagia, 661
Menstruation, disorders of, 661
Menstruation, vicarious, 666
Mentagra, 727
Mental disorders, 346
Metritis, chronic, 670
Metrorrhagia, 683
Migraine, 400
Miliaria, 230
Milk-abscess, 708
Milk, delayed appearance of, 707.
Miscarriage, 697
Mollities ossium, 742
Molluscum, 724
Morbilli, 221
Mouth, diseases of, 460
Muco-enteritis acute, 459 ; pseudo-membranous, 489
Mumps, 466
Myalgia, 738
Myelitis, 368
Myopia, 443
Myositis 737
Myxoedema, 614

N

Naevus 783
Nails, diseases of, 732
Nasal catarrh, 530
Necrosis, 742
Nephritis, albuminosa, 618 ; suppurativa, 641
Nervous debility, 391
Nervous system, diseases of, the, 334, 346, 366, 380, 392, 754.
Nettle-rash, 712
Neuralgia, 393 ; sub-occipital, 327 testis, 649 ; ovarian, 657
Neuritis, 392
Neuroses, the, 47, 380
Neurasthenia, 391
Nictitation, 413
Night-blindness, 437
Nipples, sore, 707
Nodes, 740
Nodular Rheumatism, 298
Noma pudendi, 781
Nose, diseases of, 524 ; bleeding of, 536 ; polypus of, 536
Nyotalopia, 437

Nymphomania, 688
Nystagmus, 443

O

Oculo-motor Paresis, 442
Œdema, glottidis, 541; pulmonum, 561
Œsophagitis, 471
Œsophagismus, 471
Œsophagus, inflammation, 471; spasmodic stricture. 471
Omodynia, 739
Onychia, 732
Opacities of cornea, 425
    Ophthalmia catarrhal, 415; neonatorum, 763; gonorrhoeal 417; strumous, 418; granular, 422; Egyptian, 422; rheumatic, 423 426
    Opposite effects of large and small doses, 157
    Orbital cellulitis 443; periostitis, 443
    Orchitis, 647
    Organon of Medicine, Hahnemann's, 12, 23
    Osteitis, 740
    Osteo-arthritis, 298
    Otalgia, 453
    Otitis externa, 449; interna, 453
    Otorrhoea, 450
    Ovarian Dropsy, 658; Neuralgia, 657
Ovaries and Menstruation, diseases of, 655
    Ovaritis, 656
    Over lactation, 708
    Ozaena, 532

P

Pain after food, 484
Palpitation, 586
Palsy, facial, 409
Pancreatitis 514
Pannus, 422
Paralysis, spinal, 369; labio-glosso laryngeal (tongue) 370; infantile, 760
Paresis, general 352; oculo-motor, 442; ani, 511
Paronychia, 732

Parturition, disorders of, 698; malpresentation during, 699; rigid os, during, 699; feeble pains, during, 700; adherent placenta in, 700; after-pains of, 701; haemorrhage after, 701: retention of urine after, 704; Haemorrhoids after 704; lochia, morbid states after, 704
Pelvic haematocele 685; cellulitis, 686; abscess, 686
Pemphigus, 717
Pericarditis 589
Perimetritis, 685
Perinaeum, torn, 704
Periositis, 789; orbital, 443
Peritonitis, 512; tubercular, 770
Perityphlitis, 490
Pernicious Anaemia, 317
Pertussis, 771
Phagedaena, 282
Pharyngitis, chronic, 470
Phlebitis, 606
Phlegmasia alba dolens, 708
Phlyctenular conjunctivitis, 421
Photophobia, 420
Phthisis pulmonalis, 563
Paysometra, 685
Piles, 505
Pityriasis, 718
Plague, 249
Plethora, 311
Pleurisy, 573
Pleurodynia, 577
Pneumonia, 552
Poisoning, symptoms from, 58
Pneumothorax, 576
Polypus aurium, 450; narium, 536; uteri, 681
Porrigo capitis, 782
Post-partum haemorrhage, 701
Pregnancy, diseases of, 692; mental disorder of, 693; headache of 693; sleeplessness of, 693; toothache of 693; salivation of, 694; vomiting of, 694; heartburn of, 694; longings of, 694; constipation of, 695; diarrhoea of, 695; pseudo-cyesis of, 695; cough

INDEX

and dyspnoea of, 695 ; bladder affections of, 695 ; albuminuria and anasarca of, 696 ; painful enlargement of womb and breast of, 696 ; pruritus pudendi of, 696 ; pain in uterus of, 697 ; false pains of, 697
Prickly heat, 713
Proctalgia, 511
Proctitis, 491
Progressive muscular atrophy, 373
Prolapsus ani, 509, 769 ; vaginae, 687
Prosopalgia, 393
Prostatitis, 653
Provings of medicines, 59
Prurigo, 713
Pruritus, 736 ; ani, 736 ; pudendi, 696, 735
Psora theory, 32
Psoriasis, 719 ; palmaris, 715
Pterygium, 422
Ptosis, 413
Puerperal convulsions, 702 ; fever, 705 ; insanity, 707
Puerperal state, disorders of, 702
Pulmonary, congestion, 560 ; cancer, 573 ; syphilis, 573
Purpura, 308
Pustule, malignant, 283
Pyaemia, 284
Pyelitis, 641

Q
Quinsy, 469

R
Ranula, 467
Raynaud's disease, 605
Red gum, 782
Relapsing fever, 244
Remittent fever, 258 ; bilious, 258 ; infantile, 752
Renal congestion, 639
Respiratory organs, diseases of, 524, 538, 552, 563, 770 ; medicines for, 524
Retina, detachment of, 443
Retinal anaesthesia, 435 ; hyperaemia, 432 ; haemorrhage 432 ; hyperaesthesia, 435

Retinitis, 432
Retraction of testicles, 652
Rheumatic Gout, 298
Rheumatism, 293, 299 ; gonorrhoeal, 299 ; of the diaphragm, 577
Rheumatoid arthritis, 298
Rhinitis, 530
Rickets, 752
Ringworm, 782
Rodent ulcer, 729
Rose cold, 534
Rubella, 223

S
Salivation, 466
Salpingitis, 660
Sarcocele, 648
Satyriasis, 649
Scabies, 735
Scalds, 747
Scarlatina, 223
Schema, Hahnemann's, 62
Sciatica, 398 ; thecal, 399
Scleritis, 423
Scleroderma neonatorum, 783
Sclerosis, multiple spinal, 370 ; lateral spinal, 370
Scrofula, 301
Scrotum, inflammation of, 654
Scurvy, 307
Sea-sickness, 488
Seborrhoea, 723
Seminal vesicles, 652
Seminal vesiculitis, 652
Septicaemia, 286
Shingles, 716
Shock, 750
Similar remedy, the selection of the, 82, 94 ; administration of, 107, 122
Similia Similibus, 38, 69 ; its limitations, 141
Single dose the, 112
Skin, diseases of, 709, 722 ; parasitic diseases of, 734
Sleep, derangements of, 362
Small-pox, 214
Sneezing, 537
Softening of the brain, 343 ; of the spinal cord, 374

Sore-throat, catarrhal, 467
Spasmodic stricture of the œsophagus, 471
Spasms, local, 406
Specifics, 77
Spermatic cord, 652
Spermatorrhoea, 650
Spinal cord, diseases of, 365
Spinal congestion, 366; irritation, 365; Meningitis, 367; Paralysis, 369; sclerosis, multiple, 370; sclerosis, lateral 370
Spinal cord, softening of the, 374
Spleen, diseases of, 610
Stammering, 764
Sterility, 650, 689
Stiff-neck, 739
Stings, 749
Stomach, disorders of, 472; ulcer of, 477; cancer of, 478
Stomatitis, 460, 763
Stone in bladder, 645
Strabismus, 443
Strains, 747
Strangury, 644, 781
Stricture of urethra, 646
Strophulus, 782
St. Vitus's Dance, 386
Stye, 412
Summer-complaint. 495, 767
Sunstroke, 749
Supra-renal capsules, 612
Sweating, morbid, 725
Sweating, sickness, 230
Sycosis, 333; menti, 727
Synovitis, 743
Syphilis, 319; secondary, 323; tertiary, 325; pulmonary, 573; infantile, 754

T

Tabes mesenterica, 779
Tape-worm, 510
Tessticle, diseases of 647; irritable, 648; Neuralgia of, 649; retraction of, 652
Tetanus, 377
Tetany, 406
Thread-worms, 510

Throat-deafness, 451
Throat, diseases of, 467
Thrush, 764
Thyroid, diseases of, 613
Tic douloureux, 393
Tic non-douloureux, 407
Tinea, 734; favosa, 734; circinata, 735; decalvans, 727; tonsurans, 782
Tinnitus aurium, 457
Tissue remedies, 90
Tongue, inflammation of, 463; Paralysis, 370; ulcers of, 464; Syphilis of, 464 Cancer of, 470
Tonsils, enlarged, 470
Toothache, 465
Torticollis, 407; 739
Totality of symptoms, 41
Tremor, 389
Tricophytina ton urans, 782
Trismus, 407; neonatorum, 783
Triturations, 125
Tubercle of urinary tract, 645
Tuberculin, kinds of, 578
Tumours, cerebral, 343
Typhlitis, 490
Typhoid, 233
Typhus, 231

U

Ulceration of bowels, 492
Ulcers, 733
Urethra, diseases of, 646; vasoular tumour of, 689
Urinary organs diseases of, 617, 628, 639
Urinary tract, tubercle of, 645
Urine suppression of, 639.
Urticaria, 712
Uterine fibroids, 679; polypi, 681; Cancer, 681
Uterus, diseases of, 670, 683; ulchrs of, 674; diselacements of, 677

V

Vaccinia, 220
Vagina, prolapsus of, 687
Vaginismus, 687
Vaginitis, 686
Valvular disease of heart, 592

Varicella, 221
Varicocele, 652
Varicosis, 607
Variola, 214
Varioloid, 214
Veins, diseases of, 606
Venereal, maladies, 319
Verruca, 722
Vertigo, 360 ; labrynthine or aural, 458
Vesiculitis, seminal, 652
Vicarious menstruation, 666
Vital force theory, 31
Vomiting 487 ; of blood, 488
Vulvitis, 688

W

Warts, 722

Waterbrash, 486
Waxy liver, 520
Weaning, 707
White leg, 708
White swelling, 744
Whitlow, 732
Whooping-cough, 771
Worms, 510
Wounds, 745
Writers cramp, 408

Y

Yellow fever, 245

Z

Zona, 716